Handbook of
Systemic Autoimmune Diseases

Volume 2

Pulmonary Involvement in Systemic Autoimmune Diseases

Handbook of Systemic Autoimmune Diseases

Series Editor: Ronald A. Asherson

Handbook of
Systemic Autoimmune Diseases

Volume 2

Pulmonary Involvement in Systemic Autoimmune Diseases

Edited by:

Athol U. Wells
Royal Brompton Hospital
Chelsea, London, United Kingdom

Christopher P. Denton
Royal Free Hospital, Centre of Rheumatology
London, United Kingdom

Series Editor

Ronald A. Asherson

2004

ELSEVIER

Amsterdam – Boston – Heidelberg – London – New York – Oxford
Paris – San Diego – San Francisco – Singapore – Sydney – Tokyo

ELSEVIER B.V.

P.O. Box 211, 1000 AE Amsterdam
The Netherlands

ELSEVIER Inc.
525 B Street, Suite 1900
San Diego, CA 92101-4495
USA

ELSEVIER Ltd
The Boulevard, Langford Lane
Kidlington, Oxford OX5 1GB
UK

ELSEVIER Ltd
84 Theobalds Road
London WC1X 8RR
UK

First edition 2004

Library of Congress Cataloging in Publication Data
A catalog record is available from the Library of Congress.

British Library Cataloguing in Publication Data
A catalogue record is available from the British Library.

ISBN: 0-444-51652-2
ISSN: 1571-5078 (Series)

Transferred to digital printing 2008

Preface

Pulmonary complications are now the most frequent cause of death in many systemic autoimmune disorders and are a major and increasing source of morbidity. In part, this may reflect better outcomes in recent decades with the development of optimal immunosuppressive protocols; patients now survive long enough to develop pulmonary problems. Thus, there is now a particular need for pulmonary evaluation to be accurate and pragmatic, whether undertaken by rheumatologists or chest physicians. However, published reviews have tended to focus upon single systemic autoimmune disorders, rather than providing detailed overviews of pulmonary involvement in systemic autoimmune disease at large. We were delighted to accept the invitation from Ronald Asherson to redress this deficiency. Our fellow-contributors, all leading clinical scientists in various specialities, were equally enthusiastic. The resulting monograph covers the field from a number of angles, with particular emphasis on four broad areas.

The first two chapters are devoted to the range of lung morphological abnormalities in systemic autoimmune diseases. Histological evaluation has long been regarded as the diagnostic cornerstone in diffuse lung disease, and recent advances in the field, notably the definition of non-specific interstitial pneumonia, have been particularly relevant to our readership. High resolution computed tomography of the lungs has revolutionised the routine clinical assessment of systemic autoimmune disease, by distinguishing between a bewildering array of possible pulmonary complications, and serving as an invaluable prognostic guide. Optimal management requires that clinicians make the best use of both disciplines, with appropriate recourse to surgical biopsy when clinical and imaging findings are inconclusive.

The next part consists of three chapters on pulmonary vascular disorders. There is a general overview of pulmonary hypertension in connective tissue disease, with Wegener's granulomatosis and other vasculitides covered separately. The detail contained within this section reflects our view that the vascular diseases are the most difficult of all pulmonary complications to detect and manage, especially when there are coexisting abnormalities in the lung interstitium.

Seven chapters are grouped in which the pulmonary complications of a variety of individual systemic disorders are reviewed. These disorders are notable for a wide variety of pulmonary disease processes, with the variable co-existence of pulmonary interstitial, pulmonary vascular and extra-pulmonic restrictive abnormalities. Accurate clinical evaluation is critically dependent upon the knowledge of the profile of each individual disease, without which logical investigation and focused management is unattainable. The chapters in this section are written with the practising clinician in mind and can be applied equally by rheumatologists and chest physicians.

Finally, the editors would like to highlight the chapter on drug induced lung disease by Philippe Camus. With an exponential expansion in treatments used in systemic autoimmune disease, iatrogenic disease has become an issue of concern. Despite an increasingly urgent need to provide guidance for clinicians, the topic has not previously been dealt with definitively. We are proud to offer the review by Camus as a reference statement in this difficult area.

Athol U. Wells
Christopher P. Denton

Series Editor

Dr Ronald A. Asherson

Dr Ronald A. Asherson, MD. FACP, MD (Hon) (London), FCP (SA), FACR, is Honorary Consultant Physician at the Rheumatic Disease Unit, Department of Medicine, University of Cape Town Health Sciences Centre in Cape Town, as well as being a Consultant Rheumatologist at the Rosebank Clinic in Johannesburg, South Africa. He is also a Visiting Professor at the Systemic Autoimmune Diseases Unit at the Hospital Clinic, Barcelona, Spain where he regularly visits and coordinates research projects.

Dr Asherson qualified in Medicine at the University of Cape Town in 1957 and, after completing his internship, became H/P to Prof. Sir Christopher Booth at the Hammersmith Hospital, London, in 1960. In 1961 he accepted a Fellowship at the Columbia Presbyterian Hospital in New York, returning in 1962 to become Registrar and then Senior Registrar at Groote Schuur Hospital in Cape Town in 1964. After 10 years as a Clinical Tutor in the Department of Medicine, he returned to the United States and was appointed as Assistant Clinical Professor of Medicine at the New York Hospital – Cornell Medical Centre under the late Professor Henry Heineman. From 1981 to 1986, he was associated with the Rheumatology Department at the Royal Postgraduate Medical School of London. It was at that time that he developed his interest in Connective Tissue Diseases and Antiphospholipid Antibodies.

In 1986 he moved to the Rayne Institute and St Thomas' Hospital in London, where he was appointed Honorary Consultant Physician and Senior Research Fellow. In 1991 he took a sabbatical at St Luke's Roosevelt Hospital Centre in New York, working with Prof. Robert Lahita. In 1992 he returned to South Africa to private practice in Johannesburg.

In 1998 he was elected as Fellow of the American College of Physicians (FACP) as well as a Founding Fellow of the American College of Rheumatology (FACR). From 1988 to 1991 he served on the Council of the Royal Society of Medicine in London. In 1992 he was co-winner of the European League Against Rheumatism (EULAR) Prize and in 1993 was the co-recipient of the International League Against Rheumatism (ILAR) Prize, both for his research on antiphospholipid antibodies. In 1994 he was elected as a Fellow of the Royal College of Physicians (FRCP) of London. In 2002 he was awarded an Honorary Doctorate in Medicine from the University of Pleven in Bulgaria.

Dr Asherson has been an invited speaker at many universities and International conferences both in the USA and in Europe. He is the author of more than 280 papers on connective tissue diseases and has contributed to more than 30 textbooks of medicine, rheumatology and surgery as well as having co-edited "*Problems in the Rheumatic Diseases*", the "*Phospholipid Binding Antibodies*", two editions of "*The Antiphospholipid Syndrome*" and "*Vascular Manifestations of the Systemic Autoimmune Diseases*". He is currently engaged in research on connective tissue diseases, particularly on the antiphospholipid syndrome together with colleagues in the USA, Spain, France and Israel mainly and is in clinical practice in South Africa. In 1999 he was the co-recipient of the Juan Vivancos Prize in Spain and in 2003 was the co-recipient of the Abbott Prize, awarded at the European League Against Rheumatism (EULAR) International Meeting, held in Lisbon, Portugal.

His original description of the "Catastrophic Antiphospholipid Syndrome" and the publishing of more than 40 papers on this new disease was rewarded by the attachment of the eponym "Asherson's Syndrome" to this condition at the November 2002 International Phospholipid Conference held in Sicily. He has established the first International Committee to study survivors of this Syndrome.

He is currently editing a series of 12 volumes entitled "*The Handbook of Systemic Autoimmune Disease*" (Elsevier, The Netherlands) and in September of 2003 was Co-Chairman of the First Latin American Congress on Autoimmunity, held in the Galapagos Islands, Ecuador. He co-chaired and participated in a Session at the Milan Conference on "Heart, Rheumatism and Autoimmunity" held in February 2004.

He was appointed to the International Advisory Board of the International Conference on Systemic Lupus Erythematosus held in New York in May of 2004 and also participated in this Meeting.

Volume Editors

Athol U. Wells

Athol Wells graduated in Medicine at the University of Otago in 1979 and turned to respiratory medicine after completing training as a general physician. From 1986 to 1989, he was a respiratory tutor specialist at Green Lane Hospital, in Auckland, New Zealand, and then moved to the Royal Brompton Hospital in London as a research fellow, initially. After returning to New Zealand in the mid 1990s, he subsequently accepted an appointment as a consultant chest physician at the Royal Brompton Hospital and is now one of two chest physicians who run the interstitial lung disease unit at that institution. He, therefore, has a 15-year expertise in the evaluation and management of the pulmonary complications of connective tissue diseases. The unit in which he works is recognised internationally as a leading world centre for lung disease in systemic autoimmune disease. His own personal research has focused on clinical science, with particular reference to prognostic evaluation, structure/function relationships and CT evaluation of interstitial lung disease at large and, especially, lung disease in systemic sclerosis. More recently, he has applied his expertise to the definition of phenotype in genetic studies. He is the author of numerous clinical studies and is widely involved in post-graduate education as a speaker and writer of review articles and book chapters.

Christopher P. Denton

Christopher Denton graduated in Medicine from Guy's Hospital in London in 1986 and undertook postgraduate training in internal medicine and rheumatology at Northwick Park, St. Thomas' and the Royal Free Hospital in London. He obtained a PhD in vascular biology at University College London in 1997 and gained his specialist accreditation in rheumatology in 1998. After further laboratory and clinical training in genetics and rheumatology as a Wellcome Advanced Fellow at the Texas Medical Centre in Houston, he returned to the UK to join the Centre for Rheumatology at the Royal Free Hospital in London, supported by a Senior Research Fellowship from the Arthritis Research Campaign (UK).

He is currently a senior lecturer in rheumatology and consultant rheumatologist in the scleroderma clinic at the Royal Free which reviews more than 1000 patients with systemic sclerosis and related disorders. He has extensive clinical and laboratory research interests in the field of scleroderma and works closely with cardiologists and respiratory physicians at the Royal Free and the Royal Brompton Hospitals to investigate and treat pulmonary complications of connective tissue disease. In 2003 Christopher Denton was elected as a Fellow of the Royal College of Physicians in London.

List of Contributors

Ronald A. Asherson
Rheumatic Diseases Unit
Department of Medicine
University of Capetown Health Sciences Centre
Groote Schuur Hospital
Capetown
South Africa

Alexander N. Bennett
The Lupus Research Unit
The Rayne Institute
St Thomas' Hospital
London SE1 7EH
UK

Carol M. Black
Centre for Rheumatology
Royal Free Hospital
London, NW3 2QG
UK

Roland M. du Bois
Interstitial Lung Disease Unit
Royal Brompton Hospital
London, SW3 6NP
UK
r.dubois@rbh.nthames.nhs.uk

Philippe Camus
Department of Pulmonary and Intensive Care
University Medical Center Le Bocage
and Medical School
Université de Bourgogne
Dijon
France
philippe.camus@chu-dijon.fr

Ricard Cervera
Systemic Autoimmune Diseases Unit
Hospital Clínic
Barcelona Catalonia
Spain

Joel David
Department of Rheumatology
Nuffield Orthopaedic Centre
Oxford OX3 7LD
UK
joeldavid@noc.anglox.nhs.uk

Garie Davies
Royal Brompton Hospital
Chelsea London
UK

David P. D'Cruz
The Lupus Research Unit
The Rayne Institute
St Thomas' Hospital
London SE1 7EH
UK
david.d'cruz@kcl.ac.uk

Jane Deng
Division of Pulmonary and
Critical Care Medicine
Department of Internal Medicine
University of Michigan Medical Center
Ann Arbor, MI
USA

Christopher P. Denton
Centre for Rheumatology
Royal Free Hospital
London, NW3 2QG
UK
c.denton@rfc.ucl.ac.uk

Sally Edmonds
Department of Rheumatology
Nuffield Orthopaedic Centre
Oxford OX3 7LD
UK

Gerard Espinosa
Systemic Autoimmune Diseases Unit
Hospital Clínic
Barcelona
Catalonia
Spain

Josep Font
Systemic Autoimmune Diseases Unit
Hospital Clínic
Barcelona Catalonia
Spain

Tomás Franquet
Department of Diagnostic Radiology
Hospital de Sant Pau
Universitat Autónoma de Barcelona
Barcelona
Spain
19429tfc@comb.es

Mario García-Carrasco
Systemic Autoimmune Diseases Unit
Hospital Clínic
Barcelona
Catalonia
Spain

Nicole S. Goh
Interstitial Lung Disease Unit
Royal Brompton Hospital
London, SW3 6NP
UK

Wolfgang L. Gross
Department of Rheumatology
University Hospital of Schleswig-Holstein
Luebeck
Germany

Rheumaklinik Bad Bramstedt
Ratzeburger Allee 160
D-23538 Luebeck
Germany
gross@rheuma-zentrum.de

Amy H. Kao
Division of Rheumatology and Clinical Immunology
University of Pittsburgh School of Medicine
Pittsburgh, PA
USA

Michael P. Keane
Division of Pulmonary, Critical Care Medicine and Hospitalists
David Geffen School of Medicine at UCLA
Los Angeles, CA
USA

Peter Lamprecht
Department of Rheumatology
University Hospital of Schleswig-Holstein
Luebeck
Germany

Rheumaklinik Bad Bramstedt
Ratzeburger Allee 160 D-23538
Luebeck
Germany

Joseph P. Lynch III
Division of Pulmonary, Critical Care Medicine
and Hospitalists
David Geffen School of Medicine at UCLA
Los Angeles, CA
USA
jplynch@mednet.ucla.edu

Susan Manzi
Division of Rheumatology and Clinical Immunology
University of Pittsburgh School of Medicine
and University of Pittsburgh Graduate School
of Public Health
Pittsburgh, PA
USA
sxm6@pitt.edu

Haralampos M. Moutsopoulos
Department of Pathophysiology
Laiko Hospital
School of Medicine
National and Kapodistrian University of Athens
Athens
Greece
hmoutsop@med.uoa.gr

Andrew G. Nicholson
Department of Histopathology
Royal Brompton Hospital
London, SW3 6NP
UK
a.nicholson@rbh.nthames.nhs.uk

Spyros A. Papiris
Department of Critical Care and Pulmonary Services
Evangelismos Hospital
School of Medicine
National and Kapodistrian University of Athens
Athens
Greece
papiris@otenent.gr

Janice M. Sabatine
Division of Rheumatology and Clinical Immunology
University of Pittsburgh School of Medicine
Pittsburgh, PA
USA

Armin Schnabel
Department of Rheumatology and Clinical Immunology
Sana Centre of Rheumatology
Bad Wildbad
Germany

Donall Tansey
Department of Histopathology
Royal Brompton Hospital
London, SW3 6NP
UK

Athol U. Wells
Royal Brompton Hospital
Chelsea
London
UK
a.wells@rbh.nthames.nhs.uk

Contents

PART I

Pathology

Handbook of Systemic Autoimmune Diseases, Volume 2
Pulmonary Involvement in Systemic Autoimmune Diseases
A.U. Wells and C.P. Denton, editors

CHAPTER 1

Lung Pathology in Connective Tissue Diseases

Donall Tansey, Andrew G. Nicholson*

Department of Histopathology, Royal Brompton Hospital, Sydney Street, London SW3 6NP, UK

1. Introduction

Pathologic changes are commonly seen in the lungs of patients with connective tissue diseases (CTDs) and, in a minority of patients, may actually be the site of initial manifestation of their systemic disease. All compartments of the lung can be affected, from pleura, airway, and alveolar parenchyma through to the pulmonary vasculature, and these anatomic regions can be affected either in isolation or in combination, producing a variety of both clinical and histological presentations. Furthermore, the histological features of CTDs need to be separated from the effects of therapy, including drug reactions and opportunistic infections, as well as any coexistent disease processes not directly associated with the CTDs. This may be difficult as, in most cases, the histologic patterns found in the lung are rarely specific for a particular CTD and are indistinguishable from those in patients without an underlying systemic disorder. Detailed clinicopathologic correlation is therefore essential when reviewing biopsy material from patients with CTDs or where a background CTD is suspected, in order to elucidate what is the likely cause of the patient's pulmonary symptoms. This review first documents the most commonly seen histologic patterns in this clinical setting and then reviews the specific disease processes in relation to the CTDs themselves.

*Corresponding author.
Tel.: +44-20-7351-8423; fax: +44-20-7351-8293
E-mail address: a.nicholson@rbh.nthames.nhs.uk
(A.G. Nicholson).

DOI: 10.1016/S1571-5078(04)02001-X

2. Overview of histologic patterns seen in collagen vascular diseases

2.1. Interstitial pneumonias

It is well known that the term 'fibrosing alveolitis' has been used to describe patients with diffuse fibrotic lung disease, both in relation to idiopathic disease and in cases associated with connective tissue diseases (Fairfax et al., 1981; Turner-Warwick, 1986, 1988; Askin, 1990). However, there have been considerable refinements in recent years in recognition of histological patterns of interstitial pneumonia, this work concentrating predominantly on patients with idiopathic disease. Thus, these data have led to a consensus classification system via an ATS/ERS sponsored committee comprising clinicians, radiologists and pathologists (Table 1) (Travis et al., 2002). Stemming from this work, terms such as 'lone cryptogenic fibrosing alveolitis', i.e. that arising without any clinical association, are preferably used as a collective clinicopathologic description of the patient's disease, whilst the histological features are categorised according to patterns of interstitial pneumonia. Usage of this system appears reproducible, in terms of pathologists making the diagnosis (Nicholson et al., in press), and provides prognostic information (Travis et al., 2002).

Table 1
Histologic patterns of interstitial pneumonias and clinicopathologic counterparts in an idiopathic setting (From Travis et al., 2002)

Histologic pattern	Clinicopathologic diagnosis
Usual interstitial pneumonia (UIP) (CFA)/Idiopathic pulmonary fibrosis (IPF)	Cryptogenic fibrosing alveolitis
Non-specific interstitial pneumonia (NSIP)	Non-specific interstitial pneumonia[a]
Organising pneumonia (OP)	Cryptogenic organising pneumonia
Diffuse alveolar damage (DAD)	Acute interstitial pneumonia
Desquamative interstitial pneumonia (DIP)	Desquamative interstitial pneumonia
Respiratory bronchiolitis (RB)	Respiratory bronchiolitis-associated Interstitial lung disease (RBILD)
Lymphocytic interstitial pneumonia (LIP)	Lymphocytic interstitial pneumonia

[a] provisional term for clinicopathologic diagnosis.

In parallel with and subsequent to this work on idiopathic disease, there has been a resurgence of interest in relation to interstitial pneumonias arising in association with CTDs, in particular determining whether the same patterns of interstitial pneumonia can be applied using the same criteria and whether they provide similar data in terms of clinicopathologic diagnosis, treatment and prognosis. Recent work has centred primarily on recognition of the pattern of non-specific interstitial pneumonia (NSIP), as until recently most of the published data preceded its recognition.

2.1.1. Non-specific interstitial pneumonia

In 1994, Katzenstein and Fiorelli used the term NSIP to describe a group of interstitial pneumonias that could not be classified according to recognised subsets at that time. They were particular in stating that there were several clinical associations (e.g. collagen vascular diseases, exposure to environmental allergens, history of acute lung injury) with NSIP. However, despite this, a histologic pattern of NSIP was associated with a greater response to treatment and a more favourable prognosis than a histologic pattern of usual interstitial pneumonia (UIP) (Katzenstein and Fiorelli, 1994). In the consensus classification system, there is an agreed histologic definition for the pattern of NSIP, subdivided into cellular and fibrotic types (Bjoraker et al., 1998). The characteristics on high-resolution computerised tomographic (HRCT) scan are also documented (Akira et al., 2000; Hartman et al., 2000; MacDonald et al., 2001; Travis et al., 2002). However, its clinical counterpart remains less well defined and the clinicopathologic entity of NSIP is regarded as provisional in the consensus classification system (Table 1) (Travis et al., 2002). However, whilst being of uncertain clinical significance in idiopathic disease, data are increasingly being reported indicating a high incidence in patients with CTDs (Douglas et al., 2001; Fujita et al., 2001; Kim et al., 2002; Bouros et al., 2002; Nicholson et al., 2002). These data are discussed in greater detail in relation to specific disorders.

Histologically, NSIP shows expansion of the interstitium by variable amounts of chronic inflammation and fibrosis, initially graded one to three (cellular, cellular and fibrosing, fibrosing) (Katzenstein and Fiorelli, 1994). Classification has been simplified to two groups, namely cellular and fibrotic NSIP (Travis et al., 2002), as survival rates for cellular and fibrosing (grade 2) and fibrotic (grade 3) patterns are similar (Fig. 1) (Nicholson et al., 2000; Travis et al., 2000). In NSIP, the interstitial abnormality, be it cellular or fibrotic, is more diffuse than in UIP and the key to distinguishing fibrotic NSIP from UIP is the relative absence of temporal heterogeneity in NSIP, in that fibroblastic foci are either absent or very scarce. A relative absence of alveolar macrophages, organising pneumonia (OP), and hyaline membranes distinguishes NSIP from other patterns (Travis et al., 2002).

2.1.2. Usual interstitial pneumonia

UIP is the most common histologic pattern seen in cases of idiopathic interstitial pneumonia. It correlates clinically with the idiopathic disorder cryptogenic fibrosing alveolitis/idiopathic pulmonary fibrosis (CFA/IPF) (American Thoracic Society, 2000), a disease typically characterised by chronic progression to death, with an average survival of 2–3 years (Bjoraker et al., 1998; American Thoracic Society, 2000; Nicholson et al., 2000; Travis et al., 2000;

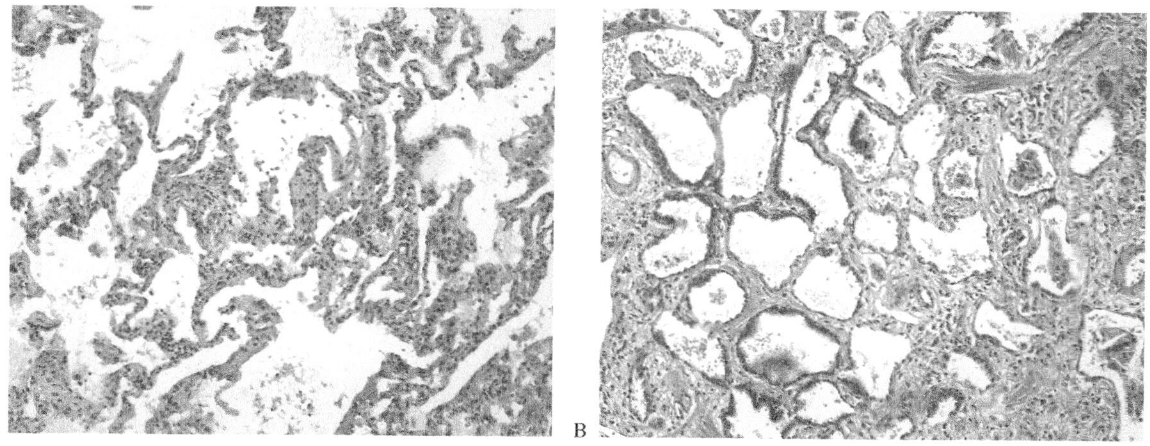

Figure 1. (A) A case of cellular NSIP where there is a mild diffuse interstitial infiltrate of chronic inflammatory cells with no interstitial fibrosis. (B) A case of fibrotic NSIP shows interstitial fibrosis that has a more diffuse distribution than UIP and also lacks fibroblastic foci.

Flaherty et al., 2002). However, although some series describe a high frequency of UIP in patients with CTDs (Tazelaar et al., 1990), most of these data precede recognition of the pattern of NSIP. Later studies have shown a much lower incidence when cases with a pattern of NSIP are recognised (Douglas et al., 2001). Nevertheless, a pattern of UIP is described in most series of patients with collagen vascular diseases with a low incidence (Douglas et al., 2001; Fujita et al., 2001; Bouros et al., 2002; Kim et al., 2002; Yamadori et al., 2002).

Histologically, UIP shows patchy established fibrosis associated with a mild to moderate non-specific chronic inflammatory cell infiltrate, being most marked in subpleural or paraseptal regions of the pulmonary acinus. The intervening lung parenchyma is normal or nearly normal. In addition, there are varying numbers of 'fibroblastic foci', these comprising an abundance of plump spindle cells and little intervening collagen, lying in continuity with areas of established interstitial fibrosis (Fig. 2). This variation in the age of the fibrosis (sometimes termed temporal heterogeneity) is a cardinal feature of UIP and the extent of these foci is associated with mortality and increased rate of disease progression in idiopathic disease (Nicholson, 2002). This has not been proven to be the case in CTDs as numbers are too small, although a comparative study of UIP in an idiopathic setting with UIP in association with CTDs showed that fibroblastic foci were more frequently found in idiopathic disease (Flaherty et al., 2003). A second study on contractility of fibroblasts in NSIP and UIP showed increased contractility in cases of UIP (Miki et al., 2000). Therefore, although fibroblastic foci may appear histologically the same in different histologic patterns and patient groups, early data suggest there may be biologic differences.

2.1.3. Organising pneumonia

Organising pneumonia (OP) is a non-specific pattern of repair seen in response to injury, usually a secondary phenomenon (one of which is an association with CTDs) (Rees et al., 1991; Wright et al., 1992), but occasionally primary when the disease is termed cryptogenic organising pneumonia (COP) (Cordier, 2000). Histologically, there is patchy filling of alveoli and bronchioles by buds of granulation tissue (also termed Masson bodies) (Fig. 3). These have a loose myxoid quality and contain little collagen, and their intra-alveolar location should distinguish them from the fibroblastic foci of UIP, which are in continuity with areas of established interstitial fibrosis. The alveolar architecture usually remains relatively normal, but there may sometimes be scarring and remodelling. Occasionally, the organising pneumonia may extend into respiratory bronchioles, which has led to the alternative term 'bronchiolitis obliterans organising pneumonia' (BOOP) being used by some groups. However,

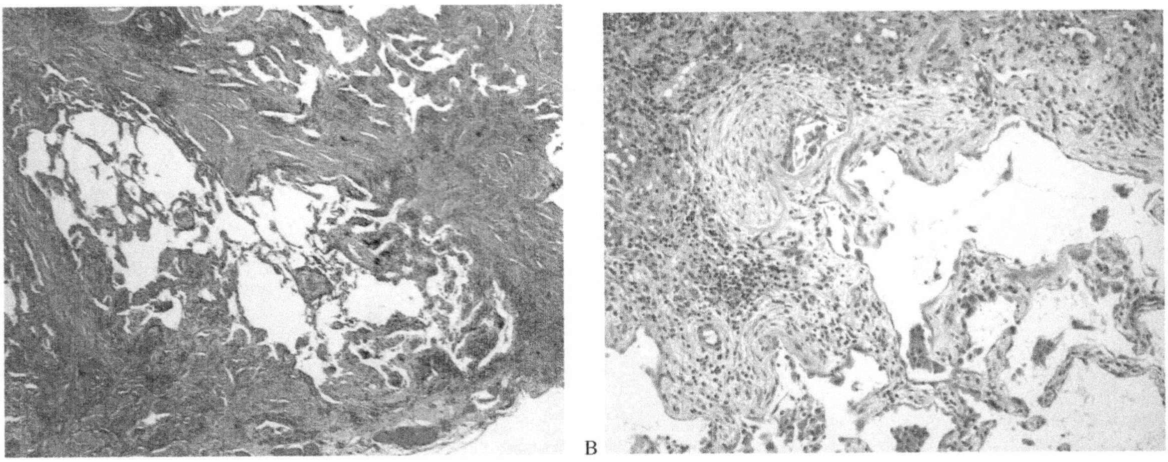

A B

Figure 2. (A) A case of UIP shows patchy, heterogenous inflammation and fibrosis with a subpleural distribution, alternating with areas of normal alveolar lung. (B) A high power view shows a fibroblastic focus adjacent to areas of established fibrosis.

the primary location of this change is within the alveoli and the consensus opinion is that OP is a more accurate term, plus it avoids confusion with constrictive obliterative bronchiolitis (OB) (see Section 2.2.3).

2.1.4. Diffuse alveolar damage

Diffuse alveolar damage (DAD) is the histological pattern seen in acute interstitial pneumonia (AIP) (Katzenstein et al., 1986) and, far more commonly, in acute respiratory distress syndrome (ARDS), one of the clinical associations for the latter being associated CTDs. Some groups have suggested the term secondary acute interstitial pneumonia for DAD in the setting of CTDs, but this has not gained acceptance (Bouros et al., 2000). Histologically, there is a marked expansion of the interstitium by a predominantly fibroblastic proliferation and an inflammatory cell infiltrate of variable intensity and content. Hyaline membranes are present in the exudative phase and intra-alveolar organisation in the organising phase (Fig. 4). Rare acute exacerbations of both NSIP and UIP may occur as terminal events, when DAD is superimposed on chronic changes (Rice et al., 2003).

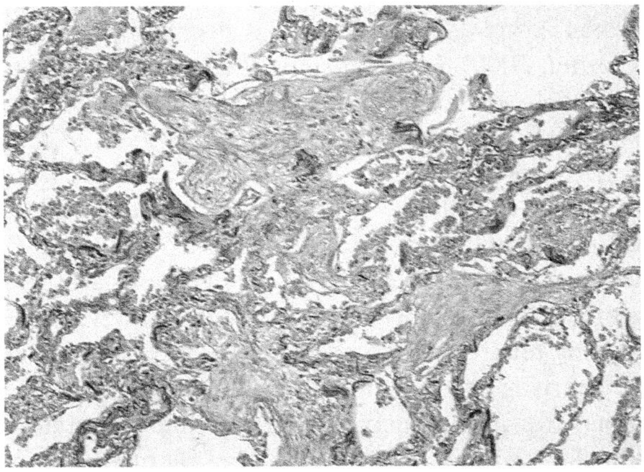

Figure 3. The histologic pattern of organising pneumonia (OP) shows patchy filling of alveoli by buds of fibroblastic tissue.

2.1.5. Lymphocytic interstitial pneumonia

Recent data suggest that lymphocytic interstitial pneumonia (LIP) is only rarely pre-neoplastic, leading to its re-inclusion in the consensus classification for idiopathic interstitial pneumonias. However, idiopathic LIP is exceptionally rare, being far more commonly associated with CTDs or immunosuppression, both acquired and congenital. Histologically, there is a diffuse dense interstitial lymphoid infiltrate comprising small round T-lymphocytes, plasma cells and histiocytes with focal B-cell aggregates (Fig. 5). LIP is readily distinguishable from other patterns of interstitial pneumonia, with the exception of cellular NSIP (although clinical data for both patterns are similar). LIP also requires distinction from non-Hodgkin's lymphomas, which can be effected

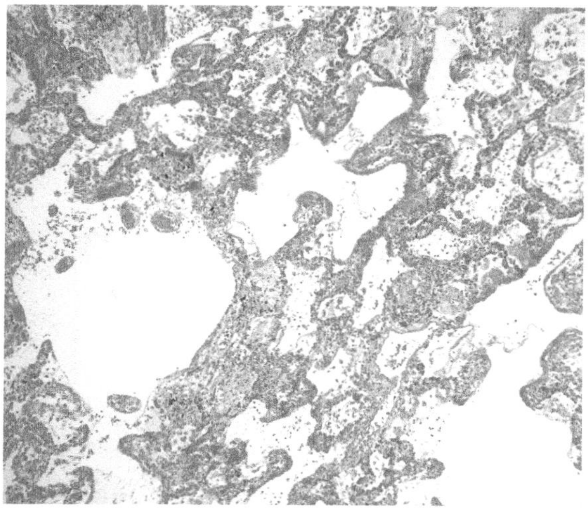

Figure 4. A case of diffuse alveolar damage (DAD) in the exudative phase. The interstitium is expanded by a few fibroblasts and a mixed inflammatory cell infiltrate, with abundant hyaline membranes lining alveoli.

through immunohistochemical and molecular analysis (Nicholson, 2002).

2.1.6. Desquamative interstitial pneumonia and respiratory bronchiolitis

Historically, desquamative interstitial pneumonia (DIP) was thought to represent an early (cellular/desquamative) phase of CFA, but the current view is much more closely associated with respiratory bronchiolitis (RB), in that smoking causes the majority of cases. Histologically, there is an accumulation of macrophages distributed diffusely within pulmonary acini, the macrophages characteristically having abundant glassy eosinophilic cytoplasm, often with a finely granular light brown pigment. The alveolar architecture is generally well maintained, although there is usually a mild chronic inflammatory cell infiltrate within the interstitium. In RB, the histologic features are very similar to DIP, other than they are centriacinar in distribution (Travis et al., 2002). Small numbers of patients with histologic patterns of both DIP and RB are reported in series relating to CTDs although, where documented, all were smokers (Carrington et al., 1978; Hakala et al., 1990; Yousem et al., 1989; Yousem, 1990; Moon et al., 1999). Therefore, these changes are likely to be unrelated to the CTD and in some cases may even be unrelated to the patient's symptoms.

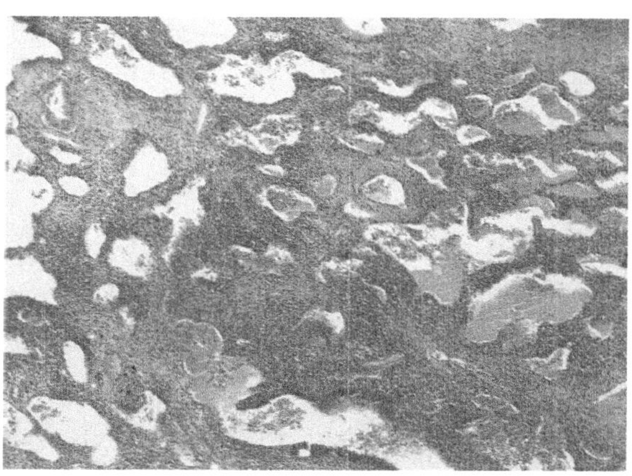

Figure 5. A case of LIP shows diffuse expansion of the interstitium by a dense infiltrate of small lymphocytes, plasma cells and histiocytes.

2.1.7. When to biopsy for interstitial pneumonias

As stated above, all patterns of interstitial pneumonia from the consensus classification are described in relation to CTDs, but there is considerable variation in incidence. Furthermore, some patients will show more than one pattern of disease (Nagao et al., 2001) and these superimposed combinations of patterns, plus other pathologies (Katzenstein and Askin, 1997; Yousem, 1990), may be distinctive for certain CTDs. However, despite these histological advances, much of these data can now be identified non-invasively, in particular through use of HRCT scanning and lung function studies, and many cases will now be diagnosed without recourse to biopsy. This is further compounded by recent data showing that there is a relative lack of prognostic data in biopsies taken from patients with CTDs (Bouros et al., 2002). Nevertheless, surgical lung biopsies are still likely to be undertaken in some patients, especially those in which there is an atypical clinical and/or radiologic presentation. This is undertaken both to identify the pattern of interstitial pneumonia and also to exclude other disorders, for example amyloidosis (Marenco et al., 1994). Many patients may also be taking immunosuppressive therapy, and biopsy may also be particularly useful in excluding both drug toxicity and opportunistic infections (Askin, 1990).

Finally, biopsies may be undertaken to investigate for associated malignancies.

2.2. Other parenchymal disorders

2.2.1. Amyloidosis

Amyloidosis is characterised by extracellular deposition of a proteinaceous substance which, when viewed under polarised light after staining with Congo red, emits a unique apple-green birefringence (Puchtler et al., 1962). Biochemically, amyloid comprises a β-pleated fibrillar structure but the exact composition of the fibrils depends on the protein from which they are derived. In respiratory tract amyloidosis, clinical disease is caused by primary or AL-type amyloid and has traditionally been classified according to the anatomical site—laryngeal, tracheobronchial or parenchymal—with further division into localised and systemic disease. This is most commonly seen in relation to Sjogren's syndrome, when it can present in association with lymphoid hyperplasia to cause cystic changes (Fig. 6) (Desai et al., 1997).

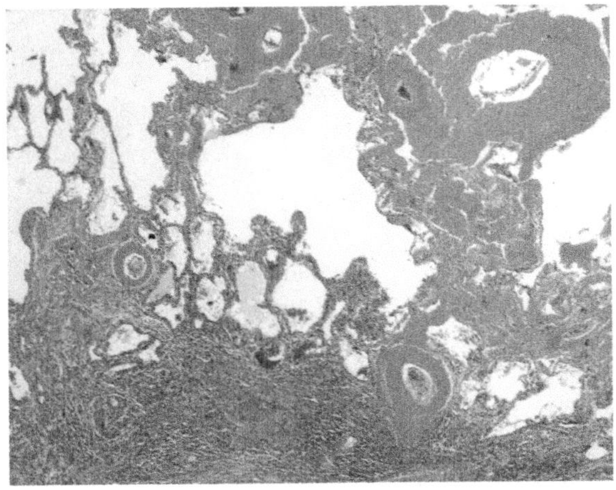

Figure 6. A case of amyloidosis is associated with lymphoid hyperplasia and air-space destruction in a patient with Sjogren's syndrome.

2.2.2. Diffuse haemorrhage

This is characterised by acute or chronic intra-alveolar haemorrhage, which may be primary or secondary, rare associations being systemic lupus erythematosus (SLE) (Myers and Katzenstein, 1986) or rheumatoid arthritis (Travis et al., 1990). Biopsy shows a combination of intra-alveolar haemorrhage and haemosiderosis. The haemosiderin, which provides evidence of previous bleeding, is largely contained within alveolar macrophages but may also impregnate elastin in blood vessel walls and can be highlighted with a Perl's stain for iron.

2.2.3. Alveolar proteinosis

This is characterised by expansion of alveoli by acellular finely granular lipoproteinaceous debris (Fig. 7). It is classified into primary and secondary type, a rare cause of secondary disease being dermatomyositis (Samuels and Warner, 1988).

2.2.4. Eosinophilic pneumonia

This is characterised by expansion of alveoli by eosinophils, macrophages and fibrinous debris, often with eosinophils involving the interstitium. There may also be focal intra-alveolar organisation and eosinophilic micro-abscesses. The differential diagnosis includes a drug reaction but eosinophilic pneumonia is described in patients with rheumatoid arthritis (Papiris et al., 1995; Kwak et al., 2003).

2.3. Airways disease

CTDs may affect both the large and small airways in relations to their walls and their lumens and, as in the

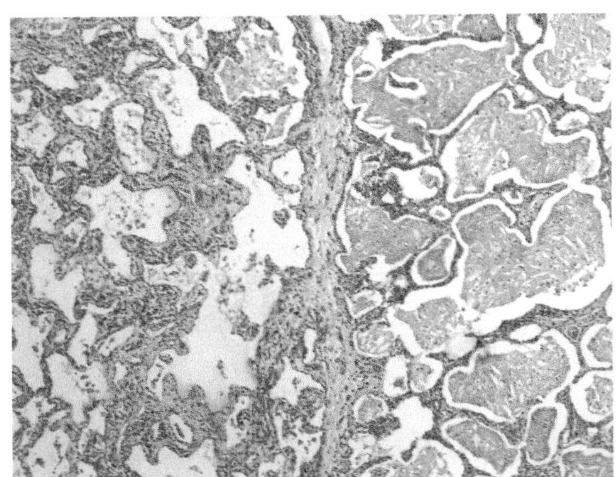

Figure 7. A case of polymyositis/dermatomyositis shows focal proteinosis superimposed upon a background of NSIP-like fibrosis.

interstitial pneumonias, the relative incidences for these histological patterns vary between disorders. The inflammatory infiltrate may be acute and chronic or chronic in CTDs and some groups use the term 'cellular bronchiolitis' as a descriptive term for such infiltrates. In some cases, a combination of patterns of bronchiolitis may be seen in the same patient (Fig. 8).

2.3.1. Chronic bronchiolitis

This term typically refers to a variably intense non-specific chronic inflammatory cell infiltrate within the bronchial or bronchiolar walls (Fig. 8). In Sjogren's syndrome, some cases show a predilection for the infiltrate to involve the seromucinous glands, leading to glandular atrophy and xerotrachea (Papiris et al., 1999).

2.3.2. Follicular bronchitis/iolitis

Follicular bronchitis/iolitis (FB) is part of the spectrum of pulmonary lymphoid hyperplasia, with FB at one end being peribronchiolar in location and LIP showing interstitial predominance. As such, LIP is part of the consensus classification for interstitial pneumonias (Travis et al., 2002) whilst FB is viewed primarily as an airways disorder. Both FB and LIP are only exceptionally found in an idiopathic setting, being most frequently seen in association with CTDs or immunosuppression. Therefore, recognition of these patterns in a patient with no recognised clinical association should precipitate investigations along these lines, particularly in children.

Histologically, FB is characterised by prominent peribronchial lymphoid follicles with a minor interstitial inflammatory component (Fig. 8). Hyperplastic follicles may also been seen in the interlobular septa and the visceral pleura. Compression of the airway lumens not infrequently leads to obstruction and a resultant intraluminal acute inflammatory cell infiltrate, plus endogenous pneumonia in some cases. FB should be distinguished from 'follicular bronchiectasis' a term used when prominent follicular hyperplasia is accompanied by marked airway dilatation, as seen in patients with conditions such as cystic fibrosis.

2.3.3. Constrictive bronchiolitis

In constrictive bronchiolitis, the damaged respiratory epithelium is replaced by chronic inflammatory granulation tissue, often laid down in a circumferential pattern with narrowing and eventual obliteration of the airway lumen. This may occur in relation to localised airway damage, such as distal to bronchiectasis, or in a diffuse fashion as seen in some CTDs (Fig. 8).

2.3.4. Bronchiectasis

Bronchiectasis is defined as a permanent abnormal dilatation of the airways, usually associated with an inflammatory cell infiltrate. Its causes are many, and include most CTDs.

2.3.5. Bronchocentric granulomatosis

Bronchocentric granulomatosis is a necrotising granulomatous process that replaces the airway walls with palisading granulomatous inflammation and fills the lumens with necrotic debris (Fig. 9). Most cases relate to allergy/infection, but rare non-infectious causes include rheumatoid arthritis (Hellems et al., 1983; Bonafede and Benatar, 1987).

2.4. Pleural disease

Pleural involvement in CTDs has been described as acute fibrinous pleuritis, organising fibrous pleuritis, chronic pleuritis and pleural fibrosis, although all these terms likely relate to the degree and intensity of active inflammation at this site (Fig. 10). Occasionally palisading granulomatous inflammation may involve the pleura in relation to rheumatoid arthritis. Marked acute inflammation may also be seen, although infection should first be excluded before diagnosing a 'sterile empyema'. Spontaneous pneumothorax has been described in patients with ankylosing spondylitis and Marfans' syndrome.

2.5. Vascular disease

2.5.1. Pulmonary hypertension

The histologic features of pulmonary hypertension typically vary in relation to the degree of raised pulmonary arterial pressure, pulmonary hypertension

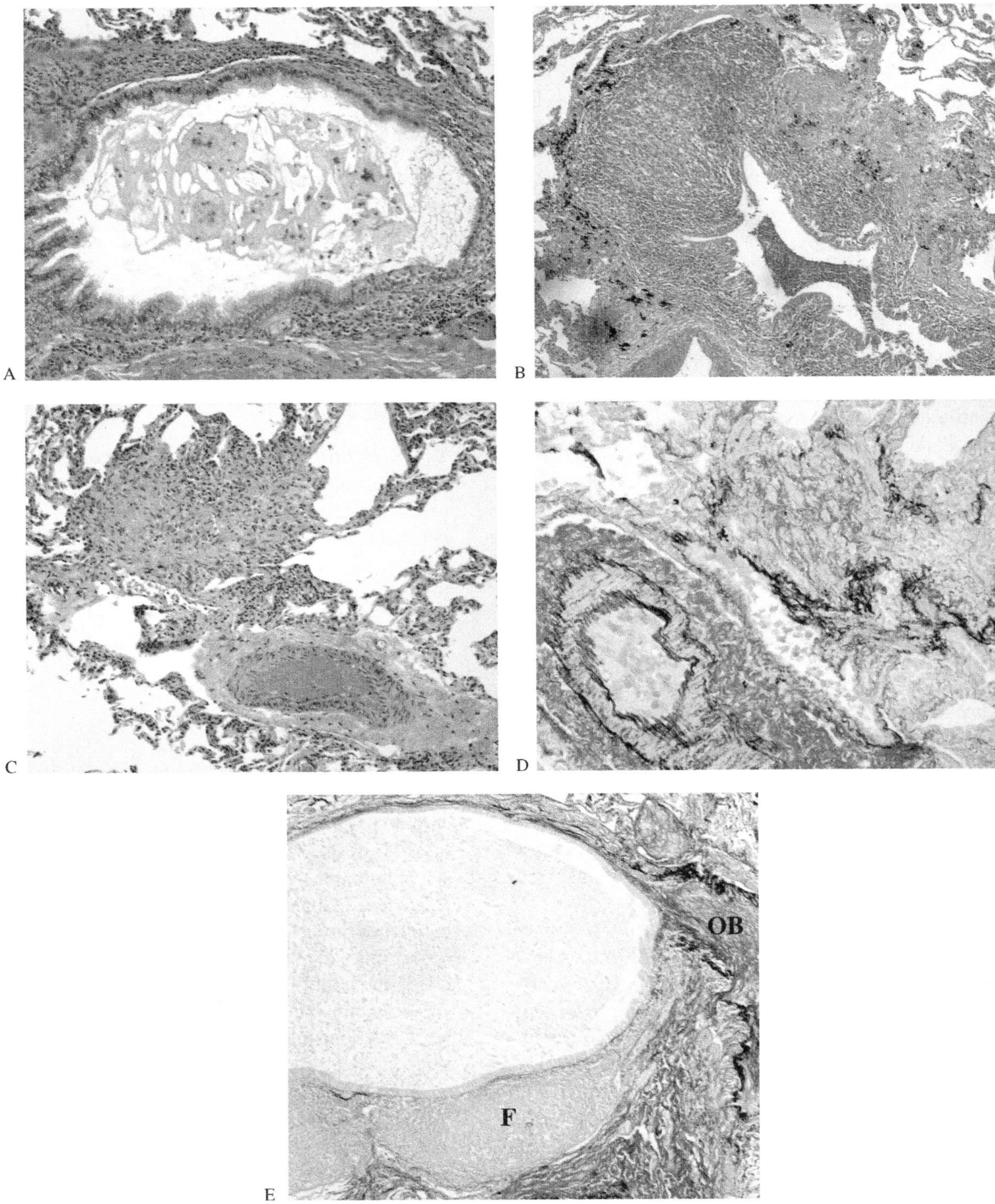
A
B
C
D
OB
F
E

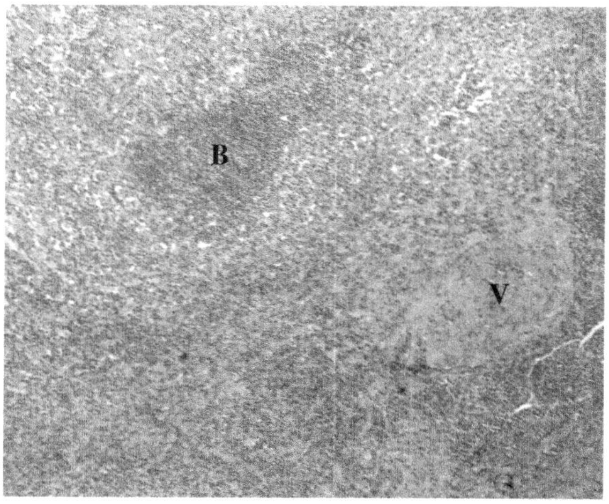

Figure 9. A case of bronchocentric granulomatosis shows palisading granulomatous inflammation destroying the airway wall with fibrinopurulent cell debris in its lumen (B). The accompanying vessel helps identify the destroyed airway (V).

defined as a mean resting pressure of above 25 mm Hg. When mild, the histological features are typically those of medial hypertrophy (Fig. 11), with progression through marked intimal hyperplasia (Fig. 11), vasculitis with fibrinoid necrosis and eventually plexogenic arteriopathy (Fig. 11), and are essentially the same as those seen in primary pulmonary hypertension. Early changes need to be distinguished from secondary changes related to an associated interstitial pneumonia.

2.5.2. Thromboembolism

Patients with SLE and the anti-phospholipid syndrome may suffer from localised thromboembolism, leading to pulmonary hypertension.

2.5.3. Vasculitis

Small vessel vasculitis may be occasionally seen in association with CTDs, most frequently SLE.

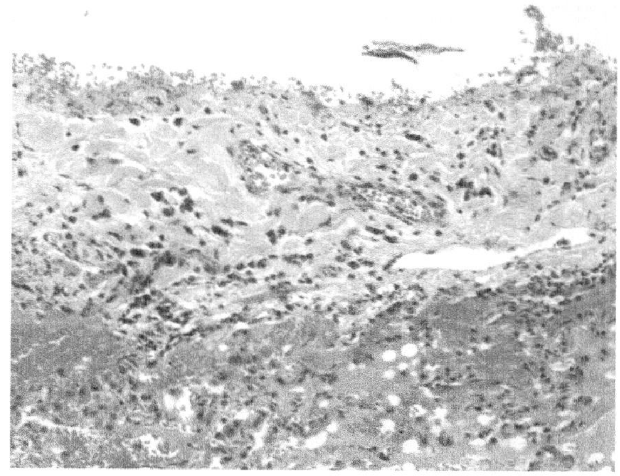

Figure 10. A case of chronic pleuritis shows fibrous thickening and mild non-specific chronic inflammation of the visceral pleura. The underlying lung is within normal limits.

2.6. Neoplasms

Evidence for an increased risk of carcinoma, lymphoma and Kaposi's sarcoma is discussed in relation to individual CTDs.

2.7. Others

Diaphragmatic and respiratory muscle dysfunction and atelectasis are also features of CTDs, particularly PM/DM and ankylosing spondylitis, respectively, although these are rarely biopsied.

3. Pathology in relation to specific connective tissue disorders

3.1. Systemic sclerosis

The most common pulmonary manifestations of scleroderma/systemic sclerosis (SSc) are the

Figure 8. (A) A case of chronic bronchiolitis shows a moderately cellular infiltrate within the bronchiolar wall. The lumen contains proteinaceous debris and macrophages. (B) In follicular bronchiolitis, prominent lymphoid follicles are present that compress airway lumens. (C) In constrictive obliterative bronchiolitis, routine H&E staining shows a nodule of fibrosis and inflammation adjacent to a small artery. (D) An EVG stain shows that this nodule is in fact the occluded airway lumen of the accompanying bronchiole. (E) In this patient with rheumatoid arthritis, both follicular bronchiolitis (F) and constrictive obliterative bronchiolitis (OB) coexist in the same patient (EVG stain).

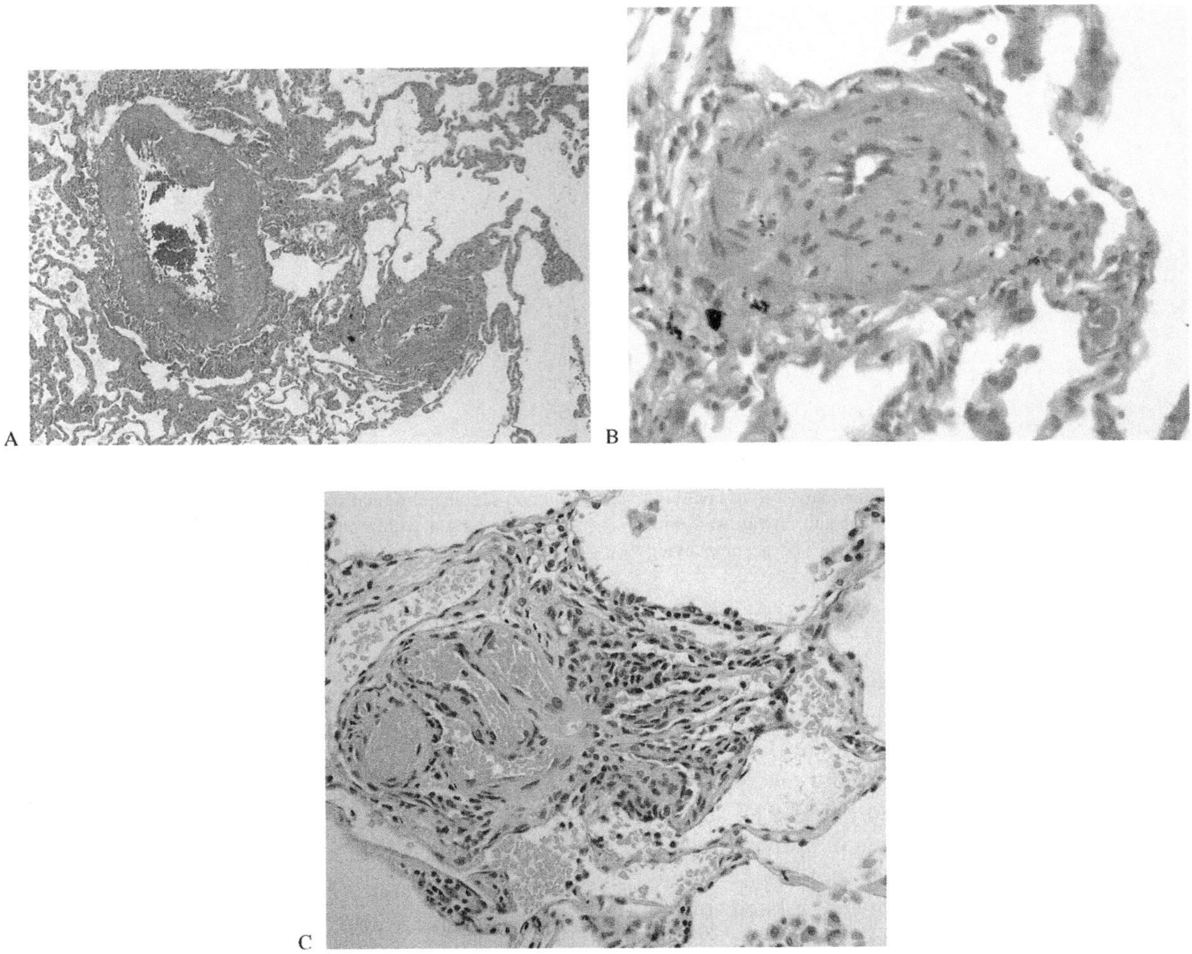

Figure 11. Features of pulmonary hypertension vary from (A) medial hypertrophy, and (B) marked intimal fibrous thickening through to (C) plexogenic lesions in the most severe cases.

interstitial pneumonias. Their prevalence at autopsy is approximately 70% (D'Angelo et al., 1969; Wiedemann and Matthay, 1989), although this figure overstates the frequency of pulmonary fibrosis in SSc in routine clinical evaluation, as a large proportion of SSc patients screened for lung disease have sub-clinical involvement or lack clinical evidence of interstitial lung disease (Harrison et al., 1989). It has long been established that a fibrosing alveolitis occurs in patients with SSc. These patients have a better prognosis and different CT appearances (Wells et al., 1994, 1997; Chan et al., 1997) when compared to patients with lone cryptogenic fibrosing alveolitis (i.e. without any associated disease process). Early studies on histological features showed no histologic differences between the two groups, other than increased lymphoid hyperplasia in those patients with SSc (Harrison et al., 1991). However, the recognition and subsequent acceptance of NSIP as a pattern of interstitial pneumonia have led to several reviews of such patients, showing an incidence of NSIP (Fig. 1) ranging from 55 to 77% of cases (Fujita et al., 2001; Bouros et al., 2002; Kim et al., 2002). The second most commonly seen pattern was UIP, although importantly the adverse prognosis that is associated with this pattern in idiopathic disease was not seen in patients with SSc. Indeed, no difference in prognosis was seen even between cellular and fibrotic variants of NSIP, with increased mortality in NSIP only being associated with lower initial DL(CO) levels, higher BAL eosinophil levels and deterioration in DL(CO) levels during the three years following biopsy (Bouros et al., 2002). Other histological patterns seen in scleroderma include DIP and RB although, as discussed earlier, it is likely that the accumulation of macrophages is related to smoking and either not relevant to symptoms or incidental to the CTD (Moon et al., 1999; Yousem, 1990). Organising pneumonia has been reported in occasional patients (Bridges et al., 1992) although, in some, the pulmonary manifestation has been attributed to penicillamine therapy. DAD in relation to presentation with ARDS in association with SSc has also been occasionally reported (Muir et al., 1997), as has the presence of sarcoid-like granulomas (Fig. 12) (Biasi et al., 1998; Bouros et al., 2002). However, whether these sarcoid-like changes relate to the SSc or are incidental is unknown.

Pulmonary hypertension is typically seen in patients with the CREST form of systemic sclerosis (calcinosis cutis, Raynaud's phenomenon, esophageal dysfunction, sclerodactyly and telangiectasia). On histology the small pulmonary arteries typically show myxoid thickening of their walls with circumferential intimal cell proliferation ('onion-skinning') (Fig. 11) (Yousem, 1990). Plexiform lesions are generally absent or scarce (Cool et al., 1997). Pulmonary hypertension has been accelerated by pregnancy (Landzberg et al., 1999). In some patients pulmonary hypertension is caused by veno-occlusive disease (Morassut et al., 1992).

Oesophageal involvement in systemic sclerosis may result in aspiration pneumonia. The histologic changes include alveolar wall necrosis, neutrophilic exudation, and pulmonary haemorrhage; the latter often shows brown discolouration due to the production of acid haematin. There is associated acute bronchitis and bronchiolitis with sloughing of the mucosa (Johnson et al., 1989). Occasional cases with isolated small airways disease have also been reported (Yousem, 1990).

There have been numerous reported cases and series of carcinoma of the lung arising on a background of SSc, suggesting an increased risk of cancer among patients. The strongest evidence for an increased risk comes from a population-based follow up study in Sweden where the standardised incidence ratio for all cancers among patient with SSc was significantly increased, including lung cancer (SIR = 2.5) (Rosenthal et al., 1993). The most commonly seen neoplasm is adenocarcinoma, not infrequently with a bronchioloalveolar pattern (Fig. 13) (Yang et al., 2001), which may provide the pathologist with significant problems in diagnosis, especially on small biopsies. Goblet cell hyperplasia in association with honeycomb change may be very difficult to distinguish from a neoplastic proliferation lining alveolar spaces (Nicholson, in press). However, although there is an increased risk to operative resection of non-small cell carcinomas on a background of pulmonary fibrosis, surgical excision remains an option in the appropriate patient (Kumar et al., 2003).

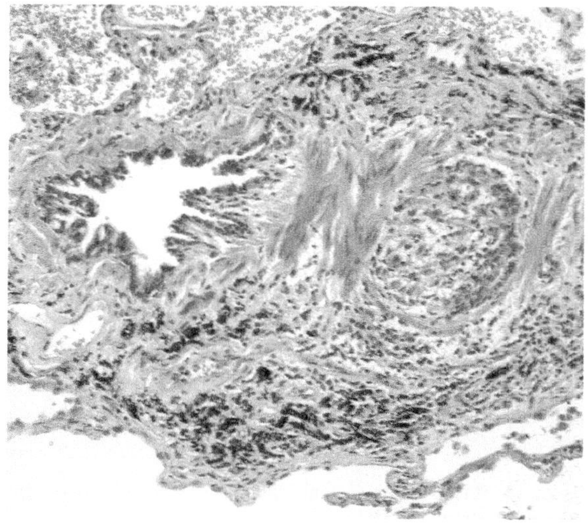

Figure 12. A patient with systemic sclerosis shows a sarcoid-like granuloma adjacent to a bronchiole.

3.2. Rheumatoid arthritis

Histologic changes in the lungs of patients with rheumatoid arthritis are diverse and may occur in isolation or superimposed upon one another. However, with the exception of rheumatoid nodules, the

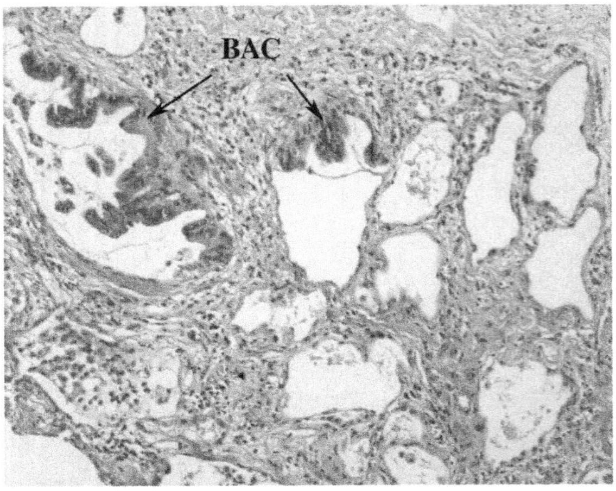

Figure 13. A case of non-specific interstitial pneumonia in systemic sclerosis is complicated by a bronchioloalveolar carcinoma.

histologic patterns do not differ from those seen in cases due to other causes. Another factor to take into account, particularly in rheumatoid arthritis, is that lung injury occurs not uncommonly as the result of drug therapy. Non-steroidal anti-inflammatory drugs (NSAIDs) can cause asthma and eosinophilic pneumonia, while the cytotoxic effects of gold and penicillamine may result in DAD and pulmonary fibrosis. The immunosuppressive effects of methotrexate may also result in varying patterns of interstitial pneumonias, as well as opportunistic infections and lymphoproliferative disease (Imokawa et al., 2000).

In terms of incidence of pulmonary manifestations of rheumatoid arthritis, pleuritis and pleural effusions are the most common. The pleural effusions may be unilateral or bilateral. Cytologic examination of the fluid typically shows elongated and multinucleated histiocytes, necrotic debris and inflammatory cells. Lipid droplets may be visible in the cytoplasm of neutrophils, similar to the ragocytes seen in the joint fluid of arthritic patients. Superimposed bacterial infection can result in empyema. Histology typically shows fibrosis with often prominent chronic inflammation including hyperplastic lymphoid follicles. Less commonly, discrete pleural rheumatoid nodules are seen or there is a linear granulomatous reaction with the mesothelium replaced by palisading histiocytes. Rarely a cavitating intrapulmonary rheumatoid nodule may result in a bronchopleural fistula and pyopneumothorax (Davies, 1966).

Clinically overt pulmonary parenchymal disease in the form of interstitial pneumonias has been reported in approximately 5% of patients with rheumatoid arthritis. All seven patterns of interstitial pneumonias from the consensus classification have been described in patients with rheumatoid arthritis and studies from the 1980s reported that UIP and organising pneumonia were relatively common (Yousem et al., 1985; Hakala et al., 1990). However, more recent data suggest that a pattern of NSIP is more common using current criteria, often with superimposed follicular bronchiolitis (Tansey et al., in press).

Rheumatoid nodules occur in approximately 25% of patients with rheumatoid arthritis, usually in those with severe disease. They typically occur in the skin over pressure points but may also form in a variety of viscera including the lungs, the heart, and the spleen. In the lungs the rheumatoid nodules are found most commonly in the subpleural regions of the upper lung zones although they may also occur within the substance of the lung and in the trachea and bronchi. Pulmonary rheumatoid nodules may be single or multiple, measure up to 7 cm across and can increase or decrease in size depending on disease activity. On histology they show a central zone of fibrinoid necrosis surrounded by a palisading rim of epithelioid histiocytes together with lymphocytes and plasma cells (Fig. 14) (Walters and Ojeda, 1986; Yousem et al., 1985). They enter the differential diagnosis of necrotising granulomas and therefore infection should be thoroughly excluded, before a diagnosis of rheumatoid nodule is made.

Caplan's syndrome is the co-existence of rheumatoid arthritis with a pneumoconioisis, typically coal worker's pneumoconiosis or silicosis. Patients develop single or multiple large necrobiotic nodules in the periphery of the lung. Similar to rheumatoid nodules, the nodular lesions in Caplan's syndrome show central necrosis surrounded by palisading histiocytes, fibroblasts and collagen. They differ from rheumatoid nodules by their large size and by the presence of circumferential bands or arcs of dust within the necrotic centres of the lesions (Helmers et al., 1991).

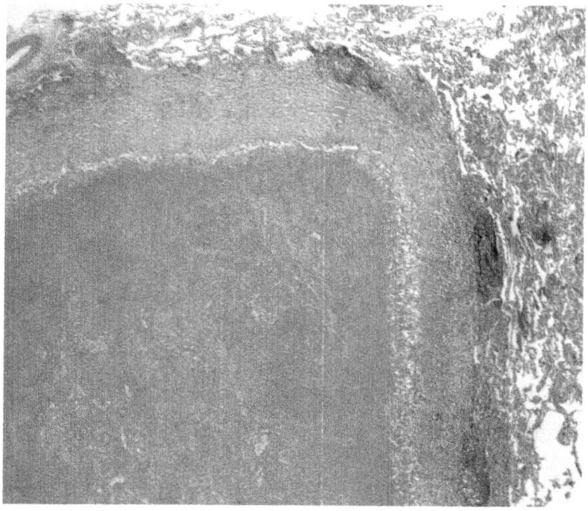

Figure 14. A rheumatoid nodule shows central necrosis surrounded by a rim of palisading histiocytes, fibrosis and mild chronic inflammation.

The airway manifestations of rheumatoid arthritis include follicular bronchiolitis and constrictive bronchiolitis, with a recent study suggesting erythromycin may be useful for the management of these diseases (Hayakawa et al., 1996). Bronchiectasis and bronchocentric granulomatosis have also been described (Bonafede and Benatar, 1987; Hellems et al., 1983). Vascular complications of rheumatoid arthritis include pulmonary hypertension, vasculitis and haemorrhage. All these histological patterns are described earlier and do not differ from when they are associated with other disorders. However, pulmonary vasculitis may occur as an autoimmune phenomenon or as a component of plexogenic pulmonary arteriopathy.

Rheumatoid interstitial lung disease is also associated with an increased risk of lung carcinoma and lymphoma, the risk being highest in patients who also smoke (Mellemkjaer et al., 1996; Symmons, 1985; Yang et al., 2001).

3.3. *Systemic lupus erythematosus*

Of all the CTDs, pleuropulmonary complications are most frequent in SLE, although infection is the most common complication and an important cause of death. It is primarily caused by opportunistic organisms in relation to the use of immunosuppressive agents in treating the disease. The opportunistic organisms include bacteria (*M. tuberculosis*, *M avium-intracellulare*), viruses (CMV, Herpes simplex, Adenovirus), fungi (*P. carinii*, *Candida*, *Aspergillus*, *C. neoformans*) and parasites (*T. gondii*) (Haupt et al., 1981; Kim et al., 1999; Keane and Lynch, 2000).

The most common non-infectious complications are pleuritis and pleural effusions (Haupt et al., 1981; Keane and Lynch, 2000). Pleural biopsy typically shows non-specific chronic inflammation or fibrosis. Pleural effusions are usually small and bilateral. The pleural fluid is usually an exudate rich in proteins (>3 g protein per 100 ml); glucose concentrations are normal. The fluid may contain lymphocytes and neutrophils together with LE cells, degenerating cells and nuclear debris. LE cells (haematoxylin bodies) are phagocytes (usually neutrophils) which have ingested effete nuclear material from other cells. The nuclear material forms large haemotoxyphilic inclusions that fill most of the cytoplasm of the neutrophil, displacing the nucleus to the periphery. Although virtually pathognomonic of SLE, LE cells are only rarely identified in pleuropulmonary material. Tubuloreticular inclusions (seen on EM of lung biopsy specimens) are also highly suggestive, although not specific, for SLE.

Pulmonary parenchymal disease in SLE most commonly takes the form of DAD (clinically termed 'acute lupus pneumonitis'), as described earlier (Cheema and Quismorio, 2000; Haupt et al., 1981; Keane and Lynch, 2000; Kim et al., 1999). Healing may be by resolution, which involves fibrinolysis and permits the lungs to return to normal, or more commonly by repair, which involves organisation of the fibrin exudate and fibrosis and leaves the lungs permanently scarred. UIP and NSIP have also been reported in SLE (Tansey et al., in press), as rarely have organising pneumonia (Min et al., 1997), amyloidosis (Marenco et al., 1994) and LIP (Yood et al., 1995).

Pulmonary vascular disease in SLE includes pulmonary hypertension and vasculitis. Pulmonary hypertension may be caused in part by a thromboembolic arteriopathy which in turn has been linked to the presence of lupus anticoagulant in the serum.

Lung biopsies may show occlusion of small pulmonary arteries by thrombi in various stages of organisation. Veno-occlusive disease has also been described (Kishida et al., 1993). Some patients develop a lymphocytic or necrotising pulmonary vasculitis with evidence of immune complex deposition. The vasculitis may be complicated by diffuse alveolar haemorrhage, which can be acute and life-threatening or chronic (Churg et al., 1980; Haupt et al., 1981; Myers and Katzenstein, 1986; Li and Tam, 1999).

Airway diseases in SLE include follicular bronchiolitis and constrictive bronchiolitis. There are also rare cases of malignant lymphoma. Renal disease is common in SLE and may lead to uraemic pulmonary oedema. Finally, myopathic changes in the respiratory muscles may produce the so-called 'shrinking lung syndrome' which is characterised radiologically by small lungs with elevated hemidiaphragms and basal atelectasis.

3.4. Polymyositis/dermatomyositis

Pulmonary disease is less common in polymyositis/dermatomyositis (PM–DM) than in other CTDs, with the most common pleuropulmonary complication being aspiration pneumonia due to weakness of the striated pharyngeal muscles and depressed cough reflex. Weakness of the intercostal muscles and diaphragm may also result in respiratory insufficiency (Lakhanpal et al., 1987). Biopsy of the intercostal muscles and diaphragm in these cases typically shows inflammation and degenerative changes in the myofibres. In dermatomyositis the inflammatory infiltrate is located predominantly around small blood vessels and in the perimysial connective tissue, and there is perifascicular muscular atrophy. In polymyositis, in contrast, there is no evidence of vascular injury; the inflammatory cells (CD8+ T-cells) are present within the endomysium directly infiltrating and damaging the muscle fibres.

In terms of interstitial pneumonias, studies have now shown that NSIP is the most common form of interstitial lung disease encountered in PM–DM patients (82% of cases) (Douglas et al., 2001; Tansey et al., in press). There is also a significant prevalence of organising pneumonia, either alone or in combination with NSIP. Other reported patterns of interstitial lung disease include DAD (Lakhanpal et al., 1987), UIP and rarely alveolar proteinosis.

Other complications include pulmonary hypertension, vasculitis and pulmonary haemorrhage (Schwarz et al., 1995). Pleuritis with pleural effusion is uncommon in PM–DM and tends to occur only in the setting of interstitial lung disease (Schwarz et al., 1976).

3.5. Sjogren's syndrome

The three most commonly seen complications of primary Sjogren's syndrome are small airways disease, often with xerotrachea (dessication of the tracheobronchial tree), interstitial pneumonias, and lymphoproliferative disease (Constantopoulos et al., 1984, 1985, 1992). In xerotrachea there is atrophy of the tracheal and bronchial submucosal glands, which results in dryness of the upper airways and the production of thick tenacious secretions. Airway clearance is impaired predisposing to bronchitis, bronchiectasis, and pneumonia, which is a major cause of death in these patients. Histologically xerotrachea is characterised by a heavy submucosal lymphoid infiltrate with destruction of the glandular tissues (Constantopoulos et al., 1984; Papiris et al., 1999).

Lymphoproliferative complications are also common in Sjogren's syndrome, although not as common as airway involvement. These include follicular bronchiolitis, LIP, and non-Hodgkin's lymphoma (Hansen et al., 1989; Ito et al., 2003). The latter is usually a marginal zone non-Hodgkin's lymphoma of mucosa-associated lymphoid (MALT) tissue.

Lung involvement is more common in secondary than in primary Sjogren's syndrome, often reflecting the pulmonary manifestations of the associated connective tissue disease. However, involvement occurs in both and patterns of disease include pleuritis, amyloidosis (Desai et al., 1997; Kobayashi et al., 1988), bullae (Desai et al., 1997; Kobayashi et al., 1988), pulmonary hypertension, and vasculitis. Interstitial pneumonia may take the form of NSIP, and more rarely UIP or more rarely organising pneumonia (Deheinzelin et al., 1996; Gardiner et al., 1993; Ito et al., 2003; Yamadori et al., 2002). Sjogren's syndrome may also rarely be associated with sarcoidosis, and they can occur together as part of the TASS (Thyroiditis, Addison's disease, Sjogren's and Sarcoidosis) Syndrome (Deheinzelin et al., 1988).

3.6. Mixed connective tissue disease (MCTD)

Pulmonary complications and their pathologic features resemble those seen in SLE, SSc and PM–DM and include interstitial pneumonia, pleuritis and pleural effusion, pulmonary hypertension, and vasculitis. The most serious complication is progressive pulmonary arterial hypertension and cor pulmonale; rapid deterioration and death can occur in spite of intensive medical intervention. In these cases the pathologic features are usually consistent with plexogenic pulmonary arteriopathy. Death due to massive alveolar haemorrhage has also been described (Hosoda et al., 1987; Prakash, 1998; Wiedemann and Matthay, 1989).

3.7. Ankylosing spondylitis

Thoracic fixation due to costovertebral ankylosis is the most common thoracic complication in these patients. Those with long-standing disease may also develop apical fibrobullous change. Lung biopsy in these cases shows variable fibrosis and lymphocytic infiltration with irregular cystic spaces lined by metaplastic epithelium. These apical cysts may rupture resulting in a spontaneous pneumothorax. They may also become secondarily colonised by *Aspergillus* sp., resulting in the formation of a saprophytic fungal ball, or colonised by opportunistic mycobacteria (Rosenow et al., 1977; Lee-Chiong, 1998).

3.8. Relapsing polychondritis

Relapsing polychondritis is a rare CTD, in which the cartilage of particularly the ears, joints and respiratory tract is chronically destroyed by a progressive inflammatory process. The disorder is associated with other CTDs in about 25% of patients. Involvement of the respiratory tract may result in life-threatening tracheobronchial obstruction and/or secondary infections. The lesions may be localised or involve the entire upper airway. Histologically there is erosion of the edges of affected cartilaginous rings by a dense infiltrate of lymphocytes, neutrophils, plasma cells and giant cells. The chondrocytes degenerate and the cartilage is eventually replaced by granulation tissue and fibrosis (Fig. 15) (Tanoue, 1992; Lee-Chiong, 1998).

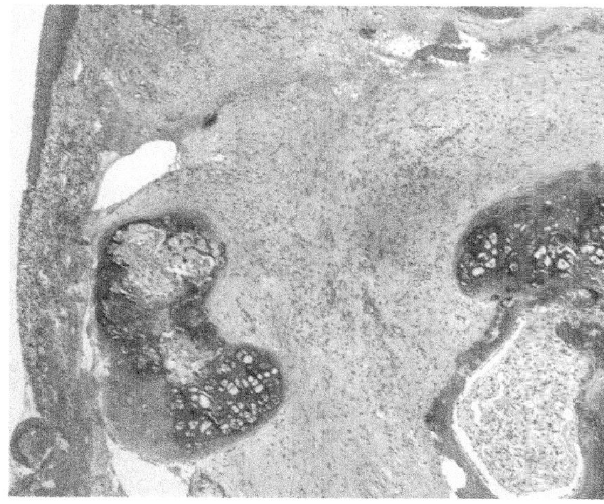

Figure 15. A case of relapsing polychondritis shows erosion of the cartilage plates with osseous metaplasia and focal replacement by fibrosis.

3.9. Cutis laxa

This may be associated with pulmonary emphysema and tracheobronchomegaly.

3.10. Marfan's syndrome

Pulmonary complications include bronchial hyperreactivity (Konig et al., 1991), recurrent pneumothoraces, and emphysema (Sharma et al., 1989).

3.11. Ehlers-Danlos syndrome

Reported pulmonary complications include pulmonary haemorrhage, recurrent pneumothoraces, and fibrous pseudotumours. There is also an association with Mounier-Kuhn's syndrome (tracheobronchomegaly) in which the large airways are dilated with saccular bulges between the tracheal and bronchial cartilages. Bronchial clearance is impaired, resulting in recurrent respiratory infections and promoting bronchiectasis in later life (Ayres et al., 1985; Corrin et al., 1990).

Key points

- Pulmonary pathology in patients with connective tissue diseases (CTDs) is not uncommon and the lung may be the site of initial manifestation of systemic disease.
- All compartments of the lung can be affected, although histologic patterns found in patients with CTDs are rarely specific for a particular disorder. Detailed clinico-radio-pathologic correlation is therefore essential to ensure that there is true cause and effect in relation to the background CTD.
- Most data precede the consensus classification for interstitial pneumonias and recent publications show that the most prevalent pattern associated with CTDs is non-specific interstitial pneumonia, as opposed to usual interstitial pneumonia in an idiopathic setting.
- Variation in prevalence of patterns of interstitial pneumonias between individual CTDs is also seen and prognostic data for interstitial pneumonias in CTDs differs from that in idiopathic setting.
- Patterns of disease often coexist in patients with CTDs and a combination of airway, pleural and/or interstitial lung disease should raise the index of suspicion for such a disorder.

References

Akira, M., Inoue, G., Yamamoto, S., Sakatani, M. 2000. Non-specific interstitial pneumonia: findings on sequential CT scans of nine patients. Thorax 55, 854.

American Thoracic Society, 2000. Idiopathic pulmonary fibrosis: diagnosis and treatment. International Consensus Statement. American Thoracic Society (ATS) and the European Respiratory Society (ERS). Am. J. Respir. Crit. Care Med. 161, 646.

Askin, F.B. 1990. Pulmonary disorders in the collagen vascular diseases. Human Pathol. 21, 465.

Ayres, J.G., Pope, F.M., Reidy, J.F., Clark, T.J. 1985. Abnormalities of the lungs and thoracic cage in the Ehlers-Danlos syndrome. Thorax 40, 300.

Biasi, D., Caramaschi, P., Carletto, A., Bambara, L.M. 1998. Localized scleroderma associated with sarcoidosis. Clin. Exp. Rheumatol. 16, 761.

Bjoraker, J.A., Ryu, J.H., Edwin, M.K., Myers, J.L., Tazelaar, H.D., Schroeder, D.A., Offord, K.P. 1998. Prognostic significance of histopathological subsets in idiopathic pulmonary fibrosis. Am. J. Respir. Crit. Care Med. 157, 199.

Bonafede, R.P., Benatar, S.R. 1987. Bronchocentric granulomatosis and rheumatoid arthritis. Br. J. Dis. Chest 81, 197.

Bouros, D., Nicholson, A.G., Polychronopoulos, V., du Bois, R.M. 2000. Acute interstitial pneumonia. Eur. Resp. J. 15, 412.

Bouros, D., Nicholson, A.G., Colby, T.V., Polychronopoulos, V., Pantelidis, P., Wells, A.U., Black, C.M., du Bois, R.M. 2002. Histopathological subsets of fibrosing alveolitis in patients with scleroderma and their relationship to natural history and treated course. Am. J. Respir. Crit. Care Med. 165, 1581.

Bridges, A.J., Hsu, K.C., Dias-Arias, A.A., Chechani, V. 1992. Bronchiolitis obliterans organizing pneumonia and scleroderma. J. Rheumatol. 19, 1136.

Carrington, C.B., Gaensler, E.A., Coutu, R.E., Fitzgerald, M.X., Gupta, R.G. 1978. Natural history and treated course of usual and desquamative interstitial pneumonia. N. Engl. J. Med. 298, 801.

Chan, T.Y.K., Hansell, D.M., Rubens, M.B., duBois, R.M., Wells, A.U. 1997. Cryptogenic fibrosing alveolitis and the fibrosing alveolitis of systemic sclerosis: Morphological differences on computed tomographic scans. Thorax 52, 265.

Cheema, G.S., Quismorio, F.P. 2000. Interstitial lung disease in systemic lupus erythematosus. Curr. Opin. Pulmonary Med. 6, 424.

Churg, A., Franklin, W., Chan, K.L., Kopp, E., Carrington, C.B. 1980. Pulmonary hemorrhage and immune-complex deposition in the lung. Complications in a patient with systemic lupus erythematosus. Arch. Pathol. Lab Med. 104, 388.

Constantopoulos, S.H., Drosos, A.A., Maddison, P.J., Moutsopoulos, H.M. 1984. Xerotrachea and interstitial lung disease in primary Sjogren's syndrome. Respiration 46, 310.

Constantopoulos, S.H., Papadimitriou, C.S., Moutsopoulos, H.M. 1985. Respiratory manifestations in primary Sjogren's syndrome. A clinical, functional, and histologic study. Chest 88, 226.

Constantopoulos, S.H., Tsianos, E.V., Moutsopoulos, H.M. 1992. Pulmonary and gastrointestinal manifestations of Sjogren's syndrome. Rheum. Dis. Clin. N. Am. 18, 617.

Cool, C.D., Kennedy, D., Voelkel, N.F., Tuder, R.M. 1997. Pathogenesis and evolution of plexiform lesions in pulmonary hypertension associated with scleroderma and human immunodeficiency virus infection. Human Pathol. 28, 434.

Cordier, J.F. 2000. Organising pneumonia. Thorax 55, 318.

Corrin, B., Simpson, C.G., Fisher, C. 1990. Fibrous pseudotumours and cyst formation in the lungs in Ehlers-Danlos syndrome. Histopathology 17, 478.

D'Angelo, W.A., Fries, J.F., Masi, A.T., Shulman, L.E. 1969. Pathologic observations in systemic sclerosis (scleroderma). A study of fifty-eight autopsy cases and fifty-eight matched controls. Am. J. Med. 46, 428.

Davies, D. 1966. Pyopneumothorax in rheumatoid lung disease. Thorax 21, 230.

Deheinzelin, D., de Carvalho, C.R., Tomazini, M.E., Barbas Filho, J.V., Saldiva, P.H. 1988. Association of Sjogren's syndrome and sarcoidosis. Report of a case. Sarcoidosis 5, 68.

Deheinzelin, D., Capelozzi, V.L., Kairalla, R.A., Barbas, F.J., Saldiva, P.H., de Carvalho, C.R. 1996. Interstitial lung disease in primary Sjogren's syndrome. Clinical–pathological evaluation and response to treatment. Am. J. Respir. Crit. Care Med. 154, 794.

Desai, S.R., Nicholson, A.G., Stewart, S., Twentyman, O.R., Flower, C.D.R., Hansell, D., M, . 1997. Benign pulmonary lymphocytic infiltration and amyloidosis: computed tomographic and pathological features in three cases. J. Thoracic Imaging 12, 215.

Douglas, W.W., Tazelaar, H.D., Hartman, T.E., Hartman, R.P., Decker, P.A., Schroeder, D.R., Ryu, J.H. 2001. Polymyositis-dermatomyositis-associated interstitial lung disease. Am. J. Respir. Crit. Care Med. 164, 1182.

Fairfax, A.J., Haslam, P.L., Pavia, D., Sheahan, N.F., Bateman, J.R., Agnew, J.E., Clarke, S.W., Turner-Warwick, M. 1981. Pulmonary disorders associated with Sjogren's syndrome. Q. J. Med. 50, 279.

Flaherty, K.R., Toews, G.B., Travis, W.D., Colby, T.V., Kazerooni, E.A., Gross, B.H., Jain, A., Strawderman, R.L. III, Paine, R., Flint, A., Lynch, J.P. III, Martinez, F.J. 2002. Clinical significance of histological classification of idiopathic interstitial pneumonia. Eur. Respir. J. 19, 275.

Flaherty, K.R., Colby, T.V., Travis, W.D., Toews, G.B., Mumford, J., Murray, S., Thannickal, V.J., Kazerooni, E.A., Gross, B.H., Lynch, J.P. III, Martinez, F.J. 2003. Fibroblastic foci in usual interstitial pneumonia: idiopathic versus collagen vascular disease. Am. J. Respir. Crit. Care Med. 167, 1410.

Fujita, J., Yoshinouchi, T., Ohtsuki, Y., Tokuda, M., Yang, Y., Yamadori, I., Bandoh, S., Ishida, T., Takahara, J., Ueda, R. 2001. Non-specific interstitial pneumonia as pulmonary involvement of systemic sclerosis. Ann. Rheum. Dis. 60, 281.

Gardiner, P., Ward, C., Allison, A., Ashcroft, T., Simpson, W., Walters, H., Kelly, C. 1993. Pleuropulmonary abnormalities in primary Sjogren's syndrome. J. Rheumatol. 20, 831.

Hakala, M., Paakko, P., Huhti, E., Tarkka, M., Sutinen, S. 1990. Open lung biopsy of patients with rheumatoid arthritis. Clin. Rheumatol. 9, 452.

Hansen, L.A., Prakash, U.B., Colby, T.V. 1989. Pulmonary lymphoma in Sjogren's syndrome. Mayo Clin. Proc. 64, 920.

Harrison, N.K., Glanville, A.R., Strickland, B., Haslam, P.L., Corrin, B., Addis, B.J., Lawrence, R., Millar, A.B., Black, C.M., Turner-Warwick, M. 1989. Pulmonary involvement in systemic sclerosis: the detection of early changes by thin section CT scan, bronchoalveolar lavage and 99 mTc-DTPA clearance. Respir. Med. 83, 403.

Harrison, N.K., Myers, A.R., Corrin, B., Soosay, G., Dewar, A., Black, C.M., Du, B.R.M., Turner-Warwick, M. 1991. Structural features of interstitial lung disease in systemic sclerosis. Am. Rev. Respir. Dis. 144, 706.

Hartman, T.E., Swensen, S.J., Hansell, D.M., Colby, T.V., Myers, J.L., Tazelaar, H.D., Nicholson, A.G., Wells, A.U., Rau, J.H., Muadhdhin, D.E., duBois, R.M., Muller, N.L. 2000. Non-specific interstitial pneumonia: Variable appearance at high-resolution chest CT. Radiology 217, 701.

Haupt, H.M., Moore, G.W., Hutchins, G.M. 1981. The lung in systemic lupus erythematosus. Analysis of the pathologic changes in 120 patients. Am. J. Med. 71, 791.

Hayakawa, H., Sato, A., Imokawa, S., Toyoshima, M , Chida, K., Iwata, M. 1996. Bronchiolar disease in rheumatoid arthritis. Am. J. Respir. Crit. Care Med. 154, 1531.

Hellems, S.O., Kanner, R.E., Renzetti, A.D. Jr. 1983. Bronchocentric granulomatosis associated with rheumatoid arthritis. Chest 83, 831.

Helmers, R., Galvin, J., Hunninghake, G.W. 1991. Pulmonary manifestations associated with rheumatoid arthritis. Chest 100, 235.

Hosoda, Y., Suzuki, Y., Takano, M., Tojo, T., Homma, M. 1987. Mixed connective tissue disease with pulmonary hypertension: a clinical and pathological study. J. Rheumatol. 14, 826.

Imokawa, S., Colby, T.V., Leslie, K.O., Helmers, R.A. 2000. Methotrexate pneumonitis: review of the literature and histopathological findings in nine patients. Eur. Respir. J. 15 (2), 373–381.

Ito, I., Nagai, S., Kitaichi, M., Nicholson, A.G., Kim, D.S., Handa, M., Mishima, M., Izumi, T. 2003. Clinical–radiological–pathological features of lung diseases in patients with primary Sjogren's syndrome. Am. J. Respir. Crit. Care Med. 167, A299.

Johnson, D.A., Drane, W.E., Curran, J., Cattau, E.L. Jr., Ciarleglio, C., Khan, A., Cotelingam, J., Benjamin, S.B. 1989. Pulmonary disease in progressive systemic sclerosis. A complication of gastroesophageal reflux and occult aspiration? Arch. Intern. Med. 149, 589.

Katzenstein, A.-L., Askin, F.B. 1997. Systemic diseases involving the lung. In: M. Katzenstein, F.B. Askin (Eds.), Surgical Pathology of Non-Neoplastic Lung Disease. Saunders, Philadelphia, PA, pp. 168–192.

Katzenstein, A.A., Fiorelli, R.F. 1994. Nonspecific interstitial pneumonia/fibrosis. Histologic features and clinical significance. Am. J. Surg. Pathol. 18, 136.

Katzenstein, A.-L., Myers, J.L., Mazur, M.T. 1986. Acute interstitial pneumonia: a clinicopathologic, ultrastructural, and cell kinetic study. Am. J. Surg. Pathol. 10 (4), 256.

Keane, M.P., Lynch, J.P. 2000. Pleuropulmonary manifestations of systemic lupus erythematosus. Thorax 55 (2), 159–166.

Kim, W.U., Kim, S.I., Yoo, W.H., Park, J.H., Min, J.K., Kim, S C., Hong, Y.S., Lee, S.H., Park, S.H., Cho, C.S., Kim, H.Y. 1999. Adult respiratory distress syndrome in systemic lupus erythematosus: causes and prognostic factors: a single center, retrospective study. Lupus 8, 552.

Kim, D.S., Yoo, B., Lee, J.S., Kim, E.K., Lim, C.M., Lee, S.D., Koh, Y., Kim, W.S., Kim, W.D., Colby, T.V., Kitaichi, M. 2002. The major histopathologic pattern of pulmonary fibrosis in scleroderma is nonspecific interstitial pneumonia. Sarcoidosis Vasc. Diffuse Lung Dis. 19, 121.

Kishida, Y., Kanai, Y., Kuramochi, S., Hosoda, Y. 1993. Pulmonary venoocclusive disease in a patient with systemic lupus erythematosus. J. Rheumatol. 20, 2161.

Kobayashi, H., Matsuoka, R., Kitamura, S., Tsunoda, N., Saito, K. 1988. Sjogren's syndrome with multiple bullae and pulmonary nodular amyloidosis. Chest 94, 438.

Konig, P., Boxer, R., Morrison, J., Pletcher, B. 1991. Bronchial hyperreactivity in children with Marfan syndrome. Pediatr. Pulmonol. 11, 29.

Kumar, P., Goldstraw, P., Yamada, K., Nicholson, A.G., Wells, A.U., Hansell, D.M., duBois, R.M., Ladas, G. 2003. Pulmonary fibrosis and lung cancer: risk and benefit analysis of pulmonary resection. J. Thorac. Cardiovasc. Surg. 125, 1321.

Kwak, J.J., Chang, J.E., Lee, J., Cho, Y.J., Sung, S.H. 2003. Chronic eosinophilic pneumonia associated with an initiation of rheumatoid arthritis. Clin. Rheumatol. 22, 240.

Lakhanpal, S., Lie, J.T., Conn, D.L., Martin, W.J. 1987. Pulmonary disease in polymyositis/dermatomyositis: a clinicopathological analysis of 65 autopsy cases. Ann. Rheum. Dis. 46, 23.

Landzberg, M.J., Ko, J., King, M.E., Roberts, D.J., Castro, M.A. 1999. A 38-year-old woman with increasing pulmonary hypertension after delivery–scleroderma overlap syndrome with pulmonary vasculopathy and malignant pulmonary hypertension accelerated during puerperium. N. Engl. J. Med. 340, 455.

Lee-Chiong, T.L. Jr. 1998. Pulmonary manifestations of ankylosing spondylitis and relapsing polychondritis. Clin. Chest Med. 19, ix, 747.

Li, E.K., Tam, L.S. 1999. Pulmonary hypertension in systemic lupus erythematosus: clinical association and survival in 18 patients. J. Rheumatol. 26, 1923.

MacDonald, S.L., Rubens, M.B., Hansell, D.M., Copley, S.J., Desai, S.R., du Bois, R.M., Nicholson, A.G., Colby, T.V., Wells, A.U. 2001. Nonspecific interstitial pneumonia and usual interstitial pneumonia: comparative appearances at and diagnostic accuracy of thin-section CT. Radiology 221, 600.

Marenco, J.L., Sanchez-Burson, J., Ruiz, C.J., Jimenez, M.D., Garcia-Bragado, F. 1994. Pulmonary amyloidosis and unusual lung involvement in SLE. Clin. Rheumatol. 13, 525.

Mellemkjaer, L., Linet, M.S., Gridley, G., Frisch, M., Moller, H., Olsen, J.H. 1996. Rheumatoid arthritis and cancer risk. Eur. J. Cancer 32A, 1753.

Miki, H., Mio, T., Nagai, S., Hoshino, Y., Nagao, T., Kitaichi, M., Izumi, T. 2000. Fibroblast contractility—usual interstitial pneumonia and nonspecific interstitial pneumonia. Am. J. Respir. Crit. Care Med. 162 (6), 2259–2264.

Min, J.K., Hong, Y.S., Park, S.H., Park, J.H., Lee, S.H., Lee, Y.S., Kim, H.H., Cho, C.S., Kim, H.Y. 1997. Bronchiolitis obliterans organizing pneumonia as an initial manifestation in patients with systemic lupus erythematosus. J. Rheumatol. 24, 2254.

Moon, J., duBois, R.M., Colby, T.V., Hansell, D.M., Nicholson, A.G. 1999. Clinical significance of respiratory bronchiolitis on open lung biopsy and its relationship to smoking related interstitial lung disease. Thorax 54, 1009.

Morassut, P.A., Walley, V.M., Smith, C.D. 1992. Pulmonary veno-occlusive disease and the CREST variant of scleroderma. Can. J. Cardiol. 8, 1055.

Muir, T.E., Tazelaar, H.D., Colby, T.V., Myers, J.L. 1997. Organizing diffuse alveolar damage associated with progressive systemic sclerosis. Mayo Clin. Proc. 72, 639.

Myers, J.L., Katzenstein, A.A. 1986. Microangiitis in lupus-induced pulmonary hemorrhage. Am. J. Clin. Pathol. 85, 552.

Nagao, T., Nagai, S., Kitaichi, M., Hayashi, M., Shigematsu, M., Tsutsumi, T., Satake, N., Izumi, T. 2001. Usual interstitial pneumonia: idiopathic pulmonary fibrosis versus collagen vascular diseases. Respiration 68, 151.

Nicholson, A.G. 2002. Classification of idiopathic interstitial pneumonias: making sense of the alphabet soup. Histopathology 41, 381.

Nicholson, A.G., Referrals in pulmonary pathology, CPD Bulletin Cellular Pathology, in press.

Nicholson, A.G., Colby, T.V., du Bois, R.M., Hansell, D.M., Wells, A.U. 2000. The prognostic significance of the histologic pattern of interstitial pneumonia in patients presenting with the clinical entity of cryptogenic fibrosing alveolitis. Am. J. Respir. Crit. Care Med. 162, 2213.

Nicholson, A.G., Colby, T.V., Wells, A.U. 2002. Histopathological approach to patterns of interstitial pneumonia in patient with connective tissue disorders. Sarcoidosis Vasc. Diffuse Lung Dis. 19, 10.

Nicholson, A.G., Gibbs, A.R., Addis, B.J., Bharucha, H., Clelland, C.A., Corrin, B., Hasleton, P.S., Kerr, K.M., Ibrahim, N.B.N., Stewart, S., Wallace, W.A.H., Wells, A.U. Interobserver variation in diffuse parenchymal lung disease. Thorax, in press.

Papiris, S.A., Maniati, M.A., Kalousis, J.V., Constantopoulos, S.H. 1995. Chronic eosinophilic pneumonia in rheumatoid arthritis. Monaldi Arch. Chest Dis. 50, 360.

Papiris, S.A., Maniati, M., Constantopoulos, S.H., Roussos, C., Moutsopoulos, H.M., Skopouli, F.N. 1999. Lung involvement in primary Sjogren's syndrome is mainly related to the small airway disease. Ann. Rheum. Dis. 58, 61.

Prakash, U.B. 1998. Respiratory complications in mixed connective tissue disease. Clin. Chest Med. 19, ix, 733.

Puchtler, H., Sweat, F., Levine, M. 1962. On the binding of Congo Red by amyloid. J. Histochem. Cytochem. 10, 355.

Rees, J.H., Woodhead, M.A., Sheppard, M.N., du, B.R. 1991. Rheumatoid arthritis and cryptogenic organising pneumonitis. Respiratory Medicine 85, 243.

Rice, A.J., Wells, A.U., Bouros, D., du Bois, R.M., Hansell, D.M., Polychronopoulos, V., Vassilakis, D., Kerr, J.R., Evans, T.W., Nicholson, A.G. 2003. Terminal diffuse alveolar damage in relation to interstitial pneumonias. An autopsy study. Am. J. Clin. Pathol. 119, 709.

Rosenow, E., Strimlan, C.V., Muhm, J.R., Ferguson, R.H. 1977. Pleuropulmonary manifestations of ankylosing spondylitis. Mayo Clin. Proc. 52, 641.

Rosenthal, A.K., McLaughlin, J.K., Linet, M.S., Persson, I. 1993. Scleroderma and malignancy: an epidemiological study. Ann. Rheum. Dis. 52, 531.

Samuels, M.P., Warner, J.O. 1988. Pulmonary alveolar lipoproteinosis complicating juvenile dermatomyositis. Thorax 43, 939.

Schwarz, M.I., Matthay, R.A., Sahn, S.A., Stanford, R.E., Marmorstein, B.L., Scheinhorn, D.J. 1976. Interstitial lung disease in polymyositis and dermatomyositis: analysis of six cases and review of the literature. Medicine (Baltimore) 55, 89.

Schwarz, M.I., Sutarik, J.M., Nick, J.A., Leff, J.A., Emlen, J.W., Tuder, R.M. 1995. Pulmonary capillaritis and diffuse alveolar hemorrhage. A primary manifestation of polymyositis. Am. J. Respir. Crit. Care Med. 151, 2037.

Sharma, B.K., Talukdar, B., Kapoor, R. 1989. Cystic lung in Marfan's syndrome. Thorax 44, 978.

Symmons, D.P. 1985. Neoplasms of the immune system in rheumatoid arthritis. Am. J. Med. 78 (1A), 22.

Tanoue, L.T. 1992. Pulmonary involvement in collagen vascular disease: a review of the pulmonary manifestations of the Marfan syndrome, ankylosing spondylitis, Sjogren's syndrome, and relapsing polychondritis. J. Thorac. Imag. 7, 62.

Tansey, D., Wells, A.U., Colby, T.V., Ip, S., Nikolakopoulou, A., du Bois, R.M., Hansell, D.M., Nicholson, A.G., Variations in histologic patterns of interstitial pneumonia between connective tissue disorders and their relationship to prognosis, Histopathology, in press.

Tazelaar, H.D., Viggiano, R.W., Pickersgill, J., Colby, T.V. 1990. Interstitial lung disease in polymyositis and dermatomyositis. Clinical features and prognosis as correlated with histologic findings. Am. Rev. Respir. Dis. 141, 727.

Travis, W.D., King, T.E., Bateman, E.D., Lynch, D.A., Capron, F., Colby, T.V., Center, D., Cordier, J.F., du Bois, R.M., Galvin, J.R., Grenier, J., Hansell, D.M., Hunninghake, G.W., Kitaichi, M., Myers, J.L., Muller, N.L., Nagai, S., Nicholson, A.G., Raghu, G., Wallaert, B. 2002. American Thoracic Society/ European Respiratory Society International Multidisciplinary Consensus Classification of the Idiopathic Interstitial Pneumonias. Am. J. Respir. Crit. Care Med. 165, 277.

Travis, W.D., Colby, T.V., Lombard, C., Carpenter, H.A. 1990. A clinicpathologic study of 34 cases of diffuse pulmonary hemorrhage with lung biopsy confirmation. Am. J. Surg. Pathol. 14 (12), 1112.

Travis, W.D., Matsui, K., Moss, J., Ferrans, V.J. 2000. Idiopathic nonspecific interstitial pneumonia: prognostic significance of cellular and fibrosing patterns—survival comparison with usual interstitial pneumonia and desquamative interstitial pneumonia. Am. J. Surg. Pathol. 24, 19.

Turner-Warwick, M. 1986. Connective tissue disorders and the lung. Aust. NZ J. Med. 16, 257.

Turner-Warwick, M. 1988. Some connective tissue disorders of the lung. Postgrad. Med. J. 64, 497.

Walters, M.N., Ojeda, V.J. 1986. Pleuropulmonary necrobiotic rheumatoid nodules. A review and clinicopathological study of six patients. Med. J. Aust. 144, 648.

Wells, A.U., Cullinan, P., Hansell, D.M., Rubens, M.B., Black, C.M., Newman-Taylor, A.J., du, B.R. 1994. Fibrosing alveolitis associated with systemic sclerosis has a better prognosis than lone cryptogenic fibrosing alveolitis. Am. J. Respir. Crit. Care Med. 149, 1583.

Wells, A.U., Hansell, D.M., Rubens, M.B., King, A.D., Cramer, D., Black, C.M., duBois, R.M. 1997. Fibrosing alveolitis in systemic sclerosis: indices of lung function in relation to extent of disease on computed tomography. Arthritis Rheum. 40, 1229.

Wiedemann, H.P., Matthay, R.A. 1989. Pulmonary manifestations of the collagen vascular diseases. Clin. Chest Med. 10, 677.

Wright, J.L., Cagle, P., Churg, A., Colby, T.V., Myers, J. 1992. Diseases of the small airways. Am. Rev. Respir. Dis. 146, 240.

Yamadori, I., Fujita, J., Bandoh, S., Tokuda, M., Tanimoto, Y., Kataoka, M., Yamasaki, Y., Yoshinouchi, T., Ohtsuki, Y., Ishida, T. 2002. Nonspecific interstitial pneumonia as pulmonary involvement of primary Sjogren's syndrome. Rheumatol. Int. 22, 89.

Yang, Y., Fujita, J., Tokuda, M., Bandoh, S., Ishida, T. 2001. Lung cancer associated with several connective tissue diseases: with a review of literature. Rheumatol. Int. 21, 106.

Yood, R.A., Steigman, D.M., Gill, L.R. 1995. Lymphocytic interstitial pneumonitis in a patient with systemic lupus erythematosus. Lupus 4, 161.

Yousem, S.A. 1990. The pulmonary pathologic manifestations of the CREST syndrome. Human Pathol. 21, 467.

Yousem, S.A., Colby, T.V., Carrington, C.B. 1985. Lung biopsy in rheumatoid arthritis. Am. Rev. Respir. Dis. 131, 770.

Yousem, S.A., Colby, T.V., Gaensler, E.A. 1989. Respiratory bronchiolitis-associated interstitial lung disease and its relationship to desquamative interstitial pneumonia. Mayo Clin. Proc. 64, 1373.

PART II

Radiologic Investigations in Connective Tissue Diseases

Handbook of Systemic Autoimmune Diseases, Volume 2
Pulmonary Involvement in Systemic Autoimmune Diseases
A.U. Wells and C.P. Denton, editors

CHAPTER 2

High Resolution Computed Tomography of the Lungs

Tomás Franquet

Associate Professor of Radiology and Director, Chest Imaging Section, Department of Diagnostic Radiology, Hospital de Sant Pau, Universitat Autónoma de Barcelona, Avda. Sant Antoni Mª Claret 167, 08025 Barcelona, Spain

The connective tissue diseases are a heterogeneous group of immunologically mediated disorders in which the lungs are an important target organ due to their abundant connective tissue. The most common form of diffuse pulmonary lung disease in patients with collagen vascular disorders is a chronic pulmonary fibrosis, indistinguishable from other causes of usual interstitial pneumonia (UIP). Rarely, the chronic pulmonary fibrosis may precede the extrapulmonary manifestations of the disease. Other complications of connective tissue diseases include esophageal dysfunction leading to recurrent aspiration and secondary infection (in scleroderma and mixed connective tissue disease (MCTD)), respiratory muscle weakness contributing to atelectasis and secondary infection (in systemic lupus erythematosus (SLE) and polymyositis (PM)), and drug-induced lung disease (methotrexate and gold treatment in rheumatoid arthritis) (Lynch and Hunninghake, 1992; Prakash, 1998; Wells, 2000). Because the pathology of chronic interstitial pneumonia takes a limited number of forms, there also are a limited number of radiographic manifestations (Gamsu, 1992; Primack and Müller, 1998; Franquet, 2001). Although of limited value in detecting early stages of disease, conventional chest radiography still remains an invaluable aid in documenting the presence of interstitial lung disease (ILD). Currently, high resolution computed tomography (HRCT) is the imaging method of choice in evaluating patients with ILD. HRCT demonstrates the presence, gross characteristics, and distribution of pulmonary disease with greater sensitivity than conventional chest radiographs and thereby may improve diagnosis. Additionally, HRCT can clarify confusing radiographic findings and direct invasive diagnostic procedures. In certain clinical circumstances, HRCT findings can suggest a specific diagnosis or indicate a potentially treatable disease (Remy-Jardin, 1994; Niimi et al., 1996; Johkoh et al., 1999a,b; Primack and Müller, 1998; Franquet, 2001).

This chapter is a general overview of the clinical features and radiologic manifestations of those connective tissue diseases that affect the lungs, including abnormalities of the interstitium, airways, blood vessels, pleura, and chest wall.

1. Rheumatoid arthritis

Rheumathoid arthritis (RA) is the most common of the connective tissue diseases, affecting about 1% of people worldwide, with a male to female ratio between 1:2 and 1:4 (Shannon and Gale, 1992; Tanoue, 1998; Wells, 2000). The disease can begin at any age, but the peak onset is in the fifth decade of life. The distribution of arthritis is usually symmetrical and diffuse. Females are affected 2–3 times more often than males. Although the most frequent clinical manifestation of RA is articular symptoms,

Tel.: +34-93-2919067; fax: +34-93-2919282
E-mail address: 19429tfc@comb.es (T. Franquet).

DOI: 10.1016/S1571-5078(04)02002-1

extra-articular manifestations occur in more than three-quarters of cases with severe involvement (Ayzemberg et al., 1983; Fortoul et al., 1985; Aquino et al., 1994; Tanoue, 1998).

The pulmonary manifestations of RA are varied and are likely to depend on multiple factors such as the stage of disease in which patients are studied, the source of patient referral, and the parameters used to define disease.

Pleural involvement, either pleural effusion or pleural thickening, is the most common thoracic manifestation of RA. Although pleural effusion is clinically evident in only 5% of cases, pleural disease (i.e. adhesions, thickening, or effusion) is found, in different autopsy series, in 38–73% of cases (Ayzemberg et al., 1983; Shannon and Gale, 1992; Ippolito et al., 1993). The effusion is usually small and unilateral but may be large and bilateral. Occasionally, pleural effusion may develop acutely in association with pericarditis or exacerbations of arthritis. However, the majority of pleural effusions resolve spontaneously.

The degree of ILD in RA does not necessarily correlate with the severity of underlying articular involvement. Interstitial pulmonary fibrosis is more common in men with seropositive disease and rheumatoid nodules with a male to female ratio of 3:1. Smoking is a risk factor for the development of pulmonary fibrosis (Tanoue, 1998). The radiographic findings are often subtle, and chest radiographs may be normal or show only discrete pleural abnormalities or fine interstitial opacities (Gamsu, 1992; Fujii et al., 1993; Remy-Jardin, 1994; Akira et al., 1999a,b). The reported prevalence of pleuropulmonary abnormalities in RA varies according to the criteria used to define disease, ranging from low rates (5%) based on chest radiographs to 41% based on abnormal physiology and up to 71% based on the presence of an alveolitis (Gamsu, 1992; Remy-Jardin, 1994; Tanoue, 1998; Akira et al., 1999a,b). Patients with high-titer rheumatoid factor are even more likely to have an abnormal chest radiograph. Clear fibrosis and honeycombing are only detected in the more severe forms of the disease. In contrast, pulmonary function tests were abnormal in 40% of patients with RA and normal chest radiography. This fact suggests that chest X-ray (CXR) is insensitive for lung disease in a significant number of patients.

Although the ILD associated with RA is histologically indistinguishable from UIP, lung fibrosis is usually slowly progressive (Yousem et al., 1985; Rees et al., 1991). Another form of interstitial pneumonia distinct from UIP, termed nonspecific interstitial pneumonia (NSIP), may also occur in RA (Katzenstein and Fiorelli, 1994). An NSIP pattern on biopsy may be the presenting manifestation, preceding the diagnosis of collagen vascular disease by several months or several years. This process is characterized by a diffuse lymphocyte and plasma cell infiltrate associated with relatively little fibrosis.

HRCT is much more sensitive than CXR for the detection of early interstitial changes. HRCT depicts findings of fibrosis (i.e. interlobular septal thickening, traction bronchiectasis and bronchiolectasis, and honeycombing) and ground-glass opacity with a characteristic peripheral lower lobe predominance (Fig. 1) (Remy-Jardin, 1994; Akira et al., 1999a,b). Other findings on computed topography (CT) include pleural thickening or effusion, small centilobular nodules, and large nodular opacities (rheumatoid nodules) (Caplan, 1953; Primack and Müller, 1998). The radiographic findings are indistinguishable from those of cryptogenic fibrosing alveolitis. However, a honeycombing pattern on HRCT is significantly less common in various collagen vascular diseases than in cryptogenic fibrosing alveolitis (Primack and Müller, 1998; Franquet, 2001).

Rheumatoid (necrobiotic) pulmonary nodules may be single or multiple and are pathologically identical

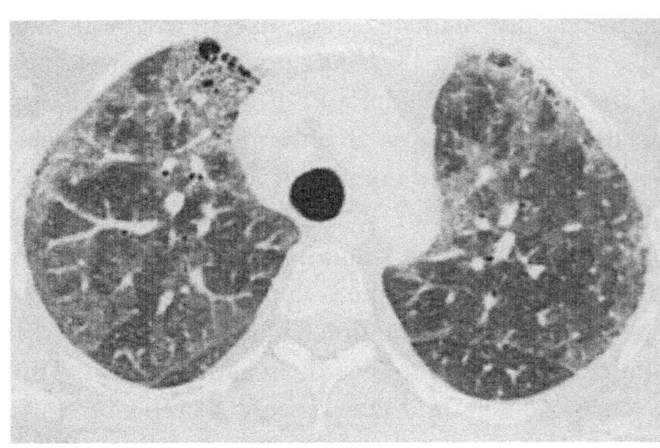

Figure 1. Rheumatoid arthritis in a 49-year-old woman. HRCT scan shows diffuse bilateral areas of patchy ground-glass opacities. Note small cyst (honeycombing) in the anterior part of both upper lobes. Open lung biopsy showed findings of mixed NSIP.

to those found in subcutaneous tissue. The nodules typically measure between 0.5 and 5 cm in size, are well circumscribed, and may cavitate (Gamsu, 1992). Pulmonary rheumatoid nodules may precede the development of systemic disease. The reported prevalence of rheumatoid nodules is variable, ranging from low rates based on CXR to 22% in a series of 77 patients evaluated by HRCT (Fig. 2) (Cortet et al., 1995). Although rheumatoid nodules are often asymptomatic, spontaneous pneumothorax due to the rupture of a cavitary necrobiotic nodule is a rare complication of RA. In asymptomatic patients, a solitary rheumatoid nodule may simulate malignancy. Caplan's syndrome is characterized by RA with pulmonary rheumatic nodules in coal miners (Caplan, 1953; Shida et al., 1996).

Airways disease is being increasingly recognized in RA and in other collagen vascular diseases (Wells, 2000). Small airways disease is difficult to diagnose with chest radiography because findings may be subtle or confusing. HRCT is well recognized as an accurate method for assessing airways diseases (Remy-Jardin, 1994; Aquino et al., 1994; Primack and Müller, 1998; Franquet, 2001). The association of bronchiectasis and RA has been found in 20–35% of patients with RA who have undergone HRCT (Remy-Jardin, 1994; Hayakawa et al., 1996; Gabbay et al., 1997). Although bronchiectasis was detected with a higher frequency in patients with respiratory symptoms, HRCT findings of bronchiectasis were identified in 8% of asymptomatic patients (Gabbay et al., 1997). Recently, it has been suggested that findings of airway obstruction in RA are only secondarily related to bronchiectasis and in fact primarily reflect the presence of obliterative bronchiolitis (OB) (Fig. 3) (Aquino et al., 1994; Hayakawa et al., 1996; Wadsworth and Hansell, 1999). OB is characterized histologically by the presence of inflammation of the walls of membranous and respiratory bronchioles and concentric narrowing of the bronchiolar lumen caused by submucosal and peribronchiolar fibrosis. The characteristic HRCT findings of OB consist of areas of decreased attenuation and vascularity with blood flow redistribution resulting in areas of increased lung attenuation and vascularity ('mosaic perfusion' pattern). Expiratory HRCT scans have proved useful in the evaluation of patients with a variety of lung diseases characterized by obstruction of airflow (Aquino et al., 1994; Remy-Jardin, 1994; Wadsworth and Hansell, 1999). Focal areas of air trapping may be present, accentuated by images obtained at the end of expiration. HRCT scans performed at end of maximal expiration enable early detection of air trapping. The extent of air trapping is a good predictor of obstructive functional deficit in these patients (Remy-Jardin, 1994; Wadsworth and Hansell, 1999).

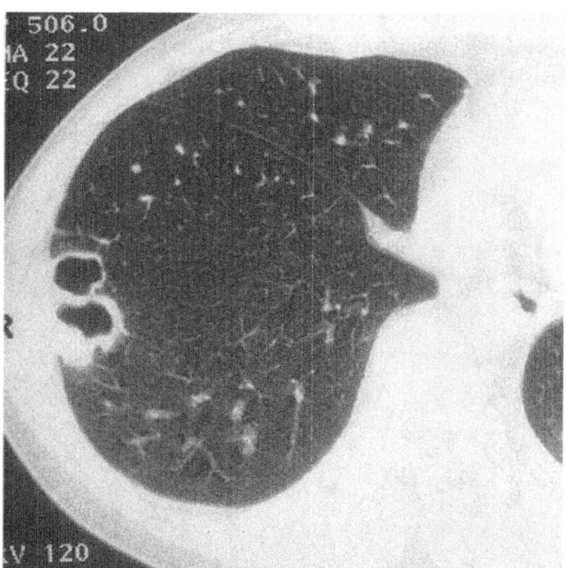

Figure 2. Necrobiotic pulmonary nodule in a 48-year-old man with longstanding rheumatoid arthritis. Close-up view of an HRCT scan demonstrates a peripheral well-defined cavitated nodule in the right lower lobe.

Occasionally, focal areas of organizing pneumonia (OP) are found in biopsy specimens of patients with RA who present radiographically with peripheral bands of air-space consolidation (Fig. 4) (Ippolito et al., 1993; Remy-Jardin, 1994). OP is a histologic description and not a specific diagnosis. Etiologies of this OP pattern include toxic fume or dust inhalation (extrinsic allergic alveolitis), post-infectious (Mycoplasma, fungal, or viral), drug toxicity (gold salts, cyclophosphamide, and methotrexate), and other different collagen vascular diseases (Diehl et al., 1996). Drug-induced pulmonary disease has been reported in 3–18% of patients with RA treated with methotrexate (Zamora et al., 1997). Methotrexate-induced pneumonitis is thought to result from an acute hypersensitivity reaction. Histopathologic findings are

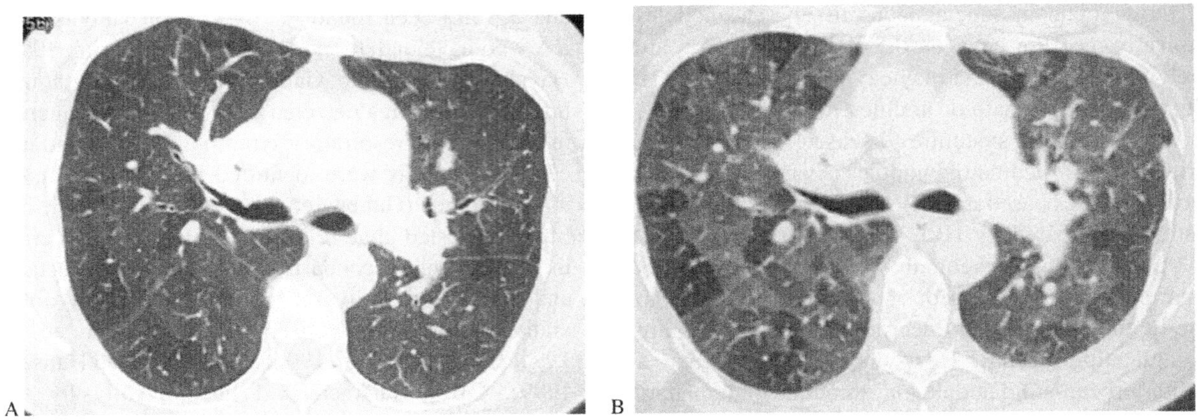

Figure 3. Obliterative bronchiolitis in a middle-aged woman with rheumatoid arthritis. (A) Inspiratory HRCT scan demonstrates a typical mosaic perfusion pattern. (B) High-resolution CT obtained at end-expiration shows patchy lobular areas of air trapping.

nonspecific and include interstitial inflammation, granuloma formation, and a diffuse pattern of alveolar damage associated with perivascular inflammation. HRCT findings may show heterogeneous or patchy areas of bilateral ground-glass opacities, centrilobular opacities, and intralobular interstitial thickening, with a predilection for the lower lung fields (Imokawa et al., 2000).

Follicular bronchiolitis, defined as lymphoid hyperplasia of the bronchus-associated lymphoid tissue (BALT), is a benign condition characterized histologically by prominent hyperplasia of peribronchial and peribronchiolar lymphoid follicles (Fortoul et al., 1985; Kinoshita et al., 1992; Howling et al., 1999). Interestingly, in a large series of 12 patients with biopsy-proven follicular bronchiolitis, 10 patients had connective tissue diseases (Hassan et al., 1995). Although symptomatic follicular bronchiolitis is rare, its recognition is important because it responds well to corticosteroid therapy. Chest radiographs typically demonstrate a heterogeneous nodular pattern. HRCT findings consist of a mixed pattern of

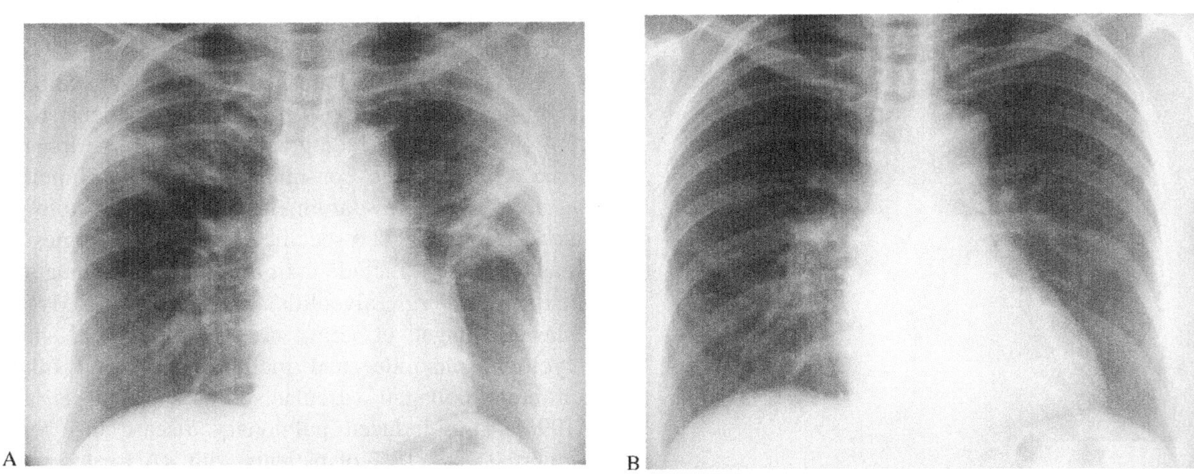

Figure 4. BOOP in a patient with rheumatoid arthritis under gold salts treatment. (A) Before steroid treatment chest radiograph shows bilateral patchy lung consolidation with associated architectural lung distortion. (B) After treatment, plain film shows complete resolution of the parenchymal opacities.

multiple small centrilobular nodules associated with patchy ground-glass opacity. The differential diagnosis of follicular bronchiolitis includes lymphocytic interstitial pneumonia (LIP), also seen with increased frequency in patients with connective tissue diseases, particularly Sjögren's syndrome (Koss et al., 1987; Desai et al., 1997; Howling et al., 1999; Johkoh et al., 1999a,b). In patients with LIP, small cysts are also a common CT finding.

Although RA is more common in women, pulmonary complications are more frequent in men (Hassan et al., 1995). Pyopneumothorax, probably due to rupture into the pleural cavity of a necrobiotic nodule, pneumomediastinum, tracheomegaly, and respiratory infection are complications occasionally associated with RA (Hindle and Yates, 1965; Patel et al., 2000).

2. Systemic lupus erythematosus

SLE is a chronic, multisystem disease of unknown origin characterized by the presence of autoantibodies against various cell nuclear antigens (Kim et al., 2000). The clinical picture of SLE is extremely variable and affected patients generally have dysfunction of multiple organ systems including the musculoskeletal system, skin, kidney, and central nervous system (Murin et al., 1998; Kim et al., 2000).

Pleuropulmonary disease will occur in more than half of patients with SLE at some point during the course of their illness (Schwab et al., 1993; Murin et al., 1998). Although pleuritis, seen either as a dry fibrinous exudate or an exudative effusion, is the most common thoracic manifestation of SLE, diverse pleuropulmonary manifestations including diaphragmatic dysfunction ('shrinking lung syndrome'), acute lupus pneumonitis, pulmonary hemorrhage, pulmonary hypertension, and diffuse ILD have been described in patients with SLE (Kim et al., 2000; Warrington et al., 2000). Subclinical involvement occurs frequently with autopsy series reporting a prevalence of up to 93%. Pericardial inflammation is less common clinically but may be found in up to 60% of patients at autopsy. The diagnosis of pericarditis may sometimes be difficult because most effusions are relatively small. The CT scan demonstrates pleural and pericardial thickening or irregularity in up to 70% of cases (Bankier et al., 1995).

Acute lupus pneumonitis is an uncommon life-threatening complication of SLE that is characterized by fever, severe hypoxemia, and diffuse pulmonary infiltrates (Braunstein et al., 1983; Schwab et al., 1993; Orens et al., 1994). Pathologically, there is interstitial edema and inflammation with intra-alveolar exudation and hyaline membrane formation corresponding to diffuse alveolar damage. The chest radiograph in acute lupus pneumonitis shows a diffuse haziness, which progresses to 'widespread opacities similar to those of pulmonary edema'.

In contrast to many other collagen vascular diseases, SLE is not commonly associated with chronic diffuse ILD. The incidence of radiographically visible lung involvement may be lower than the true incidence because the radiograph may fail to show small parenchymal abnormalities. In one study of 48 patients with serologically proved SLE but no clinical evidence of pulmonary involvement, only three (6%) presented with some radiographic abnormalities. Seventeen (38%) of the 45 patients who had normal radiographs had abnormal findings on HRCT. The most common abnormalities were interlobular septal thickening, small rounded areas of consolidation, and areas of ground-glass attenuation (Bankier et al., 1995; Fenlon et al., 1996). Pulmonary fibrosis resembling idiopathic pulmonary fibrosis (IPF) is seen on HRCT in 30–35% of patients (Primack and Müller, 1998). Ground-glass opacity and areas of consolidation may be due to OP (Gammon et al., 1992; Min et al., 1997). Findings of airways disease such as bronchial wall thickness and bronchiectasis may be seen in 20% of patients with SLE (Bankier et al., 1995; Fenlon et al., 1996).

Diffuse alveolar hemorrhage (DAH) is a rare but dramatic complication of SLE (Zamora et al., 1997). High-titer anti-DNA and other clinical evidence for active SLE (for example, serositis, rash, and polyarthritis) are present in more than 90% of cases. Lung biopsy studies demonstrate nonspecific findings of intra-alveolar hemorrhage and capillaritis. Other diseases or clinical situations in which pulmonary capillaritis may occasionally be discovered on lung biopsy include: PM, antiphospholipid antibody syndrome, RA, Sjögren's syndrome, and progressive systemic sclerosis (SSc). Clinical features of the syndrome of DAH are variable, ranging from minimal hemoptysis to fulminant respiratory failure. With severe alveolar hemorrhage, mortality exceeds 30% (Schwab et al., 1993; Zamora et al., 1997). The radiographic appearance of DAH is that of nonspecific diffuse air-space consolidation. HRCT scans can show patchy bilateral and/or diffuse areas of ground-glass attenuation with superimposed interlobular septal thickening giving an appearance of a 'crazy-paving' pattern (Fig. 5) (Fenlon et al., 1996; Kim et al., 2000). Although similar changes may be seen in patients with pulmonary edema, lipoid pneumonia, alveolar proteinosis, and PCP infection, in the correct clinical context these findings are strongly suggestive of DAH (Bankier et al., 1995; Fenlon et al., 1996; Kim et al., 2000). However, the distinction between these entities sometimes requires bronchoscopy with bronchioalveolar lavage (BAL).

A subset of patients with SLE may have an increased incidence of recurrent venous and/or arterial thrombosis (Wells, 2000). The so-called antiphospholipid antibody syndrome is defined by the occurrence of thrombotic events and the presence of autoantibodies against phospholipids (Zamora et al., 1997; Prakash, 1998; Wells, 2000). Although pulmonary thromboembolism and pulmonary hypertension are the most common complications, microvascular pulmonary thrombosis, pulmonary capillaritis, and alveolar hemorrhage have also been reported (Zamora et al., 1997). The antiphospholipid antibody syndrome occurs most frequently in patients with high titer IgG anti-cardiolipin antibodies or lupus anticoagulant. Although initially described with SLE, it has also been found in other rheumatic diseases, malignancies, hematologic disorders, and viral infections. The mechanisms of this thrombotic diathesis are uncertain, but these autoantibodies bind to target antigens on endothelial cells, platelets or coagulation factors producing a hypercoagulable state (Wells, 2000; Prakash, 1998).

Infection is the most common pulmonary complication in SLE. It is estimated that at least 50% of them will suffer a severe infectious episode during the course of the disease (Prakash, 1998). Patients receiving high doses of corticosteroids or cytotoxic agents, or with renal disease, are especially susceptible to pulmonary infection. The usual bacterial and opportunistic pathogens, mycobacterial and nocardial infections seem to be particularly important in patients with SLE (Fig. 6) (Mok et al., 1997). Acute syndromes such as DAH and acute pneumonitis must be differentiated from infectious complications.

SLE is also associated with increased risk of malignancy, with lymphoma being the most common (Murin et al., 1998). Recognition of this association is important since lymphoma can mimic an exacerbation of SLE with adenopathy, fever, malaise, and splenomegaly.

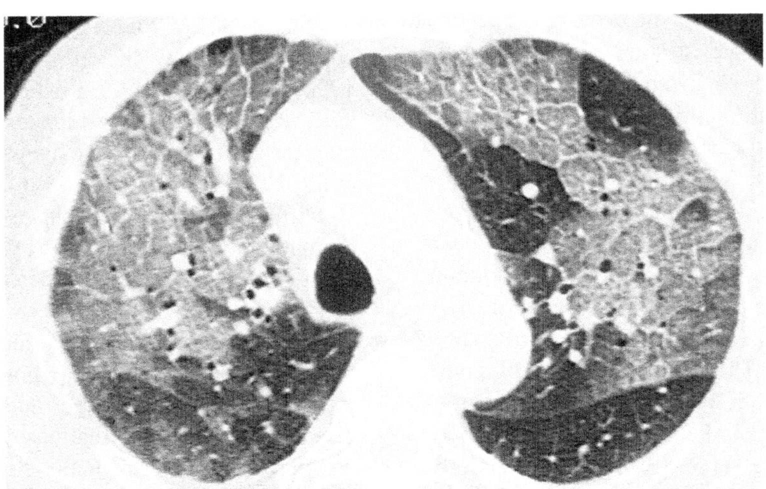

Figure 5. A 53-year-old woman with SLE and diffuse pulmonary hemorrhage. HRCT scan shows extensive bilateral ground-glass opacities with superimposed thickening of the interlobular septa with a 'crazy-paving' appearance.

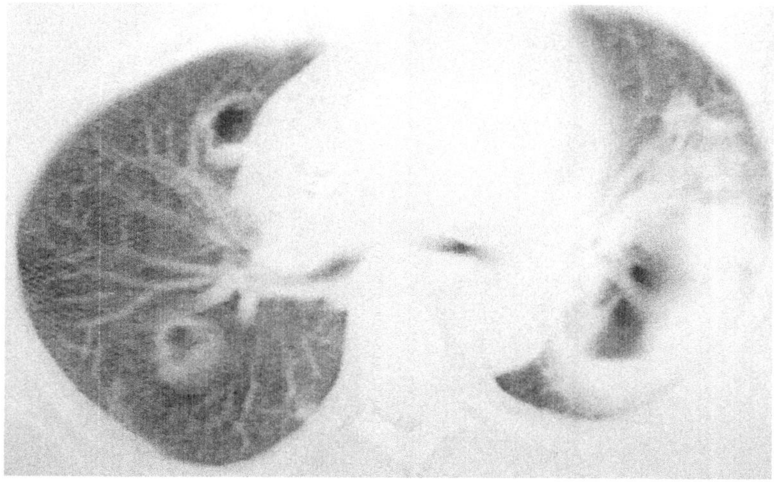

Figure 6. Nocardia infection causing multiple ill-defined cavitary nodules in a patient with systemic lupus erythematosus. Note multiple air-fluid levels in the abscess cavities.

3. Progressive systemic sclerosis (SSc) (scleroderma)

SSc is an uncommon inflammatory-fibrotic disease of the skin (scleroderma) and some internal organs. Morbidity and mortality are related directly to the extent and severity of visceral involvement. The CREST syndrome is a limited form of scleroderma (subcutaneous calcinosis, Raynaud's phenomenon, esophageal dysmotility, sclerodactyly, and telangiectasias). Raynaud's phenomenon is the initial complaint in about 70% of patients. Similar changes occur in the vasculature of the heart, lung, kidneys, and gastrointestinal tract and contribute to the dysfunction of these organs (D'Angelo et al., 1969; Taorimina et al., 1981; Minai et al., 1998).

Although ILD is the most common complication of SSc, occurring in up to 75% of cases, in the majority of patients the interstitial lung pathology is subclinical, being completely asymptomatic in the early stages like most other ILDs (D'Angelo et al., 1969). As with other collagen vascular diseases, the incidence of radiographically recognizable ILD is variable. In patients with long-standing disease, pulmonary fibrosis may occur. Although advanced pulmonary disease is easily detectable on chest radiographs, the limited role of chest radiography in the detection of earlier stages of lung involvement has also been well documented. HRCT is the method of choice for evaluating early parenchymal involvement (Silver et al., 1976; Arroliga et al., 1992; Bhalla et al., 1993; Remy-Jardin et al., 1993; Chan et al., 1997).

The HRCT findings of interstitial fibrosis in SSc include ground-glass attenuation, subpleural reticular opacities, traction bronchiectasis and bronchiolectasis, architectural distortion, pleural thickening or effusion, and centrilobular micronodules (follicular bronchiolitis) in a predominantly peripheral and basilar distribution (Fig. 7) (Fortoul et al., 1985; Remy-Jardin et al., 1993; Primack and Müller, 1998).

SSc follows a less aggressive course and has a better prognosis than IPF. NSIP is the histologic pattern that is seen in the majority of patients with SSc. A UIP pattern occurs in 8% of cases. HRCT findings in patients who have SSc are ground-glass opacities, reticular linear opacities, and subpleural and diffuse honeycombing. Mediastinal lymphadenopathy is seen in 40–58% of patients (Wechsler et al., 1996), with a significant positive relationship between lymphadenopathy and the presence of interstitial disease (Bergin and Castellino, 1990; Wechsler et al., 1996; Niimi et al., 1996).

In addition to interstitial fibrosis, SSc is commonly associated with pulmonary vasculitis and pulmonary hypertension. Pulmonary hypertension may

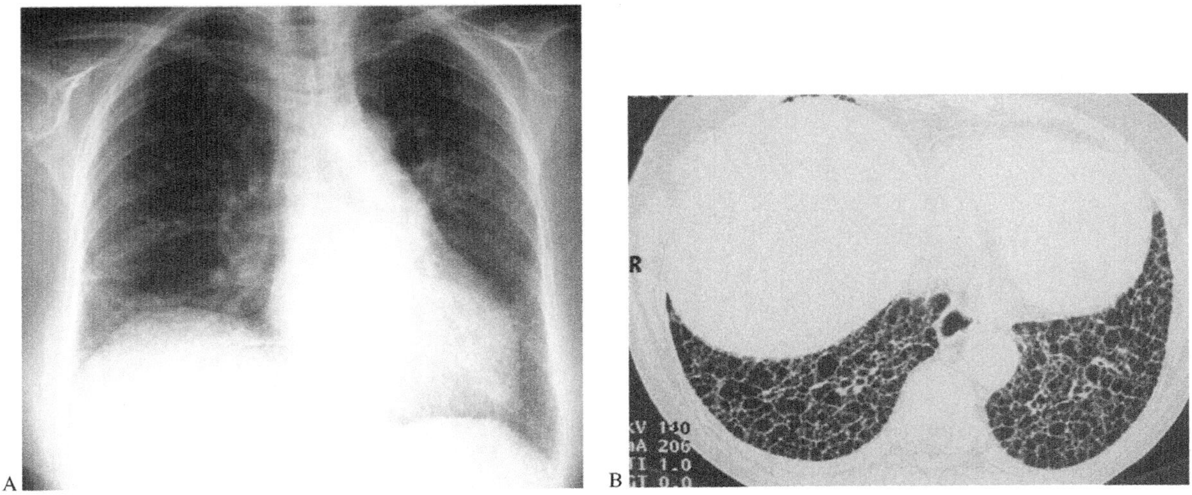

Figure 7. Chest radiograph in a patient who has progressive systemic sclerosis. (A) Bilateral ill-defined opacities are present in both lung bases. (B) Corresponding CT scan shows typical features of interstitial lung fibrosis (honeycombing). Dilatation of the esophagus is also noted.

occur independently of the degree of pulmonary fibrosis (Lynch and Hunninghake, 1992; Prakash, 1998). On chest radiographs an enlargement of the pulmonary arteries is observed (Wells, 2000). HRCT imaging can show enlargement of the pulmonary arteries and a bilateral diffuse mosaic pattern of lung attenuation due to regions of hyperemia and oligemia (Arroliga et al., 1992; Remy-Jardin et al., 1993; Primack and Müller, 1998).

Esophageal dilatation is demonstrated on CT in 80% of patients with ILD (Bhalla et al., 1993). Esophageal dilatation and dysmotility predispose to aspiration pneumonitis and bronchiolitis. Aspiration pneumonia appears to be a serious pulmonary complication in patients with SSc, PM, and dermatomyositis (DM), and is an important cause of morbidity in such patients. On HRCT, aspiration bronchiolitis can be diagnosed by the presence of tubular or branched bronchioles distended with air or mucus. Patchy areas of consolidation may also be observed in association with bronchiolitis due to transbronchial spread of aspirated material into peribronchial alveolar space (Warrick et al., 1991; Bhalla et al., 1993; Remy-Jardin et al., 1993; Primack and Müller, 1998).

The prevalence of lung cancer is increased in patients with SSc. Adenocarcinoma has been associated with concomitant lung disorders that produce focal or diffuse fibrosis. Interestingly, although bronchioloalveolar cell carcinoma (BACC) accounts for less than 10% of primary lung tumors, up to 50% of localized or diffuse forms of BACC are associated with previous scarring in the lung as occurring in IPF, RA, and SSc (Roumm and Medsger, 1985).

4. Sjögren's syndrome

Sjögren's syndrome (SS) is a chronic, inflammatory, autoimmune disorder characterized by the triad of keratoconjunctivitis sicca, xerostomia, and, in up to 50% of cases, a connective tissue disorder. SS that only involves gland inflammation (sicca syndrome) is referred to as primary SS (Lynch and Hunninghake, 1992; Prakash, 1998; Wells, 2000). Secondary SS not only involves gland inflammation, but is associated with a connective tissue disease, such as RA, SLE, or scleroderma (Deheinzelin et al., 1996; Franquet et al., 1997a,b; Cain et al., 1988).

The natural history and frequency of respiratory involvement in primary SS remains a subject of considerable controversy due to the differences in studied populations (primary, secondary, or mixed Sjögren's patients) and the methods used to study the respiratory system, which vary from predominantly clinical to mainly functional. It is not surprising, therefore, that the prevalence of pulmonary abnormalities in SS range from 9 to 75% (Cain et al., 1988). Lung abnormalities in secondary SS are often dominated by associated autoimmune disease and, as such, are difficult to distinguish from those that characterize SS itself (Strimlan et al., 1976).

The frequency of lung involvement in patients with primary SS is difficult to ascertain and varies according to whether clinical, radiologic, functional or pathologic criteria are used to diagnose lung disease (Franquet et al., 1997a,b; Cain et al., 1988; Franquet et al., 1999). It is characterized both by manifestations of the associated rheumatic disease (secondary form of SS) and by lesions related more specifically to SS itself (Fig. 8). In early studies, radiographic analyses were made on the basis of conventional radiographs only and no distinction was established between the primary and the secondary form of SS (Strimlan et al., 1976). Various forms of pulmonary complications have been reported in patients with primary SS, including interstitial fibrosis (Fig. 9), small airways disease (Franquet et al., 1997a,b), lymphocytic interstitial pneumonitis (LIP) (Desai et al., 1997; Johkoh et al., 1999a,b), pseudolymphoma and lymphoma (Hansen et al., 1989; Franquet et al., 1997a,b), lung adenocarcinoma (Takabatake et al., 1999), atelectasis, bronchiectasis (Franquet et al., 1997a,b), and pulmonary hypertension.

ILD occurs in 4–52% of patients and is more common in secondary SS or in patients with primary disease with extraglandular features such as Raynaud's, renal disease, or intermittent purpura (Strimlan et al., 1976; Franquet et al., 1997a,b). The most common HRCT findings in SS consist of ground-glass opacity, findings of fibrosis, centrilobular nodular opacities, and lung cysts (Franquet et al., 1997a,b).

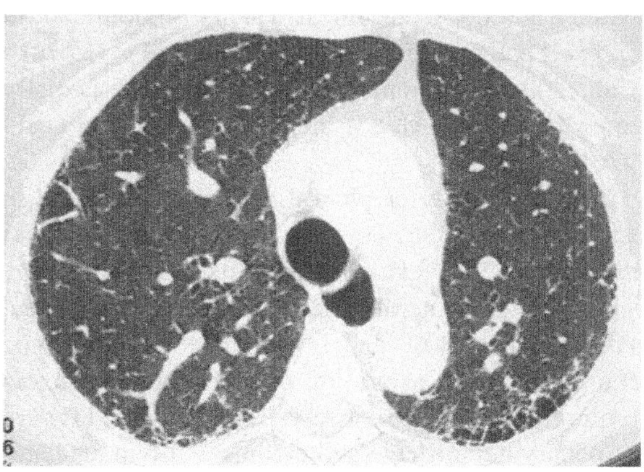

Figure 8. A 64-year-old woman with scleroderma. HRCT scan through the lung bases shows typical features of interstitial lung fibrosis. Note the dilatation of the upper esophagus.

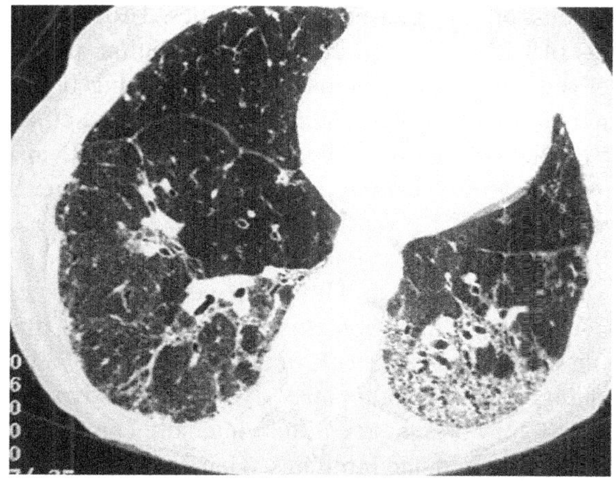

Figure 9. A 59-year-old woman with Sjögren's syndrome. HRCT scan through the lung bases again shows typical features of interstitial lung fibrosis with a patchy distribution of mild reticular opacities in the right lower lobe and extensive honeycombing, traction bronchiectasis, and marked loss of lung volume in the left lower lobe.

Lymphoid infiltration of extranodal sites are prominent features of SS (Koss et al., 1987; Hansen et al., 1989; Nicholson et al., 1995; Deheinzelin et al., 1996; Desai et al., 1997; Johkoh et al., 1999a,b). These lesions include LIP, mucosa associated lymphoid tissue lymphoma or MALTOMA (Hansen et al., 1989; Franquet et al., 1997a,b), and amyloidosis (Desai et al., 1997).

LIP is a benign lymphoproliferative disorder characterized by a diffuse interstitial proliferation of small lymphocytes and plasma cells that have been described in patients with SS, AIDS, autoimmune thyroid disease, or Castleman's disease (Nicholson et al., 1995; McGuiness et al., 1995; Johkoh et al., 1999a,b). Narrowing of both large and small airways by a lymphocytic mucosal infiltration has been documented and may account for obstructive ventilatory changes noted at pulmonary function testing (Deheinzelin et al., 1996). The radiographic manifestations of LIP are nonspecific, ranging from interstitial reticular opacities to nodular opacities. HRCT findings of LIP include ground-glass attenuation, poorly defined centrilobular nodules, and thickening of the interstitium along the lymphatic vessels (Koss et al., 1987; Johkoh et al., 1999a,b). Multiple cystic airspaces have also been typically described in patients with LIP (Fig. 10) (Desai et al., 1997; Meyer et al., 1997).

Moreover, patients with SS have a high risk of developing primary non-Hodgkin lymphoma of the lung (Hansen et al., 1989; Franquet et al., 1997a,b). Radiographically, pulmonary lymphoma associated with SS may present as a diffuse interstitial process or as multiple nodular infiltrates (Hansen et al., 1989; Franquet et al., 1997a,b). In a series of 50 patients with primary SS, one patient (2%) had multiple ill-defined pulmonary opacities with an associated air-bronchogram visible on CT (Franquet et al., 1997a,b). Lung biopsy obtained by thoracotomy demonstrated a low grade B-cell lymphoma (BALTOMA).

The prevalence of subclinical bronchiolitis in SS is therefore uncertain. Air trapping on expiratory HRCT has been found in asymptomatic patients with normal pulmonary function tests (Franquet et al., 1999). This finding may represent obstructive bronchiolitis due to submucosal lymphoid infiltration or fibrotic obstruction of small airways, but could also result from mucous plugging (Franquet et al., 1999).

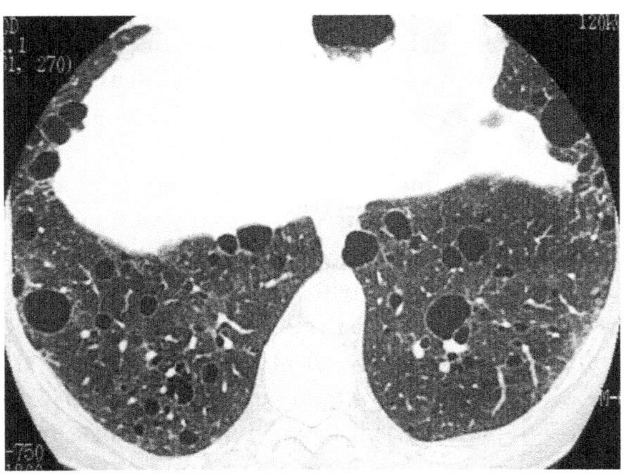

Figure 10. Lymphocytic interstitial pneumonia in a patient with Sjögren's syndrome. HRCT scan demonstrates bilateral thin-walled cystic lesions in the lower lobes in a random distribution.

5. Mixed connective tissue disease

MCTD, or overlap syndrome, is a chronic inflammatory autoimmune disease of unknown origin that has a combination of SLE, scleroderma or SSc, and PM/DM (Gamsu, 1992; Prakash, 1992, 1998). Patients with this pattern of illness have features of each of these three diseases. They also typically have very high quantities of antinuclear antibodies (ANAs) and antibodies to ribonucleoprotein (anti-RNP) detectable in their blood. MCTD can occur at any age, with the average age of onset in the third decade. Eight out of 10 patients are women. Diagnosis of MCTD as a different entity from lupus or RA is difficult. The syndrome is characterized by joint pain, muscle weakness, cardiac, lung and skin manifestations, kidney disease, and dysfunction of the esophagus. The symptoms of many of these patients eventually evolve to become dominated by features of one of three component illnesses, most commonly scleroderma. It is now known that certain patients can have overlap syndromes that involve any combination of the connective tissue diseases (Prakash, 1992, 1998; Lynch and Hunninghake, 1992; Wells, 2000).

ILD and pulmonary hypertension are the most common thoracic manifestations of MCTD. In a Mayo Clinic series, ILD was noted in 21% of cases (Prakash et al., 1985). The predominant abnormalities on HRCT scans consist of ground-glass attenuation, intralobular reticular opacity, subpleural small nodules, and nonseptal linear opacity predominant in the lower and peripheral lung fields (Fig. 11) (Kozuka et al., 2001). Pulmonary hypertension is especially seen when features of SSc are prominent (Silver et al., 1976).

Pleural effusion or pleural thickening is noted in less than 10% of cases and occurs in patients with predominant SLE features. The effusions are typically right-sided or bilateral. The incidence of esophageal involvement is 80% and is associated with chronic reflux and risk of aspiration pneumonitis. Other less common thoracic manifestations of MCTD are pulmonary hemorrhage and mediastinal lymphadenopathy (Prakash et al., 1985; Prakash, 1992; Niimi et al., 1996; Primack and Müller, 1998). Ill-defined centrilobular opacities were uncommon and may

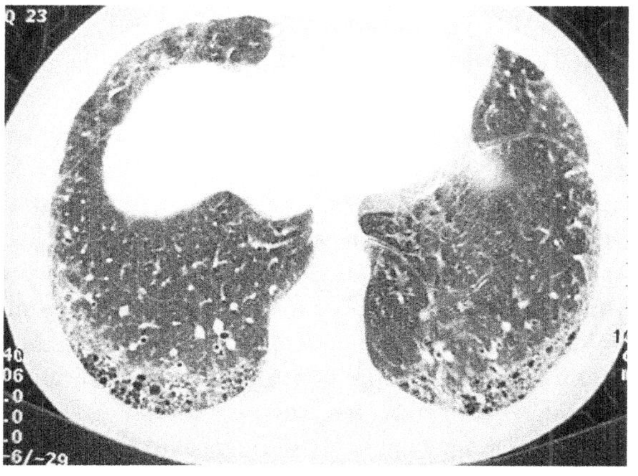

Figure 11. A 56-year-old woman with mixed connective tissue disease. HRCT scan shows bilateral reticular opacities, ground-glass attenuation and honeycombing predominantly in the subpleural lung regions.

reflect vascular or small airways disease in this population.

6. Polymyositis and dermatomyositis

PM is an idiopathic inflammatory myopathy with systemic manifestations, mediated by autoimmune and cellular mechanisms. PM and DM are similar disorders that differ in the predominance of skin or muscle involvement. Young and middle-aged women are more apt to be affected than men. The onset of PM/DM in patients over 50 years may be the result of an underlying malignancy (colon, breast, prostate, lung, or uterus) (Dickey and Myers, 1984; Airio et al., 1995; Ikezoe et al., 1996; Akira et al., 1999a,b).

Thoracic involvement is common in PM/DM, resulting in: (a) direct involvement of the respiratory muscles, (b) interstitial pneumonitis, and (c) aspiration pneumonia secondary to pharyngeal muscle weakness (Dickey and Myers, 1984; Shannon and Gale, 1992).

The radiographic findings of interstitial fibrosis in patients who have PM/DM are indistinguishable from those seen in patients with IPF, and consist of a symmetrical, predominantly basal, reticular or reticulonodular pattern (Fig. 12) (Dickey and Myers, 1984; Ikezoe et al., 1996; Akira et al., 1999a,b). In one series of 25 patients, 23 had abnormal HRCT findings

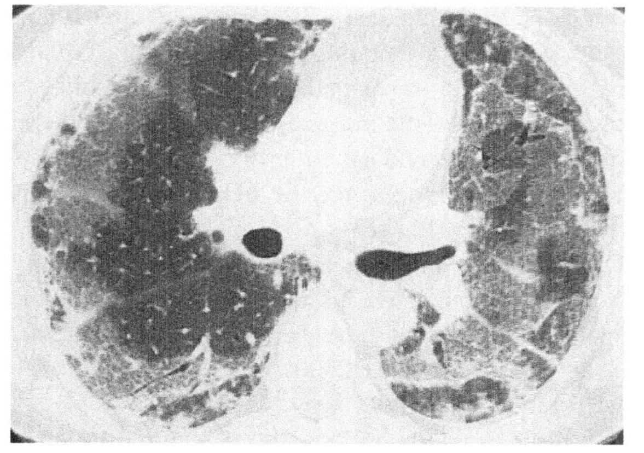

Figure 12. A 46-year-old man with PM. HRCT scan shows bilateral areas of consolidation. The consolidation has a subpleural distribution.

including ground-glass attenuation (92%), linear opacities (92%), air-space consolidation (52%), small nodules (28%), and honeycombing (16%) (Ikezoe et al., 1996). From the results of HRCT-pathologic correlation, eight patients who had localized air-space consolidation had bronchiolitis obliterans organizing pneumonia, two patients with diffuse ground-glass opacity with air-space consolidation had diffuse alveolar damage, and four patients

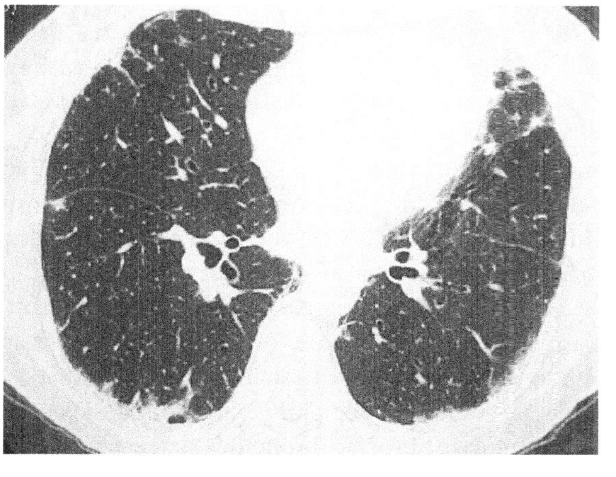

Figure 13. A 42-year-old woman with PM/DM. Abnormalities predominate in the subpleural area. Ground-glass opacity is superimposed on the abnormal reticulation. The fine reticular pattern visible largely reflects intralobular interstitial thickening. The distinction between normal and abnormal lung parenchyma is clearly visible in the right lung. Bilateral small areas of consolidation are also visible in a subpleural distribution.

with honeycombing had UIP (Ikezoe et al., 1996). Although the HRCT findings in patients with PM/DM are similar to those in patients with other collagen vascular diseases, the presence of areas of subpleural consolidation secondary to bronchiolitis obliterans organizing pneumonia may be helpful in the differential diagnosis (Fig. 13).

Spontaneous pneumomediastinum is a rare complication of connective tissue diseases. Most of the reported associations have been with DM, systemic lupus, and RA (Wells, 2000; Prakash, 1998; Lynch and Hunninghake, 1992).

Aspiration pneumonia has been reported to occur in 15–20% of patients (Ikezoe et al., 1996).

7. Ankylosing spondylitis

Those most commonly affected by ankylosing spondylitis are young men between 20 and 40 years of age, 90% of whom are HLA-B27 positive (Lynch and Hunninghake, 1992; Tanoue, 1992; Prakash, 1998; Wells, 2000). Although the exact prevalence of pulmonary disease is rare and remains to be determined, the prevalence of pulmonary disease ranges from 0 to 30% of patients (Crompton et al., 1974; Rosenow et al., 1977; Casserly et al., 1997; Fenlon et al., 1997; Lee-Choing, 1998). The cause of pulmonary involvement remains controversial but it probably develops in patients with severe bone changes. Radiographic manifestations are variable and dependent on the chronicity of the disease (Rosenow et al., 1977; Mayberry et al., 2000). The earliest manifestation of the disease is thought to be bilateral apical scarring. These radiographic changes may mimic those of chronic tuberculosis with apical fibrocavitary changes and cyst formation (Fig. 13). Additional radiographic abnormalities such as nonapical fibrosis, bronchiectasis, paraseptal emphysema, and tracheobronchomegaly have also been documented (Crompton et al., 1974). Bone changes, consisting of symmetric marginal syndesmophytes ('bamboo spine'), are usually visible on the thoracic spine of patients with ankylosing spondylitis who have pleuropulmonary abnormalities.

8. Parenchymal lung diseases other than fibrosing alveolitis

The diagnosis of parenchymal lung diseases other than fibrosing alveolitis poses a particular challenge to the clinician, as several additional complicating features may appear in a patient with connective tissue diseases. Drug-induced lung disease, opportunistic infections and malignancy may complicate the clinical course of these patients. In many cases, they present with nonspecific constitutional or respiratory complaints and symptoms may be minimal or absent. In these circumstances, the only evidence of an ongoing pulmonary process may be an abnormal chest radiograph.

8.1. Diffuse alveolar damage associated with connective diseases

A form of rapidly progressive disease resembling the Hamman-Rich syndrome ('accelerated stage') may occur in patients with DM/PM, RA and SSc. A similar syndrome ('acute lupus pneumonitis') is seen in up to 2% of patients with SLE. Diffuse alveolar damage, OP, cellular interstitial pneumonitis, or a combination of these are the underlying histologic findings. The clinical picture is characterized by a severe acute respiratory failure that often requires assisted mechanical ventilation (Kondoh et al., 1993; Akira et al., 1997). Infection is an important differential diagnosis and must be ruled out in all patients before considering the diagnosis of diffuse alveolar damage. A chest radiograph shows bilateral alveolar infiltrates which can be patchy or densely consolidated. HRCT shows a combination of ground-glass opacification, air-space consolidation, bronchial dilatation, and architectural distortion (Johkoh et al., 1999a,b). Because of the difficulty in distinguishing rapidly progressive interstitial pneumonitis from an infectious pneumonia, a bronchoalveolar lavage and sometimes an open lung biopsy are often warranted. Other possible diagnoses are DAH and acute eosinophilic lung disease.

8.2. Drug-induced lung disease

Drug-induced pulmonary toxicity represents a significant clinical problem in patients with connective tissue diseases. A large number of drugs have been implicated in causing lung damage (Everts et al., 1973; Sostman et al., 1976; Wolfe et al., 1983; Cooper et al., 1986; Rossi et al., 2000). However, a definitive diagnosis of a drug reaction is difficult to establish because the clinical, radiologic, and histologic findings are usually nonspecific. Most pulmonary drug reactions remain suspected rather than proven. Methotrexate is currently used as an anti-inflammatory agent in the treatment of RA and psoriasis. Methotrexate-induced interstitial pneumonitis is the most frequently encountered pulmonary toxicity in RA. As many as 10% of patients receiving methotrexate will develop pulmonary toxicity (Cooper et al., 1986). Moreover, in a previously reported series, more than half of the patients with methotrexate pneumonitis had RA (Camus et al., 2001). No correlation with cumulative dose has been reported. The mechanism of methotrexate-induced lung injury is unknown. Chemotherapeutic drugs can result in four main types of lung reaction: interstitial pneumonitis and fibrosis, hypersensitivity reaction, acute respiratory distress syndrome, and OP (Padley et al., 1992; Ellis et al., 2000). The manifestations of pulmonary toxicity are better visualized on HRCT than on a chest radiograph. The HRCT findings reflect the histologic findings and range from subtle hazy areas of increased density (ground-glass opacities) to patchy or homogeneous air-space consolidation (Padley et al., 1992; Ellis et al., 2000). Interstitial pneumonitis and fibrosis result in ground-glass and irregular opacities that tend to involve the basal lung zones. A hypersensitivity reaction to methotrexate can result in extensive bilateral air-space consolidation. Acute respiratory distress syndrome and an organizing pneumonia-like reaction can also result in subpleural areas of consolidation. The pattern and distribution of parenchymal abnormalities on HRCT scan are indistinguishable from those of cryptogenic organizing pneumonia (COP). In a significant number of cases, the consolidation involves mainly the peripheral or peribronchial lung regions (Primack and Müller, 1998; Franquet, 2001). Other findings include nodular or ground-glass opacities, and bronchial dilatation, most frequently seen in the periphery of the lung (Oikonomou and Hansell, 2002). Pulmonary toxicity has also been described in gold salts, D-penicillamine, nonsteroidal anti-inflammatory agents ($NSAID_S$), and sulphasalazine (Camus et al., 1982; Khalil et al., 1993; Rosenow and Limper, 1995; Tomioka and King, 1997).

Parenchymal abnormalities induced by drugs are often difficult to distinguish from more common illnesses or causes of acute exacerbation of an ongoing illness such as infection, hemorrhage, heart failure, or malignancy. In methotrexate-induced lung disease, the clinical onset is relatively acute and new mixed alveolar infiltrates may appear on a chest radiograph (Primack and Müller, 1998; Franquet, 2001). A definitive diagnosis may be established on the basis of: an appropriate history of exposure, pulmonary opacities on chest radiograph or HRCT, and exclusion of other pulmonary diseases, especially infections (Camus et al., 2001).

OB, characterized by airflow obstruction, is a well-recognized cause of progressive obstructing lung disease in patients with RA. This complication has been recognized as a consequence of either penicillamine or gold salts therapy; however, many cases have appeared in the absence of either treatment (Wolfe et al., 1983). A chest radiograph is usually normal or shows only hyperinflation. The characteristic HRCT findings consist of a 'mosaic perfusion' pattern with areas of decreased attenuation and vascularity and other areas showing increased attenuation and blood flow redistribution (Aquino et al., 1999). CT is much more sensitive than radiography, highlighting the distribution of the areas of air trapping.

8.3. Opportunistic infections

Pulmonary infections are somewhat increased in connective tissue diseases and may complicate the clinical course of RA, SLE, and ankylosing spondylitis. Infections may be related to the immunologic defects conditioned by the disease or its therapy. The degree of neutropenia may predict the severity of the infection and affect the prognosis. Respiratory tract infection is an important cause of mortality in patients with RA (Mutru et al., 1976). Previous series have reported that pulmonary infection was the cause of death in 15–19% of patients with RA (Mutru et al., 1976; Koota et al., 1977). Etiologic agents include *Streptococcus*, *Staphylococcus*, gram-negative bacteria including *Pseudomonas*, and fungi (dermatomycosis, onychomycosis) (Myllykangas-Luosujarvi et al., 1995). Fungal infection in RA patients is promoted by methotrexate and corticosteroids. A clinical diagnosis of infectious pneumonia can be made in light of a compatible clinical picture, along with suggestive chest radiographic features. Radiologically, the most common finding of infectious pneumonia is a focal air-space consolidation. Although the diagnosis is based on radiograph appearance, it is important for clinicians to appreciate that patients with pulmonary infiltrates on the chest radiograph may have a noninfectious process. Thus, the differential diagnosis should also include other disorders such as OP and bronchioloalveolar carcinoma.

Infection is also the commonest pulmonary complication in SLE, accounting for about 50% of pleuropulmonary manifestations. Patients under a high dose of steroid administration or cytotoxic agents, or with renal disease, are especially susceptible to pulmonary infection. Bacterial pathogens cause more than 90% of the infectious episodes in SLE patients (Staples et al., 1974; Petri, 1998). A chest radiograph shows unilateral or bilateral pulmonary areas of consolidation that usually involve the lower lung zones. Thin-section CT is more sensitive than radiographs in the detection and assessment of pulmonary complications associated with connective tissue diseases. Pulmonary nocardiosis has been well described in SLE patients treated with corticosteroids. Radiographically, it usually presents as lung nodules, which are often cavitated. Other infections occasionally described in patients with SLE include tuberculosis and other mycobacterial infections, *Pneumocystis carinii*, *Rhodococcus* spp., and *Pseudomonas* spp. Acute lupus pneumonitis, hemorrhage, ARDS, and OP can result in similar radiologic findings (Onomura et al., 1991; Wiederman and Matthay, 1992; Bankier et al., 1995; Primack and Müller, 1998; Franquet, 2001).

In patients with ankylosing spondylitis, cavities may develop within distorted fibrotic apical tissue. Secondary superinfection of these cavities with Aspergillus has been described in some of these patients (Casserly et al., 1997; Fenlon et al., 1997). Life-threatening hemoptysis is an occasional complication of mycetoma formation within cavities and may be controlled by bronchial artery embolization (Franquet et al., 2004).

Aspiration pneumonia needs to be considered in patients with pharyngeal muscle weakness and esophageal motor disturbances (DePaso, 1991). Recurrent aspiration of oral-pharyngeal contents is frequent among patients with PM/DM and pulmonary systemic sclerosis. Aspiration pneumonia is the most important cause of mortality in patients with PM/DM. The radiologic manifestations of aspiration pneumonia consist of unilateral or bilateral segmental areas of air-space consolidation in the dependent lung zones (Kennedy et al., 1981; Lee et al., 1995). Associated bronchiolitis can also result from aspiration episodes. On thin-section CT, aspiration bronchiolitis is characterized by tubular or branched bronchioles which reflect the presence of bronchiolar dilatation with associated mucous impaction and infection. Patchy areas of consolidation may be observed in association with bronchiolitis due to transbronchial spread of aspirated material into peribronchial space.

Exogenous lipoid pneumonia is most often due to the aspiration of mineral oil in patients with esophageal disorders or gastroesophageal reflux, but may also be due to the aspiration of oily nose drops or to inhalation of oil-based sprays. Lipoid pneumonia may be an incidental finding on chest radiography of an asymptomatic patient. Lipoid pneumonia can result in a variety of patterns, depending on the amount of aspirated substance (Kennedy et al., 1981; Lee et al., 1995). Chest CT may demonstrate focal areas of fat attenuation in the consolidation, or a 'crazy-paving' pattern consisting of ground-glass consolidation with superimposed septal lines (Franquet et al., 1997a,b).

8.4. Malignancy

Different studies have provided evidence of an increased incidence of lung cancer in patients with connective tissue disease (Yang et al., 2001; Hill et al., 2003). Lung cancer arises in previously damaged or fibrotic tissue and is frequently of the bronchioloalveolar (BACC) or adenocarcinoma type rather than the more common squamous cell type. Although BACC accounts for less than 10% of primary lung tumors, up to 50% of BACC is associated with

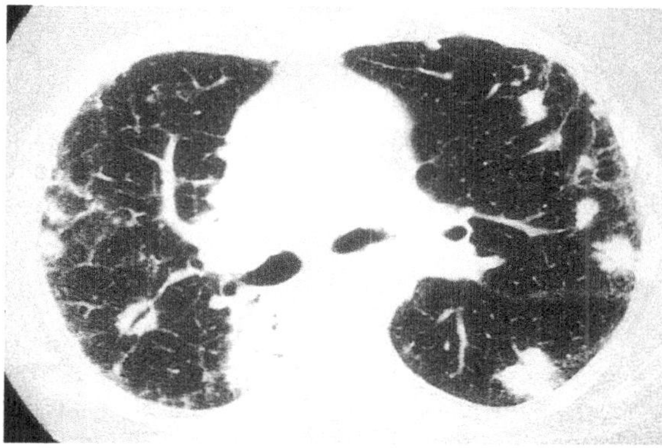

Figure 14. HRCT in a 56-year-old woman with progressive systemic sclerosis and associated lung carcinoma. The HRCT scan shows a bilateral fine reticular pattern in a patchy and subpleural distribution. Multiple peripheral nodules representing multifocal bronchiolo-alveolar cell carcinoma are also seen. Note that an air-bronchogram is visible within some of the nodules.

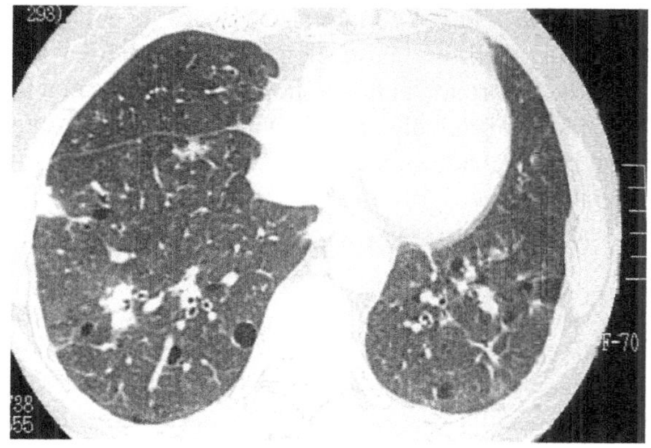

Figure 15. A 62-year-old woman with Sjögren's syndrome. HRCT scan shows a bilateral thin-walled cystic lesions in a random distribution. Multiple ill-defined pulmonary nodules representing MALT lymphoma are visible. Note extensive areas of ground-glass opacity in the lower lung zones.

previous scarring in the lung (Fig. 14) (Yang et al., 2001; Hill et al., 2003). Occupations such as construction work, coal work, and sugarcane farming, and chronic interstitial disease, especially in patients with scleroderma, are associated with an increased incidence of bronchioloalveolar carcinoma.

LIP is a benign process frequently seen in RA and SS. The CT features consist of ground-glass opacification, air-space consolidation, poorly defined centrilobular nodules, and cystic-air spaces (Johkoh et al., 1999a,b). The formation of cystic dilated air spaces may be related to peribronchiolar lymphoid hyperplasia. Additionally, patients with RA, SLE, and SS are at increased risk of developing hematologic malignancies, especially lymphomas (Hansen et al., 1989; Li et al., 1990; Cordier et al., 1993; Franquet et al., 1997a,b). Up to 70% of primary lymphomas of the lung are BALT lymphomas. In one study of 50 patients with primary SS, one patient (2%) had BALT lymphoma (Franquet et al., 1997a,b). Radiographically, the most common findings are solitary or multiple pulmonary nodules or multiple areas of patchy consolidation (Fig. 15) (Matteson and Ike, 1990). However, air-space consolidations may be also associated with areas of OP (Lee et al., 1997; Koyama et al., 2001).

PM/DM is associated with increased incidence of lung cancer, cancer of the stomach and ovaries, and lymphomas (Sigurgeirsson et al., 1992). The diagnosis of cancer may precede, coincide, or follow the diagnosis of PM/DM and it significantly affects prognosis (Zantoss et al., 1994).

8.5. Concurrent processes that might be masked by DPLD

Several studies have reported enlarged mediastinal nodes in association with a variety of chronic ILDs and connective tissue disease (Niimi et al., 1996; Bhalla et al., 1993). The detection of lymphadenopathy in these patients can be the cause of considerable clinical concern. However, it should be emphasized that enlarged mediastinal lymph nodes do not necessarily indicate the presence of an associated malignancy. The cause of enlargement of the mediastinal lymph nodes is not yet understood and usually represents a reactive hyperplasia.

Bronchiectasis can be a frequent finding in patients with RA. HRCT studies show that up to 30% of patients with RA have bronchiectasis unassociated with ILD. This rate of occurrence is more frequent than in other connective tissue diseases. Consequently, in RA patients with bronchiectasis, recurrent pulmonary infections may occur (bronchiectasis can be morphologically classified into three types: cylindric, varicose, and cystic). Traction bronchiectasis is a distinct type of bronchial dilatation occurring in patients who have pulmonary fibrosis because of traction by fibrous tissue on the bronchial wall. On HRCT, bronchiectasis should be differentiated from traction bronchiectasis in which underlying lung parenchyma is not affected by fibrotic disease.

8.6. HRCT in relation to key clinical issues

The patient-effective radiation dose from a postero-anterior chest radiograph is approximately 0.05 mSv. Conversely, conventional chest CT and spiral CT pitch 1 results in an effective patient dose of approximately 7.0 mSv, 140 times that of a single-view chest radiograph. CT is an invaluable cross-sectional imaging technique in the assessment of pulmonary, mediastinal and chest wall abnormalities. The introduction of helical single-detector row computed tomography and more recently multi-detector row CT has greatly increased the clinical indications for CT. The increase in population radiation exposure from CT has been of concern to radiologists, medical physicists, and govern regulators. It has been shown that three low-dose, thin-section CT sections provide an effective dose comparable to that of posteroanterior chest radiography (0.05 mSv), with no significant loss of diagnostic accuracy in ILD (Lee et al., 1994; Mayo et al., 2003).

Although the rate of pulmonary disease progression is variable, the great majority of connective tissue diseases are relentlessly progressive. Clinical and physiologic deterioration in a patient with connective tissue disease most often represents disease progression. Pulmonary function tests and HRCT are the most useful noninvasive diagnostic methods for detection and follow-up, as well as assessing the response to therapy of an ILD. Radiologists and medical practitioners must be attentive to their responsibility to maintain an appropriate balance between diagnostic image and radiation dose (Lee et al., 1994; Mayo et al., 2003).

Key points

- Due to its abundant connective tissue, the lungs are an important target organ in connective tissue diseases. However, because the pathology of chronic interstitial pneumonia takes a limited number of forms, there are also a limited number of radiographic manifestations.
- In rheumatoid arthritis, the degree of ILD does not necessarily correlate with the severity of underlying articular involvement.
- Expiratory HRCT scans have proved useful in the evaluation of patients with a variety of lung diseases characterized by obstruction of airflow.
- Infection is the most common pulmonary complication in SLE. In contrast to many other collagen vascular diseases, SLE is not commonly associated with chronic diffuse ILD.
- NSIP is the histologic pattern that is seen in the majority of patients with SSc. A usual interstitial pneumonitis (UIP) pattern occurs in 8% of cases.
- Lymphoid infiltration of extranodal sites are prominent features of SS. Pulmonary lesions associated with SS are LIP, mucosa associated lymphoid tissue lymphoma or MALTOMA and amyloidosis.
- A form of rapidly progressive disease resembling the Hamman-rich syndrome ('accelerated stage') may occur in patients with DM/PM, RA and SSc. This acute form must be distinguished from infectious pneumonia, alveolar hemorrhage and acute eosinophilic lung disease.
- Drug-induced pulmonary toxicity represents a significant clinical problem in patients with connective tissue diseases.
- Pulmonary function tests and HRCT are the most useful noninvasive diagnostic methods for detection and follow-up as well as assessing the response to therapy of an ILD.

References

Airio, A., Pukkala, E., Isomaki, H. 1995. Elevated cancer incidence in patients with dermatomyositis: a population based study. J. Rheumatol. 22, 1300.

Akira, M., Hamada, H., Sakatani, M., et al. 1997. CT findings during phase of accelerated deterioration in patients with idiopathic pulmonary fibrosis. AJR 168, 79.

Akira, M., Hara, H., Sakatani, M. 1999a. Interstitial lung disease in association with polymyositis–dermatomyositis: long-term follow-up CT evaluation in seven patients. Radiology 210, 333.

Akira, M., Sakatani, M., Hara, H. 1999b. Thin-section CT findings in rheumatoid arthritis associated lung disease: CT patterns and their courses. J. Comput. Assist. Tomogr. 23, 941.

Aquino, S.L., Webb, W.R., Golden, J. 1994. Bronchiolitis obliterans associated with rheumatoid arthritis: findings on HRCT and dynamic expiratory CT. J. Comput. Assist. Tomogr. 18, 555.

Aquino, S.L., Webb, R.W., Golden, J. 1999. Bronchiolitis obliterans associated with rheumatoid arthritis: findings on HRCT and dynamic expiratory CT. J. Comput. Assist. Tomogr. 18, 555.

Arroliga, A.C., Podell, D.N., Mathay, R.A. 1992. Pulmonary manifestations of scleroderma. J. Thorac. Imaging 7, 30.

Ayzemberg, O., Reiff, D.B., Levin, L. 1983. Bilateral pneumothoraces and pleural effusions complicating rheumatoid lung disease. Thorax 38, 159.

Bankier, A.A., Kiener, H.P., Wiesmayr, M.N., Fleischmann, D., Kontrus, M., Herold, C.J., Graninger, W., Hubsch, P. 1995. Discrete lung involvement in systemic lupus erythematosus: CT assessment. Radiology 196, 835.

Bergin, C., Castellino, R.A. 1990. Mediastinal lymph node enlargement on CT scans in patients with usual interstitial pneumonitis. AJR 54, 251.

Bhalla, M., Silver, R.M., Shepard, J.A.O., McLoud, T.C. 1993. Chest CT in patients with scleroderma: prevalence of asymptomatic esophageal dilatation and mediastinal lymphadenopathy. AJR 161, 269.

Braunstein, E.M., Weissman, B.N., Sosman, J.L., Schur, P.H. 1983. Radiologic findings in late-onset systemic lupus erythematosus. AJR 140, 587.

Cain, H.C., Noble, P.W., Matthay, R.A. 1988. Pulmonary manifestations of Sjögren's syndrome. Clin. Chest Med. 19, 687.

Camus, P., Reybet-Degat, Justrabo, E., Jeannin, L.D. 1982. Penicillamine-induced severe pneumonitis. Chest 81, 376.

Camus, Ph., Foucher, P., Bonniaud, Ph., Ask, K. 2001. Drug induced infiltrative lung disease. Eur. Respir. J. 18 (Suppl. 32), 93s.

Caplan, A. 1953. Certain unusual radiographic appearances in the chest of coal-miners suffering from rheumatoid arthritis. Thorax 8, 19.

Casserly, I.P., Fenlon, H.M., Breatnach, E., Sant, S.M. 1997. Lung findings on high-resolution computed tomography in idiopathic ankylosing spondylitis: correlation with clinical findings, pulmonary function testing and plain radiography. Br. J. Rheumatol. 36, 677.

Chan, T.Y.K., Hansell, D.M., Rubens, M.B., du Bois, R.M., Wells, A.U. 1997. Cryptogenic fibrosing alveolitis of systemic sclerosis: morphological differences on computed tomographic scans. Thorax 52, 265.

Cooper, J.A. Jr., White, D.A., Matthay, R.A. 1986. Drug-induced pulmonary disease. 2. Noncytotoxic drugs. Am. Rev. Respir. Dis. 133, 488.

Cordier, J.F., Chailleux, E., Lauque, D., Reynaud-Gaubert, M., Dietemann-Molard, A., Dalphin, J.C., Blanc-Jouvan, F., Loire, R. 1993. Primary pulmonary lymphomas. Chest 103, 201.

Cortet, B., Flipo, R.M., Remy-Jardin, M., Coquerelle, P., Duquesnoy, B., Remy, J., Delcambre, B. 1995. Use of high resolution computed tomography of the lungs in patients with rheumatoid arthritis. Ann. Rheum. Dis. 54, 815.

Crompton, G.K., Cameron, S.J., Langlands, A.O. 1974. Pulmonary fibrosis, pulmonary tuberculosis, and ankylosing spondylitis. Br. J. Dis. Chest 68, 51.

D'Angelo, W.A., Fries, J.F., Masi, A.T., Shulman, L.E. 1969. Pathologic observations in systemic sclerosis (scleroderma): a study of fifty-eight autopsy cases and fifty-eight matched controls. Am. J. Med. 46, 428.

Deheinzelin, D., Capelozzi, V.L., Kairalla, R.A., Barbas Filho, J.V., Saldiva, P.H., de Carvalho, C.R. 1996. Interstitial lung disease in primary Sjögren's syndrome: clinical–pathological evaluation and response to treatment. Am. J. Respir. Crit. Care Med. 154, 794.

DePaso, W.J. 1991. Aspiration pneumonia. Clin. Chest Med. 12, 269.

Desai, S.R., Nicholson, A.G., Stewart, S., Twentyman, O.M., Flower, C.D., Hansell, D.M. 1997. Benign pulmonary lymphocytic infiltration and amyloidosis: computed tomographic and pathologic features in three cases. J. Thorac. Imaging 12, 215.

Dickey, B.F., Myers, A.R. 1984. Pulmonary disease in polymyositis/dermatomyositis. Semin. Arthritis Rheum. 14, 60.

Diehl, J.L., Gisselbrecht, M., Meyer, G., Israel-Biet, D., Sors, H. 1996. Bronchiolitis obliterans organising pneumonia associated with chlamydial infection. Eur. Respir. J. 9, 1320.

Ellis, S.J., Joanne, R., Cleverley, J.R., Müller, N.L. 2000. Drug-induced lung disease: high-resolution CT findings. AJR 175, 1019.

Everts, C.S., Wescott, J.L., Bragg, D.G. 1973. Methotrexate therapy and pulmonary disease. Radiology 107, 539.

Fenlon, H.M., Doran, M., Sant, S.M., Breatnach, E. 1995. High-resolution CT in systemic lupus erythematosus. AJR 166, 301.

Fenlon, H.M., Casserly, I., Sant, S.M., Breatnach, E. 1997. Plain radiographs and thoracic high-resolution CT in patients with ankylosing spondylitis. AJR 168, 1067.

Fortoul, T.I., Cano-Valle, F., Oliva, E., Barrios, R. 1985. Follicular bronchiolitis in association with connective tissue diseases. Lung 163, 305.

Franquet, T. 2001. High-resolution CT of lung disease related to collagen vascular disease. Radiol. Clin. North Am. 39, 1171.

Franquet, T., Giménez, A., Bordes, R., Rodríguez-Arias, J.M., Castella, J. 1997a. The crazy paving pattern in exogenous lipoid pneumonia: CT-pathologic correlation. AJR 170, 315.

Franquet, T., Giménez, A., Monill, J.M., Diaz, C., Geli, C. 1997b. Primary Sjögren's syndrome and associated lung disease: CT findings in 50 patients. AJR 169, 655.

Franquet, T., Díaz, C., Domingo, P., Gimenez, A., Geli, C. 1999. Air-trapping in primary Sjögren's syndrome: correlation of expiratory CT with pulmonary function tests. J. Comput. Assist. Tomogr. 23, 169.

Franquet, T., Müller, N.L., Flint, J.D. 2004. A patient with ankylosing spondylitis and recurrent hemoptysis. Eur. Respir. J. 23, 488.

Fujii, M., Adachi, S., Shimizu, T., Hirota, S., Sako, M., Kono, M. 1993. Interstitial lung disease in rheumatoid arthritis: assessment with high-resolution computed tomography. J. Thorac. Imaging 8, 54.

Gabbay, E., Tarala, R., Will, R., Carroll, G., Adler, B., Cameron, D., Lake, F.R. 1997. Interstitial lung disease in recent onset rheumatoid arthritis. Am. J. Rev. Respir. Crit. Care Med. 156, 528.

Gammon, R.B., Bridges, T.A., al-Nezir, H., Alexander, C.B., Kennedy, J.I. Jr. 1992. Bronchiolitis obliterans organizing pneumonia associated with systemic lupus erythematosus. Chest 102, 1171.

Gamsu, G. 1992. Radiographic manifestations of thoracic involvement by collagen vascular diseases. J. Thorac. Imaging 7, 1.

Hansen, L.A., Prakash, U.B., Colby, T.V. 1989. Pulmonary lymphoma in Sjögren's syndrome. Mayo Clin. Proc. 64, 920.

Hassan, W.U., Keaney, N.P., Holland, C.D., Kelly, C.A. 1995. High resolution computed tomography of the lung in lifelong non-smoking patients who have rheumatoid arthritis. Ann. Rheum. Dis. 54, 308.

Hayakawa, H., Sato, A., Imokawa, S., Toyoshima, M., Chida, K., Iwata, M. 1996. Bronchiolar disease in rheumatoid arthritis. Am. J. Respir. Crit. Care Med. 154, 1531.

Hill, C.L., Nguyen, A.M., Roder, D., Roberts-Thomson, P. 2003. Risk of cancer in patients with scleroderma: a population based cohort study. Ann. Rheum. Dis. 62, 728.

Hindle, W., Yates, D.A.H. 1965. Pyopneumothorax complicating rheumatoid lung disease. Ann. Rheum. Dis. 24, 57.

Howling, S.J., Hansell, D.M., Wells, A.U., Nicholson, A.G., Flint, J.D., Muller, N.L. 1999. Follicular bronchiolitis: thin-section CT and histologic findings. Radiology 212, 637.

Ikezoe, J., Johkoh, T., Kohno, N., Takeuchi, N., Ichikado, K., Nakamura, H. 1996. High resolution CT findings in patients with polymyositis and dermatomyositis. J. Thorac. Imaging 11, 250.

Imokawa, S., Colby, T.V., Leslie, K.O., Helmers, R.A. 2000. Methotrexate pneumonitis: review of the literature and histopathological findings in nine patients. Eur. Respir. J. 15, 373.

Ippolito, J.A., Palmer, L., Spector, S., Kane, P.B., Gorevic, P.D. 1993. Bronchiolitis obliterans organizing pneumonia and rheumatoid arthritis. Semin. Arthritis Rheum. 23, 70.

Johkoh, T., Müller, N.L., Taniguchi, H., Kondoh, Y., Akira, M., Ichikado, K., Ando, M., Honda, O., Tomiyama, N., Nakamura, H. 1999a. Acute interstitial pneumonia: thin-section CT findings in 36 patients. Radiology 211, 859.

Johkoh, T., Müller, N.L., Pickford, H.A., Hartman, T.E., Ichikado, K., Akira, M., Honda, O., Nakamura, H. 1999b. Lymphocytic interstitial pneumonia: thin-section CT findings in 22 patients. Radiology 212, 567.

Katzenstein, A.L., Fiorelli, R.F. 1994. Nonspecific interstitial pneumonia/fibrosis: features and clinical significance. Am. J. Surg. Pathol. 18, 136.

Kennedy, J.D., Costello, P., Balikian, J.P., Herman, P.G. 1981. Exogenous lipoid pneumonia. AJR 136, 1145.

Khalil, H., Molinary, E., Stoller, J.K. 1993. Diclofenac (Voltaren)-induced eosinophilic pneumonitis: case report and review of the literature. Arch. Intern. Med. 153, 1649.

Kim, J.S., Lee, K.S., Koh, E.M., Kim, S.Y., Chung, M.P., Han, J. 2000. Thoracic involvement of systemic lupus erythematosus: clinical, pathologic, and radiologic findings. J. Comput. Assist. Tomogr. 24, 9.

Kinoshita, M., Higashi, T., Tanaka, C., Tokunaga, N., Ichikawa, Y., Oizumi, K. 1992. Follicular bronchiolitis associated with rheumatoid arthritis. Intern. Med. 31, 674.

Kondoh, Y., Taniguchi, H., Kawabata, Y., Iwata, K., Tajima, T., Mitomi, T. 1993. Acute exacerbation in idiopathic pulmonary fibrosis. Analysis of clinical and pathologic findings in three cases. Chest 103, 1808.

Koota, K., Isomaki, H., Mutru, O. 1977. Death rate and causes of death in RA patients during a period of five years. Scand. J. Rheumatol. 6, 241.

Koss, M.N., Hochholzer, L., Langloss, J.M., Wehunt, W.D., Lazarus, A.A. 1987. Lymphoid interstitial pneumonia: clinicopathological findings in 18 cases. Pathology 19, 178.

Koyama, M., Johkoh, T., Honda, O., Mihara, N., Kozuka, T., Tomiyama, N., Hamada, S., Nakamura, H. 2001. Pulmonary involvement in primary Sjögren's syndrome. Spectrum of pulmonary abnormalities and computed tomographic findings in 60 patients. J. Thorac. Imaging 16, 290.

Kozuka, T., Johkoh, T., Honda, O., Mihara, N., Koyama, M., Tomiyama, N., Hamada, S., Nakamura, H., Ichikado, K. 2001. Pulmonary involvement in mixed connective tissue disease. High-resolution CT findings in 41 patients. J. Thorac. Imaging 16, 94.

Lee, K.S., Primack, S.L., Staples, C.A., Mayo, J.R., Aldrich, J.E., Müller, N.L. 1994. Chronic infiltrative lung disease: comparison of diagnostic accuracies of radiography and low- and conventional-dose thin-section CT. Radiology 191, 669.

Lee, K.S., Müller, N.L., Hale, V., Newell, J.D.J., Lynch, D.A., Im, J.G. 1995. Lipoid pneumonia: CT findings. J. Comput. Assist. Tomogr. 19, 48.

Lee, K.S., Kim, Y., Primack, S.L. 1997. Imaging of pulmonary lymphomas. AJR 168, 339.

Lee-Choing, T.L. Jr. 1998. Pulmonary manifestations of ankylosing spondylitis and relapsing polychondritis. Clin. Chest Med. 19, 747.

Li, G., Hansmann, M.L., Zwingers, T., Lennert, K. 1990. Pulmonary lymphomas of the lung: morphological, immunohistochemical and clinical features. Histopathology 16, 519.

Lynch, J.P. III, Hunninghake, G.W. 1992. Pulmonary complications of collagen vascular disease. Annu. Rev. Med. 43, 17.

Matteson, E.L., Ike, R.W. 1990. Bronchiolitis obliterans organizing pneumonia and Sjögren's syndrome. J. Rheumatol. 17, 676.

Mayberry, J.P., Primack, S.L., Müller, N.L. 2000. Thoracic manifestations of systemic autoimmune diseases: radiographic and high-resolution CT findings. RadioGraphics 20, 1623.

Mayo, J.R., Aldrich, J., Müller, N.L. 2003. Radiation exposure at chest CT: a statement of the Fleischner society. Radiology 228, 15.

McGuiness, G., Scholes, J.V., Jagirdar, J.S., Lubat, E., Leitman, B.S., Bhalla, M., McCauley, D.I., Garay, S.M., Naidich, D.P. 1995. Unusual lymphoproliferative disorders in nine adults with HIV or AIDS: CT and pathologic findings. Radiology 197, 59.

Meyer, C.A., Pina, J.S., Taillon, D., Godwin, J.D. 1997. Inspiratory and expiratory high-resolution CT findings in a patient with Sjögren's syndrome and cystic lung disease. AJR 168, 101.

Min, J.K., Hong, Y.S., Park, S.H., Park, J.H., Lee, S.H., Lee, Y.S., Kim, H.H., Cho, C.S., Kim, H.Y. 1997. Bronchiolitis obliterans organizing pneumonia as an initial manifestation in patients with systemic lupus erythematosus. J. Rheumatol. 24, 2254.

Minai, O.A., Dweik, R.A., Arroliga, A.C. 1998. Manifestations of scleroderma pulmonary disease. Clin. Chest Med. 19, 713.

Mok, C.C., Yuen, K.Y., Lau, C.S. 1997. Nocardiosis in systemic lupus erythematosus. Sem. Arthritis Rheum. 26, 675.

Murin, S., Wiedemann, H.P., Matthay, R.A. 1998. Pulmonary manifestations of systemic lupus erythematosus. Clin. Chest Med. 19, 641.

Mutru, O., Koota, K., Isomaki, H. 1976. Causes of death in autopsied RA patients. Scand. J. Rheumatol. 5, 239.

Myllykangas-Luosujarvi, R.A., Aho, K., Isomaki, H.A. 1995. Mortality in rheumatoid arthritis. Semin. Arthritis Rheum. 25, 193.

Nicholson, A.G., Wotherspoon, A.C., Diss, T.C., Hansell, D.M., Du Bois, R., Sheppard, M.N., Isaacson, P.G., Corrin, B. 1995. Reactive pulmonary lymphoid disorders. Histopathology 26, 405.

Niimi, H., Kang, E.Y., Kwong, J.S., Carignan, S., Müller, N.L. 1996. CT of chronic infiltrative lung disease: prevalence of mediastinal lymphadenopathy. J. Comput. Assist. Tomogr. 20, 305.

Oikonomou, A., Hansell, D.H. 2002. Organizing pneumonia. Eur. Radiol. 12, 1486.

Onomura, K., Nakata, H., Tanaka, Y., Tsuda, T. 1991. Pulmonary hemorrhage in patients with systemic lupus erythematosus. J. Thorac. Imaging 6, 57.

Orens, J.B., Martinez, F.J., Lynch, J.P. 3rd 1994. Pleuropulmonary manifestations of systemic lupus erythematosus. Rheum. Dis. Clin. North Am. 20 (1), 159.

Padley, S.P.G., Adler, B., Hansell, D.M., Müller, N.L. 1992. High-resolution computed tomography of drug-induced lung disease. Clin. Radiol. 46, 232.

Patel, A., Kesler, B., Wise, R.A. 2000. Persistent pneumomediastinum in interstitial fibrosis associated with rheumatoid arthritis. Chest 117, 1809.

Petri, M. 1998. Infections in systemic lupus erythematosus. Rheum. Dis. Clin. North. Am. 24, 423.

Prakash, U.B.S. 1992. Lungs in mixed connective tissue disease. J. Thorac. Imaging 7, 55.

Prakash, U.B. 1998. Respiratory complications in mixed connective tissue disease. Clin. Chest Med. 19, 733.

Prakash, U.B.S., Luthra, H.S., Divertie, M.B. 1985. Intrathoracic manifestations in mixed connective tissue disease. Mayo Clin. Proc. 60, 813.

Primack, S.L., Müller, N.L. 1998. Radiologic manifestations of the systemic autoimmune diseases. Clin. Chest Med. 19, 573.

Rees, J.H., Woodhead, M A., Sheppard, M.N., du Bois, R.M. 1991. Rheumatoid arthritis and cryptogenic organising pneumonitis. Respir. Med. 85, 243.

Remy-Jardin, M. 1994. Lung changes in rheumatoid arthritis: CT findings. Radiology 193, 375.

Remy-Jardin, M., Remy, J., Wallaert, B., Bataille, D., Hatron, P.Y. 1993. Pulmonary involvement in progressive systemic sclerosis: sequential evaluation with CT, pulmonary function tests, and bronchoalveolar lavage. Radiology 188, 499.

Rosenow, E.C., Limper, A.H. 1995. Drug-induced pulmonary disease. Semin. Respir. Infect. 10, 86.

Rosenow, E.C., Strimlan, C.V., Muhn, J.R., Ferguson R.H. 1977. Pleuropulmonary manifestations of ankylosing spondilytis. Mayo Clin. Proc. 52, 641.

Rossi, S., Erasmus, J.J., McAdams, H.P., Sporn, T.A , Goodman, P.C. 2000. Pulmonary drug toxicity: radiologic and pathologic manifestations. RadioGraphics 20, 1245.

Roumm, A.D., Medsger, T.A. Jr. 1985. Cancer and systemic sclerosis: an epidemiologic study. Arthritis Rheum. 28, 1336.

Schwab, E.P., Schummacher, H.R. Jr., Freundlinch, E., Callegari, P.E. 1993. Pulmonary hemorrhage in systemic lupus erythematosus. Sem. Arthritis Rheum. 23, 8.

Shannon, T.M., Gale, M.E. 1992. Noncardiac manifestations of rheumatoid arthritis in the thorax. J. Thorac. Imaging 7, 19.

Shida, H., Chiyotani, K., Honma, K., Hosoda, Y., Nobechi, T., Morikubo, H., Wiot, J.F. 1996. Radiologic and pathologic characteristics of mixed dust pneumoconiosis. RadioGraphics 16, 483.

Sigurgeirsson, B., Lindelof, B., Edhag, O., Allander, E. 1992. Risk of cancer in patients with polymyositis or dermatomyositis: a population-based study. N. Engl. J. Med. 326, 363.

Silver, T.M., Farber, S.J., Bole, G.G., Martel, W. 1976. Radiological features of mixed connective tissue disease and scleroderma—systemic lupus erythematosus overlap. Radiology 120, 269.

Sostman, H., Matthay, R., Putman, C., Smith, G. 1976. Methotrexate-induced pneumonitis. Medicine (Baltimore) 55. 371.

Staples, P., Gerding, D., Decker, J., Gordon, R.S. Jr. 1974. Incidence of infections in systemic lupus erythematosus. Arthritis Rheum. 17, 1.

Strimlan, C.V., Rosenow, E.C. 3rd, Divertie, M.B., Harrison, E.G. Jr. 1976. Pulmonary manifestations of Sjögren's syndrome. Chest 70, 354.

Takabatake, N., Sayama, T., Shida, K., Matsuda, M., Nakamura, H., Tomoike, H. 1999. Lung adenocarcinoma in lymphocytic interstitial pneumonitis associated with primary Sjögren's syndrome. Respirology 4, 181.

Tanoue, L.T. 1992. Pulmonary involvement in collagen vascular disease: a review of the pulmonary manifestations of the Marfan syndrome, ankylosing spondylitis, Sjögren's syndrome, and relapsing polychondritis. J. Thorac. Imaging 7, 62.

Tanoue, L.T. 1998. Pulmonary manifestations of rheumatoid arthritis. Clin. Chest Med. 19, 667.

Taorimina, V.J., Miller, W.T., Gefter, W.B., Epstein, D.M. 1981. Progressive systemic sclerosis subgroups: variable pulmonary features. AJR 137, 277.

Tomioka, R., King, T.E. Jr. 1997. Gold-induced pulmonary disease clinical features, outcome, and differentiation from rheumatoid luna disease. Am. J. Respir. Crit. Care Med. 155, 1011.

Wadsworth, S.J., Hansell, D.M. 1999. High resolution computed tomography (HRCT) of the lung in rheumatoid arthritis. Imaging 11, 53.

Warrick, J.H., Bhalla, M., Schabel, S.I., Silver, R.M. 1991. High resolution computed tomography in early scleroderma lung disease. J. Rheumatol. 18, 1520.

Warrington, K.J., Moder, K.G., Brutinel, W.M. 2000. The shrinking lung syndrome in systemic lupus erythematosus. Mayo Clin. Proc. 75, 467.

Wechsler, R.J., Steiner, R.M., Spirn, P.W., Rubin, S., Salazar, A.M., Shah, R., Russell, K., Jimenez, S., Varga, J. 1996. The relationship of thoracic lymphadenopathy in diffuse and limited systemic sclerosis: CT findings. AJR 167, 101.

Wells, A.U. 2000. Lung disease in association with connective tissue diseases. Eur. Respir. Mon. 14, 137.

Wiederman, H.P., Matthay, R.A. 1992. Pulmonary manifestations of systemic lupus erythematosus. J. Thorac. Imaging 7, 1.

Wolfe, F., Schurle, D.R., Lin, J.J., Polland, S.M., Smith, T.W., Montgomery-Short, R., James, D.L. 1983. Upper and lower airway disease in penicillamine treated patients with rheumatoid arthritis. J. Rheumatol. 10, 406.

Yang, Y., Fujita, J., Tokuda, M., Bandoh, S., Ishida, T. 2001. Lung cancer associated with several connective tissue diseases: with a review of literature. Rheumatol. Int. 21, 106.

Yousem, S.A., Colby, T.V., Carrington, C.B. 1985. Lung biopsy in rheumatoid arthritis. Am. Rev. Respir. Dis. 131, 770.

Zamora, M.R., Warner, M.L., Tuder, R., Schwarz, M.I. 1997. Diffuse alveolar hemorrhage and systemic lupus erythematosus. Clinical presentation, histology, survival, and outcome. Medicine (Baltimore) 76, 192.

Zantoss, D., Zhang, Y., Felson, D. 1994. The overall and temporal association of cancer with polymyositis and dermatomyositis. J. Rheumatol. 21, 1855.

PART III

Pulmonary Hypertension

Handbook of Systemic Autoimmune Diseases, Volume 2
Pulmonary Involvement in Systemic Autoimmune Diseases
A.U. Wells and C.P. Denton, editors

CHAPTER 3

Pulmonary Arterial Hypertension in Connective Tissue Disease

Christopher P. Denton*, Carol M. Black
Centre for Rheumatology, Royal Free Hospital, London NW3 2QG, UK

1. Introduction

As with many of the major organ-based complications of rheumatic disease, there has been a substantial growth in understanding of pathogenesis and improvements in management of pulmonary hypertension by drawing upon the considerable progress that has been made addressing this complication in other contexts and in cases of idiopathic or primary pulmonary hypertension (PPH). The first important consideration is one of terminology. Pulmonary hypertension can occur for several reasons and consensus amongst experts as to the correct terminology and classification has been an important milestone. The mechanisms by which pulmonary hypertension can arise that are relevant to rheumatic disease are listed in Table 1. These mechanisms need to be considered in the context of the rheumatic disease in which they occur and also in the light of recent classification systems that have been revised and reviewed.

The principles of management of pulmonary hypertension depend upon the underlying disease. In cases of severe interstitial lung fibrosis with hypoxia and pulmonary hypertension, the management is that of the underlying interstitial disease and treatment of hypoxia. In cases of pulmonary vasculitis, treatments should include immunosuppression and corticosteroids. Thromboembolic disease can arise in a number of ways. Pulmonary embolism can complicate intercurrent illness, venous stasis, and operative procedures, or may be a manifestation of a thrombotic tendency. Of the latter, the most important cases are those with antiphospholipid antibody syndrome. Pulmonary venoocclusive disease is another important cause for pulmonary hypertension that should be excluded during the initial investigation of suspected cases.

Clinically, the most important group of patients with rheumatic disease and pulmonary hypertension are those with systemic sclerosis (SSc). It is now appreciated that many patients with scleroderma appear to have a pulmonary vasculopathy. This may be part of a more general vascular disease and correlates, for example, with the presence of renal hypoperfusion. In SSc-associated pulmonary hypertension, advances in therapy have been made possible by applying treatments developed for PPH to scleroderma-associated disease. This is logical as the pathology of both conditions appears to be very similar, with evidence of fibroproliferative occlusion of the pulmonary arterial tree associated on occasion with vasospasm. The latter appears less frequent than in idiopathic disease but can still, on occasion, be associated with improvements in cardiac output. Many of the studies of new therapies for pulmonary arterial hypertension (PAH) have included patients with SSc-associated disease and so some comparative efficacy data are available. Overall, these results have supported inclusion of such patients but suggest that SSc-associated cases may do less well than those with idiopathic disease.

*Corresponding author.
Tel./fax: +44-20-7794-0432
E-mail address: c.denton@medsch.ucl.ac.uk (C.P. Denton).

DOI: 10.1016/S1571-5078(04)02003-3

Table 1
Mechanisms for pulmonary hypertension in scleroderma

Pulmonary arterial hypertension
Vasospasm
Proliferative changes (predominant)
Pulmonary vasculitis
Thromboembolic disease
Pulmonary embolism—e.g. antiphospholipid antibody syndrome
Chronic venous thromboembolic disease
Pulmonary fibrosis
Pulmonary venous hypertension
Myocarditis
Concurrent coronary artery disease
Myocardial fibrosis

There have been major clinical advances over the past 5 years in the management of PAH, both within and outside the context of connective tissue diseases (CTDs). In particular, there have now been several clinical trials confirming efficacy for parenteral or inhaled prostacyclin analogues and also for an oral endothelin receptor antagonist. These therapies are now licensed for use in primary or CTD-associated PAH in many countries.

The earliest reports of PAH as a complication of scleroderma are of historical interest (Young and Mark, 1978; Sackner et al., 1966), but it has almost certainly been an under-recognised complication and may well have often been misdiagnosed as interstitial pulmonary fibrosis (IPF). It is likely that cases of cardiac involvement from SSc are, on occasion, attributable to decompensated PAH. There has been an excess of cardiac mortality in almost all published series of SSc survival and a substantial proportion of deaths may have resulted from unrecognised pulmonary vascular disease or secondary cardiac problems.

2. Prevalence

There is a wide range in reported frequency of PAH in SSc. This probably results from differences in diagnostic criteria and patient populations examined. The best data come from cardiac catheter studies, although these may underdiagnose the prevalence, as most patients must present a clinical suspicion of PAH in order to proceed to this invasive test. Our own data suggest a prevalence of 12–15% in a hospital-based cohort (Mukerjee et al., 2003). This is within the published range of 5–50% of SSc cases (Magdiliano et al., 2002).

A key factor in studies of prevalence and natural history in SSc-associated pulmonary hypertension is the way in which PAH is diagnosed. This includes the methods used to detect PAH, notably Doppler echocardiography, pulmonary function tests or right heart catheterisation (RHC). Refinements including stress echocardiography have also been evaluated. Some studies have used lower thresholds than others and this is generally reflected by higher frequency of PAH and better outcome overall. It has been suggested that isolated low Dlco measurements over a long period of observation may be especially predictive of evolving PAH in SSc (Steen and Medsger, 2003) and this may reflect progression of a chronic sublinical pulmonary vasculopathy.

The relationship between the severity or pattern of SSc and PAH is unclear. The isolated form is associated with classical limited cutaneous systemic sclerosis (lcSSc) (previously termed CREST syndrome) and with anticentromere ACA reactivity (Steen and Medsger, 2003; Mitri et al., 2003). It is also seen in dcSSc associated with anti fibrillarin autoantibodies (U3RNP) (Sacks et al., 1996). Overlap syndromes may also be associated with PAH through other mechanism such as antiphospholipid antibody syndrome or lupus vasculitis (Tanaka et al., 2002).

3. Survival

Outcome in SSc is largely determined by the pattern and severity of internal organ-based manifestations. For some complications, such as accelerated phase hypertension and scleroderma renal crisis, there are robust clinical tools for diagnosis and the clinical presentation is inevitable relatively soon after onset of the involvement. For others, diagnosis is dependent upon more sophisticated assessment methods and presentation can be insidious. Thus cardiorespiratory involvement from SSc can arise due to cardiac complications (fibrosis, inflammatory cardiomyopathy, systemic hypertension, haemodynamically significant pericardial effusion), respiratory involvement (interstitial lung disease) or pulmonary hypertension. Together, these account for most cases of SSc-related mortality but it is pulmonary hypertension that has benefited from substantial advances over the past several years in appreciation of its diagnosis, definition of clinical patterns and especially from progress. The development of novel therapies appears to improve the clinical symptoms and may reduce mortality in advanced cases. Pulmonary hypertension is a relatively common complication, although its exact prevalence is unclear. Most hospital-based series suggest that PAH occurs in around 10–15% (Coghlan and Mukerjee, 2001). Three patterns of PAH should be considered. First, there are cases, especially complicating lcSSc, in which there is severe isolated PAH. Secondly, there are cases of PAH complicating IPF. Finally, there may be a third type of pulmonary vascular disease occurring in SSc that reflects the vascular pathology of the disease and results in a more indolent pulmonary process. This would potentially account for those individuals who appear to have very slowly progressive PAH in the context of lcSSc and those who have a secondary pulmonary vascular component in the context of relatively mild fibrosis, distinct from the severe interstitial process seen in true secondary PAH. It is noteworthy that secondary PAH in other forms of lung fibrosis is only seen at the last stages of disease associated with very extensive tissue destruction and especially with hypoxia. Thus, as described elsewhere in this volume there are important differences between SSc-associated lung fibrosis and cryptogenic fibrosing alveolitis (CFA), also termed IPF. Likewise, although there are similarities between idiopathic or familial primary PAH and SSc-associated isolated PAH these do not apply to all cases. Definition of the pathology and natural history of PAH in SSc is an important goal for current clinical research. Drawing an analogy with other aspects of the disease, clinical heterogeneity seems likely and it may ultimately be possible to sub-classify this complication, just as the patterns of lung fibrosis, skin involvement or severity of Raynaud's phenomenon may be segregated.

A number of reports have confirmed that PAH in SSc has a major impact on survival and outcome. In a recent study (Kawut et al., 2003), the survival of patients with SSc-related PAH was shown to be substantially worse that those with similar baseline haemodynamics and primary PAH. This difference may reflect comorbidity such as lung fibrosis or other life-threatening involvements but is also consistent with observations that the pathology of these two conditions may be different. A pivotal study by Koh et al., examined a small number of cases but determined a median survival of 50% at 12 months if PAH was present (Koh et al., 1996). Here, PAH diagnosis was based upon echocardiography. A study from our own unit suggested differences in survival according to the level of PAH by echo-Doppler at diagnosis (MacGregor et al., 2001). Pressures remained static in most cases but the mortality among those with a single pressure reading of 30 mm Hg or higher was 20% at 20 months. An increased mortality risk was associated with high initial pressures and rising pressures. Rapid pressure rises occurred more frequently in limited than in diffuse SSc.

These simple studies probably overlook important differences between SSc-PAH patients. As discussed above it is likely that different patterns of disease have varying natural histories and this may reflect fundamental differences between patient subsets and or pathogenic process. It is clear that advanced PAH is progressive and has a high mortality and likely that this can be improved using advanced modern therapy, by analogy with PPH. It is less clear how milder forms progress and whether the difference in natural history suggested by cohort studies reflects earlier diagnosis or different progression. This is an important question for future examination.

4. Aetiopathogenesis of PAH in CTD

Unlike skin disease, studies of biology and pathogenetic mechanism in PAH are hampered by the relative inaccessibility of lung tissue for histological and cell culture analysis. Moreover, whereas biopsies may be performed in some patients with active interstitial lung disease to aid diagnosis and classification, this cannot be justified in cases of SSc-associated PAH due to the risk of haemorrhage. Direct examination of lesional tissue is, therefore, only possible in surgical resection specimens or at autopsy. There is inherently a bias towards established or end-stage pathology from such studies and relatively little information concerning early events. The aetiology of PAH in SSc is likely to be complex and multifactorial. There are major pathological and histological similarities between SSc-associated PAH and primary PAH but differences also exist. The initial lesion is unclear but a plausible sequence of events involves a predisposed individual and genetic predisposition. There is likely to be a balance between protective or predisposing alleles at a number of loci that interact either at the level of gene expression or via gene products. In primary PAH and especially cases of familial PAH, this appears to involve mutations in a member of the TGFβ superfamily of receptors (Lane et al., 2000; Thomson et al., 2000). BMPR2 mutations in either the intracellular kinase domain or the long cytoplasmic tail are implicated in approximately 50% of familial cases (Rudarakanchana et al., 2002). A smaller number of familial cases are associated with mutations in the Alk1 receptor, an accessory TGFβ receptor (Trembath et al., 2001; Trembath 2001). Although studies have not suggested that either of these loci are involved as susceptibility alleles for SSc-associated PAH (Morse et al., 2002), it is recognised that altered expression of TGFβ superfamily receptors, interacting proteins or downstream signalling molecules occurs in SSc and some, although not other, studies have associated TGFβ1 single nucleotide polymorphisms (SNPs) with SSc or its clinical subsets (Crilly et al., 2002). Recent reports have linked fibrillin SNP haplotypes with idiopathic or clustered SSc (Tan et al., 2001) and TGFβ2 linked microsatellite markers with SSc (Susol et al., 2000). Thus, there is a body of evidence implicating potentially systemic alterations in the TGFβ family ligand-receptor axis with SSc. However, there is also a prominent vascular phenotype in SSc and this is manifest in the skin by telangiectasis, and on mucosal surfaces, for example, as angiodysplastic lesions or gastric antral venous ectasia (GAVE) (Watson et al., 1996). In addition, there is evidence of widespread endothelial cell (EC) activation or damage in SSc and this may be the earliest lesion in this disease (Yamane et al., 2000). Furthermore, markers of EC activation have been reported to be elevated in SSC-associate PAH, suggesting the possibility that early EC pathology may be important in SSc-related PAH (Stratton et al., 2000, 1998). Finally, the end-stage lesion of PAH is microvascular luminal obliteration/attenuation with medial and adventitial fibrosis and with proliferative lesions and intimal hyperplasia. This may be somewhat distinct from the endothelial lesions in primary PAH that have been shown to be clonal and which are associated with a characteristic plexiform lesion in primary PAH. These features have, however, been much less extensively studied in SSc-associated disease and data are conflicting. It is very likely that SSc-associated PAH in some clinical contexts such as isolated PAH may be more similar histologically and even mechanistically to primary PAH. In other contexts, SSc-related PAH may be quite different from primary PAH, as the latter sometimes demonstrates haploinsufficiency of the BMPR2 gene (Machado et al., 2001). Primary proliferative abnormalities within the pulmonary arterial wall have been suggested to contribute to the characteristic endothelial lesions in PAH and so altered expression or function of TGFβ superfamily members may be highly relevant. Interestingly, the histology of digital arteries is very similar to that of PAH, with medial and advential fibrosis leading to structural luminal narrowing (Yi et al., 2000). There are also some histological similarities between PAH and the vascular changes of hypertensive renal scleroderma crisis, although the rate of progression is much more acute in SRC. This may reflect the higher pressures involved, differences between the pulmonary and renal microvasculature or other pathogenic factors. Although the vascular manifestations of SSc may all have a vasospastic element, it does not seem likely that reversible vasospasm is the major process underlying established lesions. Defects in the balance of vasoconstrictors and vasodilators may be important and it is notable that effective agents in the treatment of these complications (prostacyclin analogues, endothelin receptor blockers and ACEIs for SRC) all have vasodilatory properties and that elevated levels of the potent vasoconstrictor ET-1 are a feature of SSc-associated PAH (Vancheeswaran et al., 1994). It has been suggested that altered sensitivity of voltage gated potassium channels in the pulmonary arterial smooth muscle may be involved in initiation or progression of primary PAH (Yuan et al., 1998). Almost all SSc patients have Raynaud's phenomenon; it is possible that defects in vasomotor regulation occur at sites other than the digital vessels. Deficiency in natural vasodilators such as endothelium-derived nitric oxide or excessive vasoconstrictors such as endothelin-1 might contribute to pathogenesis. It is possible that the less severely involved vessels may be responsive to vasodilatation and that some of the short-term benefits of therapy occur in this way. It is very unlikely to be a prominent longer-term mechanism for PAH, as the time-course of improvement is generally over days or weeks and some form of structural remodelling is much more likely. It is interesting that endothelin receptor blockade is antifibrotic (Shi-Wen et al., 2001) and also that iloprost appears to downregulate expression of a potentially important downstream profibrotic mediator, connective tissue growth factor (CTGF) (Stratton et al., 2001). It seems likely that down-regulation of profibrotic factors is an important aspect of therapy and perhaps explains the time-course for improvement in patients treated with advanced PAH therapies such as prostacyclin analogues and the apparent clinical benefit even in cases when pulmonary vasoresponsiveness cannot be demonstrated on acute challenge.

Recent data have suggested that a more general defect in TGFβ signalling may underlie other cases of PAH. Expression of angiopoeitin or its receptor TIE2 have been demonstrated to be reduced in PAH samples. Moreover, a link between this ligand-receptor axis and expression of BMPR1 has been suggested, thereby unifying the presence of defects in the BMP signalling pathway in patients with PAH (Du et al., 2003). Further studies are needed to determine whether these abnormalities may be extrapolated into other causes of pulmonary hypertension, although a recent animal model overexpressing angiopoetin developed histological and haemodynamic evidence of pulmonary hypertension (Sullivan et al., 2003).

5. Clinical manifestations

The clinical features attributed to pulmonary hypertension are similar in the context of CTD to those in other clinical situations. Thus, breathlessness, especially on exertion, is generally the first symptom. In taking a history it is important to precisely define the nature, duration and severity of dyspnoea and its impact on function. Patients with CTD may have other musculoskeletal or vascular causes for breathlessness or other pathologies such as anaemia, cardiac disease or interstitial lung disease or pleural effusion. These features are dealt with elsewhere in this book. Another cardinal symptom is chest pain, due to right ventricular angina. The nature and distribution of this pain may be atypical and it is important to try and avoid confusion with symptoms of oesophagitis or oesophageal spasm which are very frequent in some CTDs such as SSc. Syncope or near-syncope can occur due to systemic hypotension and features of right heart failure with ankle or sacral oedema can be elicited. On examination, signs of an accentuated pulmonary component of the second heart sound, right ventricular parasternal heave or elevated right-sided filling pressure (JVP) may confirm the presence of significant PAH. However, most cases of early PAH are likely to be asymptomatic and signs will develop later than symptoms. This makes it crucial to elicit a full and appropriate history in all cases of CTD in which a diagnosis of PAH may be entertained. Other disease features should also be noted, such as clinical evidence of vasculitis or scleroderma, or suggestions of a predisposition to thrombosis, such as the rash of livedo reticularis that is often associated with antiphospholipid antibody syndrome.

The heterogeneous nature of pulmonary hypertension is illustrated by the current classification of disorders leading to pulmonary hypertension (Table 2). These conditions are differential diagnoses for PAH-complicating SSc. As discussed above, PAH in SSc has probably been underdiagnosed in the past. Clinical features probably occur relatively late in the natural history. It has been suggested that pulmonary vascular disease can occur in SSc without necessarily progressing to haemodynamically significant pulmonary hypertension (Magdiliano et al., 2002). This may account for the frequent observation of mildly impaired Dlco and Kco in SSc patients despite normal Doppler-echocardiography. It is unclear whether these cases represent early disease or a subset with more indolent progression and this should be defined better in prospective series that are currently being collected. The earliest symptom is probably exertional breathlessness or reduced exercise capacity. Symptomatically this may lead to dyspnoea on exertion, commonly first noted when climbing stairs or hills. Later this can occur at rest. There are, of course, important other reasons for dyspnoea in SSc (anaemia or interstitial pulmonary disease or mechanical

Table 2
World Health Organisation Diagnostic classification of pulmonary hypertension (1998)

Pulmonary arterial hypertension
Primary pulmonary hypertension
Sporadic
Familial
Related to:
Connective tissue disease
Congenital systemic to pulmonary shunts
Portal hypertension
HIV infection
Drugs/toxins
Anorexigens
Other
Persistent pulmonary hypertension of the newborn
Other
Pulmonary venous hypertension
Left-sided atrial or ventricular heart disease
Left-sided valvular heart disease
Extrinsic compression of central pulmonary veins
Fibrosing mediastinitis
Adenopathy/tumors
Pulmonary veno-occlusive disease
Other
Pulmonary Hypertension associated with disorders of the respiratory system and/or hypoxemia
Chronic obstructive pulmonary disease
Interstitial lung disease
Sleep disordered breathing
Alveolar hypoventilation disorders
Chronic exposure to high altitude
Neonatal lung disease
Alveolar-capillary dysplasia
Other
Pulmonary hypertension due to chronic thrombotic and/or embolic disease
Thromboembolic obstruction of proximal pulmonary arteries
Obstruction of distal pulmonary arteries
Pulmonary embolism (thrombus, tumour, ova/parasites, foreign material)
In situ thrombosis
Sickle cell disease
Pulmonary hypertension due to disorders directly affecting the pulmonary vasculature
Infammatory
Schistosomiasis
Sarcoidosis
Other
Pulmonary capillary haemangiomatosis

restriction in ventilation) and for diminished exercise tolerance (e.g. general constitutional symptoms, musculoskeletal disease, cardiac or intrinsic lung manifestations). Other symptoms that occur at later stages are chest pain due to right ventricular angina and syncope or near syncope on exertion due to reduced cardiac reserve. Late-stage disease leads to features of right-sided cardiac failure including ankle swelling. Operationally PAH can be graded into fours groups based upon modified New York Heart Association criteria. The widely used Class I to IV classification is summarised in Table 3.

In established disease, clinical examination can be confirmatory with features of loud pulmonary second sound due to accelerated valve closure, parasternal heave due to right ventricular strain and signs of elevated right-sided filling pressures (elevated JVP and prominent jugular venous pulsation), together with fluid retention (ankle/sacral oedema, ascites). Tachypnoea at rest or central cyanosis (peripheral cyanosis is very common in SSc due to Raynaud's phenomenon) are late events. Anecdotal evidence suggests that patients with significant isolated PAH in lcSSc often have extensive and increasing cutaneous vascular lesions.

Although these clinical features are important, emphasis should be upon pre-clinical or early diagnosis and, therefore, depends upon other investigation. Traditionally, most emphasis has been placed upon a combination of PFT and Doppler-echocardiography supplemented by ECG, although changes are likely to be present on Echo before the ECG

Table 3
1998 World Health Organisation functional classification of pulmonary hypertension (modified after the New York Heart Association functional classification)

Class I	Patients with pulmonary hypertension but without resulting limitation of physical activity. Ordinary physical activity does not cause undue dyspnoea or fatigue, chest pain or near syncope
Class II	Patients with pulmonary hypertension resulting in slight limitation of physical activity. They are comfortable at rest. Ordinary physical activity causes undue dyspnoea, fatigue, chest pain or near syncope
Class III	Patients with pulmonary hypertension resulting in marked limitation of physical activity. They are comfortable at rest. Ordinary physical activity causes undue dyspnoea or fatigue, chest pain or near syncope
Class IV	Patients with pulmonary hypertension with inability to carry out any physical activity without symptoms. These patients manifest signs of right heart failure. Dyspnoea and/or fatigue may even be present at rest. Discomfort is increased by any physical activity

becomes abnormal. The most typical PFT abnormality in isolated PAH is a reduction in CO transfer factor (Tlco or Dlco) with preservation of lung volumes. Kco (Krogue coefficient, defined by Dlco/alveolar volume) is generally proportionately reduced in these cases but longitudinal studies suggest that Dlco is probably less subject to variation. In SSc, the Kco is of most value in excluding significant intrinsic pulmonary disease in patients showing a restrictive pattern of respiratory impairment due to chest wall pathology such as diffuse skin involvement or thoracic muscle weakness. In such cases, Kco generally will be much higher than the Dlco or FVC. It is of some value in assessing patients with mixed pulmonary vascular and fibrotic disease since Kco will tend to be higher than Dlco if there is predominant pulmonary vascular disease but reduced if changes are the result of interstitial pathology (Bouros et al., 2002). However, it has been observed that isolated and often transient changes in CO diffusing capacity are quite common in SSc. The explanation for this is unclear but may relate to altered regulation of ventilation and perfusion resulting in ventilation:perfusion mismatch. Pulmonary function tests, therefore, must be interpreted in the clinical context and repeated if results seem inconsistent. Tobacco smoking, it should be noted, will also lead to a depressed transfer factor. Echocardiography has been shown to be a useful tool for PAH assessment. There may be structural changes on the Echo suggesting elevated PAP such as increased pulmonary acceleration time, altered movement of the interventricular septum, impaired right ventricular function or pulmonary outflow dilatation. It is often possible to estimate the peak (systolic) pulmonary artery pressure (PAP) by combining echocardiography with Doppler assessment of the regurgitant blood jet velocity through the tricuspid valve. Accuracy of the measurement varies, assessment is operator dependent and a mild degree of regurgitation may be especially hard to assess. Doppler-echocardiography is most reliable when performed by an experienced observer. In this case it has a high sensitivity and specificity for detecting PAH. We have previously compared echocardiographic assessment with RHC in 33 SSc patients in whom routine clinical assessment had raised strong suspicion of PHT (pulmonary hypertension). Sixty-four percent of these patients had PHT (PASP (pulmonary artery systolic pressure) at least 30 mm Hg) on RHC, and echocardiography correctly identified 19 of these (sensitivity 90%). Of the 12 patients without PHT on RHC, nine were correctly identified by echocardiography (specificity 75%). The five incorrectly classified patients all had PASP in the borderline normal/abnormal range (Denton et al., 1997). Overall there is a strong correlation between Doppler estimated peak PAP and that determined at right heart catheter but in practice this is influenced by extreme values and in the clinically important range of 30–45 mm peak pressure has false positive or negative rates of around 30% compared to RHC (Mukerjee et al., 2002). Attempts to improve diagnostic sensitivity have been assessed. Most promising are stress tests, especially including echo assessment during or immediately after exercise. The former requires specialised equipment but has produced promising data (Chemla et al., 2001); the latter has only been used so far in small studies, but may be useful. It is possible that alternative forms of cardiac provocation may ultimately be more useful. Dopamine stress testing does not appear to be especially additive to regular tests with normal responses present in more than 30% of patients with exercise induced PAH by right heart catheter (Mukerjee et al., 2002). It is possible that alternative forms of cardiac provocation may ultimately be more useful, particularly as dobutamine may have specifically beneficial effects on pulmonary haemodynamics that compensate for the cardiac stress associated with acute administration (Vizza et al., 2001).

6. Diagnostic investigations

There are now well-established diagnostic criteria for PAH. Clinical features and simple investigations such as ECG, Doppler-echocardiogram and pulmonary function tests are useful and also assist with important differential diagnoses such as cardiac involvement or interstitial lung fibrosis. Other causes for PHT must be excluded and ventilation:perfusion (V:Q) scans or CT pulmonary angiogram (CTPA) are important. Additional cardiac tests might also be needed to exclude coronary arterial or intrinsic cardiac disease. Inflammatory myocarditis is often associated with elevated CKMB and troponin levels. Gated cardiac MRI appears to be a valuable research tool that may be applied to the diagnosis of both cardiac and pulmonary vascular disease through its effects on cardiac cavity and muscle mass (Boxt, 1999) and movement. One study in a mixed group of PAH cases has shown that a calculated ventricular mass index (VMI) provides an accurate means of estimating PAP non-invasively, and compared the results with conventional Doppler echocardiography and invasive measurement. A total of 26 subjects referred for investigation of pulmonary hypertension were studied by MRI and echocardiography within 2 weeks of cardiac catheterisation. Sensitivity and specificity for pulmonary hypertension were 84 and 71%, respectively, for the MRI, compared with 89 and 57% for echocardiography. The calculated VMI provides an accurate and practical means of estimating PAP non-invasively in pulmonary hypertension and may provide a more accurate estimate than Doppler echocardiography. This may be because it reflects the right ventricular response to sustained pulmonary hypertension over a long period and is not influenced by short-term physiological variables affecting echocardiography, such as heart rate, posture, hydration status and oxygen supplementation (Saba et al., 2002). MRI has also proven useful for assessing cardiac involvement in SSc (Karwatowski et al., 2000), with a recent study showing that duration of SSc correlated with left ventricular mass ($r = 0.7$, $p < 0.05$), the coefficient of variation of velocity ($r = 0.63$, $p < 0.05$), and inversely with the mean left ventricular diastolic long-axis velocity ($r = -0.63$, $p < 0.05$). The authors concluded that there was a relationship between duration of scleroderma and both left ventricular mass and diastolic function, which may result from increased myocardial fibrosis. The value of echo-Doppler, dobutamine stress echocardiography and exercise testing is discussed above.

Current criteria define PAH as a resting mean PAP above 25 mm Hg or an exercise mean PAP of greater than 30 mm Hg by RHC (Denton et al., 1997). These levels are accepted internationally and precise definition is important for comparison of cohorts and standardisation of therapy. However, there are many causes for PAH based upon these criteria and these must be further excluded in order to confirm true SSc-related PAH. Diastolic dysfunction is associated with left ventricular disease and so pulmonary venous hypertension leading to secondary PHT is an important exclusion. A currently accepted classification system for PAH is shown in Table 3 (Gibbs, 2001).

There have been several recent studies evaluating the potential of N-terminal propeptide of brain natriuretic peptide (BNP) as a potential early marker of right ventricular dysfunction in PAH in SSc (Nagaya et al., 2000). These data have been reported in abstract form and suggest that, as in PPH, this marker may be a useful tool for evaluating or screening patients at risk of developing significant PAH. Potential pitfalls include the need for detailed longitudinal studies and discriminating the potential effects of left ventricular dysfunction. Other neuropeptide mediators are also under evaluation.

7. Invasive haemodynamic testing: rheumatological perspective

Although RHC remains the definitive tool for diagnosis and assessment of PAH, it has limitations in rheumatology. These relate to its applicability to supplement screening tools that are less invasive. Thus, a subset of patients that are suspected to have PAH based upon clinical, echocardiographic or lung function test data proceeds to RHC. This is an invasive test that may be especially risky in patients with a complex multisystem disease such as SSc or another CTD. A major goal is defining better the criteria that should lead to RHC in order to maximise sensitivity and specificity.

RHC remains the gold standard for investigation of PAH in all contexts, although significant thromboembolic disease should be excluded by $V{:}Q$ scan or CTPA. This might be an indication for a filter to be inserted or other specific interventions including embolectomy. The advantages of RHC include the direct measurement of PAP, the determination of mean PAP which is used for defining true PAH, and the ability to perform a stress test to identify exercise induced PAH that might be associated with normal pressures at rest. Also, vasodilator challenge can be performed to assess pulmonary vascular responsiveness. In SSc-PAH, this is rarely positive and does not appear to associate with outcome. In PPH, it has been

Table 4
Principal investigations recommended in the assessment of pulmonary hypertension

Doppler echocardiography
Qualitative assessment
Enlarged right atrium and ventricle
Right ventricular hypertrophy
D-shaped left ventricular cavity with interventricular septum flattening in systole
Diminished atrial wave of the pulmonary valve
Mid-systolic closure or notching of pulmonary valve
Haemodynamic assessment
Tricuspid regurgitation velocity (most accurate echocardiographic technique for estimating peak PAP
Right ventricular outflow tract flow acceleration time
Pulmonary artery systolic flow acceleration time
Right ventricular ejection time
Right ventricular index of myocardial performance
Timing of mid systolic deceleration of right ventricular ejection
Right ventricle long axis function (marker of overall right ventricular systolic function)
Pulmonary function tests
Full spirometry and CO diffusion studies necessary to differentiate obstructive or restrictive pathology. Express data as % predicted, corrected for haematocrit. Reduction in transfer factor the most sensitive test for pulmonary vascular disease, especially if disproportionately severe compared with reduced FVC. FEV1, FVC, TLC, Dlco, Kco should all be assessed
Right heart catheterisation
The following variables should be measured:
Right atrial pressure
Right ventricular systolic and end-diastolic pressure
Pulmonary artery systolic, diastolic and mean pressure
Pulmonary capillary wedge pressure
Systemic and pulmonary arterial oxygen saturation
Cardiac output
Vasodilator testing
Recommended using intravenous iloprost/epoprostanol or adenosine or inhaled nitric oxide
Positive if >10 mm Hg fall in mean PAP and no change or increase in cardiac output

suggested that responsive patients might benefit from high dose vasodilator therapy with calcium channel blockers, although this is controversial (Rich et al., 1992). Also, RHC allows accurate measurement of cardiac index, a measure of cardiac output corrected for body size, pulmonary vascular resistance and other indices. These appear to have important prognostic value when related to outcome or survival (Raffy et al., 1996). Currently, in the UK, it is regarded as mandatory to have RHC information in order to commence advanced PAH therapy such as prostacyclin or bosentan (Gibbs, 2001). In situations where coexistent left ventricular disease is suspected, it may be useful to perform a left heart catheter and coronary angiogram at the same time as the RHC. The range of investigations central to accurate assessment of PAH in SSc is listed in Table 4.

8. Treatment of PAH

Treatments for pulmonary hypertension in CTD have progressed in parallel with those for idiopathic pulmonary hypertension and also benefited from more consistent and rigorous methods of classification of PHT. Thus, causes such as thromboembolism or chronic pulmonary veno-occlusive disease require specific treatment. It is suggested that cases of PAH in lupus may respond to treatment with immunosuppression but this is unclear. The benefits of long-term oxygen treatment in cases of PAH associated with hypoxia and of anticoagulation in all cases in whom there is no contraindication is clear.

The development of treatments of proven efficacy for PAH is a major medical advance (Sanchez et al., 1999). Historically, pulmonary hypertension therapies were confined to treatment with vasodilators, including calcium channel blockers, which were modestly effective in some patients (Rich et al., 1992). Oxygen was provided, either intermittently for exertional dyspnoea or as long-term (16 h per day) low-flow oxygen via nasal specula, aiming to reduce or reverse hypoxia-induced pulmonary vasodilation (Roberts et al., 2001). Right heart failure was treated conventionally, although care to avoid over-diuresis was important as viable systemic perfusion was only feasible if there were relatively high right-sided filling pressures. End-stage pulmonary hypertension was sometimes amenable to heart-lung transplantation, although donor organ availability generally limited this option to younger patients with primary PHT or a small number of other isolated cardiopulmonary conditions. A recent report of 12 patients with SSc-associated PAH concluded, however, that the benefits were comparable to patients with other chronic acquired lung disease and that SSc patients should not be denied this approach if conventional criteria for eligibility were fulfilled (Kobo et al., 2001).

The development of long-term parenteral prostacyclin analogue infusions was originally envisioned as a 'bridge to transplantation', but many patients felt much improved with this therapy and elected not to proceed to surgery (D'Alonzo et al., 1991). There were some series using intermittent bolus infusions, especially in the context of CTD where this approach had been in use to treat critical digital ischaemia and severe Raynaud's phenomenon, but these approaches were generally less successful (Mok et al., 1999). Early studies suggested profound clinical benefit from continuous parenteral prostacyclin alaloges such as epoprostenol in PAH, without excessive treatment-associated complications. In a pivotal early open study, continuous intravenous prostacyclin was administered by portable infusion pump at doses determined by acute responses during baseline catheterisation in 10 patients. Six of 10 prostacyclin-treated patients who completed the 8-week study period had reductions in mean PAP of greater than 10 mm Hg, whereas only one of nine in the conventional treatment group had a similar response ($P = 0.057$) (Rubin et al., 1990). Based upon the results of uncontrolled studies, a prospective placebo-controlled clinical trial was designed, involving patients with PPH who were treated for 16 weeks. The results were dramatic, with improved exercise capacity in the 41 patients treated with epoprostenol compared with a decrease in the 40 patients treated with conventional therapy alone. Indexes of the quality of life were improved only in the epoprostenol group. Hemodynamics improved at 12 weeks in the epoprostenol-treated patients. The changes in mean PAP for the epoprostenol and control groups were a drop of 8% and a rise of 3%, respectively ($P < 0.001$). More importantly, eight patients died during the study, all of whom had been randomly assigned to conventional therapy. There was improvement in exercise capacity with treatment but also significant mortality benefit even in this small study (Barst et al., 1996). This landmark trial was later repeated in patients with CTD-associated hypertension and positive results were obtained. Exercise capacity improved on epoprostenol (median distance walked in 6 min, 316 m at 12 weeks compared with 270 m at baseline) but decreased with conventional therapy (192 m at 12 weeks compared with 240 m at baseline). The difference between treatment groups in the median distance walked at week 12 was 108 m ($P < 0.001$), although unlike the similar primary PAH trial, no mortality benefit was seen in SSc-associated PAH treated with epoprostenol (Badesch et al., 2000). More recent studies have also shown benefit for the subcutaneous prostacyclin analogue treprostinil (Simonneau et al., 2002) and for nebulised agents given by inhalation (Olschewski et al., 2002). The robust nature of these responses provides important proof of concept support that prostacyclin metabolism and signalling is important in the pathogenesis of PAH.

Another agent that showed strong promise in an early trial is the orally active endothelin receptor blocker, bosentan. This drug was originally developed for more common forms of cardiovascular disease but was serendipitously tested in pulmonary hypertension with remarkable benefit. The first serious controlled trial used a similar trial design to that used to evaluate parenteral prostacyclin and similar beneficial effects on exercise capacity were observed for oral bosentan (Channick et al., 2001). A more recent extensive trial for bosentan therapy in both primary and CTD-associated PAH was strongly positive BREATHE-1) (Rubin et al., 2002). In this double-blind, placebo-controlled study of 213 patients with PAH (primary or associated with CTD), after 16 weeks patients treated with bosentan had an improved 6-min walking distance; the mean difference between the placebo group and the combined bosentan groups was 44 m ($P < 0.001$). Bosentan also improved the Borg dyspnea index and WHO functional class and increased the time to clinical worsening. Recent data suggest that a similar benefit is obtained for SSc-associated PAH treated with bosentan to that observed in primary pulmonary hyperetension, based upon subgroup analysis of the patients enrolled into the placebo-controlled 351 and 352 clinical trials.

In North America and Europe, licensed therapies for PAH now include parenteral prostacyclin analogues (epoprostanol and iloprost, and remodulin) and oral bosentan. Other studies to refine and integrate these therapies are presently underway, including selective phosphodiesterase inhibitors such as sildenafil (Ghofrani et al., 2002). The major limitation to these treatments is the very high annual cost of advanced therapies for pulmonary hypertension. Other major issues are developing appropriate and reliable strategies for early identification of PAH in CTD. This represents a unique at-risk population with the potential for much earlier detection of PAH than is possible in sporadic primary PAH. Methods of accurate risk stratification and early assessment are very much needed. Whether earlier initiation of therapies will ultimately have a bigger impact on outcome, and especially survival, remains to be determined. Other specific problems include line sepsis and the catastrophic effect of pump failure and acute withdrawal of prostanoids in established patients (Albert and Hague, 1997) and the general problems of long-term ambulatory central venous catheterisation.

9. Current best-practice management of PAH in SSc

With established therapies and formalised assessment protocols, there is now an accepted standard of practice for SSc-associated PAH and this is summarised in the algorithm shown in Fig. 1. These care pathways are likely to be refined and modified but represent a tremendous advance upon the available approaches of just a few years ago and reflect consensus amongst rheumatologists, cardiologists and respiratory physicians in the UK. A major goal at present is education of patients and the medical community and integration of care between pulmonologists, cardiologists and rheumatologists. Specialised centres should coordinate management of these cases after RHC. If therapeutic benefit of earlier treatment is shown, decentralisation of care may become essential. Non-invasive methods for accurately diagnosing PAH in at-risk populations are actively being developed. There are now established protocols and clinical support infrastructure to allow effective administration of advanced therapies for SSc-associated PAH. Surgical options remain, notably atrial septostomy (Allcock et al., 2001) and transplantation for end-stage disease (Rosas et al., 2000). The major focus over the next few years should, however, be definition of identification of early stage pulmonary vascular disease with prevention rather than treatment of Class III and IV disease.

Currently it is our practice to have a low threshold for performing invasive diagnostic testing by RHC with formal exercise challenge and assessment of acute vasodilator response. This is undertaken in any SSc patient with unexplained breathlessness, disproportionate reduction in Dlco compared to FVC (compared with % predicted), an elevated pressure (peak PA 40 mm Hg above right atrial pressure) on echo-Doppler or in an individual with pulmonary fibrosis where secondary PAH was suspected clinically. For mild PAH, usually Class II patients who have exercise-induced disease, warfarin is commenced. Patients with PAH at rest are treated with warfarin and high dose calcium channel blockers if they are responsive on acute vasodilator challenge. Catheterisation and haemodynamic studies are repeated at 6-monthly intervals in these patients. When moderate PAH develops (usually Class III), with mPAP above 35 mm Hg at rest irrespective of the presence of pulmonary fibrosis, warfarin and bosentan are used. Severe PAH (mean PAP above 45 mm Hg) is treated with long-term prostacyclin therapy. These will be Class III or IV cases. Those with fibrosis are likely to have more intrapulmonary $V:Q$ mismatch and it is our current practice to treat these individuals with oral sildenafil or inhaled iloprost.

10. Monitoring and screening for pulmonary hypertension in scleroderma

Monitoring of all patients with SSc with, at least, annual Doppler-echocardiogram and pulmonary function testing is an appropriate minimum standard of observation of these patients, although this is not yet universally practised. Once the diagnosis has been made, it is important that the disease is monitored. Although some centres perform repeated RHC studies, this is invasive and probably follow-up is most practically done by serial Doppler-echocardiography every 3–6 months depending upon clinical change and also by symptom severity and exercise capacity. The 6-min walk test (the ultimate walking distance) has been established as a reproducible simple clinical measure of exercise capacity in PAH and this associates with progression and survival. It is widely used as the primary end point in clinical PAH

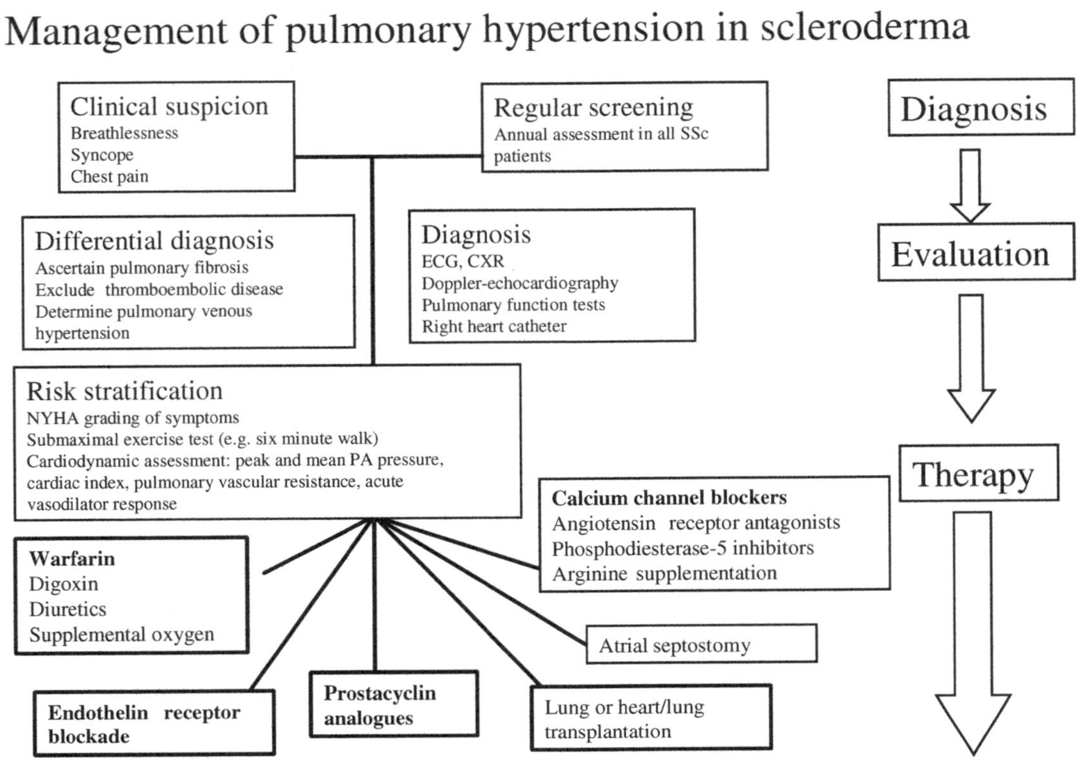

Figure 1. Current management of pulmonary arterial hypertension. This algorithm incorporates consensus guidelines recently established in the UK by cardiologists, rheumatologists and respiratory physicians. It reflects current practice in our own centre.

interventional trials (Demers et al., 2001) although not yet validated for SSc-associated PAH. It should be regularly performed in all patients using a marked 50 m course. There are defined levels of encouragement and patients decide when the test is complete unless they exceed 500 m. Some centres perform arterial desaturation tests using arterialised ear lobe blood sampling or pulse oximetry.

11. The future

Despite advances in management of advanced pulmonary hypertension there are still many challenges. It is important that appropriate comparative studies are developed to confirm the benefit of treatments in CTD-associated pulmonary hypertension. Also the place of combination therapies needs to be better defined. There is some promise from preliminary studies in PPH that phosphodiesterase-5 inhibitors may be useful and even synergistic with endothelin receptor antagonists but this remains to be confirmed. In addition, it is possible to assess the potential benefit of treating earlier stage disease in CTD-associated PAH, especially SSc-associated pulmonary hypertension, as these patients can now be screened prospectively and potentially diagnosed in Class I or II. Finally, it is plausible that the treatments that are used to treat PAH in CTD, especially scleroderma, may benefit other aspects of the disease as well as the pulmonary vasculature. This is the case for preliminary data from the RAPIDS-1 trial of bosentan as a preventative treatment for scleroderma-associated ischaemic digital ulcers, and clinical trials to evaluate bosentan as a potential treatment for interstitial lung fibrosis, based upon the potent profibrotic activity of endothelin-1 in vitro, are currently underway. In addition there is a substantial body of evidence that prostacyclin analogues may have beneficial effects upon the expression of profibrotic mediators in SSc (Mayes, 2003).

There is also pressing need to develop better and more integrated services for patients with CTD-associated PAH. This will allow appropriate access to advanced methods of assessment and medical treatments. It is important that criteria for response to treatment, thresholds for changing treatments and referral for surgical intervention are as standardised and consistent as possible. Critically ill patients may benefit from atrial septostomy (see above). Referral for transplantation is made according to other disease manifestations, but should not be delayed. Overall, there have been significant developments in the options for therapy in this important complication of SSc and other CTDs. This has promoted awareness amongst specialists but there is a need for effective networks in secondary and tertiary care to ensure that patients are screened regularly, that facilities for timely evaluation by RHC exist and that the evolving repertoire of advanced therapies for PAH can be used in an effective way.

Key points

- Pulmonary hypertension is a major complication of CTD and occurs in up to 10% of SSc cases.
- All patients with SSc should be screened annually for PAH. Both Doppler echo and lung function can be misleading.
- Advanced therapies for PAH seem to be effective in SSc-associated disease, although the magnitude of effect may be less than seen with PPH.
- Cardiac output and exercise capacity predict survival in PAH.
- In well-selected cases lung or heart-lung transplantation can be very effective.
- Few SSc PAH cases demonstrate vasodilator response at RHC. In those that demonstrate improvement in cardiac output during an acute vasodilator challenge it is logical to try treatment with vasodilators such as high dose calcium channel blockers.

References

Albert, N.M., Hague, K. 1997. Managing patients with primary pulmonary hypertension: prostacyclin therapy. Am. J Crit. Care. 6, 274–280. Review.

Allcock, R.J., O'Sullivan, J.J., Corris, P.A. 2001. Palliation of systemic sclerosis-associated pulmonary hypertension by atrial septostomy. Arthritis Rheum. 44, 1660–1662.

Badesch, D.B., Tapson, V.F., McGoon, M.D., Brundage, B.H., Rubin, L.J., Wigley, F.M., Rich, S., Barst, R.J., Barrett, P.S., Kral, K.M., Jobsis, M.M., Loyd, J.E., Murali, S., Frost, A., Girgis, R., Bourge, R.C., Ralph, D.D., Elliott, C.G., Hill N.S., Langleben, D., Schilz, R.J., McLaughlin, V.V., Robbins I.M., Groves, B.M., Shapiro, S., Medsger, T.A. Jr. 2000. Continuous intravenous epoprostenol for pulmonary hypertension due to the scleroderma spectrum of disease. A randomized, controlled trial. Ann. Intern. Med. 132, 425–434.

Barst, R.J., Rubin, L.J., Long, W.A., McGoon, M.D., Rich, S., Badesch, D.B., Groves, B.M., Tapson, V.F., Bourge, R.C., Brundage, B.H., et al. 1996. A comparison of continuous intravenous epoprostenol (prostacyclin) with conventional therapy for primary pulmonary hypertension. The Primary Pulmonary Hypertension Study Group. N. Engl. J. Med. 334, 296–302.
The first major trial to confirmsurvival benefit of intravenous prostacyclin for primary PAH. The trial template has since been adapted for most studies of novel therapies.

Bouros, D., Wells, A.U., Nicholson, A.G., Colby, T.V., Polychronopoulos, V., Pantelidis, P., Haslam, P.L., Vassilakis, D.A., Black, C.M., du Bois, R.M. 2002. Histopathologic subsets of fibrosing alveolitis in patients with systemic sclerosis and their relationship to outcome. Am. J. Respir. Crit Care Med. 165, 1581–1586.

Boxt, L.M. 1999. Radiology of the right ventricle. Radiol. Clin. North. Am. 37, 379–400.

Channick, R.N., Simonneau, G., Sitbon, O., Robbins, I.M., Frost, A., Tapson, V.F., Badesch, D.B., Roux, S., Rainisio, M., Bodin, F., Rubin, L.J. 2001. Effects of the dual endothelin-receptor antagonist bosentan in patients with pulmonary hypertension: a randomised placebo-controlled study. Lancet 358, 1119–1123.

Chemla, D., Castelain, V., Herve, P., Lecarpentier, Y., Brimioulle, S. 2002. Haemodynamic evaluation of pulmonary hypertension. Eur. Respir. J. 20, 1314–1331.

Coghlan, J.G., Mukerjee, D. 2001. The heart and pulmonary vasculature in scleroderma: clinical features and pathobiology. Curr. Opin. Rheumatol. 13, 495–499.

Crilly, A., Hamilton, J., Clark, C.J., Jardine, A., Madhok, R. 2002. Analysis of transforming growth factor beta1 gene polymorphisms in patients with systemic sclerosis. Ann. Rheum. Dis. 61, 678–681.

D'Alonzo, G.E., Barst, R.J., Ayers, S.M., et al. 1991. Survival in patients with primary pulmonary hypertension. Ann. Int. Med. 115, 343–349.

Demers, C., McKelvie, R.S., Negassa, A., Yusuf, S. 2001. Reliability, validity, and responsiveness of the six-minute walk test in patients with heart failure. Am. Heart J. 142, 698–703.

Denton, C.P., Cailes, J.B., Phillips, G.D., Wells, A.U., Black, C.M., Bois, R.M. 1997. Comparison of Doppler-echocardiography and right heart catheterization to assess pulmonary hypertension in systemic sclerosis. Br. J. Rheumatol. 36, 239–243.

Du, L., Sullivan, C.C., Chu, D., Cho, A.J., Kido, M., Wolf, P.L., Yuan, J.X., Deutsch, R., Jamieson, S.W., Thistlethwaite, P.A. 2003. Signaling molecules in nonfamilial pulmonary hypertension. N. Engl. J. Med. 348, 500–509.

Ghofrani, H.A., Wiedemann, R., Rose, F., Schermuly, R.T., Olschewski, H., Weissmann, N., Gunther, A., Walmrath, D., Seeger, W., Grimminger, F. 2002. Sildenafil for treatment of lung fibrosis and pulmonary hypertension: a randomised controlled trial. Lancet 360, 895–900.

Gibbs, S. 2001. Recommendations on the management of pulmonary hypertension in clinical practice. British Cardiac Society Guidelines and Medical Practice Committee, and approved by the British Thoracic Society and the British Society of Rheumatology. Heart 86, I1–I13.

A major step forward in management of PAH has been the establishment of consensus guidelines agreed by cardiologists, respiratory physicians and rheumatologists. This has allowed recommended best-practice to be stated and facilitates best use of new therapies for established PAH.

Karwatowski, S.P., Chronos, N.A., Sinclair, H., Forbat, S.M., St John Sutton, M.G., Black, C., Underwood, S.R., Pennell, D.J. 2000. Effect of systemic sclerosis on left ventricular long-axis motion and left ventricular mass assessed by magnetic resonance. J. Cardiovasc. Magn. Reson. 2, 109–117.

Kawut, S.M., Taichman, D.B., Archer-Chicko, C.L., Palevsky, H.I., Kimmel, S.E. 2003. Hemodynamics and survival in patients with pulmonary arterial hypertension related to systemic sclerosis. Chest 123, 344–350.

Kobo, M., Vensak, J., Dauber, J., Keenan, R., Griffith, B., McCurry, K. 2001. Lung transplantation in patients with scleroderma. J. Heart Lung Transplant. 20, 174.

Koh, E.T., Lee, P., Gladman, D.D., Abu-Shakra, M. 1996. Pulmonary hypertension in systemic sclerosis: an analysis of 17 patients. Br. J. Rheumatol. 35, 989–993.

Lane, K.B., Machado, R.D., Pauciulo, M.W., Thomson, J.R., Phillips, J.A., Loyd, J.E., Nichols, W.C., Trembath, R.C. 2000. Heterozygous germline mutations in BMPR2, encoding a TGF-beta receptor, cause familial primary pulmonary hypertension. The International PPH Consortium. Nature Genet. 26, 81–84.

In this landmark study a series of mutations in the BMPR2 were associated with familial pulmonary hypertesion. This was the first confirmation that bmp signalling may be relevant to PAH.

MacGregor, A.J., Canavan, R., Knight, C., Denton, C.P., Davar, J., Coghlan, J., Black, C.M. 2001. Pulmonary hypertension in systemic sclerosis: risk factors for progression and consequences for survival. Rheumatology 40, 453–459.

Machado, R.D., Pauciulo, M.W., Thomson, J.R., Lane, K.B., Morgan, N.V., Wheeler, L., Phillips, J.A. 3rd, Newman, J., Williams, D., Galie, N., Manes, A., McNeil, K., Yacoub, M., Mikhail, G., Rogers, P., Corris, P., Humbert, M., Donnai, D., Martensson, G., Tranebjaerg, L., Loyd, J.E., Trembath, R.C., Nichols, W.C. 2001. BMPR2 haploinsufficiency as the inherited molecular mechanism for primary pulmonary hypertension. Am. J. Hum. Genet. 68, 92–102.

Magdiliano, M., Isenberg, D.A., Hillson, J. 2002. Pulmonary hypertension in autoimmune rheumatic diseases. Arthritis Rheum. 46, 1997–2009.

Mayes, M.D. 2003. Endothelin and endothelin receptor antagonists in systemic rheumatic disease. Arthritis Rheum. 48, 1190–1199.

Mitri, G.M., Lucas, M., Fertig, N., Steen, V.D., Medsger, T.A. Jr. 2003. A comparison between anti-Th/To- and anticentromere antibody-positive systemic sclerosis patients with limited cutaneous involvement. Arthritis Rheum. 48, 203–209.

Mok, M.Y., Tse, H.F., Lau, C.S. 1999. Pulmonary hypertension secondary to systemic lupus erythematosus: prolonged survival following treatment with intermittent low dose iloprost. Lupus 8, 328–331.

Morse, J., Barst, R., Horn, E., Cuervo, N., Deng, Z., Knowles, J. 2002. Pulmonary hypertension in scleroderma spectrum of disease: lack of bone morphogenetic protein receptor 2 mutations. J. Rheumatol. 29, 2379–2381.

Mukerjee, D., St. George, D., Knight, C., Davar, J., Wells, A.U., Du Bois, R.M., Black, C.M., Coghlan, J.G. 2002. Accuracy of noninvasive tests in the evaluation of pulmonary arterial hypertension in a large population of patients with systemic sclerosis. European Society of Cardiology, Berlin.

Mukerjee, D., St. George, D., Coleiro, B., Knight, C., Denton, C.P., Davar, J., Black, C.M., Coghlan, J.G. 2003. Prevalence and outcome in systemic sclerosis associated pulmonary arterial hypertension: application of a registry approach. Ann. Rheum. Dis. 62, 1088–1093.

Nagaya, N., Nishikimi, T., Uematsu, M., Satoh, T., Kyotani, S., Sakamaki, F., Kakishita, M., Fukushima, K., Okano, Y., Nakanishi, N., Miyatake, K., Kangawa, K. 2000. Plasma brain natriuretic peptide as a prognostic indicator in patients with primary pulmonary hypertension. Circulation 22; 102, 865–870.

Olschewski, H., Simonneau, G., Galie, N., Higenbottam, T., Naeije, R., Rubin, L.J., Nikkho, S., Speich, R., Hoeper, M.M., Behr, J., Winkler, J., Sitbon, O., Popov, W., Ghofrani, H.A., Manes, A., Kiely, D.G., Ewert, R., Meyer, A., Corris, P.A., Delcroix, M., Gomez-Sanchez, M., Siedentop, H., Seeger, W. 2002. Inhaled iloprost for severe pulmonary hypertension. N. Engl. J. Med. 347, 322–329.

Raffy, O., Azarian, R., Brenot, F., Parent, F., Sitbon, O., Petitpretz, P., Herve, P., Duroux, P., Dinh-Xuan, A.T., Simonneau, G. 1996. Clinical significance of vasodilator response during short-term infusion of prostacyclin in primary pulmonary hypertension. Circulation 93, 484–488.

Rich, S., Kaufman, R., Levy, P. 1992. The effects of high doses of calcium channel blockers on survival in primary pulmonary hypertension. N. Engl. J. Med. 327, 76–81.

Roberts, D.H., Lepore, J.J., Maroo, A., Semigran, M.J., Ginns, L.C. 2001. Oxygen therapy improves cardiac index and pulmonary vascular resistance in patients with pulmonary hypertension. Chest 120, 1547–1555.

Rosas, V., Conte, J.V., Yang, S.C., Gaine, S.P., Borja, M., Wigley, F.M., White, B., Orens, J.B. 2000. Lung transplantation and systemic sclerosis. Ann. Transplant. 5, 38–43.

Rubin, L.J., Mendoza, J., Hood, M., McGoon, M., Barst, R., Williams, W.B., Diehl, J.H., Crow, J., Long, W. 1990. Treatment of primary pulmonary hypertension with continuous intravenous prostacyclin (epoprostenol). Ann. Intern. Med. 112, 485–491.

Rubin, L.J., Badesch, D.B., Barst, R.J., Galie, N., Black, C.M., Keogh, A., Pulido, T., Frost, A., Roux, S., Leconte, I., Landzberg, M., Simonneau, G. 2002. Bosentan therapy for pulmonary arterial hypertension. N. Engl. J. Med. 346, 896–903.
The second of two pivotal trials comparing placebo with bosentan. Effectiveness was clearly shown and SSc patients demonstrated qualitatively similar treatment effect to those with primary PAH.

Rudarakanchana, N., Flanagan, J.A., Chen, H., Upton, P.D., Machado, R., Patel, D., Trembath, R.C., Morrell, N.W. 2002. Functional analysis of bone morphogenetic protein type II receptor mutations underlying primary pulmonary hypertension. Hum. Mol. Genet. 11, 1517–1525.

Saba, T.S., Foster, J., Cockburn, M., Cowan, M., Peacock, A.J. 2002. Ventricular mass index using magnetic resonance imaging accurately estimates pulmonary artery pressure. Eur. Respir. J. 20, 1519–1524.

Sackner, M.A., Heinz, E.R., Steinberg, A.J. 1966. The heart in scleroderma. Am. J. Cardiol..

Sacks, D.G., Okano, Y., Steen, V.D., Curtiss, E., Shapiro, L.S., Medsger, T.A. Jr. 1996. Isolated pulmonary hypertension in systemic sclerosis with diffuse cutaneous involvement: association with serum anti-U3RNP antibody. J. Rheumatol. 23, 639–642.

Sanchez, O., Humbert, M., Sitbon, O., et al. 1999. Treatment of pulmonary hypertension secondary to connective tissue diseases. Thorax 54, 273–277.

Shi-Wen, X., Denton, C.P., Dashwood, M.R., Holmes, A.M., Bou-Gharios, G., Pearson, J.D., Black, C.M., Abraham, D.J. 2001. Fibroblast matrix gene expression and connective tissue remodeling: role of endothelin-1. J. Invest. Dermatol. 116, 417–425.

Simonneau, G., Barst, R.J., Galie, N., Naeije, R., Rich, S., Bourge, R.C., Keogh, A., Oudiz, R., Frost, A., Blackburn, S.D., Crow, J.W., Rubin, L.J. 2002. Continuous subcutaneous infusion of treprostinil, a prostacyclin analogue, in patients with pulmonary arterial hypertension: a double-blind, randomized, placebo-controlled trial. Am. J. Respir. Crit. Care Med. 165, 800–804.

Steen, V., Medsger, T.A. Jr. 2003. Predictors of isolated pulmonary hypertension in patients with systemic sclerosis and limited cutaneous involvement. Arthritis Rheum. 48, 516–522.

Stratton, R.J., Coghlan, J.G., Pearson, J.D., Burns, A., Sweny, P., Abraham, D.J., Black, C.M. 1998. Different patterns of endothelial cell activation in renal and pulmonary vascular disease in scleroderma. QJM 91, 561–566.

Stratton, R.J., Pompon, L., Coghlan, J.G., Pearson, J.D., Black, C.M. 2000. Soluble thrombomodulin concentration is raised in scleroderma associated pulmonary hypertension. Ann. Rheum. Dis. 59, 132–134.

Stratton, R., Shiwen, X., Martini, G., Holmes, A., Leask, A., Haberberger, T., Martin, G.R., Black, C.M., Abraham, D. 2001. Iloprost suppresses connective tissue growth factor production in fibroblasts and in the skin of scleroderma patients J. Clin. Invest. 108, 241–250.
This study provides a mechanism for the presumed effect of prostacyclin analogues on vasculopathy by downregulating the potential mediator CTGF.

Sullivan, C.C., Du, L., Chu, D., Cho, A.J., Kido, M., Wolf, P.L., Jamieson, S.W., Thistlethwaite, P.A. 2003. Induction of pulmonary hypertension by an angiopoietin 1/TIE2/serotonin pathway. Proc. Natl Acad. Sci. USA 100, 12331–12336.

Susol, E., Rands, A.L., Herrick, A., McHugh, N., Barrett, J.H., Ollier, W.E., Worthington, J. 2000. Association of markers for TGFbeta3, TGFbeta2 and TIMP1 with systemic sclerosis. Rheumatology 39, 1332–1336.

Tan, F.K., Wang, N., Kuwana, M., Chakraborty, R., Bona, C.A., Milewicz, D.M., Arnett, F.C. 2001. Association of fibrillin 1 single-nucleotide polymorphism haplotypes with systemic sclerosis in Choctaw and Japanese populations. Arthritis Rheum. 44, 893–901.

Tanaka, E., Harigai, M., Tanaka, M., Kawaguchi, Y., Hara, M., Kamatani, N. 2002. Pulmonary hypertension in systemic lupus erythematosus: evaluation of clinical characteristics and response to immunosuppressive treatment. J. Rheumatol. 29, 282–287.

Thomson, J.R., Machado, R.D., Pauciulo, M.W., Morgan, N.V., Humbert, M., Elliott, G.C., Ward, K., Yacoub, M., Mikhail, G., Rogers, P., et al. 2000. Sporadic primary pulmonary hypertension is associated with germline mutations of the gene encoding BMPR-II, a receptor member of the TGF-beta family. J. Med. Genet. 37, 741–745.

Trembath, R.C. 2001. Mutations in the TGF-beta type 1 receptor, ALK1, in combined primary pulmonary hypertension and hereditary haemorrhagic telangiectasia, implies pathway specificity. J. Heart Lung Transplant. 20, 175.

Trembath, R.C., Thomson, J.R., Machado, R.D., Morgan, N.V., Atkinson, C., Winship, I., Simonneau, G., Galie, N., Loyd, J.E., Humbert, M., Nichols, W.C., Morrell, N.W., Berg, J., Manes, A., McGaughran, J., Pauciulo, M., Wheeler, L. 2001. Clinical and molecular genetic features of pulmonary hypertension in patients with hereditary hemorrhagic telangiectasia. N. Engl. J. Med. 345, 325–334.

Vancheeswaran, R., Magoulas, T., Efrat, G., Wheeler-Jones, C., Olsen, I., Penny, R., Black, C.M. 1994. Circulating endothelin-1 levels in systemic sclerosis subsets—a marker of fibrosis or vascular dysfunction? J. Rheumatol. 21, 1838–1844.

Vizza, C.D., Rocca, G.D., Roma, A.D., Iacoboni, C., Pierconti, F., Venuta, F., Rendina, E., Schmid, G., Pietropaoli, P., Fedele, F. 2001. Acute hemodynamic effects of inhaled nitric oxide, dobutamine and a combination of the two in patients with mild to moderate secondary pulmonary hypertension. Crit. Care. 5, 355–361.

Watson, M., Hally, R.J., McCue, P.A., Varga, J., Jimenez, S.A. 1996. Gastric antral vascular ectasia (watermelon stomach) in patients with systemic sclerosis. Arthritis Rheum. 39, 341–346.

Yamane, K., Ihn, H., Asano, Y., Yazawa, N., Kubo, M., Kikuchi, K., Soma, Y., Tamaki, K. 2000. Clinical and laboratory features of scleroderma patients with pulmonary hypertension. Rheumatology 39, 1269–1271.

Yi, E.S., Kim, H., Ahn, H., Strother, J., Morris, T., Masliah, E., Hansen, L.A., Park, K., Friedman, P.J. 2000. Distribution of obstructive intimal lesions and their cellular phenotypes in chronic pulmonary hypertension. A morphometric and immunohistochemical study. Am. J. Respir. Crit. Care Med. 162, 1577–1586.

Young, R.H., Mark, G.J. 1978. Pulmonary vascular changes in scleroderma. Am. J. Med. 64, 998–1004.

Yuan, J.X., Aldinger, A.M., Juhaszova, M., Wang, J., Conte, J.V. Jr., Gaine, S.P., Orens, J.B., Rubin, L.J. 1998. Dysfunctional voltage-gated K+ channels in pulmonary artery smooth muscle cells of patients with primary pulmonary hypertension. Circulation 98, 1400–1406.

PART IV

Vasculitides

Handbook of Systemic Autoimmune Diseases, Volume 2
Pulmonary Involvement in Systemic Autoimmune Diseases
A.U. Wells and C.P. Denton, editors

CHAPTER 4

Wegener's Granulomatosis: A Pulmonary Perspective

Peter Lamprecht[a,b], Armin Schnabel[c], Wolfgang L. Gross[a,b,*]

[a]*Department of Rheumatology, University Hospital of Schleswig-Holstein, Campus Luebeck, Ratzeburger Allee 160, D-23538 Luebeck, Germany*

[b]*Rheumaklinik Bad Bramstedt, Oskar-Alexander-Strasse 26, D-24576 Bad Bramstedt, Germany*

[c]*Department of Rheumatology and Clinical Immunology, Sana Centre of Rheumatology, Baden-Württemberg, König-Karl-Strasse 5, D-75323 Bad Wildbad, Germany*

1. Introduction

Wegener's granulomatosis is a chronic inflammatory disease that affects the respiratory tract, the kidneys and a multitude of other organ systems. It was one of the first vasculitides to be recognized as a separate entity by Friedrich Wegener in the 1930s. Although the aetiology remains unknown, much has been learned about the nature of the disease and its clinical course. The dismal prognosis, if untreated, has improved dramatically with the introduction and progressive refinement of immunosuppressive treatment. The discovery of antineutrophil cytoplasmic antibodies (ANCA) directed against proteinase 3 (PR3-ANCA), a constituent of neutrophil granulocytes and monocytes, not only facilitated clinical diagnosis but also paved the way for insight into the pathogenesis.

Wegener's granulomatosis affects the respiratory tract in the form of granulomatous disease, vasculitis or a combination of the two. A spectrum of clinical manifestations originates from either of the two components. This makes Wegener's granulomatosis one of the most complex but also one of the most fascinating vasculitides encountered in pulmonary medicine.

*Corresponding author.
Tel.: +49-4192-902576; fax: +49-4192-902389
E-mail address: gross@rheuma-zentrum.de (W.L. Gross).

DOI: 10.1016/S1571-5078(04)02004-5

2. Prevalence

The disease was described by F. Wegener as a separate entity at the beginning of the 1930s. H. Klinger had reported one patient before but was unaware of the new entity (Klinger, 1931; Wegener, 1939). Generally accepted classification criteria and a definition of Wegener's granulomatosis were developed about 15 years ago (Table 1). A prevalence of 3/100 000 has been reported for the US-state of New York (Cotch et al., 1996). Data on prevalence from other regions of the world are subject to ongoing epidemiological studies. Moreover, variants of the disease may cause underestimates of the 'real' prevalence of Wegener's granulomatosis. Carrington and Liebow (1966) introduced the term 'limited' Wegener's granulomatosis to characterize patients with a predominant involvement of the lungs in the absence of kidney involvement. Some patients may present with isolated meningo-cerebral inflammation or ophthalmic involvement without renal manifestations or ANCA (Reinhold-Keller et al., 2001).

The European Vasculitis Study Group (EUVAS) refined the term 'limited' Wegener's granulomatosis in order to define disease stages based on clinical and pathological considerations. 'Localized' Wegener's granulomatosis is defined as Wegener's granulomatosis restricted to the upper and/or lower respiratory tract. 'Early systemic' Wegener's granulomatosis includes any organ involvement except renal or

Table 1
Definition and classification criteria of Wegener's granulomatosis according to the Chapel Hill Consensus (CHC) (Jennette et al., 1994) and American College of Rheumatology (ACR) (Leavitt et al., 1990)

CHC definition	ACR classification criteria
Granulomatous inflammation involving the respiratory tract, and necrotizing vasculitis affecting small to medium-sized vessels (i.e. capillaries, venules, arterioles, and arteries)	Nasal or oral inflammation Abnormal chest radiograph
Necrotizing glomerulonephritis is common	Nephritic urinary sediment
Cytoplasmic-pattern ANCA (C-ANCA) with antigen specificity for proteinase 3 (PR3-ANCA) are a very sensitive marker for Wegener's granulomatosis	Granulomatous inflammation on biopsy

The ACR classification criteria were developed by comparing 85 patients with Wegener's granulomatosis with 722 control patients. At least two out of the four criteria are present in Wegener's granulomatosis. The presence of any two or more criteria yields a sensitivity of 88.2% and a specificity of 92.0% (Leavitt et al., 1990).

imminent vital organ failure. Finally, 'generalized' Wegener's granulomatosis includes renal involvement and/or imminent organ failure. Two other subgroups, namely 'severe renal' and 'refractory' disease, were defined to cover the spectrum of Wegener's granulomatosis and microscopic polyangiitis, another ANCA-associated vasculitis (Table 2) (Jayne, 2001).

In most patients, the disease progresses to generalized Wegener's granulomatosis. However, in a smaller fraction of patients the disease remains 'localized' or 'early systemic' for a long time for as yet unknown reasons. It seems that the pathophysiological chain of events leading to generalized Wegener's granulomatosis is somehow interrupted or 'frozen' (*formes frustes*) in these patients.

3. Epidemiology

Wegener's granulomatosis is a worldwide disease. It is encountered in children as well as in elderly people, but the peak incidence is in the fourth and fifth decades with females and males equally affected (Hoffman et al., 1992; Reinhold-Keller et al., 2000; Abdou et al., 2002). Its incidence ranges between $2.9/10^6$/year and $10.6/10^6$/year depending on the

Table 2
Clinical subgrouping of Wegener's granulomatosis (WG) and microscopic polyangiitis (MPA) according to the definitions of the European Vasculitis Study Group (EUVAS)

Subgroup	Disease	Organ involvement	Constitutional symptoms[a]	Presence of ANCA
Localized	WG	Upper and/or lower respiratory tract	No	±
Early systemic	WG, MPA	Any except renal or imminent organ failure[b]	Yes	Usually +
Generalized	WG, MPA	Renal with serum creatinine <500 μmol/l and/or other imminent organ failure[b]	Yes	+
Severe renal	WG, MPA	Renal with serum creatinine >500 μmol/l	Yes	+
Refractory	WG, MPA	Progressive disease despite therapy with corticosteroids and cyclophosphamide	Yes	±

[a] Fever, night sweats, weight loss, malaise, and fatigue.
[b] Includes progressive lung, eye, nervous system, or gastrointestinal involvement. +, present; −, not present (According to Jayne, 2001).

Table 3
Incidence rates of Wegener's granulomatosis in different European regions

	UK	Spain	Norway	Germany
Incidence cases/10^6/year	10.6	2.9–4.9	8.0	5.5–7.0

Koldingsnes and Nossent, 2000; Watts et al., 2001; Reinhold-Keller et al., 2002; Gonzalez-Gay et al., 2003.

geographic region (Table 3) (Carruthers et al., 1996; Reinhold-Keller et al., 2002). A prevalence of 3.0×10^5 has been reported for the US-state of New York (Cotch et al., 1996). It is debated whether there is an increase in the incidence or an increased awareness of Wegener's granulomatosis. New and better diagnostic procedures, including the determination of ANCA and imaging procedures such as magnetic resonance imaging (MRI) of the head, may have helped to establish an earlier and more accurate diagnosis of Wegener's granulomatosis in many cases (Carruthers et al., 1996). Moreover, new diagnostic procedures have also improved the diagnosis of variants of the disease such as *formes frustes* limited to single organs (Carrington and Liebow, 1966; Jayne, 2001).

4. Aetiology/Pathology

Wegener's granulomatosis is an organ- and/or life-threatening autoimmune disease of as yet unknown aetiology, characterized by granulomatous lesions and a necrotizing vasculitis. Pulmonary-renal syndrome is common (Jennette and Falk, 1997; Savage et al., 1997). A highly specific autoantibody, PR3-ANCA, is detected in about 95% of the patients with generalized Wegener's granulomatosis, but only in about 50% of the patients with localized Wegener's granulomatosis. A few patients with Wegener's granulomatosis may present with myeloperoxidase (MPO)-ANCA or have no detectable ANCA (Nölle et al., 1989).

One of the key questions with respect to the pathophysiology of Wegener's granulomatosis is how granulomatous lesions, autoimmune vasculitis and PR3-ANCA evolve and give rise to distinct features such as granulomas of the respiratory tract or orbita and rapidly progressive glomerulonephritis. Infections such as *Staphylococcus aureus*, other environmental influences or 'Wegener's autoantigen' PR3 itself are thought to play a role in triggering and/or maintaining disease activity in Wegener's granulomatosis on the basis of a genetic predisposition to an exaggerated Th1-type response early in the disease process (Popa et al., 2002; Sneller, 2002).

A new hypothesis suggests that a complimentary peptide coded by the antisense DNA strand of PR3 elicits their cognate antibody, which in turn evokes an anti-idiotype of this antibody with specificity for the autoantigen, i.e. PR3-ANCA (Pendergraft et al., 2004).

4.1. Genetic background

One hypothesis suggests that there is an inverse relationship between the intensity of genetic predisposition and the time necessary to develop an autoimmune disease. Disease-causing and disease-modifying genes may determine the eventual risk of developing an autoimmune disease. The delayed onset of an autoimmune disease suggests that the net genetic abnormality may be quite subtle. Multiple genetic abnormalities in a biological pathway may finally give rise to a complex autoimmune disease (Lipsky, 2001). Genetic abnormalities may also be relevant in the development of Wegener's granulomatosis. As with Lipsky's (2001) considerations for systemic lupus erythematosus, it can be argued that over time, subtle genetic abnormalities might also result in an increasing deviation of cellular immune responses giving rise to granulomatous lesions and an autoimmune vasculitis characteristic of Wegener's granulomatosis. Ethnic differences may influence the prevalence of genetic determinants. So far, no particularly penetrant single genetic factor has been identified in Wegener's granulomatosis, suggesting that combinations of various factors rather than single factors may be operative. Moreover, clustering of Wegener's granulomatosis in relatives has rarely been reported (Munian et al., 1986).

4.1.1. HLA-association

MHC class I and II molecules bind peptide fragments from foreign antigens and potential autoantigens and present them on the cell surface for recognition by the appropriate $CD8^+$ and $CD4^+$ T-cells, respectively. Polymorphism of the MHC molecules determines which amino acid sequences preferentially bind to the peptide binding groove, through specific anchor residues. Thus, the MHC genotype restricts the antigen specificity of T-cells. Since T-cells are involved in autoimmune responses, several human autoimmune diseases such as rheumatoid arthritis, ankylosing spondylitis, and systemic lupus erythematosus have been found to be associated with certain MHC genotypes (Janeway et al., 2001).

An analysis of HLA alleles of a patient population from Southern Germany found HLA-DRB1*04 to be over-represented in patients with end-stage renal disease and HLA-DRB1*13 and HLA-DQB1*0603 under-represented. A protective role of HLA-DRB1*13 was postulated, but study results may have been biased by over- and under-representation of HLA alleles within that particular region of Germany (Gencik et al., 1999). A number of studies suggest an association of Wegener's granulomatosis with distinct HLA-alleles such as HLA-DR1 or HLA-DR2 (Elkon et al., 1983; Papiha et al., 1992), but other studies failed to establish an association between HLA alleles and Wegener's granulomatosis (Zhang et al., 1995). The fact that approximately half of normal Caucasian individuals are HLA-DR2 positive might explain why no particular narrow HLA phenotype has been identified to convey susceptibility to Wegener's granulomatosis. Therefore, other factors than the HLA phenotype may be more important for the development of Wegener's granulomatosis (Peen and Williams, 2000).

4.1.2. Polymorphism of cytokine and signal transducer genes

No clear-cut association has been established between polymorphisms of tumour necrosis factor α (TNF-α) and Wegener's granulomatosis (Mascher et al., 1997). Analysis of a biallelic polymorphism at position −1082 of the promoter region of the interleukin 10 (IL-10) gene showed a significant shift to genotype AA in Wegener's granulomatosis patients. This genotype is associated with blunted IL-10 secretion from activated macrophages and certain T-cell subsets. Lower IL-10 secretion may favour skewing of the immune response towards a T-helper 1 (Th1)-type pattern (Muraközy et al., 2001).

A single nucleotide polymorphism at position −318 of the promoter region of CTLA-4 (CD152) was found to be associated with Wegener's granulomatosis. CTLA-4 is an inducible negative regulator of T-cell activation (Giscombe et al., 2002). Recently, familial Crohn's disease has been shown to be associated with a NOD2 gene mutation. NOD proteins are pattern-recognition receptors that bind endotoxin intracellularly. Crohn's disease is a granulomatous disease characterized by the predominance of a Th1-type cytokine response. However, an analysis of NOD2 gene mutations found no association with Wegener's granulomatosis (Newman et al., 2003).

4.1.3. Genes involved in proteinase 3 (PR3) expression and regulation

Genetic factors may also play a role in the interaction of neutrophil granulocytes, PR3-ANCA and endothelial cells. An association of protease inhibitor, e.g. alpha-1-antitrypsin, deficiency with PR3-ANCA-associated vasculitis has been observed. Over-expression of the PiZ and PiZZ alleles results in subnormal concentrations of alpha-1-antitrypsin (Esnault et al., 1993; Griffith et al., 1996). This can provide an explanation for increased circulating levels of proteinase 3 and up-regulated tissue levels of secretory leukocyte proteinase inhibitor in Wegener's granulomatosis, the latter being an important local protease inhibitor in the upper respiratory tract (Ohlsson et al., 2003).

TNF-α and IL-8 primed neutrophil granulocytes translocate PR3 from intracellular granules to the neutrophil membrane. Subsequent binding of PR3-ANCA enables Fc gamma receptor (Fcγ-R) mediated neutrophil activation (Csernok et al., 1994). ANCA preferentially engage the Fcγ-RIIIb (CD16) and Fcγ-RIIa (CD32) expressed on neutrophils (Porges et al., 1994; Kocher et al., 1998). Whereas some studies found an influence of alleles of Fcγ-RIIa (H131/R131) and Fcγ-RIIIb (NA1/NA2) on disease severity, relapses and/or the organ pattern (Wainstein et al., 1996; Edberg et al., 1997; Dijstelbloem et al., 1999), another study argued against this effect (Tse et al., 1999).

High constitutive expression of PR3 on the surface of neutrophil granulocytes may also predispose individuals to Wegener's granulomatosis

(Csernok et al., 1993; Muller Kobold et al., 1998). An association of Wegener's granulomatosis with the A-564G polymorphism in the PR3 promoter region affecting a putative transcription factor-binding site has been reported recently (Gencik et al., 1999).

4.2. Environmental influences

4.2.1. Silica

Case-control studies by Gregorini et al. (1993) and Nuyts et al. (1995) suggest a role for silica (inorganic mineral form of silicone) and silicone (synthetic polymers with a SiO backbone) in the pathogenesis of ANCA-associated rapidly progressive glomerulonephritis and Wegener's granulomatosis, respectively. Silicates activate T-cells by a superantigen-like mechanism via T-cell receptor (TCR) Vβ chain stimulation. They also activate macrophages in vitro, and might inactivate alpha 1 antitrypsin. Thus, silica may contribute to an exaggerated immune response in predisposed individuals. Other occupational exposures have not been shown to be associated with Wegener's granulomatosis so far (Cohen Tervaert et al., 1998).

4.2.2. Drugs

Drug induced ANCA-positive vasculitis may occasionally mimic Wegener's granulomatosis. Antithyroid drugs, especially propylthiouracil, but also methimazole and carbimazole, can cause ANCA-positive cutaneous vasculitis and glomerulonephritis in rare cases. Other drugs such as hydralazine, minocycline and penicillamine may also induce ANCA-positive vasculitis. Usually MPO-ANCA are detected in such cases, but occasionally PR3-ANCA are also detected (reviewed by Merkel (1998)). Propylthiouracil induces MPO-ANCA in a cat model. Reactive metabolites of propylthiouracil are thought to modify MPO itself, resulting in the generation of antibodies directed against MPO in this model (Waldhauser and Uetrecht, 1996). Activated neutrophil granulocytes and MPO may also play a role in the generation of potential cytotoxic products from other drugs (Jiang et al., 1994).

4.2.3. Malignancy

An association between Wegener's granulomatosis and malignancy has been observed. In one study renal cell carcinoma was diagnosed in 7 of 23 patients with malignant disease before or simultaneously with Wegener's granulomatosis. PR3 has been found in a renal cancer cell line and might induce autoimmune phenomena (Tatsis et al., 1999).

4.2.4. *Staphylococcus aureus* and other infections

In Wegener's granulomatosis, symptoms of respiratory tract infections often precede or accompany initial symptoms. Chronic nasal carriage of *S. aureus* is approximately three times higher in Wegener's granulomatosis than in healthy and disease controls (Stegeman et al., 1994; Gadola et al., 1997). Nasal carriage of *S. aureus* constitutes a risk factor for disease exacerbation. Prophylactic treatment with trimethoprim-sulfamethoxazole reduces respiratory and non-respiratory tract infections and the risk of relapses in Wegener's granulomatosis (Stegeman et al., 1996). Trimethoprim-sulfamethoxazole may also induce remissions in localized Wegener's granulomatosis (DeRemee et al., 1985; Reinhold-Keller et al., 1996). Sera from patients with Wegener's granulomatosis recognize endothelial bound *S. aureus* acid phosphatase. This observation led to the hypothesis that staphylococcal acid phosphatase might act as a planted antigen and induce vasculitis in susceptible individuals (Brons et al., 2000).

S. aureus B-cell superantigens such as staphylococcal protein A might also play a role in stimulating autoreactive PR3 producing B-cells within granulomatous lesions of the respiratory tract (Popa et al., 2002; Voswinkel et al., 2002). Neutrophil granulocytes are found in granulomatous lesions in Wegener's granulomatosis. During active disease they display features of antigen-presenting cells such as the expression of MHC-class II molecules, CD80 and CD86 and may present antigen to T-cells (Iking-Konert et al., 2001). *S. aureus* can survive inside neutrophil granulocytes under certain conditions (Gresham et al., 2000). High affinity PR3-ANCA producing autoreactive B-cells might be induced by PR3 or cross-reacting microbial epitopes within granulomatous lesions (Brockmann et al., 2002; Popa et al., 2002; Voswinkel et al., 2002). Subsequent expansion of autoreactive PR3 producing B-cells may be a consequence of *S. aureus* B-cell superantigen activity. The superantigenic activity of staphylococcal protein A is induced by binding to membrane bound immunoglobulin heavy chain subunits encoded by V_H3 family genes. The V_H3 gene family is over-expressed in autoreactive PR3-ANCA producing B-cells isolated from the circulation and from granulomatous lesions in Wegener's granulomatosis (Sibilia et al., 1997; Popa et al., 2002; Voswinkel et al., 2002). Whereas these studies suggest *S. aureus* superantigen activity on B-cells, conflicting results have been reported with regard to the evidence of skewing of T-cell receptor Vβ usage indicative of T-cell superantigen mediated expansion of T-cells (Grunewald et al., 1998; Popa et al., 2002, 2003).

Several studies suggested an association of viral infections with Wegener's granulomatosis. So far, no clear evidence of such an association has been established. Recent case-control studies have excluded an association between Parvo B19 virus infection and Wegener's granulomatosis (Nikkari et al., 1995; Eden et al., 2003). However, such serological studies do not exclude subversion of the immune system by viruses or other infectious agents through other, as yet unknown, mechanisms in susceptible individuals.

4.3. Granulomatous lesions

The granulomatous lesions seen in Wegener's granulomatosis show a wide morphological spectrum. Because of this, and because the pattern is often irregular, this form of tissue injury is usually referred to as 'granulomatous lesion' rather than 'granuloma'. The lesions display different morphologies, such as neutrophilic microabscesses, necrotizing palisading granulomas, and epitheloid cell granulomas (Fig. 1). Granulomatous lesions of the respiratory tract of both localized and generalized Wegener's granulomatosis are characterized by $CD4^+$ T-cells, $CD8^+$ T-cells, histiocytes, $CD20^+$ B lymphocytes, $CD68^+$ macrophages, and $CD68^+$ multinucleated giant cells. The central necrosis may be confluent or may show the irregular serpiginous pattern known as 'geographic' necrosis. A palisade of epitheloid histiocytes may arrange around the necrotic foci. The centre of the necrosis is acelluar or, in some instances, contains polymorphonuclear leukocytes. Apart from the respiratory tract, granulomatous lesions may be found in virtually any organ, e.g. retroorbital tissues or meninges (Fienberg, 1989; Lieberman and Churg, 1991; Müller et al., 2003). However, renal granulomas are rare (Bajema et al., 1998).

The earliest lesions in the lung are foci of swollen collagen fibres representing apparent tissue injury and/or necrosis. In the next stage, mononuclear histiocytes migrate to the vicinity of the necrosis. Neutrophil granulocytes, lymphocytes, epitheloid cells and multinucleated giant cells appear subsequently. Finally, the histiocytes become orientated in a palisading manner about the central necrosis area. Granulomatous lesions in the lung can be found in the vicinity of inflamed vessels, but also at extravascular sites (Fienberg, 1989; Lieberman and Churg, 1991). Fienberg (1989) suggested that Wegener's granulomatosis starts as granulomatous disease in the respiratory tract and systemic vasculitis develops subsequently. However, early foci of fibrinoid necrosis could also be a consequence of necrotizing capillaritis. PR3 from neutrophil granulocytes, the target antigen of ANCA in Wegener's granulomatosis, has recently been found within or around fibrinoid necrotic lesions in the kidney. However, PR3 was absent in a considerable number of necrotic lesions

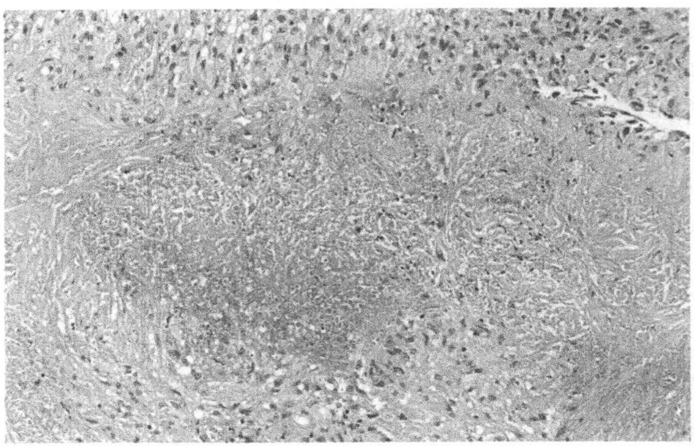

Figure 1. Nasal mucosa biopsy in Wegener's granulomatosis. Hematoxylin and eosin staining shows geographic necrosis bordered by histiocytes. Original magnification × 400 (from Müller et al., 2003).

(Bajema et al., 2001). Thus, it still is a matter of debate whether PR3-ANCA could give rise to granulomatous lesions. Alternatively, autoreactive B-cells are stimulated within granulomatous lesions and produce PR3 (see Section 4.2.4). Since granulomatous lesions in the lung are found both close to and distant from inflamed vessels, there might also be a staged development of granulomatous lesions. Moreover, rare cases of ANCA-negative Wegener's granulomatosis have been reported (Reinhold-Keller et al., 2001).

Abundant IFN-γ expression and CD26 (optional Th1-type marker) expression on $CD4^+$ T-cells is seen in granulomatous lesions of the respiratory tract in localized Wegener's granulomatosis, but not in generalized Wegener's granulomatosis (Müller et al., 2000; Balding et al., 2001). Predominance of Th1-type chemokine receptor CCR5 expression on T-cells may favour stronger recruitment of Th1-type cytokine secreting cells into inflammatory lesions in localized Wegener's granulomatosis, as compared to generalized Wegener's granulomatosis. In generalized Wegener's granulomatosis, but not in localized Wegener's granulomatosis, a fraction of Th2-type $CCR3^+$ T-cells are found in the circulation and in tissue lesions (Balding et al., 2001; Lamprecht et al., 2003a,b). The CC chemokine RANTES (regulated on activation normal T-cell expressed and secreted/CCL5) is expressed in granulomatous lesions of the respiratory tract. RANTES is one of the ligands for both CCR5 and CCR3 (Coulomb-L'Hermine et al., 2001). Peripheral blood T-cells and monocytes produce Th1-type cytokines such as interferon (IFN)-γ in Wegener's granulomatosis (Ludviksson et al., 1998; Csernok et al., 1999; Lamprecht et al., 2002a,b), but secrete higher amounts of IFN-γ in localized Wegener's granulomatosis, as compared to generalized Wegener's granulomatosis (Müller et al., 2000). Changes in the cytokines balance may cause or accompany disease progression.

T-cells play an important role in granuloma formation and the induction of necrotic centres in animal models and in vitro studies (Table 4). In Wegener's granulomatosis, certain T-cell subsets seem to be particularly important. T-cells remain activated during clinical remission of the disease, in contrast to B-cells (Popa et al., 1999). In Wegener's granulomatosis, circulating T-cells lacking the co-stimulatory molecule CD28 are expanded (Schlesier et al., 1995; Moosig et al., 1998). In granulomatous lesions, T-cells also lack CD28 expression (Lamprecht et al., 2001). The Th1-type $CD28^-$ T-cell subset displays features of effector memory T-cells. The expansion of $CD28^-$ T-cells appears to start early in the disease process and is already evident in localized Wegener's granulomatosis (Lamprecht et al., 2003a,b). In generalized Wegener's granulomatosis, expansion of $CD28^-$ T-cells correlates with organ involvement (Moosig et al., 1998; Lamprecht et al., 2003a,b). Circulating peripheral blood as well as granuloma $CD4^+$ T-cells lacking the costimulatory molecule CD28 are a major source of Th1-type cytokine secretion, which is mainly restricted to tumour necrosis factor (TNF)-α and interferon (IFN)-γ (Komocsi et al., 2002). Th1-type CCR5 expression is seen on $CD28^-$ T-cells. A lower CCR5 expression on $CD4^+CD28^-$ T-cells in generalized Wegener's granulomatosis, as compared to localized Wegener's granulomatosis, suggests further differentiation of this T-cell subset during disease progression. These effector memory T-cells might contribute to granuloma formation and maintenance of disease activity through their cytokine secretion and bystander activation of autoreactive B- and T-cell subsets (Lamprecht et al., 2003a,b; Winek et al., 2004). Apart from T-cells, macrophages and

Table 4
Findings from animal models and in vitro studies concerning the role of T-cells in granuloma formation

Model	Main finding	Reference
Granuloma formation in animal model	T-cells and IFN-γ are crucial for the formation of granulomas	Ehlers et al. (2001)
	Activated $CD4^+$ Th1-type T-cells induce transformation from unspecific microabscesses to granuloma	Mielke et al. (1997)
In vitro model of granuloma formation	Activated T-cells induce necrotic centers in granulomas	Heinemann et al. (1997)

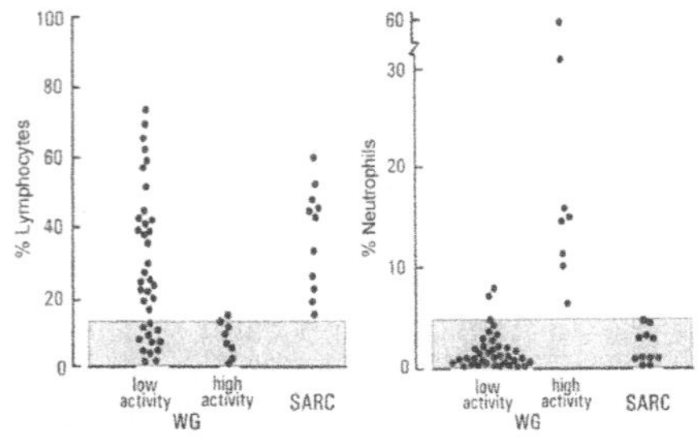

Figure 2. Bronchoalveolar lavage neutrophil and lymphocyte count in Wegener's granulomatosis and pulmonary sarcoidosis, presented as percentage of total cells. Radiographic and high-resolution CT features of Wegener's granulomatosis of low activity suggested predominantly granulomatous lung disease, whereas pulmonary highly active patients had florid pneumonitis.

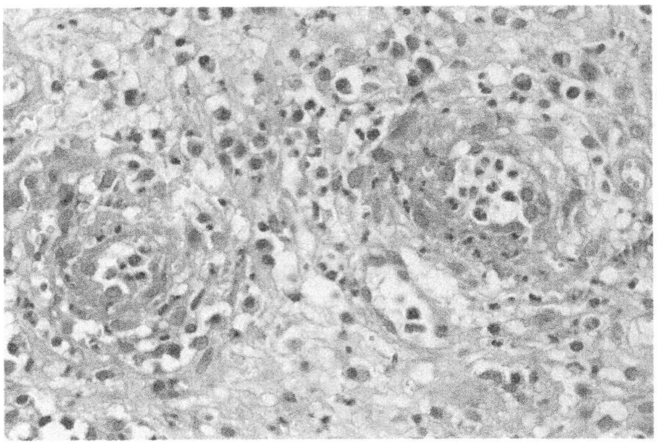

Figure 3. Nasal mucosa biopsy in Wegener's granulomatosis. Hematoxylin and eosin staining shows venules with fibrinoid necrosis and a mixed inflammatory infiltration of vessel walls, i.e. vasculitis. Neutrophil granulocytes are seen in the vessel and close to endothelial cells. Original magnification × 630 (from Müller et al., 2003).

monocytes are other important sources of Th1-Type cytokine production in Wegener's granulomatosis (Ludviksson et al., 1998; Lamprecht et al., 2002a,b; Müller et al., 2003). As mentioned above (Section 4), aberrant Th1-type responses might play a role during the initiation of the disease process (Sneller, 2002).

The bronchoalveolar lavage (BAL) cell profile in patients with the radiologic findings of granulomatous lung disease features elevated lymphocytes in the presence of normal granulocytes (Fig. 2) (Schnabel et al., 1999a–c). More than 90% of the lymphocytes are $CD3^+$ mature T-cells. A disproportionate elevation of $CD4^+$ cells in the BAL, compared with the blood, results in an elevated CD4/CD8 ratio in approximately two-thirds of these patients (Schnabel et al., 1999a–c). Purified $CD4^+$ and $CD8^+$ BAL T-cells and T-cell lines generated from pulmonary active Wegener's granulomatosis patients with a lymphocytic BAL cell profile were found to secrete interferon-γ (IFNγ) in excess of interleukin 4 (IL-4), i.e. a Th1-type cytokine pattern (Csernok et al., 1999). The same pattern was found in lesional tissue and in blood lymphocytes and monocytes (Csernok et al., 1999; Ludviksson et al., 1998; Lamprecht et al., 2002a,b).

4.4. Vasculitis

In Wegener's granulomatosis, necrotizing vasculitis predominantly affects small vessels and medium-sized vessels, i.e. capillaries, venules, arterioles, and arteries (Jennette et al., 1994). Endothelial cells are the targets of the initial injury. The earliest changes affect the vascular endothelium with swelling, necrosis and deadherence. Lysed neutrophil granulocytes are found within affected vessels (Fig. 3). In the lung capillaries, venules, and arterioles are infiltrated by polymorphonuclear leukocytes. Pulmonary microvascular necrotizing vasculitis (capillaritis) is the cause of pulmonary haemorrhage. In the kidney, rupture of the basement membrane subsequent to neutrophil degranulation gives rise to glomerular capillary thrombosis followed by segmental necrosis of the tuft. Necrotic material, blood, and fibrin spill into the Bowman's space. As a consequence, accumulation and proliferation of monocytes and parietal (Bowman's) epithelial cells with the formation of crescents is seen. The growing crescent compresses the capillary tuft, leading to segmental and global loss of circulation through the glomerulus (reviewed by Lieberman and Churg (1991) and Harper and Savage (2000)).

In Wegener's granulomatosis, the histological picture of vasculitis is polymorphic. Apart from necrotizing vasculitic lesions, leukocytoclastic vasculitis of the skin may be seen as cutaneous vasculitis manifestation. Necrotizing granulomatous arteritis involving medium-sized vessels is commonly found close to large necrotizing granulomatous foci in the lung. Non-granulomatous fibrinoid necrosis is rare in the lung but may affect bronchial arteries. Finally, vasculitis morphologically identical to that seen in polyarteritis, in terms of both size of the vessels involved and the presence of fibrinoid necrosis, may be seen in Wegener's granulomatosis (reviewed by Lieberman and Churg (1991) and Harper and Savage (2000)). The vasculitis is 'pauci-immune' because few or no immunoglobulin and/or complement deposits are detected in glomerular lesions and at other sites. However, in one study immune-complex deposits were reported to be prevalent in cutaneous vasculitis of Wegener's granulomatosis (Brons et al., 2001). Based on the finding of immune deposits along glomerular capillary walls in early lesions of MPO-ANCA-induced vasculitis in an animal model (Brouwer et al., 1993; Foucher et al., 1999), the same group hypothesized that early immune deposits might be degraded. This provides an explanation for pauci-immune lesions seen during later stages (Brons et al., 2001).

Several in vitro and animal models using different approaches support the concept that an interaction of PR3-ANCA with primed neutrophil granulocytes results in premature degranulation of neutrophil granulocytes, subsequent endothelial cell damage and leukocyte recruitment (Tables 5 and 6, Fig. 4). The existing animal models do not exactly mirror Wegener's granulomatosis or provide true 'Wegener's mice', but they offer reproducible, controlled conditions in which specific pathomechanisms can be analysed. The induction of an immune-complex mediated vasculitis rather than a pauci-immune vasculitis in some models, the induction of MPO- rather than PR3-ANCA and the absence of granulomatous lesions are some of the differences to the human disease (Yang et al., 1994; Specks, 2000; Neumann et al., 2003).

Pulmonary biopsy specimens commonly feature more advanced stages of Wegener's granulomatosis lung disease (Mark et al., 1988; Travis et al., 1990).

Table 5
Summary of findings in different animal models supporting the concept that ANCA are involved in the pathogenesis of autoimmune vasculitis in Wegener's granulomatosis (WG) and microscopic polyangiitis (MPA)

Main finding	Reference
SCG/Kj mice spontaneously develop crescentic glomerulonephritis, systemic vasculitis, and P-ANCA. Presence of glomerular immune deposits differs from the pauci-immune pattern found in human WG and MPA	Neumann et al. (2003)
Crescentic glomerulonephritis and systemic necrotizing vasculitis is induced in Rag2 (−/−) mice lacking T- and B-cells after transfer of splenocytes from MPO (−/−) knockout mice immunized with MPO. Similar lesions are induced in Rag2 (−/−) mice and wild-type C57BL/6J (intact immune system) mice receiving anti-MPO IgG (MPO-ANCA)	Xiao et al. (2002)
Mice immunized with human ANCA develop anti-human ANCA and anti-anti-human ANCA (mouse ANCA) as well as perivascular mononuclear cell infiltrates in the lungs and glomerular pathology	Blank et al. (1995) and Tomer et al. (1995)
Similar approach to Brouwer et al. (1993). In contrast, immune complex-mediated glomerulonephritis was found	Yang et al. (1994)
Brown Norway rats immunized with MPO develop MPO-ANCA. Subsequent perfusion of a kidney or lung with a lysosomal enzyme extract results in crescentic glomerulonephritis, vasculitis and pulmonary tissue injury. Immune deposits are seen in early glomerular lesions	Brouwer et al. (1993) and Foucher et al. (1999)
Brown Norway rats treated with mercuric chloride ($HgCl_2$) develop MPO-ANCA and a necrotizing vasculitis including leukocytoclastic vasculitis of the gut	Esnault et al. (1992) and Qasim et al. (1995)

MPO, myeloperoxidase.

Table 6
Summary of findings from different in vitro studies supporting the concept of ANCA-induced neutrophil degranulation and subsequent endothelial damage in Wegener's granulomatosis and microscopic polyangiitis

Main finding	Reference
Release of neutrophilic PR3 results in its uptake in endothelial cells and activation of distinct signaling proapoptotic events	Preston et al. (2002a,b)
PR3 enhances endothelial MCP-1 production and induces increased adhesion of neutrophil granulocytes to endothelial cells by upregulating ICAM-1	Taekema-Roelvink et al. (2001)
ANCA stabilize adhesion and promote migration of flowing neutrophil granulocytes on endothelial cells activated with TNF-α	Radford et al. (2001)
Production of IL-8 by ANCA-stimulated neutrophil granulocytes with the intravascular compartment inhibits neutrophil transmigration and, thus, may contribute to endothelial damage by premature neutrophil degranulation	Cockwell et al. (1999)
PR3 is also constitutively expressed on the cell surface of neutrophil granulocytes and high expression is associated with relapses in Wegener's granulomatosis	Muller Kobold et al. (1998)
TNF-α primed neutrophil granulocytes stimulated with PR3-ANCA and arachidonic acid secrete superoxide and leukotriene 4. PR3-ANCA also activate endothelial cells	Grimminger et al. (1996) and Sibelius et al. (1998)
TNF-α and IL-8 induce translocation of PR3 from azurophilic granules on the cell surface of neutrophil granulocytes where PR3 becomes accessible for PR3-ANCA	Csernok et al. (1994)
ANCA induce the release of primary granule contents from neutrophil granulocytes in a dose-dependent manner. Primung with TNF-α results in translocation of MPO on the cell surface and enhance degranulation	Falk et al. (1990)

PR3, proteinase 3; MCP-1, monocyte chemoattractant protein-1; ICAM-1, intercellular cell adhesion molecule-1.

Capillaries, arteries and veins are infiltrated by mononuclear cells more often than by granulocytes. Tissue eosinophilia is seen in up to 60% of pulmonary specimens. Foci of capillaritis with acute or chronic haemorrhage are found in approximately 40% of specimens from open lung biopsy (Travis et al., 1991).

4.4.1. ANCA in the pathogenesis of vasculitis

ANCA were first described in the early 1980s as a cause of diffuse granular cytoplasmic immunofluorescence staining on ethanol-fixed neutrophils (C-ANCA pattern) (Fig. 5). PR3 was found to be the principal target antigen for C-ANCA (Gross et al., 1992). PR3-ANCA is highly specific for Wegener's granulomatosis. C-ANCA is found in more than 90% of patients with generalized Wegener's granulomatosis, approximately 50% of those with localized Wegener's granulomatosis, 5% of patients with microscopic polyangiitis and 50% or less of patients with Churg–Strauss syndrome (Gross et al., 1992; Hoffman and Specks, 1998). In rare instances, C-ANCA is found in chronic bacterial infections and in cryoglobulinaemic patients.

ANCA reacting with MPO and producing a perinuclear immunofluorescence staining pattern (P-ANCA) (Fig. 5) are found mainly in patients with microscopic polyangiitis and those with pauci-immune glomerulonephritis, the renal limited form of the former disease (Gross et al., 1992; Hoffman and Specks, 1998). Approximately 70% of these patients have P-ANCA, as opposed to approximately 5% of the Wegener's granulomatosis patients.

Several lines of evidence suggest that PR3-ANCA and MPO-ANCA are not only markers of disease but also are implicated in the pathogenesis of the ANCA-associated vasculitides (Kallenberg et al., 1990). The ANCA-cytokine-sequence-theory holds that neutrophils translocate the target antigens for ANCA to the cell surface when they are primed by inflammatory

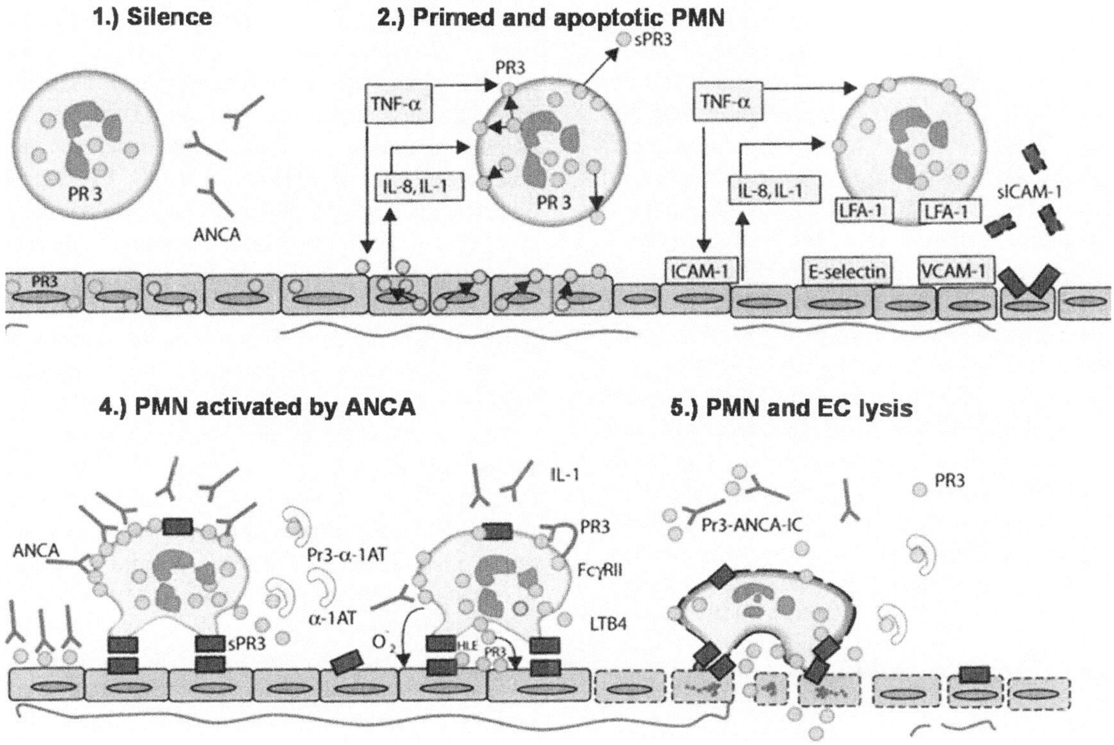

Figure 4. Pathophysiological model of ANCA-induced neutrophil degranulation and subsequent endothelial damage and leukocyte recruitment.

cytokines. The primed cells are fully activated by binding of ANCA to their respective target antigen, this resulting in adhesion to endothelial cells, degranulation and oxidative burst activity, which are thought to initiate the inflammatory response (Gross et al., 1992).

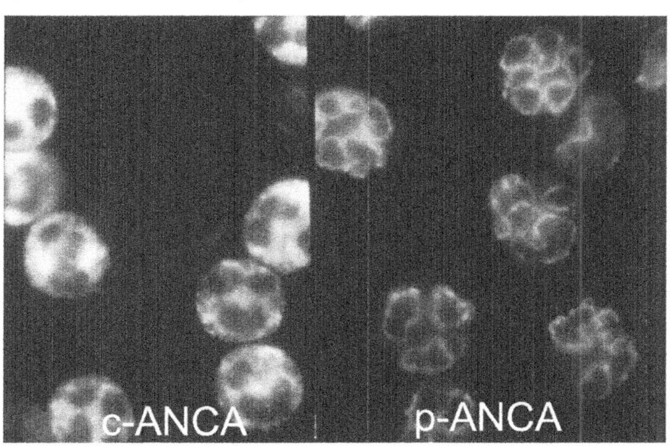

Figure 5. Detection of ANCA by indirect immunofluorescence. A C-ANCA pattern is seen on the left, a P-ANCA pattern on the right.

The idea that neutrophils are paramount in the initiation of vasculitic injury is supported by the abundance of this cell species in highly active tissue lesions. MPO, which is a readily detected marker of neutrophil degranulation, is abundant in inflammatory lesions in the kidneys (Brouwer et al., 1994; Mrowka et al., 1995) and in orbital tissue (Trocme et al., 1991). Elevated levels of MPO, together with eosinophil cationic protein, were also measured in the BAL fluid in pulmonary active Wegener's granulomatosis and declined in response to clinically effective immunosuppression (Schnabel et al., 1999a–c).

Physiologically, PR3 is largely confined to myeloid cells (Hoffman and Specks, 1998). However, recent studies on inflammatory tissues found PR3 also in non-myeloid cells. Specifically, these are vascular endothelial cells (Mayet et al., 1993), renal tubular and glomerular cells (Schwarting et al., 2000), and resident pulmonary cells (Brockmann et al., 2002). The expression of PR3 was found to be upregulated in pneumocytes type I and II in lung tissue from pulmonary active Wegener's granulomatosis patients (Brockmann et al., 2002). Moreover, PR3 can adhere to endothelial surfaces and can be taken up by endothelial cells, arguably via receptor-mediated endocytosis (van der Geld et al., 2001). This suggests that not only neutrophils but also a broader spectrum of cell types may be the target of ANCA-mediated immune injury. Alternatively, PR3 might exert a direct toxic effect on these cells by use of its proteolytic properties (Preston et al., 2002a,b).

By engaging their target antigen, ANCA can also promote the release of inflammatory mediators from neutrophils. ANCA binding to neutrophils enhances the transcription of IL-1β, IL-8, and cyclooxygenase 2 genes (Yang et al., 2001). Phagocytosis of apoptotic neutrophils by macrophages elicits the release of proinflammatory cytokines if the apoptotic cells are opsonized by ANCA, whereas the uptake of non-opsonized cells lacks this effect (Moosig et al., 2000).

5. Clinical manifestations

In the majority of cases, Wegener's granulomatosis takes a biphasic course (Gross et al., 1992). Initial disease is confined to the respiratory tract (so-called localized WG). Prototypical disease starts in the upper respiratory tract with chronic rhinitis, sinusitis or mastoiditis. Patients complain of chronic discharge that is often putride or sanguinolent, and crusting discharge is common. The histopathological basis of this chronic progressive disorder is granulomatous inflammation. It is a destructive process that can lead to collapse of the nasal cartilaginous structures, resulting in saddle nose deformity, and the destruction of the osseous membranes between the nasal cavity, the sinuses and the orbit (Hoffman et al., 1992). Orbital disease can lead to proptosis, impaired bulbar motility, and optic nerve injury. Granulomatous, osteodestructive rhinitis or sinusitis should always stimulate a strong suspicion of Wegener's granulomatosis. The destruction of the cartilaginous and osseous structures is readily detected by computed tomography (CT) or MRI (Fig. 6) (Muhle et al., 1996).

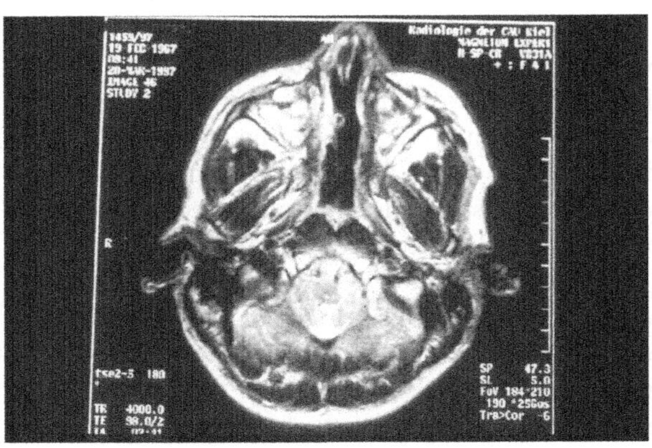

Figure 6. Maxillar sinus opacification and destruction of the nasal septum, conchae and parts of the lateral walls of the nasal cavity in Wegener's granulomatosis. MRI scan.

Occasionally, initial disease manifests with granulomatous disease of the lower respiratory tract (Katzenstein and Locke, 1995). Nodules or irregular masses in the chest radiograph without accompanying upper respiratory tract disease prompt suspicion of neoplastic or infectious lung disease until their true nature is disclosed by biopsy.

Characteristically, constitutional symptoms are absent in localized WG. The same applies to the serologic markers of inflammation. The erythrocyte sedimentation rate (ESR) and C-reactive protein (CRP) are only marginally elevated, if at all, and ANCA is detected in only half of the patients.

Localized WG can persist for many years, but most untreated patients appear to progress to generalized disease within several months or a few years. In generalized disease, the signs and symptoms of systemic vasculitis are superimposed upon granulomatous disease (Hoffman et al., 1992). Symptoms in other organs beyond the respiratory tract are mostly in the form of non-granulomatous inflammation. The most common disease manifestations outside the respiratory tract are glomerulonephritis; scleritis or episcleritis; polyneuropathy or mononeuropathy; arthralgia, arthritis or myalgia; cutaneous vasculitis; digital gangrene; perimyocarditis or coronariitis; and focal encephalitis (Hoffman et al., 1992; Reinhold-Keller et al., 2000). Necrotizing small-vessel vasculitis is the hallmark lesion in these organ manifestations, but ischaemia due to inflammatory involvement of intermediate or large arteries can occur. Constitutional symptoms are prominent in generalized disease, as are the serologic markers of

Table 7
Synopsis of granulomatous and vasculitis respiratory tract disease in Wegener's granulomatosis

Granulomatous disease
Upper respiratory tract: rhinitis, sinusitis, mastoiditis, subglottic stenosis
Lower respiratory tract: nodules, masses, septal, non-septal lines, ulcerative tracheitis, bronchitis, inflammatory pseudotumours, stenosing/obliterative bronchitis
Vasculitic disease
Pneumonitis, pulmonary capillaritis/diffuse alveolar haemorrhage

inflammation. More than 90% of these patients are positive for ANCA (Tables 7 and 8).

5.1. Granulomatous lung disease

Pulmonary Wegener's granulomatosis can be either granulomatous or vasculitic. Most patients seen in clinical practise do not show either disease expression in its pure form but rather a combination of the two. Nonetheless, a separate discussion of the two facets of the disease promotes an understanding of the diversity of clinical manifestations and the reconciliation of seemingly contradictory findings.

Single or multiple nodules or masses are the most common finding in granulomatous pulmonary disease

Table 8
Organ system involvement in Wegener's granulomatosis at diagnosis and throughout the disease

	At diagnosis (%)	Throughout disease (%)
Upper respiratory tract	73–93	92–99
Kidneys	18–54	70–77
Lower respiratory tract	45–55	66–85
Ophthalmic	15–40	52–61
Cardiac	13	8–25
Peripheral nervous system	21	15–40
Central nervous system	6	8–11
Gastrointestinal tract	3	6
Cutaneous	13–21	33–46
Musculo-skeletal	32–61	67–77

According to Hoffman et al. (1992) and Reinhold-Keller et al. (2000).

(Fig. 7) (Cordier et al., 1990; Hoffman et al., 1992; Reuter et al., 1998). Cavitation is fairly common and is detected more often in CT scans than on plain radiography (Reuter et al., 1998; Attali et al., 1998). Computed tomography proved also to be more sensitive in the detection of nodules than plain radiography. However, many of the small nodules that are detected by CT but evade plain radiography proved to be unresponsive to immunosuppression and appear therefore to be cicatricial. Nodules exceeding 3 cm and cavitating nodules generally recede in response to immunosuppression and thus reflect active inflammatory disease, whereas small nodules without cavitation are heterogeneous in their response to treatment (Attali et al., 1998; Komocsi et al., 2002).

The introduction of high-resolution computed tomography (HRCT) further augmented the spectrum of pulmonary lesions in Wegener's granulomatosis (Reuter et al., 1998; Komocsi et al., 2002). In addition to nodules and masses, HRCT discloses septal and non-septal thickening, focal ground-glass opacities, centrilobular interstitial thickening, bronchial wall thickening and, less commonly, bronchiectasis (Fig. 8). Only ground-glass opacities are invariably responsive to immunosuppression, whereas septal and non-septal lines are heterogeneous in their response to treatment, suggesting that they can be either active inflammatory or cicatricial (Komocsi et al., 2002). In aggregate, HRCT is obviously more sensitive in the detection of parenchymal lung disease than plain radiography, but offers little extra value in the distinction between active and inactive disease. In contrast, the nodules and masses that are detected by plain radiography regularly respond to immunosuppression, which marks them as inflammatory active.

The clinical symptoms of nodular lung disease are often unimpressive. Complaints like cough, hemoptysis or dyspnoea are the exception rather than the rule. Spirometry is commonly of no help in detecting or monitoring nodular lung disease. Granulomatous inflammation is also a common feature of tracheobronchial disease. This is discussed below.

5.2. Vasculitic lung disease

Vasculitic lung disease is commonly associated with highly active systemic disease. Radiographically, it

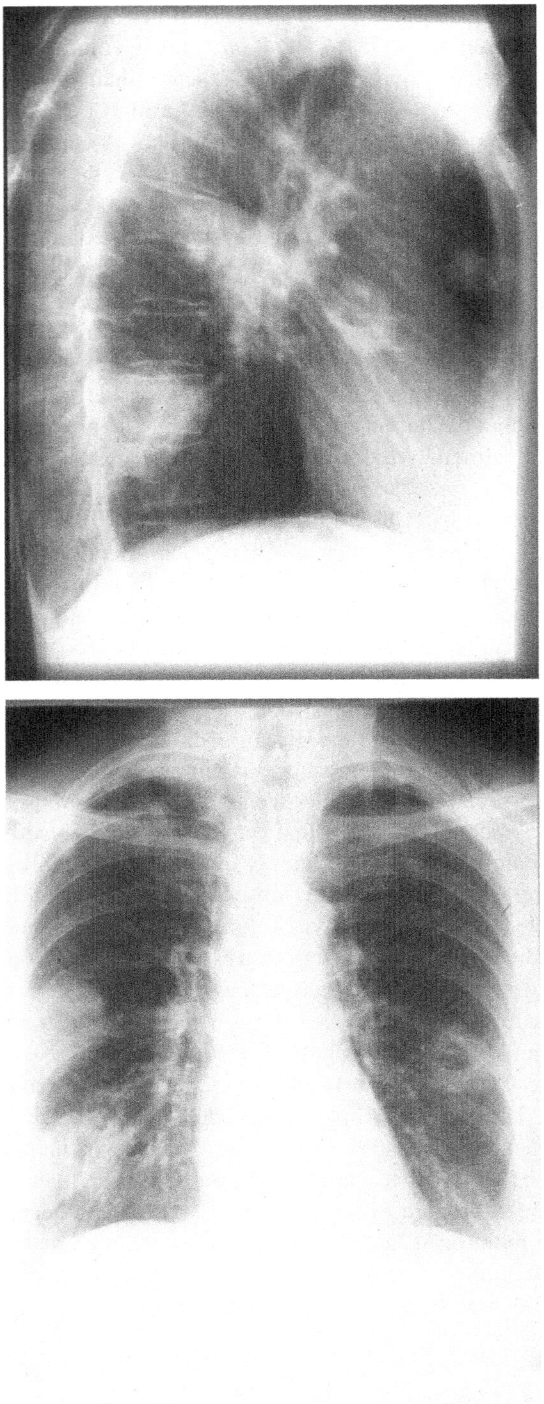

A

B

Figure 7. Chest radiograph with multiple cavitating and non-cavitating nodules in Wegener's granulomatosis.

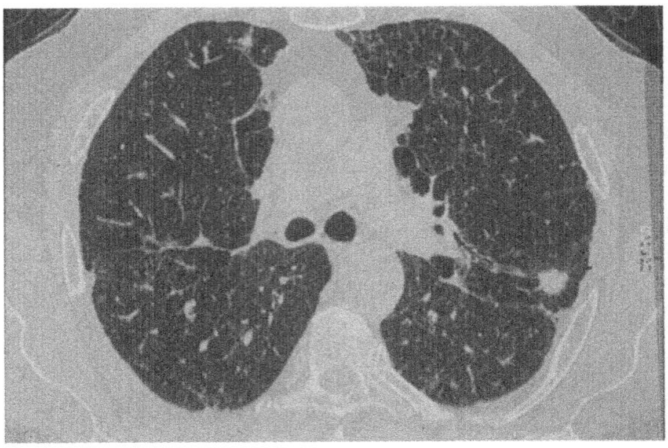

Figure 8. Subcarinal high-resolution CT section in Wegener's granulomatosis, showing small nodules, septal and non-septal lines, suggestive of granulomatous lung disease.

features localized or disseminated poorly defined opacities (Fig. 9) (Cordier et al., 1990). The underlying histopathology is an alveolitis with thickening of the alveolar septae by a mixed inflammatory infiltrate and airspace filling with granulocytes and mononuclear cells, accompanied by florid small-vessel vasculitis (Yoshikawa and Watanabe, 1985) (Table 9). The clinical picture of highly active Wegener's granulomatosis pneumonitis is dramatic. It includes progressive malaise, dyspnoea and cough that commonly evolve over a

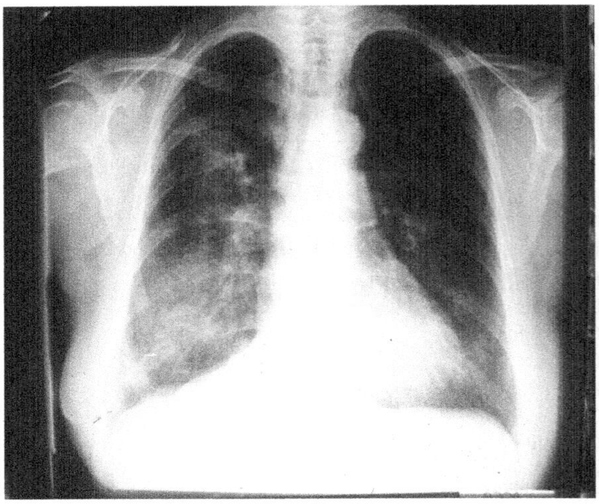

Figure 9. Chest radiograph in florid pneumonitis due to Wegener's granulomatosis, showing bilateral ill-defined opacities.

Table 9
Histopathologic features of pulmonary capillaritis

Deposition of erythrocytes or haemosiderin in the pulmonary interstitium
Fibrinoid necrosis in pulmonary vessels
Alveolar capillary occlusion by fibrin thrombi
Interstitial neutrophilia and leukocytoklasia with nuclear dust
Fibrin clots attached to alveolar septa

couple of days. Occasionally, the clinical picture may develop within a few hours. Hypoxemia without carbon dioxide retention is common and the clinical condition can deteriorate rapidly when accompanying renal failure due to glomerulonephritis leads to fluid overload (Yoshikawa and Watanabe, 1985; Cordier et al., 1990).

The pulmonary findings of Wegener's granulomatosis pneumonitis can be indistinguishable from infectious pneumonitis. Microbiologic studies should therefore be vigorously pursued and treatment must target conventional bacterial agents as well as opportunistic agents. The presence of multisystem disease and of ANCA in most patients aids the diagnosis of Wegener's granulomatosis but they do not, in themselves, rule out coexisting infection.

5.3. Pulmonary capillaritis—diffuse alveolar haemorrhage

Pulmonary capillaritis leading to the syndrome of diffuse alveolar haemorrhage (DAH) is a variant of vasculitic lung disease. (Travis et al., 1990; Bosch et al., 1994). The clinical and radiographic appearance of clinically manifest capillaritis is that of vasculitic lung disease, on which is superimposed the syndrome of DAH. The full-blown picture of DAH is characterized by dyspnoea, diffuse alveolar opacities, and a low or decreasing haemoglobin level (Specks, 2001). Radiographically, the perihilar regions tend to be more intensely affected than the lung periphery and in most instances the disorder is bilateral (Fig. 10).

The extent of the histopathological features of capillaritis is quite variable. It ranges from scattered foci of parenchymal bleeding to widespread haemorrhage (Travis et al., 1990). This is paralleled by the range of clinical expressions, from subclinical to

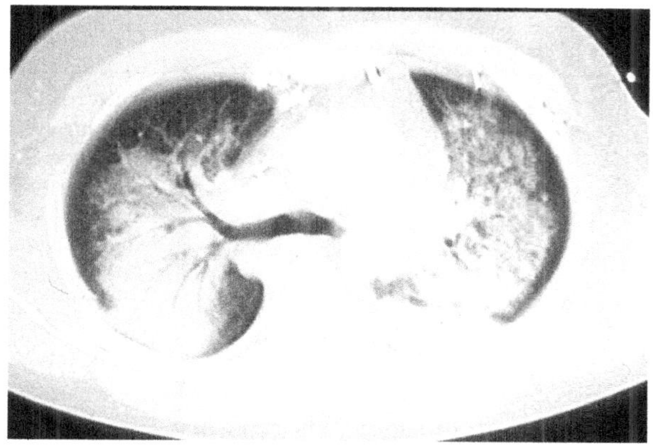

Figure 10. Diffuse alveolar haemorrhage due to Wegener's granulomatosis. A pulmonary CT section at the level of the main carina shows centrally accentuated parenchymal opacities with an air bronchogramm on the right side.

severe, life-threatening disease (Specks, 2001). In mild forms of the disease, haemoptysis and dyspnoea may not be present. These patients may have scattered soft opacities in the chest radiograph or even a normal chest film. On bronchoscopy, there is no overt blood in the bronchial tree, but BAL yields a reddish or brownish fluid containing erythrocytes, siderophages or a combination of the two (Schnabel et al., 1999a–c). At the severe end of the spectrum are the patients with overt haemoptysis, extensive dense opacities on the chest radiograph, haemorrhagic material spilling from multiple bronchial orifices, circulatory instability due to volume loss and rapidly evolving anaemia (Hayworth et al., 1985; Ter Maaten et al., 1996). Patients experiencing this life-threatening disorder may report a premonitory phase with repeated bouts of blood-streaked sputum. This calls for careful evaluation of Wegener's granulomatosis patients presenting with a recent history of haemoptysis.

Clinically manifest DAH is commonly accompanied by intense constitutional symptoms and strikingly elevated ESR and CRP (Hayworth et al., 1985; Ter Maaten et al., 1996). Patients with isolated DAH due to Wegener's granulomatosis have been encountered, but in the vast majority of cases DAH occurs in the setting of multi-organ disease. Most patients with overt DAH have a pulmonary-renal syndrome, i.e. a combination of pulmonary capillaritis and glomerulonephritis (Bosch et al., 1994; Travis et al., 1990; Ter Maaten et al., 1996).

Table 10
Causes of the pulmonary–renal syndrome

Common causes	ANCA associated vasculitides, Wegener's granulomatosis, microscopic polyangiitis rarely Churg-Strauss syndrome	60%
	Goodpastures syndrome, systemic lupus erythematosus (SLE)	20–30%
Rare causes	Cryoglobulinaemic vasculitis, Henoch-Schönlein disease, Behçet's disease, rheumatoid vasculitis, collagen diseases other than SLE, antiphospholipid syndrome, thrombotic thrombocytopenic purpura, drug-induced disease: penicillamine hydralazine, propylthiouracil	10%

The latter is commonly a rapidly progressive type of disease, the underlying histopathology being a pauci-immune crescentic glomerulonephritis. The coincidence of these two organ manifestations in an individual patient is an important diagnostic feature, strongly suggesting a vasculitic origin and virtually excluding other aetiologies of pulmonary bleeding, among which are coagulation disorders, neoplasia, valvular heart disease, vascular malformations and veno-occlusive disease (Specks, 2001).

A limited number of other immune diseases can evoke a pulmonary-renal syndrome (Table 10). ANCA-associated vasculitides account for approximately 60% of the cases, Goodpasture's syndrome and systemic lupus erythematosus for approximately 20–30% and the remainder is made up of a variety of conditions, several of which have other serologic markers (e.g. distinctive ANA specificities, anti-cardiolipin antibodies, cryoglobulins). Large retrospective studies demonstrate that 80–90% of the patients with pulmonary-renal syndrome feature autoantibodies or other immune markers (Niles et al., 1996; Gallagher et al., 2002). Serologic testing therefore greatly facilitates a tentative diagnosis of the underlying disorder and thereby hastens targeted treatment. The presence of IgM plus IgG ANCA was found to be strongly associated with DAH (Esnault et al., 1992), but immunoglobulin isotype-specific ANCA tests are not routinely available in most clinical laboratories.

The formerly dismal prognosis of DAH and the pulmonary-renal syndrome has improved. The two conditions are still amongst the leading causes of intensive care unit treatment in vasculitis patients. Early mortality formerly amounted to 70% but dropped to 35–45% in recent series (Niles et al., 1996; Gallagher et al., 2002). Early in the course, refractory hypoxaemia due to vasculitic damage is the prevailing cause of death, whereas late fatalities relate mostly to infectious complications.

5.4. Airway disease

Wegener's granulomatosis can affect any segment of the upper and lower airways. The introduction of bronchoscopy into the care of Wegener's granulomatosis patients disclosed airway involvement in a substantial proportion of the patients, ranging between 26 and 59% (Cordier et al., 1990; Daum et al., 1995; Schnabel et al., 1997). In addition to a non-specific tracheobronchitis, a number of characteristic lesions are encountered in Wegener's granulomatosis patients. These comprise, in decreasing order of frequency:

1. Ulcerative tracheitis or bronchitis with or without mucosal bleeding.
2. Inflammatory nodules and pseudotumours (Fig. 11).
3. Segmental stenosis.

The most common complaints in affected patients are non-productive cough or cough with small amounts of blood-streaked sputum; dyspnoea on exertion; and stridor or wheezing. Grossly productive cough is uncommon in Wegener's granulomatosis and gives rise to the suspicion that an infectious complication is involved. The sensitivity of the chest radiograph for detecting tracheobronchial disease is low. The roentgenographically detected sequelae of stenosing airway disease, namely segmental, lobar or one-sided loss of volume, generally reflect advanced disease with high-grade stenosis (Fig. 12). The same applies to spirometry, the sensitivity of which is poor in the event of non-stenosing disease or stenotic disease of peripheral airways.

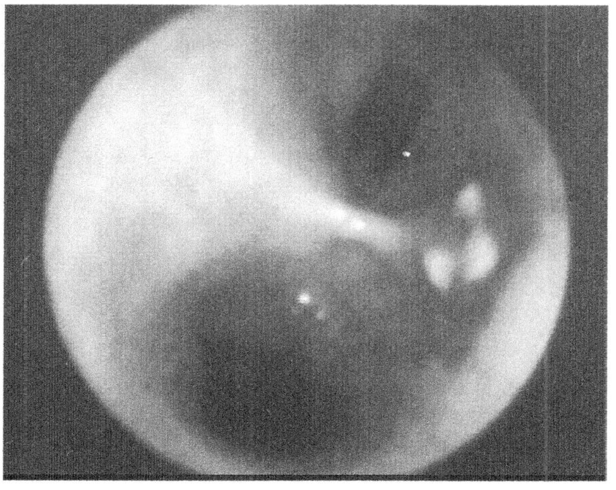

Figure 11. Bronchoscopic view of granulomatous nodules at the main carina in Wegener's granulomatosis.

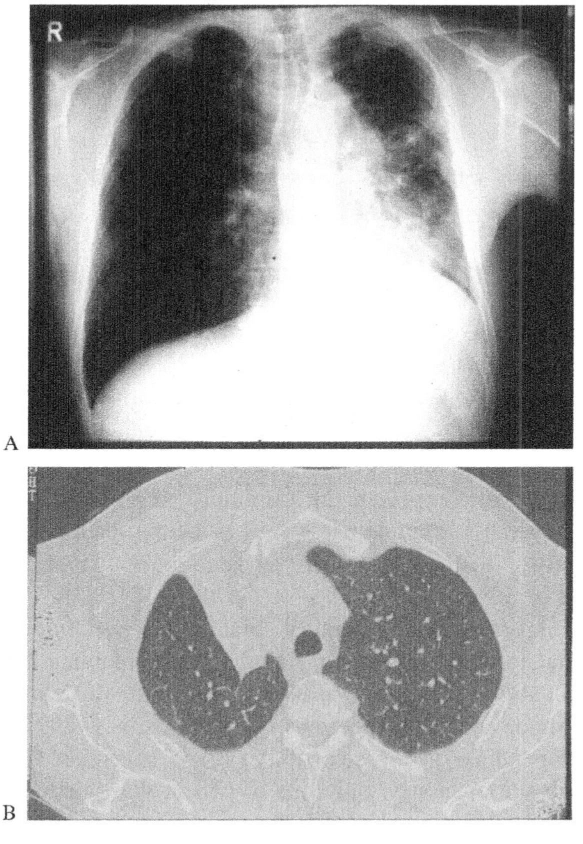

Figure 12. Stenosing and obliterative airway disease in Wegener's granulomatosis. The radiograph on the left (A) shows loss of volume of the right (B) lung to due stenosis of the to main stem bronchus; the apical CT section on the right shows segmental atelactasis.

A peculiar lesion in Wegener's granulomatosis is subglottic stenosis. It is encountered in 10–23% of Wegener's granulomatosis patients (Lebovics et al., 1992; Daum et al., 1995; Langford et al., 1996). A sexual preponderance is not apparent, but patients with a disease onset at young age appear to be more often affected than patients with disease of late onset (Lebovics et al., 1992; Langford et al., 1996). Characteristically, the lesion is located 3–5 cm below the glottis, leading to concentric or eccentric stenosis (Fig. 13). In addition to cough and hoarseness, patients complain of dyspnoea and inspiratory stridor. The flow-volume curve on spirometry shows inspiratory and expiratory limitation of flow (Langford et al., 1996; Daum et al., 1995) (Fig. 14). In advanced disease, segmental stenosis of the proximal trachea is visible in the chest radiograph. Less advanced lesions are visualized accurately by spiral CT (Screaton et al., 1998), but laryngoscopy or bronchoscopy remain the methods of choice for evaluation and monitoring.

Subglottic stenosis can develop in the absence of other disease manifestations of Wegener's granulomatosis; in rare instances, it is the presenting feature of Wegener's granulomatosis. In one series, only half the patients presenting with tracheal stenosis had concomitant systemic disease activity (Langford et al., 1996). It is also of note that in many instances the lesion responds poorly to systemic treatment. In the aforementioned series, half the patients were diagnosed with this lesion whilst receiving immunosuppressive treatment.

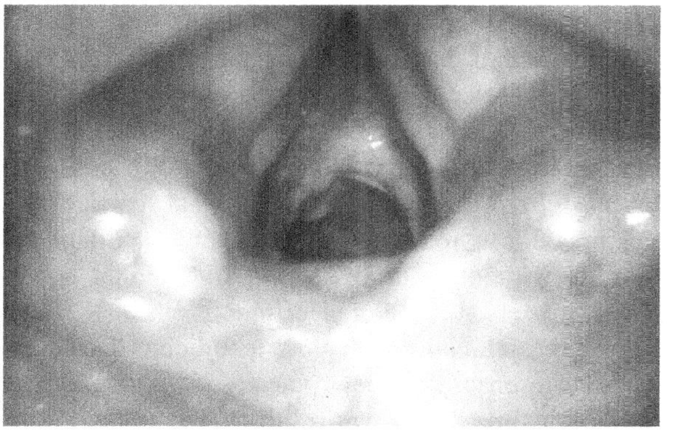

Figure 13. Laryngoscopic view of subglottic stenosis due to Wegener's granulomatosis.

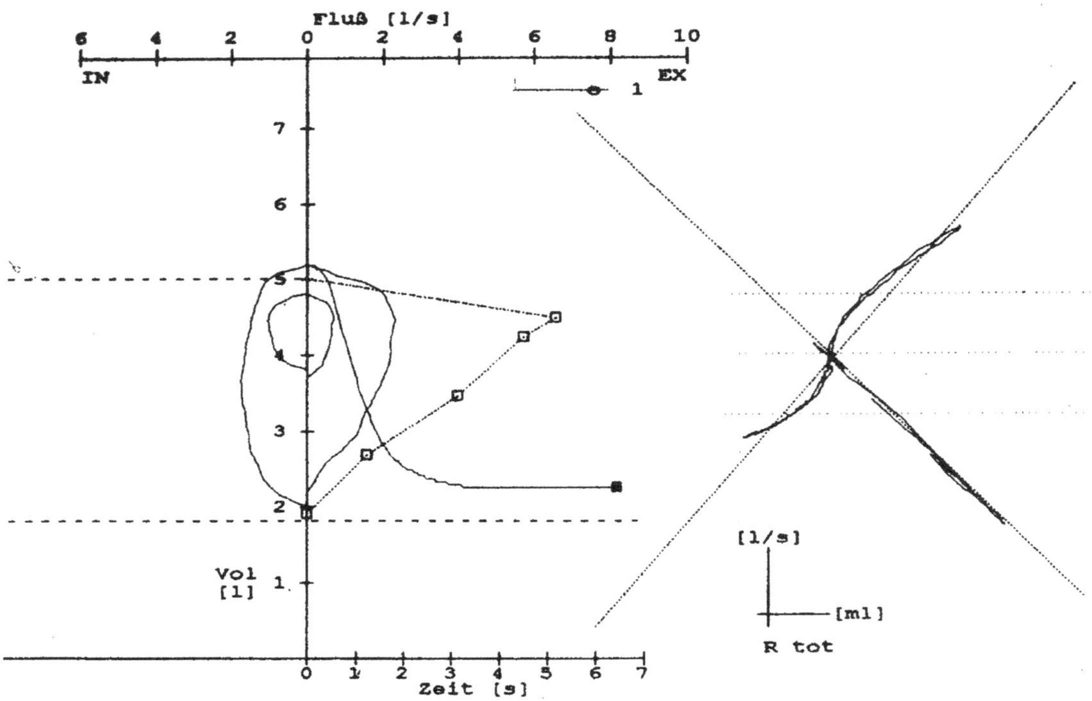

Figure 14. Flow–volume curve and body plethysmographic tracing in a patient with high-grade subglottic stenosis due to Wegener's granulomatosis, showing inspiratory and expiratory limitation of flow.

Subglottic stenosis commonly takes a progressive course that, before the introduction of effective treatment, resulted in the need for tracheostomy in many patients (McDonald et al., 1982; Lebovics et al., 1992). Topical treatment has been applied in the form of mechanical removal of tissue, ablation by laser, irradiation, rigid bronchoscopic dilatation, stenting and reconstructive surgery. Commonly, these interventions provided only relief of limited duration and it has been emphasized that thermal ablation by laser can further compromise the local situation by excessive scarring (Hoffmann et al., 2003). Encouraging results were obtained by laryngoscopically applied intralesional corticosteroid injections, followed by mechanical dilatation with or without microdissection of lesional tissue (Langford et al., 1996; Hoffmann et al., 2003). Repeated application of this technique has been reported to ensure tracheal patency over progressive periods of time and it can result in decannulation in patients who failed to improve with other forms of topical treatment.

6. Diagnostic investigations

6.1. Biopsy procedures

A compatible clinical picture in association with a positive PR3-ANCA test provides strong evidence in favour of a diagnosis of Wegener's granulomatosis. However, experienced clinicians maintain that Wegener's granulomatosis is a clinico-pathologic entity, histopathological verification of which is imperative.

From a histopathological point of view, a definitive diagnosis of Wegener's granulomatosis requires the coexistence of three principal features: vasculitis, granuloma, and necrosis (Travis et al., 1991). Depending on the size of the tissue specimen and the site of biopsy, only one or two of these features may be found, which renders the biopsy suggestive but not conclusive (Devaney et al., 1990). Nonetheless, non-diagnostic but suggestive histological appearances can provide crucial diagnostic support when associated with a typical clinical picture and positive ANCA serology.

Open or thoracoscopic lung biopsy has long been considered to be the biopsy method of choice in Wegener's granulomatosis with pulmonary involvement (Mark et al., 1988; Hoffman et al., 1992; Travis et al., 1991). The high diagnostic yield needs to be balanced against its invasive nature and the associated risks. Transbronchial biopsy yields diagnostically helpful specimens if targeted to radiographically abnormal lung segments or endoscopically visualized tracheobronchial lesions (Lombard et al., 1990; Daum et al., 1995; Schnabel et al., 1997). By contrast, transbronchial biopsy of the minor interstitial changes that are detected by HRCT adds little (Schnabel et al., 1997). Image-guided percutaneous core needle biopsy can also result in adequate tissue specimens, but experience with this technique is limited (Carruthers et al., 2000).

Most patients with Wegener's granulomatosis lung disease have concomitant upper respiratory tract involvement (Hoffman et al., 1992; Reinhold-Keller et al., 2000). Endoscopic biopsy from lesions within the nasal cavity and biopsy from sinusoidal lesions visualized by CT or MRI (Muhle et al., 1996) yield a high number of adequate specimens (Reinhold-Keller et al., 2000; Schnabel et al., 1997). The histopathological triad of vasculitis, granuloma, and necrosis is found in only a minority of specimens (Devaney et al., 1990). However, either granuloma or vasculitis in an upper respiratory tract biopsy in association with a clinical picture suggestive of Wegener's granulomatosis and a PR3-ANCA confers a high degree of diagnostic confidence. Alternative biopsy sites are the kidney, the skin, and skeletal muscle, provided that lesional tissue is sampled (Hoffman et al., 1992; Reinhold-Keller et al., 2000).

6.2. Bronchoalveolar lavage

Granulomatous and vasculitic lung disease in Wegener's granulomatosis is associated with distinct BAL cell profiles. Bronchoalveolar lavage lymphocytosis is commonly found in patients with the radiological features of granulomatous lung disease (Schnabel et al., 1999a–c). Approximately two-thirds of these patients have an elevated CD4/CD8 ratio. A depressed CD4/CD8 ratio in the BAL fluid is rare in Wegener's granulomatosis patients and demands careful exclusion of an alternative aetiology, particularly viral or fungal infection.

Patients with diffuse dense opacities in the chest radiograph, reflecting vasculitic lung disease, generally have BAL neutrophilia with or without accompanying lymphocytosis (Schnabel et al., 1999a–c). The magnitude of the BAL neutrophilia in Wegener's granulomatosis vasculitic disease depends on the severity of the disease and can overlap broadly with the range of neutrophilia seen in bacterial infection. Microbiological examination of the BAL material is therefore indispensable.

Highly-active DAH features haemorrhagic discharge from multiple bronchial orifices. Less severe forms of DAH feature only localized traces of endobronchial blood or entirely lack visible blood. Fractionated BAL yields progressively reddish fluid in the event of active bleeding (Fig. 15), or progressively brownish fluid in the event of remote bleeding (Schnabel et al., 1999a–c; Specks, 2001). On microscopical examination, erythrocytes abound in the former. In patients with protracted or remote alveolar bleeding, siderophages are found in numbers that range from a few percent to 90% (Schnabel et al., 1999a–c). Siderophages are alveolar macrophages that stain positive for iron in the Prussian blue stain (Fig. 16). Patients with more than 5% siderophages in the BAL fluid usually have clinical and serologic evidence of active systemic and pulmonary disease.

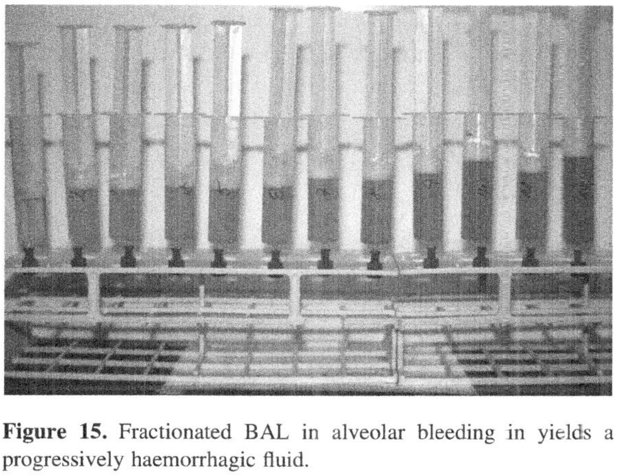

Figure 15. Fractionated BAL in alveolar bleeding in yields a progressively haemorrhagic fluid.

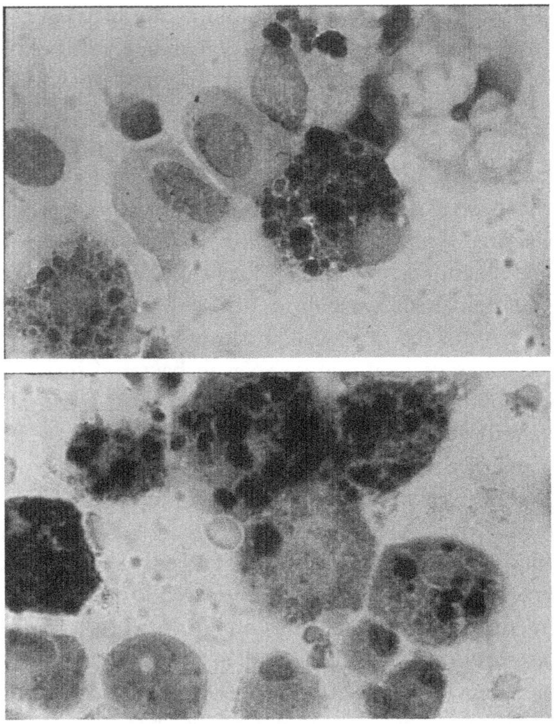

A

B

Figure 16. Microscopic view of cytocentrifuge preparations from BAL fluid in a patient with recent alveolar bleeding. The macrophages contain brownish material on May–Grünwald–Giemsa staining (A), which on Prussian blue staining (B) gives an intense blue colour, marking them as siderophages.

6.3. Diagnosis, staging, and scoring

In 1992, the Chapel-Hill Conference generated definitions for the most common vasculitic entities (Jennette et al., 1994). In 1990, classification criteria were provided by a working party of the American College of Rheumatology (Leavitt et al., 1990) (Table 1). These were intended not to be diagnostic criteria but to aid in the distinction between vasculitic entities.

The European Community Systemic Vasculitis Study Group (EUVAS) proposed five clinical subgroups for the ANCA-associated vasculitides that are presented in Table 2 (Jayne, 2001). The rationale was that treatment should be adapted to the initial extent and severity of the disease to improve outcome and minimize treatment toxicity. Subsequent therapeutic trials were designed to establish standard and best alternative treatment regimens for these subgroups.

Several scoring systems were proposed for the assessment of disease activity. The Birmingham Vasculitis Activity Score (BVAS) became widely accepted and evolved to be a current standard (Luqmani et al., 1994). In its most recent form, the BVAS also distinguishes between clinical features of worsening vasculitis and features of stable disease (Stone et al., 2001a,b). Definitions of remission and relapse proposed by EUVAS are mainly based on the BVAS. The disease extent index (DEI) gives an assessment at organ of involvement attributable to active disease (de Groot et al., 2001a,b).

A further category of disease severity is irreversible damage resulting from either disease or treatment. The systemic necrotizing vasculitis damage index (SNVDI) is applicable to Churg–Strauss syndrome and polyarteritis nodosa (Abu-Shakara et al., 1994), whereas the vasculitis damage index (VDI) is also applicable to other vasculitides (Exley et al., 1997). The BVAS, VDI, and the Short Form 36 (SF-36), which is a generic measure of function, were combined to give the vasculitis integrated total assessment log (VITAL) (Bacon et al., 1995). This provides a global picture of disease activity, damage, and the resulting functional status.

7. Treatment

A breakthrough in the treatment of Wegener's granulomatosis was the introduction of cyclophosphamide by Fauci et al. (1983). In contrast to corticosteroid monotherapy, which had only a marginal effect on disease outcome, intense immunosuppression by cyclophosphamide improved the long-term prognosis profoundly. However, the cost is substantial treatment-associated morbidity (Hoffman et al., 1992). This prompted an ongoing search for safer therapies and safer administration of available drugs.

Current remission-inducing treatment consists of intense immunosuppression of limited duration, which is followed by less intense maintenance treatment. As a standard regimen in full-blown disease, data from the EUVAS group now suggest cyclophosphamide 2.0 mg/kg body weight/day for induction of remission, for approximately 3–6 months, and subsequent maintenance treatment with azathioprine 2.0 mg/kg body weight/day (Jayne et al., 2003).

In patients with early systemic disease, i.e. without renal involvement and without immediately organ-threatening disease (NORAM study), methotrexate 0.3 mg/kg body weight/week proved to be equally effective to daily oral cyclophosphamide in the induction of remission (de Groot et al., 2001a,b). However, termination of treatment at month 12 was associated with a relapse rate of 69% in the methotrexate arm compared with 45% in the cyclophosphamide arm. Together with previous studies, the NORAM study suggests that methotrexate can replace daily oral cyclophosphamide for induction of remission, but the treatment needs to be extended beyond 12 months.

At the severe end of the disease spectrum, cyclophosphamide remains indispensable (Reinhold-Keller et al., 1994). The studies addressing the question whether intravenous pulse cyclophosphamide is a viable alternative for daily oral therapy, the potential advantage of the former regimen being lesser cumulative doses and, hopefully, less treatment-associated toxicity, are inconclusive (de Groot et al., 2001a,b). Results from the CYCLOPS study are expected to clarify this issue (Jayne, 2001).

Patients with advanced renal failure at the initiation of treatment have particularly poor renal and overall survival. The addition of either plasmapheresis or methylprednisolone pulse therapy to daily oral cyclophosphamide have been examined in the MEPEX study (Gaskin and Pusey, 2001). The addition of plasmapheresis resulted in better preservation of renal function than the addition of methylprednisolone pulses. However, mortality was high in both study arms (25%) and the question of whether organ involvement other than renal also benefits from plasma exchange has not been addressed.

High-dose intravenous immunoglobulin treatment has been employed as salvage therapy in difficult-to-treat Wegener's granulomatosis patients. Responses proved to be unpredictable and ranged between 30 and 70% (Richter et al., 1995; Jayne et al., 2000). Further trials involved monoclonal antibodies against CD52 (Campath-1H) or CD4 positive cells and anti-thymocyte globulin (Lockwood et al., 1993; Jayne, 2001). Recently published experience with TNF-α antagonists, i.e. infliximab or etanercept, in refractory Wegener's granulomatosis is promising (Stone et al., 2001a,b; Lamprecht et al., 2002a,b).

A number of drugs were used for maintenance of remission. In the CYCAZAREM study, azathioprine 2.0 mg/kg body weight/day was compared with cyclophosphamide 1.5 mg/kg body weight/day with respect to its ability to maintain remission (Jayne et al., 2003). During a follow-up period of 18 months, the two regimens were equally effective, rates of relapse being 15.5% in the former and 13.7% in the latter.

The optimal duration of maintenance treatment awaits further clarification. To this end, the REMAIN study examines whether maintenance treatment with azathioprine plus low-dose prednisolone given up to 42 months after primary diagnosis is more effective than the same regimen given up to 22 months after diagnosis (Jayne, 2001). Results from further studies are awaited which compare methotrexate with either leflunomide or azathioprine and azathioprine with mycophenolate mofetil.

Very interesting, although incompletely understood, is the beneficial effect of co-trimoxazole in Wegener's granulomatosis (DeRemee, 1988). Clinical observations suggest that this drug can retard the progression from localized to systemic disease and a placebo-controlled study demonstrates its remission-maintaining effect (Stegeman et al., 1996). This drug is particularly attractive for its favourable tolerability.

Table 11 summarizes the current evidence. Corticosteroids are generally added to any of the aforementioned immunosuppressives. A prednisolone dose of 0.8–1.0 mg/kg body weight/day is given initially, followed by tapering to a maintenance dose of 5–7.5 mg. Mega-doses of corticosteroids commonly have a beneficial effect in immediately organ-threatening disease, such as florid pneumonitis or highly-active capillaritis, although experimental evidence to this effect is missing.

7.1. Treatment toxicity

A large proportion of treatment toxicity in Wegener's granulomatosis is attributable to cyclophosphamide and corticosteroids. In the cohort from the National Institutes of Health that comprised mainly patients diagnosed and treated in the 1970s and 1980s (Hoffman et al., 1992), toxicity attributable to

Table 11
Therapy of Wegener's granulomatosis (WG)

Stage	Therapy	Dose	Reference	Evidence
Induction therapy				
Localized WG	Cotrimoxazole	2 × 960 mg/day p.o.	Reinhold-Keller et al. (1996)	IIa/A
Early systemic WG	Methotrexate	0.3 mg/kg/week i.v.	Langford et al. (1996)	IIb/A
Generalized WG	Cyclophosphamide	2 mg/kg/day p.o.	Hoffman et al. (1992)	IIb/A
	Cyclophosphamide	15–20 mg/kg/3–4 weeks i.v.	Haubitz et al. (1998)	Ib/A
Maintenance therapy				
Generalized WG	Azathioprine	2 mg/kg/day p.o.	Jayne et al. (2003)	I-b/A
Generalized WG	Methotrexate	0.3 mg/kg/week i.v.	Langford et al. (1996)	II-b/B
Generalized WG	Leflunomide	30 mg/day p.o.	Metzler et al. (2004)	III/C
Generalized WG	Cyclosporine A	2.5–5 mg/kg/day p.o.	Haubitz et al. (1998)	III/C
Generalized WG	Mycophenolate mofetil	2 g/day p.o.	Nowack et al. (1999)	III/C
Generalized WG/ Early systemic WG	Cotrimoxazole	2 × 960 mg/day p.o.	Stegeman et al. (1996)	I-b/A
Escalation therapy				
Refractory WG	Cyclophosphamide	2–4 mg/kg/day p.o.	Hoffman et al. (1992)	II-b/B
Refractory WG	Etanercept	25 mg/2 × week s.c.	Stone et al. (2001a,b)	II-b/B
Refractory WG	Infliximab	5 mg/kg/every 4–6 weeks i.v.	Lamprecht et al. (2002)	II-b/B
Refractory WG	Rituximab	375 mg/m^2/every 4 weeks i.v.	Specks et al. (2001)	III/B
Refractory WG	Intravenous immunoglobulin	0.4 g/kg/day i.v. for 5 days	Jayne and Lockwood (1996)	II-b/A
Refractory WG	Anti-thymocyte globuline	5 mg/kg i.v. for 10 days		III/C
Refractory WG	Anti-CD4 (YNB 46.1 or hIgG1CD4) and/or anti-CD52 (hIgG1CD52 = Campath-1H)	20 mg i.v. for 5–12 days and/or 2–40 mg i.v. for 5–8 days	Lockwood et al. (1993)	III/C
Refractory WG	15-Deoxyspergualin	0.5 mg/kg/day for 2–3 weeks, 6 cycles	Birck et al. (2003)	IIb/C

Stages according to Jayne et al. (2000) (see Table 2). Levels of evidence: I-a, supported by meta-analysis; I-b, at least one randomized, controlled study; II-a, at least one good controlled study; II-b, at least one good, virtually experimental study; III, at least one good descriptive study; IV, clinical experience or consensus; Strength of evidence: A, strong evidence, support; B, satisfactory evidence, support; C, weak evidence, support; D, good evidence, reject; E, strong evidence, reject.

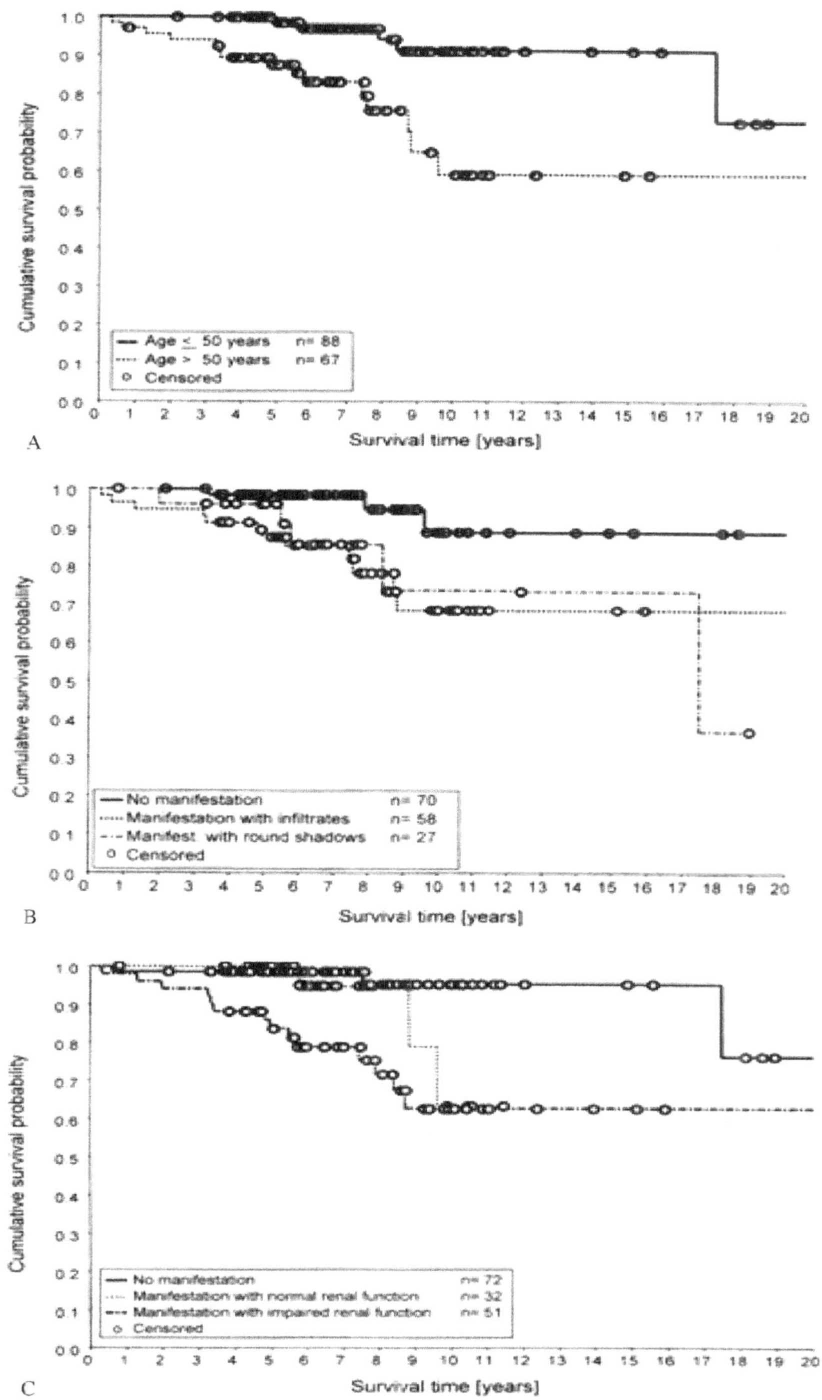

Figure 17. Kaplan–Meier graphs depicting survival in Wegener's granulomatosis, depending on (A) age at diagnosis, (B) lung involvement at diagnosis and (C) kidney involvement at diagnosis (from Reinhold-Keller et al., 2000).

cyclophosphamide was dominated by chemocystitis (43%), bladder cancer (2.8%), myelodysplasia (2%) and, in a subset of women in the fertile age, amenorrhoea (57%). A 2.4 overall increase in malignant neoplasia and an 11-fold increase in lymphomas were observed. Serious infections were observed in 46% of the patients and included mainly conventional bacterial agents, but also mycobacteria, *Pneumocystis carinii*, other fungi and cutaneous zoster. Pneumonias accounted for 39% of the serious infections. In this study, daily prednisolone given over extended periods of time in substantial doses emerged as a principal risk factor for infections and a substantial reduction in infectious complications was documented in a later study that adhered to rapid dose reduction (Reinhold-Keller et al., 2000). Prophylaxis with low-dose co-trimoxazole against *P. carinii* has been advocated if higher doses of corticosteroids over extended periods of time are inevitable (Ognibene et al., 1995; Yale and Limper, 1996).

7.2. Long-term outcome

Before the introduction of cyclophosphamide into the treatment of Wegener's granulomatosis, the mean survival was only 5 months. Survival in the Luebeck cohort, which comprises 155 consecutive Wegener's granulomatosis patients treated in the 1990s, was 88% after 10 years and the estimated median survival after diagnosis was 21.7 years. Age over 50 years, pulmonary involvement, and renal involvement at diagnosis were found to be significant predictors of survival time (Fig. 17), hazard ratios of all-cause mortality being 5.45, 3.75, and 4.45 in these conditions.

Relapses after effective treatment remain a continuing problem. In the aforementioned study, the rate of relapses among the patients followed for at least 5 years amounted to 71%. The NIH study, which comprised a comparable patient cohort, reported 50% relapses. The latter cohort was treated with higher cumulative doses of cyclophosphamide and corticosteroids. Obviously, this blunted the number of relapses, but it was also associated with a higher number of severe infections (46 versus 26% in the Luebeck cohort).

Organ damage that accumulates over time is common in Wegener's granulomatosis patients, this resulting from either the disease itself or the treatment. Chronic renal insufficiency, hearing loss, nasal deformities, tracheal stenosis, and loss of vision make up a large share of disease-related permanent damage. Treatment-related morbidity has been outlined above. Chronic sinus dysfunction and pulmonary insufficiency often relate to the combined effects of disease and medication.

In aggregate, these figures signify that the management of Wegener's granulomatosis is a long-term endeavour, a central aspect of which is to strike a balance between the need to prevent accumulating damage originating from chronic-progressive disease and the importance of avoiding treatment-related morbidity.

Key points

- Pulmonary involvement is common in Wegener's granulomatosis.
- Wegener's granulomatosis affects the respiratory tract in the form of granulomatous disease, vasculitis, or a combination of the two.
- Infections such as *S. aureus*, other environmental influences, or 'Wegener's autoantigen' proteinase 3 (PR3) itself are thought to play a role in triggering and/or maintaining disease activity in Wegener's granulomatosis on the basis of a genetic predisposition to an exaggerated Th1-type response.
- The detection of ANCA directed against proteinase 3 (PR3-ANCA) is highly specific for Wegener's granulomatosis.
- The diagnosis is based on clinical presentation, detection of PR3-ANCA, and bioptic findings.
- BAL and imaging techniques may support the diagnosis by alveolitis and diffuse alveolar haemorrhage subsequent to inflammation and capillaritis.
- Standard treatment in organ- and life-threatening full-blown disease consists of cyclophosphamide 2.0 mg/kg body weight/-day for the induction of remission, for approximately 3–6 months, and subsequent maintenance treatment with azathioprine 2.0 mg/kg body weight/day.

References

Abdou, N.I., Kullman, G.J., Hoffman, G.S., Sharp, G.C., Specks, U., McDonald, T., Garrity, J., Goeken, J.A., Allen, N.B. 2002. Wegener's granulomatosis: survey of 701 patients in North America. Changes in outcome in the 1990s. J. Rheumatol. 29, 309.

Abu-Shakara, M., Smythe, H., Lewtas, J., Badley, E., Weber, D., Keystone, E. 1994. Outcome of polyarteritis nodosa and Churg–Strauss syndrome. An analysis of twenty-five patients. Arthritis Rheum. 37, 1798–1803.

Attali, P., Begum, R., Ben Romdhane, H., Valere, D., Guillevin, L., Brauner, M.W. 1998. Pulmonary Wegener's granulomatosis: changes and follow-up CT. Eur. Radiol. 8, 1009–1113.

Bacon, P.A., Moots, R., Exley, A., Luqmani, R., Rasmussen, N. 1995. VITAL (Vasculitis Integrated Total Assessment Log) assessment of vasculitis. Clin. Exp. Rheumatol. 13, 275–278.

Bajema, I.M., Hagen, E.C., Ferrario, F., Waldherr, R., Noel, L.H., Hermans, J., van der Woude, F.J., Bruijn, J.A. 1998. Renal granulomas in systemic vasculitis. EC/BCR project for ANCA-assay standardization. Clin. Nephrol. 48, 16.

Bajema, I.M., Hagen, E.C., De Herr, E., van der Woude, F.J., Bruijn, J.A. 2001. Colocalization of ANCA-antigens and fibrinoid necrosis in ANCA-associated vasculitis. Kidney Int. 60, 2025.

Balding, C.E.J., Howie, A.J., Drake-Lee, A.B., Savage, C.O.S. 2001. Th2 dominance in nasal mucosa in patients with Wegener's granulomatosis. Clin. Exp. Immunol. 125, 332.

Birck, R., Warnatz, K., Lorenz, H.M., Choi, M., Haubitz, M., Grunke, M., Peter, H.H., Kalden, J.R., Gobel, U., Drexler, J.M., Hotta, O., Nowack, R., Van der Woude, F.J. 2003. 15-Deoxyspergualin in patients with refractory ANCA-associated systemic vasculitis: a six-month open-label trial to evaluate safety and efficacy. J. Am. Soc. Nephrol. 14, 440.

Blank, M., Tomer, Y., Stein, M., Kopolovic, J., Wiik, A., Meroni, P.L., Conforti, G., Shoenfeld, Y. 1995. Immunization with anti-neutrophil cytoplasmic antibody (ANCA) induces the production of mouse ANCA and perivascular lymphocyte infiltration. Clin. Exp. Immunol. 102, 120.

Bosch, X., Lopez-Soto, A., Mirapeix, E., Font, J., Ingelmo, M., Urbano-Marquez, A. 1994. Antineutrophil cytoplasmatic autoantibody-associated alveolar capillaritis in patients presenting with pulmonary hemorrhage. Arch. Pathol. Lab. Med. 118, 517–522.

Brockmann, H., Schwarting, A., Kriegsmann, J., Petrow, P., Gaumann, A., Müller, K.M., Galle, P.R., Mayet, W. 2002. Proteinase-3 as the major autoantigen of c-ANCA is strongly expressed in lung tissue of patients with Wegener's granulomatosis. Arthritis Res. 4, 220.

Brons, R.H., Bakker, H.I., Van Wijk, R.T., Van Dijk, N.W., Muller Kobold, A.C., Limburg, P.C., Manson, W.L., Kallenberg, C.G., Cohen Tervaert, J.W. 2000. Staphylococcal acid phosphatase binds to endothelial cells via charge interaction; a pathogenic role in Wegener's granulomatosis? Clin. Exp. Immunol. 119, 566.

Brons, R.H., de Jong, M.C., de Boer, N.K., Stegeman, C.A., Kallenberg, C.G., Cohen Tervaert, J.W. 2001. Detection of immune deposits in skin lesions of patients with Wegener's granulomatosis. Ann. Rheum. Dis. 60, 1097.

Brouwer, E., Huitema, M.G., Klok, P.A., de Weerd, H. Tervaert, J.W., Weening, J.J., Kallenberg, C.G. 1993. Antimyeloperoxidase-associated proliferative glomerulonephritis: an animal model. J. Exp. Med. 177, 905.

Brouwer, E., Huitema, M.G., Mulder, A.H.L., Heeringa, P., Van Goor, H., Tervaert, J.W.C., Weening, J.J., Kallenberg, C.G.M. 1994. Neutrophil activation in vitro and in vivo in Wegener's granulomatosis. Kidney Int. 45, 1120–1131.

Carrington, C.B., Liebow, A.A. 1966. Limited forms of angiitis and granulomatosis of Wegener's type. Am. J. Med. 41, 497.

Carruthers, D.M., Watts, R.A., Symmons, D.P., Scott, D.G. 1996. Wegener's granulomatosis—increased incidence or increased recognition? Br. J. Rheumatol. 35, 142.

Carruthers, D.M., Connor, S., Howie, A.J., Exley, A.R., Raza, K., Bacon, P.A., Guest, P. 2000. Percutaneous image-guided biopsy of lung nodules in the assessment of disease activity in Wegener's granulomatosis. Rheumatology 39, 776–782.

Cockwell, P., Brooks, C.J., Adu, D., Savage, C.O.S. 1999. Interleukin-8: a pathogenetic role in antineutrophil cytoplasmic autoantibody-associated glomerulonephritis. Kidney Int. 55, 852.

Cohen Tervaert, J.W., Stegeman, C.A., Kallenberg, C.G.M. 1998. Silicon exposure and vasculitis. Curr. Opin. Rheumatol. 10, 12.

Cordier, J.-F., Valeyre, D., Guillevin, L., Loire, R., Brechot, J.-M. 1990. Pulmonary Wegener's granulomatosis. Chest 97, 906–912.

Cotch, M.F., Hoffman, G.S., Yerg, D.E., Kaufman, G.I., Targonski, P., Kaslow, R.A. 1996. The epidemiology of Wegener's granulomatosis: estimates of the five-year period prevalence, annual mortality and geographic disease distribution from population-based data sources. Arthritis Rheum. 39, 87.

Coulomb-L'Hermine, A., Capron, F., Zhou, W., Piard, F., Galateau, F., Laurent, P., Crevon, M.C., Galanaud, P., Emilie, D. 2001. Expression of the chemokine RANTES in pulmonary Wegener's granulomatosis. Hum. Pathol. 32, 320.

Csernok, E., Schmitt, W.H., Ernst, M., Bainton, D.F., Gross, W.L. 1993. Membrane surface proteinase 3 expression and intracytoplasmic immunoglobuline on neutrophils from patients with ANCA-associated vasculitides. Adv. Exp. Med. Biol. 336, 45.

Csernok, E., Ernst, M., Schmitt, W., Bainton, D.F., Gross, W.L. 1994. Activated neutrophils express proteinase 3 on their plasma membrane in vitro and in vivo. Clin. Exp. Immunol. 95, 244.

Csernok, E., Trabandt, A., Müller, A., Wang, G.C., Moosig, F., Paulsen, J., Schnabel, A., Gross, W.L. 1999. Cytokine profiles in Wegener's granulomatosis: predominance of type 1 (Th1) in the granulomatous inflammation. Arthritis Rheum. 42, 742.

Daum, T.E., Specks, U., Colby, T.V., Edell, E.S., Brutinel, M.W., Prakash, D.B.S., DeRemee, R.A. 1995. Tracheobronchial involvement in Wegener's granulomatosis. Am. J. Respir. Crit. Care Med. 151, 522.

de Groot, K., Adu, D., Savage, C.O., European Vasculitis Study Group 2001a. The value of pulse cyclophosphamide in ANCA-associated vasculitis: meta-analysis and critical review. Nephrol. Dial. Transplant. 16, 2018.

de Groot, K., Gross, W.L., Herlyn, K., Reinhold-Keller, E. 2001b. Development and validation of a disease extent index for Wegener's granulomatosis. Clin. Nephrol. 55 (1), 31.

DeRemee, R.A. 1988. The treatment of Wegener's granulomatosis with trimethoprim/sulfamethoxazole: illusion or vision? Arthritis Rheum. 31, 1068–1074.

DeRemee, R.A., McDonald, T.J., Weiland, L.H. 1985. Wegener's granulomatosis: observation on treatment with antimicrobial agents. Mayo Clin. Proc. 60, 27.

Devaney, K.O., Travis, W.D., Hoffman, G., Leavitt, R., Lebovics, R., Fauci, A.S. 1990. Interpretation of head and neck biopsies in Wegener's granulomatosis. Am. J. Surg. Pathol. 14, 555–564.

Dijstelbloem, H.M., Scheepers, R.H., Oost, W.W., Stegeman, C.A., van der Pol, W.L., Sluiter, W.J., Kallenberg, C.G., van de Winkel, J.G., Tervaert, J.W. 1999. Fcgamma receptor polymorphisms in Wegener's granulomatosis: risk factors for disease relapse. Arthritis Rheum. 42, 1823.

Edberg, J.C., Wainstein, E., Wu, J., Csernok, E., Sneller, M.C., Hoffman, G.S., Keystone, E.C., Gross, W.L., Kimberly, R.P. 1997. Analysis of FcgammaRII gene polymorphisms in Wegener's granulomatosis. Exp. Clin. Immunogenet. 14, 183.

Eden, A., Mahr, A., Servant, A., Radjef, N., Amard, S., Mouthon, L., Garbarg-Chenon, A., Guillevin, L. 2003. Lack of association between B19 or V9 erythrovirus infection and ANCA-positive vasculitides: a case-control study. Rheumatology 42, 660.

Ehlers, S., Benini, J., Held, H.D., Röck, C., Alber, G., Uhlig, S. 2001. $\alpha\beta$ TCR+ cells and IFNγ, but not iNOS are critical for granuloma necrosis in a mouse model for mycobacteria-induced pulmonary immunopathology. J. Exp. Med. 194, 1847–1859.

Elkon, K.B., Sutherland, D.C., Rees, A.J., Hughes, G.R.V., Batchelor, J.R. 1983. HLA frequencies in systemic vasculitis. Increase in HLA-DR2 in Wegener's granulomatosis. Arthritis Rheum. 26, 102.

Esnault, V.L., Mathieson, P.W., Thiru, S., Oliveira, D.B., Lockwood, M.C. 1992. Autoantibodies to myeloperoxidase in brown Norway rats treated with mercuric chloride. Lab. Invest. 67, 114.

Esnault, V.L.M., Testa, A., Audrain, M., Roge, C., Hamidou, M., Barrier, J.H., Sesboue, R., Martin, J.P., Lesavre, P. 1993. Alpha 1 antitrypsin genetic ploymorphism in ANCA-positive systemic vasculitis. Kidney Int. 43, 1329.

Exley, A.R., Bacon, P.A., Luqmani, R.A. 1997. Development and initial validation of the vasculitis damage index for the standardized clinical assessment of damage in the systemic vasculitides. Arthritis Rheum. 40, 371–380.

Falk, R.J., Terrell, R.S., Charles, L.A., Jennette, J.C. 1990. Antineutrophil cytoplasmic autoantibodies induce neutrophils to degranulate and produce oxygen radicals in vitro. Proc. Natl Acad. Sci. USA 87, 4115.

Fauci, A.S., Haynes, B.F., Katz, P., Wolff, S.M. 1983. Wegener's granulomatosis: prospective clinical and therapeutic experience with 85 patients for 21 years. Ann. Int. Med. 98, 76–85.

Fienberg, R. 1989. A morphologic and immunohistologic study of the evolution of the necrotizing palisading granuloma of pathergic (Wegener's) granulomatosis. Semin. Respir. Med. 10, 126.

Foucher, P., Heeringa, P., Petersen, A.H., Huitema, M.G., Brouwer, E., Tervaert, J.W., Prop, J., Camus, P., Weening, J.J., Kallenberg, C.G. 1999. Antimyeloperoxidase-associated lung disease. An experimental model. Am. J. Respir. Crit. Care Med. 160, 987.

Gadola, S., Sahly, H., Reinhold-Keller, E., Hellmich, B., Paulsen, J., Gross, W.L. 1997. Nasal carriage of *Staphylococcus aureus* in patients with Wegener's granulomatosis (WG), rheumatoid arthritis (RA), and polyposis nasi (PN) (*abstract*). Sarcoidosis Vasc. Diffuse Lung Dis. 14 (Suppl. 1), 29.

Gallagher, H., Kwan, J.T., Jayne, D.R. 2002. Pulmonary renal syndrome: a 4-year, single center experience. Am. J. Kidney Dis. 39, 42–47.

Gaskin, G., Pusey, C.D. 2001. Plasmapheresis in antineutrophil cytoplasmic antibody-associated systemic vasculitis. Ther. Apher. 5, 176–181.

Gencik, M., Borgmann, S., Zahn, R., Albert, E., Sitter, T., Epplen, J.T., Fricke, H. 1999. Immunogenetic risk factor for antineutrophil cytoplasmic antibody (ANCA) associated systemic vasculitis. Clin. Exp. Immunol. 117, 412.

Giscombe, R., Wang, X., Huang, D., Lefvert, A.K. 2002. Coding sequence 1 and promoter single nucleotide polymorphisms in the CTLA-4 gene in Wegener's granulomatosis. J. Rheumatol. 29, 950.

Gonzalez-Gay, M.A., Garcia-Porrua, C., Guerrero, J., Rodriguez-Ledo, P., Llorca, J. 2003. The epidemiology of the primary systemic vasculitides in northwest Spain: implications of the Chapel Hill Consensus Conference definitions. Arthritis Rheum. 49, 388.

Gregorini, G., Ferioli, A., Donato, F., Tira, P., Morassi, L., Tardanico, R., Lancini, L., Maiorca, R. 1993. Association between silica exposure and necrotizing crescentic glomerulonephritis with p-ANCA and anti-MPO antibodies: a hospital based case-control study. Adv. Exp. Med. Biol. 336, 435.

Gresham, H.D., Lowrance, J.H., Caver, T.E., Wilson, B.S., Cheung, A.L., Lindberg, F.P. 2000. Survival of *Staphylococcus aureus* inside neutrophils contributes to infection. J. Immunol. 164, 3713.

Griffith, M., Lovegrove, J., Gaskin, G., Whitehouse, D., Pusey, C. 1996. C-antineutrophil cytoplasmic antibody positivity in vasculitis patients is associated with the Z allele of alpha-1-antitrypsin, and p-antineutrophil cytoplasmic antibody positivity with the S allele. Nephrol. Dial. Transplant. 11, 438.

Grimminger, F., Hattar, K., Papavassilis, C., Temmesfeld, B., Csernok, E., Gross, W.L., Seeger, W., Sibelius, U. 1996. Neutrophil activation by anti-proteinase 3 antibodies in Wegener's granulomatosis: role of exogenous arachidonic acid and leukotriene B4 generation. J. Exp. Med. 184, 1567.

Gross, W.L., Schmitt, W.H., Csernok, E. 1992. ANCA and associated diseases: immunodiagnostic and pathogenetic aspects. Clin. Exp. Immunol. 91, 1–12.

Grunewald, J., Halapi, E., Wahlstrom, J., Giscombe, R., Nityanand, S., Sanjeevi, C., Lefvert, A.K. 1998. T-cell expansions with conserved T-cell receptor beta chain motifs in the peripheral blood of HLA-DRB1*0401 positive patients with necrotizing vasculitis. Blood 92, 3737.

Harper, L., Savage, C.O.S. 2000. Pathogenesis of ANCA-associated systemic vasculitis. J. Pathol. 190, 349.

Haubitz, M., Schellong, S., Gobel, U., Schurek, H.J., Schaumann, D., Koch, K.M., Brunkhorst, R. 1998. Intravenous pulse administration of cyclophosphamide versus daily oral treatment in patients with antineutrophil cytoplasmic antibody-associated vasculitis and renal involvement: a prospective, randomized study. Arthritis Rheum. 41 (10), 1835–1844.

Hayworth, S.J., Savage, C.O.S., Carr, D., Hughes, J.M.B., Rees, A.J. 1985. Pulmonary haemorrhage complicating Wegener's granulomatosis and microscopic polyarteritis. Br. Med. J. 290, 1775–1778.

Heinemann, D.E.H., Peters, J.H., Gahr, M. 1993. A human in vitro granuloma model using heat killed candida albicans cells immobilized on plastic culture wells. Scand. J. Immunol. 45, 596–604.

Hoffman, G.S., Specks, U. 1998. Antineutrophil cytoplasmic antibodies. Arthritis Rheum. 41, 1521–1537.

Hoffman, G.S., Kerr, G.S., Leavitt, R.Y., Hallahan, C.W., Lebovics, R.S., Travis, W.D., Rottem, M., Fauci, A.S. 1992. Wegener's granulomatosis: an analysis of 158 patients. Ann. Intern. Med. 116, 488.

Hoffmann, G.S., Thomas-Golbanov, C.K., Chan, J., Akst, L.M., Eliachar, I. 2003. Treatment of subglottic stenosis, due to Wegener's granulomatosis, with intralesional corticosteroids and dilation. J. Rheumatol. 30, 1017–1021.

Iking-Konert, C., Vogt, S., Radsak, M., Wagner, C., Hänsch, G.M., Andrassy, K. 2001. Polymorphonuclear neutrophils in Wegener's granulomatosis acquire characteristics of antigen presenting cells. Kidney Int. 60, 2247.

Janeway, C.A., Travers, P., Walport, M., Shlomchik, M. 2001. Immunobiology. The immune system in healthy and disease, 5th ed., Garland Publishing, New York, NY.

Jayne, D., European Vasculitis Study Group (EUVAS) 2001. Update on the European Vasculitis Study Group trials. Curr. Opin. Rheumatol. 13, 48.

Jayne, D.R., Lockwood, C.M. 1996. Intravenous immunoglobulin as sole therapy for systemic vasculitis. Br. J. Rheumatol. 35, 1150.

Jayne, D.R., Chapel, H., Adu, D., Misbah, S., O'Donoghue, D., Scott, D., Lockwood, C.M. 2000. Intravenous immunoglobulin for ANCA-associated systemic vasculitis with persistent disease activity. QJM 93 (7), 433–439.

Jayne, D., Rasmussen, N., Andrassy, K., Bacon, P., Cohen Tervaert, J.W., Dadoniene, J., Ekstrand, A., Gaskin, G., Gregorini, G., de Groot, K., Gross, W.L., Hagen, E.C., Mirapeix, E., Pettersson, E., Siegert, C., Sinico, A., Tesar, V., Westman, K., Pusey, C. 2003. A randomized trial of maintenance therapy for vasculitis associated with antineutrophil cytoplasmic autoantibodies. N. Engl. J. Med. 349, 36.

Jennette, J.C., Falk, R.J. 1997. Small-vessel vasculitis. N. Engl. J. Med. 337, 1512.

Jennette, J.C., Falk, R.J., Andrassy, K., Bacon, P.A., Churg, J., Gross, W.L., Hagen, E.C., Hoffman, G.S., Hunder, G.G., Kallenberg, C.G., McCluskey, R.T., Sinico, R.A., Rees, A.J., van Es, L.A., Waldherr, R., Wiik, A. 1994. Nomenclature of systemic vasculitides. Proposal of an international consensus conference. Arthritis Rheum. 37, 187.

Jiang, X., Khursigara, G., Rubin, R.L. 1994. Transformation of lupus-inducing drugs to cytotoxic products by activated neutrophils. Science 266, 810.

Kallenberg, C.G.M., Cohen Tervaert, J.W., Stegeman, C.A. 1990. Criteria for disease activity in Wegener's granulomatosis: a requirement for longitudinal clinical studies. APMIS 19, 37–39.

Katzenstein, A.L., Locke, W.K. 1995. Solitary lung lesions in Wegener's granulomatosis. Pathologic findings and clinical significance in 25 cases. Am. J. Surg. Pathol. 19, 545–552.

Klinger, H. 1931. Grenzformen der Periarteriitis nodosa Frankfurt. Ztschr. f. Path. 42, 455.

Kocher, M., Edberg, J.C., Fleit, H.B., Kimberly, R.P. 1998. Antineutrophil cytoplasmic antibodies preferentially engage Fc gammaRIIIb on human neutrophils. J. Immunol. 161, 6909.

Koldingsnes, W., Nossent, H. 2000. Epidemiology of Wegener's granulomatosis in Northern Norway. Arthritis Rheum. 43, 2481.

Komocsi, A., Lamprecht, P., Csernok, E., Müller, A., Holl-Ulrich, K., Seitzer, U., Moosig, F., Schnabel, A., Gross, W.L. 2002. Peripheral blood and granuloma $CD4^{+}CD28^{-}$ T-cells are a major source of IFN-γ and TNF-α in Wegener's granulomatosis. Am. J. Pathol. 160, 1717.

Lamprecht, P., Moosig, F., Csernok, E., Seitzer, U., Schnabel, A., Müller, A., Gross, W.L. 2001. CD28 negative T cells are enriched in granulomatous lesions of the respiratory tract in Wegener's granulomatosis. Thorax 56, 751.

Lamprecht, P., Kumanovics, G., Müller, A., Csernok, E., Komosci, A., Trabandt, A., Gross, W.L., Schnabel, A. 2002a. Elevated monocytic IL-12 and TNF-α production in Wegener's granulomatosis is normalized by cyclophosphamide and corticosteroid therapy. Clin. Exp. Immunol. 128, 181.

Lamprecht, P., Voswinkel, J., Lilienthal, T., Nölle, B., Heller, M., Gross, W.L., Gause, A. 2002b. Effectiveness of TNF-α blockade with infliximab in refractory Wegener's granulomatosis. Rheumatology 41, 1303.

Lamprecht, P., Erdmann, A., Müller, A., Csernok, E., Reinhold-Keller, E., Holl-Ulrich, K., Feller, A.C., Brühl, H., Gross W.L. 2003a. Heterogeneity of CD4+ and CD8+ memory T cells in localized and generalized Wegener's granulomatosis. Arthritis Res. Ther. 5, R25.

Lamprecht, P., Brühl, H., Erdmann, E., Holl-Ulrich, K., Csernok, E., Seitzer, U., Mack, M., Feller, A.C., Reinhold-Keller, E., Gross, W.L., Müller, A. 2003b. Differences in CCR5 expression on peripheral blood $CD4^{+}CD28^{-}$ T-cells and in granulomatous lesions between localized and generalized Wegener's granulomatosis. Clin. Immunol. 108, 1.

Langford, C.A., Sneller, M.C., Hallahan, C.W., Hoffmann, G.S., Kammerer, W.A., Talar-Williams, C., Fauci, A.S., Lebovics, R.S. 1996. Clinical features and therapeutic management of subglottic stenosis in patients with Wegener's granulomatosis. Arthritis Rheum. 39, 1754–1760.

Leavitt, R.Y., Fauci, A.S., Bloch, D.A., Michel, B.A., Hunder, G.G., Arend, W.P., Calabrese, L.H., Fries, J.F., Lie, J.T., Lightfoot, R.W. Jr., Masi, A.T., McShane, D.J., Mills, J.A., Wallace, S.L., Zvaifler, N.J. 1990. The American College of Rheumatology 1990 criteria for the classification of Wegener's granulomatosis. Arthritis Rheum. 33, 1101.

Lebovics, R.S., Hoffmann, G., Leavitt, R.Y., Kerr, G.S., Travis, W.D., Kammerer, W., Hallahan, C., Rottem, M., Fauci, A.S. 1992. The management of subglottic stenosis in patients with Wegener's granulomatosis. Laryngoscope 102, 1341–1345.

Lieberman, K., Churg, A. 1991. Wegener's granulomatosis. In: A. Churg, J. Churg (Eds.), Systemic Vasculitis. Igaku Shoin Medical Publishers, Tokyo, p. 79.

Lipsky, P. 2001. Systemic lupus erthematosus: an autoimmune disease of B cell hyperactivity. Nat. Immunol. 2, 764.

Lockwood, C.M., Thiru, S., Isaacs, J.D., Hale, G., Waldmann, H. 1993. Long-term remission of intractable systemic vasculitis with monoclonal antibody therapy. Lancet 341, 1620.

Lombard, C.M., Duncan, S.R., Rizk, N.W., Colby, T.V. 1990. The diagnosis of Wegener's granulomatosis from transbronchial biopsy specimens. Hum. Pathol. 21, 838–842.

Ludviksson, B.R., Sneller, M.C., Chua, T.S., Talar-Williams, C., Langford, C.A., Ehrhardt, R.O., Fauci, A.S., Strober, W. 1998. Active Wegener's granulomatosis is associated with HLA-DR+ CD4+ T cells exhibiting an unbalanced Th1-type T cell cytokine pattern: reversal with IL-10. J. Immunol. 160, 3602.

Luqmani, R.A., Bacon, P.A., Moots, R.J., Janssen, B.A., Pall, A., Emery, P. 1994. Birmingham vasculitis activity score (BVAS) in systemic necrotizing vasculitis. QJM 87, 671–678.

Mark, E.J., Matsubara, O., Tan-Liu, N.S., Fienberg, R. 1988. The pulmonary biopsy in the early diagnosis of Wegener's (pathergic) granulomatosis: a study based on 35 open lung biopsies. Hum. Pathol. 19, 1065–1071.

Mascher, B., Schmitt, W.H., Csernok, E., Tatsis, E., Reil, A., Gross, W.L., Seyfarth, M. 1997. Polymorphism in the tumor necrosis factor genes in Wegener's granulomatosis. Exp. Clin. Immunogenet. 14, 226.

Mayet, W.J., Csernok, E., Szymkowiak, C., Gross, W.L., Meyer zum Büschenfelde, K.H. 1993. Human endothelial cells express proteinase 3, the target antigen of anticytoplasmic antibodies in Wegener's granulomatosis. Blood 82, 1221–1229.

McDonald, T.J., Neel, H.B., DeRemee, R.A. 1982. Wegener's granulomatosis of the subglottis and the upper portion of the trachea. Ann. Otol. Rhiol. Laryngol. 91, 588–592.

Merkel, P.A. 1998. Drugs associated with vasculitis. Curr. Opin. Rheumatol. 10, 45.

Metzler, C., Lamprecht, P., Fink, C.O., Gross, W.L., Reinhold-Keller, E. 2004. Maintenance of remission with leflunomide in Wegener's granulomatosis. Rheumatology 43, 315–320.

Mielke, M.E., Peters, C., Hahn, H. 1997. Cytokines in the induction and expression of T-cell-mediated granuloma formation and protection in the murine model of listeriosis. Immunol. Rev. 158, 79–93.

Moosig, F., Csernok, E., Wang, G., Gross, W.L. 1998. Costimulatory molecules in Wegener's granulomatosis (WG): lack of expression of CD28 and preferential up-regulation of its ligands B7-1 (CD80) and B7-2 (CD86) on T cells. Clin. Exp. Immunol. 114, 113.

Moosig, F., Csernok, E., Kumanovics, G., Gross, W.L. 2000. Opsonization of apoptotic neutrophils by anti-neutrophil cytoplasmic antibodies (ANCA) leads to enhanced uptake by macrophages and increased release of TNF-alpha. Clin. Exp. Immmunol. 122, 499–503.

Mrowka, C., Csernok, E., Gross, W.L., Feucht, H.E., Bechtel, U., Thoenes, G.H. 1995. Distribution of the granulocyte serine proteinases proteinase 3 and elastase in human glomerulonephritis. Am. J. Kidney Dis. 25, 253–261.

Muhle, C., Reinhold-Keller, E., Richter, Ch., Duncker, G., Beigel, A., Brinkmann, G., Gross, W.L., Heller, M. 1996. MRI of the nasal cavity, the paranasal sinuses and orbits in Wegener's granulomatosis. Eur. Radiol. 7, 566–570.

Müller, A., Trabandt, A., Glockner-Hofmann, K., Seitzer, U., Csernok, E., Schönermarck, U., Feller, A.C., Gross, W.L. 2000. Localized Wegener's granulomatosis: predominance of CD26 and IFN-γ expression. J. Pathol. 192, 113.

Müller, A., Holl-Ullrich, K., Feller, A.C., Gross, W.L., Lamprecht, P. 2003. Immune phenomena in localized and generalized Wegener's granulomatosis. Clin. Exp. Rheumatol. 21 (Suppl. 32), 549–554.

Muller Kobold, A.C., Kallenberg, C.G., Tervaert, J.W. 1998. Leukocyte membrane expression of proteinase 3 correlates with disease activity in patients with Wegener's granulomatosis. Br. J. Rhuematol. 37, 901.

Munian, M., Moreno, J., Campora, R. 1986. Wegener's granulomatosis in two sisters. Ann. Rheum. Dis. 45, 417.

Muraközy, G., Gäde, K.I., Ruprecht, B., Gutzeit, O., Schürmann, M., Schnabel, A., Schlaak, M., Gross, W.L., Müller-Quernheim, J. 2001. Gene polymorphism of immunoregulatory cytokines and angiotensin-converting enzyme in Wegener's granulokatosis. J. Mol. Med. 79, 665.

Neumann, I., Birck, R., Newman, M., Schnulle, P., Kriz, W., Nemoto, K., Yard, B., Waldherr, R., Van Der Woude, F.J. 2003. SCG/Kinjoh mice: a model of ANCA-associated crescentic glomerulonephritis with immune deposits. Kidney Int. 64, 140.

Newman, B., Rubin, L.A., Siminovitch, K.A. 2003. NOD2/CARD15 gene mutation is not associated with susceptibility to Wegener's granulomatosis. J. Rheumatol. 30, 305.

Nikkari, S., Vainionpää, R., Toivanen, P., Gross, W.L., Mistry, N., Csernok, E., Szpirt, W., Baslund, B., Wiik, A. 1995. Wegener's granulomatosis and parvovirus B19 infection. Arthritis Rheum. 38, 1175.

Niles, J.L., Bottinger, E.P., Saurins, G.R. 1996. The syndrome of lung hemorrhage and nephritis is usually an ANCA-associated condition. Arch. Intern. Med. 156, 440–445.

Nölle, B., Specks, U., Lüdemann, J., Rohrbach, M., De Remee, R., Gross, W.L. 1989. Anticytoplasmic autoantibodies: their immunodiagnostic value in Wegener's granulomatosis. Ann. Intern. Med. 111, 28–40.

Nowack, R., Gobel, U., Klooker, P., Hergesell, O., Andrassy, K., van der Woude, F.J. 1999. Mycophenolate mofetil for maintenance therapy of Wegener's granulomatosis and microscopic polyangiitis: a pilot study in 11 patients with renal involvement. J. Am. Soc. Nephrol. 10, 1965.

Nuyts, G.D., van Vlem, E., de Vos, A., Daelemans, R.A., Rorive, G., Elseviers, M.M., Schurgers, M., Segaert, M., d'Haese, P.C., de Broe, M.E. 1995. Wegener's granulomatosis is associated to exposure to silicon compounds: a case-control study. Nephrol. Dial. Transplant. 10, 1162.

Ognibene, F.P., Shelhamer, J.H., Hoffman, G.S., Kerr, G.S., Reda, D., Fauci, A., Leavitt, R.Y. 1995. *Pneumocystis carinii* pneumonia: a major complication of immunosuppressive therapy in patients with Wegener's granulomatosis. Am. J. Respir. Crit. Care Med. 151, 795–799.

Ohlsson, S., Falk, R., Yang, J.J., Ohlsson, K., Segelmark, M., Wieslander, J. 2003. Increased expression of the secretory leukocyte proteinase inhibitor in Wegener's granulomatosis. Clin. Exp. Immunol. 131, 190.

Papiha, S.S., Murty, G.E., Ad'Hia, A., Mains, B.T., Venning, M. 1992. Association of Wegener's granulomatosis with HLA antigens and other genetic markers. Ann. Rheum. Dis. 51, 246.

Peen, E., Williams, R.C. Jr. 2000. What you should know about PR3-ANCA, structural aspects of antibodies to proteinase 3 (PR3). Arthritis Res. 2, 255.

Pendergraft, W.F. III, Preston, G.A., Shah, R.R., Tropsha, A., Carter, C.W. Jr., Jennette, J.C., Falk, R.J. 2004. Autoimmunity is triggered by cPR-3(105–201), a protein complementary to human autoantigen proteinase-3. Nat. Med. 10, 72.

Popa, E.R., Stegeman, C.A., Bos, N.A., Kallenberg, C.G., Tervaert, J.W. 1999. Differential B- and T-cell activation in Wegener's granulomatosis. J. Allergy Clin. Immunol. 103, 885.

Popa, E.R., Stegeman, C.A., Kallenberg, C.G.M., Cohen Tervaert, J.W. 2002. *Staphylococcus aureus* and Wegener's granulomatosis. Arthritis Res. 4, 77.

Popa, E.R., Stegeman, C.A., Bos, N.A., Kallenberg, C.G., Tervaert, J.W. 2003. Staphylococcal superantigens and T cell expansions in Wegener's granulomatosis. Clin. Exp. Immunol. 132 (3), 496–504.

Porges, A.J., Redecha, P.B., Kimberly, W.T., Csernok, E., Gross, W.L., Kimberly, R.P. 1994. Antineutrophil cytoplasmic antibodies engage and activate human neutrophils via Fc gamma RIIa. J. Immunol. 153, 1271.

Preston, G.A., Zarella, C.S., Pendergraft, W.F., Rudolph, E.H., Yang, J.J., Sekura, S.B., Jennette, J.C., Falk, R.J. 2002a. Novel effects of neutrophil-derived proteinase 3 and elastase on the endothelium involve *in vivo* cleavage of NF-κB and proapoptotic changes in JNK, ERK, and p38 MAPK signaling pathways. J. Am. Soc. Nephrol. 13, 2840.

Preston, G.A., Yang, J.J., Xiao, H., Falk, R.J. 2002b. Understanding the pathogenesis of ANCA: where are we today? Cleveland Clin. J. Med. 69 (Suppl. 2), SII51–SII54.

Qasim, F.J., Thiru, S., Mathieson, P.W., Oliveira, D.B. 1995. The time course and characterization of mercuric chloride-induced immunopathology in the brown Norway rat. J. Autoimmun. 8, 193.

Radford, D.J., Luu, N.T., Hewins, P., Nash, G., Savage, C.O.S. 2001. Antineutrophil antibodies stabilize adhesion and promote migration of flowing neutrophils on endothelial cells. Arthritis Rheum. 44, 2851.

Reinhold-Keller, E., Kekow, J., Schnabel, A., Schmitt, W.H., Heller, M., Beigel, A., Duncker, G., Gross, W.L. 1994. Influence of disease manifestation and antineutrophil cytoplasmic antibody titer on the response to pulse cyclophosphamide therapy in patients with Wegener's granulomatosis. Arthritis Rheum. 37, 919–924.

Reinhold-Keller, E., de Groot, K., Rudert, H., Nölle, B., Heller, M., Gross, W.L. 1996. Response to trimethoprim/sulfamethoxazole in Wegener's granulomatosis depends on the phase of disease. Q. J. Med. 89, 15.

Reinhold-Keller, E., Beuge, N., Latza, U., De Groot, K., Rudert H., Noelle, B., Heller, M., Gross, W.L. 2000. An interdisciplinary approach to the care of patients with Wegener's granulomatosis. Long-term outcome in 155 patients. Arthritis Rheum. 43, 1021.

Reinhold-Keller, E., de Groot, K., Holl-Ulrich, K., Arlt, A.C., Heller, M., Feller, A.C., Gross, W.L. 2001. Severe CNS manifestations as the clinical hallmark in generalised Wegener's granulomatosis consistently negative for antineutrophil cytoplasmic antibodies (ANCA). A report of 3 cases and a review of the literature. Clin. Exp. Rheumatol. 19, 541.

Reinhold-Keller, E., Herlyn, K., Wagner-Bastmeyer, R., Gutfleisch, J., Peter, H.H., Raspe, H.H., Gross, W.L. 2002. No difference in the incidences of vasculitides between north and south Germany: first results of the German vasculitis register. Rheumatology 41, 540.

Reuter, M., Schnabel, A., Wesner, F., Tetzlaff, K., Risheng, Y., Gross, W.L., Heller, M. 1998. Pulmonary Wegener's granulomatosis. Chest 114 (2), 500–506.

Richter, C., Schnabel, A., Csernok, E., De Groot, K., Reinhold-Keller, E., Gross, W.L. 1995. Treatment of anti-neutrophil cytoplasmic antibody (ANCA)-associated systemic vasculitis with high-dose intravenous immunoglobulin. Clin. Exp. Immunol. 101 (1), 2–7.

Savage, C.O.S., Harper, L., Adu, D. 1997. Primary systemic vasculitis. Lancet 349, 553.

Schlesier, M., Kaspar, T., Gutfleisch, J., Wolff-Vorbeck, G., Peter, H.H. 1995. Activated CD4$^+$ and CD8$^+$ T-cell subsets in Wegener's granulomatosis. Rheumatol. Int. 14, 213.

Schnabel, A., Holl-Ulrich, K., Dalhoff, K., Reuter, M., Gross, W.L. 1997. Efficacy of transbrochial biopsy in pulmonary vasculitis. Eur. Respir. J. 10, 2738–2743.

Schnabel, A., Csernok, E., Braun, J., Gross, W.L. 1999a. Activation of neutrophils, eosinophils and lymphocytes in the lower respiratory tract in Wegener's granulomatosis. Am. J. Respir. Crit. Care Med. 161, 399–405.

Schnabel, A., Reuter, M., Müller-Quernheim, J., Gross, W.L. 1999b. Bronchoalveolar lavage cell profiles in Wegener's granulomatosis. Respir. Med. 93, 498–506.

Schnabel, A., Reuter, M., Csernok, E., Richter, C., Gross, W.L. 1999c. Subclinical alveolar bleeding in pulmonary vasculitides: correlation with indices of disease activity. Eur. Respir. J. 14, 118–124.

Schwarting, A., Hagen, D., Odenthal, M., Brockmann, H., Dienes, H.P., Wandel, E., Rumpelt, H.J., Meyer zum Büschenfelde, K.H., Mayet, W.J. 2000. Proteinase 3 mRNA expressed by human glomerular epithelial cells correlates with crescent formation in patients with Wegener's granulomatosis. Kidney Int. 57, 2412–2422.

Screaton, N.J., Sivasothy, P., Flower, C.D.R., Lockwood, C.M. 1998. Tracheal involvement in Wegener's granulomatosis: evaluation using spiral CT. Clin. Radiol. 53, 809–815.

Sibelius, U., Hattar, K., Schenkel, A., Noll, T., Csernok, E., Gross, W.L., Mayet, W.J., Piper, H.M., Seeger, W., Grimminger, F. 1998. Wegener's granulomatosis: anti-proteinase 3 antibodies are potent inductors of human endothelial cell signaling and leakage response. J. Exp. Med. 187, 497.

Sibilia, J., Benlagha, K., Vanhille, P., Ronco, P., Brouet, J.C., Mariette, X. 1997. Structural analysis of human antibodies tp proteinase 3 from patients with Wegener's granulomatosis. J. Immunol. 159, 712.

Sneller, M.C. 2002. Granuloma formation, implications for the pathogenesis of vasculitis. Cleveland Clin. J. Med. 69 (Suppl. 2), SII-S40.

Specks, U. 2000. Are animal models of vasculitis suitable tools? Curr. Opin. Rheumatol. 12, 11.

Specks, U. 2001. Diffuse alveolar hemorrhage syndromes. Curr. Opin. Rheumatol. 13, 12–17.

Specks, U., Fervenza, F.C., McDonald, T.J., Hogan, M.C.E. 2001. Response of Wegener's granulomatosis to anti-CD20 chimeric monoclonal antibody therapy. Arthritis Rheum. 44, 2836.

Stegeman, C.A., Cohen Tervaert, J.W., Sluiter, W.J., Manson, W.L., de Jong, P.E., Kallenberg, C.G.M. 1994. Persistent carriage of *Staphylococcus aureus* and relapse rate of Wegener's granulomatosis. Ann. Intern. Med. 120, 12.

Stegeman, C.A., Cohen Tervaert, J.W., de Jong, P.E., Kallenberg, C.G.M. 1996. Trimethoprim-sulfamethoxazole (co-trimoxazole) for the prevention of relapses of Wegener's granulomatosis. N. Engl. J. Med. 335, 16.

Stone, J.H., Uhlfelder, M.L., Hellmann, D.B., Crook, S., Bedocs, N.M., Hoffman, G.S. 2001a. Etanercept combined with conventional treatment in Wegener's granulomatosis: a six-month open-label trial to evaluate safety. Arthritis Rheum. 44, 1149.

Stone, J.H., Hoffman, G.S., Merkel, P.A. 2001b. A disease-specific activity index for Wegener's granulomatosis. Modification of the Birmingham Vasculitis Activity Score. International Network for the Study of the Systemic Vasculitides (INSSYS). Arthritis Rheum. 44, 912–920.

Taekema-Roelvink, M.E., Kooten, C., Kooij, S.V., Heemskerk, E., Daha, M.R. 2001. Proteinase 3 enhances endothelial monocyte chemoattractant protein-1 production and induces increased adhesion of neutrophils to endothelial cells by upregulating intercellular cell adhesion molecule-1. J. Am. Soc. Nephrol. 12, 932.

Tatsis, E., Reinhold-Keller, E., Steindorf, K., Feller, A.C., Gross, W.L. 1999. Wegener's granulomatosis associated with renal cell carcinoma. Arthritis Rheum. 42, 751.

Ter Maaten, J.C., Franssen, C.F.M., Gans, R.O.B., Strack van Schijndel, R.J.M., Hoorntje, S.J. 1996. Respiratory failure in ANCA-associated vasculitis. Chest 110 (2), 357–362.

Tomer, Y., Gilburd, B., Blank, M., Lider, O., Hershkoviz, R., Fishman, P., Zigelman, R., Meroni, P.L., Wiik, A., Shoenfeld, Y. 1995. Characterization of biologically active antineutrophil cytoplasmic antibodies induced in mice. Pathogenetic role in experimental vasculitis. Arthritis Rheum. 38, 1375.

Travis, W.D., Colby, T.V., Lombard, C., Carpenter, H.A. 1990. A clinicopathologic study of 34 cases of diffuse pulmonary hemorrhage with lung biopsy confirmation. Am. J. Surg. Pathol. 14, 1112–1125.

Travis, W.D., Hoffman, G.S., Leavitt, R.Y., Pass, H.I., Fauci, A.S. 1991. Surgical pathology of the lung in Wegener's granulomatosis. Am. J. Surg. Pathol. 15, 315–333.

Trocme, S.D., Bartley, G.B., Campbell, R.J., Gleich, G.J., Leiferman, K.M. 1991. Eosinophil and neutrophil degranulation in ophthalmic lesions of Wegener's granulomatosis. Arch. Ophtalmol. 109, 1585–1589.

Tse, W.Y., Abadeh, S., McTiernan, A., Jefferis, R., Savage, C.O.S., Adu, D. 1999. No association between neutrophil FcγRIIa allelic polymorphism and anti-neutrophil cytoplasmic antibody (ANCA)-positive systemic vasculitis. Clin. Exp. Rheumatol. 117, 198–205.

van der Geld, Y.M., Limburg, P.C., Kallenberg, C.G. 2001. Proteinase 3, Wegener's autoantigen: from gene to antigen. J. Leukoc. Biol. 69, 177–190.

Voswinkel, J., Müller, A., Lamprecht, P., Gross, W.L., Gause, A. 2002. Does ANCA formation result from an antigen-triggered immune response in Wegener's endonasal inflamed tissue? Cleveland Clin. J. Med. 69 (Suppl. 2), SII-S159.

Wainstein, E., Edberg, J.C., Csernok, E., Sneller, M.C., Hoffman, G.S., Keystone, E.C., Gross, W.L., Kimberly, R.P. 1996. Fcγ RIIIB alleles predict renal dysfunction in Wegener's granulomatosis. Arthritis Rheum. 39, S210.

Waldhauser, L., Uetrecht, J. 1996. Antibodies to myeloperoxidase in propylthiouracil-induced autoimmune disease in the cat. Toxicology 114, 155.

Watts, R.A., Gonzalez-Gay, M.A., Lane, S.E., Garcia-Porrua, C., Bentham, G., Scott, D.G. 2001. Geoepidemiology of systemic vasculitis: comparison of the incidence in two regions of Europe. Ann. Rheum. Dis. 60, 170.

Wegener, F. 1939. Ueber eine eigenartige rhinogene Granulomatose mit besonderer Beteiligung des Arteriensystems und der Nieren. Beitr. Pathol. Anat. 102, 36.

Winek, J., Mueller, A., Csernok, E., Gross, W.L., Lamprecht, P. 2004. Frequency of proteinase 3 (PR3)-specific autoreactive T-cells determined by cytokine flow cytometry in Wegener's granulomatosis. J. Autoimmun. 22, 79.

Xiao, H., Heeringa, P., Hu, P., Liu, Z., Zhao, M., Aratani, Y., Maeda, N., Falk, R.J., Jennette, J.C. 2002. Antineutrophil cytoplasmic autoantibodies specific for myeloperoxidase cause glomerulonephritis and vasculitis in mice. J. Clin. Invest. 110, 955.

Yale, S.H., Limper, A.H. 1996. *Pneumocystis carinii* pneumonia in patients without acquires immunodeficiency syndrome: associated illnesses and prior corticosteroid therapy. Mayo Clin. Proc. 71, 5–13.

Yang, J.J., Jennette, J.C., Falk, R.J. 1994. Immune complex glomerulonephritis is induced in rats immunized with heterologous myeloperoxidase. Clin. Exp. Immunol. 97, 466.

Yang, J.J., Preston, G.A., Pendergraft, W.F. 2001. Internalization of proteinase 3 is concomitant with endothelial cell apoptosis and internalization of myeloperoxidase with generation of intracellular oxidants. Am. J. Pathol. 158, 581–592.

Yoshikawa, Y., Watanabe, T. 1985. Pulmonary lesions in Wegener's granulomatosis: a clinicopathologic study of 22 autopsy cases. Hum. Pathol. 17, 401–410.

Zhang, L., Jayne, D., Zhao, M., Lockwood, C., Oliveira, D. 1995. Distribution of MHC class II alleles in primary systemic vasculitis. Kidney Int. 47, 294.

Handbook of Systemic Autoimmune Diseases, Volume 2
Pulmonary Involvement in Systemic Autoimmune Diseases
A.U. Wells and C.P. Denton, editors

CHAPTER 5

Vasculitic Syndromes other than Wegener's Granulomatosis

Alexander N. Bennett, David P. D'Cruz*

The Lupus Research Unit, The Rayne Institute, St Thomas' Hospital, London SE1 7EH, UK

1. Introduction

Pulmonary vasculitis can be seen in a variety of conditions. It is seen in primary systemic vasculitides: giant cell arteritis (GCA), Takayasu's arteritis (TA), polyarteritis nodosa (PAN), Wegener's granulomatosis, Churg–Strauss syndrome, microscopic polyangiitis, Henoch-Schönlein purpura and Behçet's disease; in autoimmune disorders: systemic lupus erythematosus (SLE), rheumatoid arthritis, systemic sclerosis; in primary lung disorders: sarcoidosis, eosinophilic pneumonia, hypersensitivity pneumonitis; and in infectious processes and lymphoproliferative disorders. These pulmonary vasculitides are obviously a heterogeneous group of diseases and are characterized by inflammation and destruction of blood vessels. Most are part of a systemic process but some are confined to the lung. Attempts have been made to classify and organize pulmonary vasculitis but because of the heterogeneity and considerable overlap no consensus has been reached. The exact pathogenesis is not known but in some syndromes such as SLE it is thought to be due to immune complex deposition and in chronic granulomatous conditions secondary to alterations in cell mediated immunity.

The classification of the primary systemic vasculitides has been a point of confusion for many years. In 1994 an international consensus conference met in Chapel Hill North Carolina, USA where they defined the vasculitides depending on the size of the vessels involved. Thus, large vessel vasculitis included TA and GCA, medium vessel vasculitis: PAN and Kawasaki disease and small vessel vasculitis: Wegener's granulomatosis, microscopic polyangiitis, Churg–Strauss syndrome, Henoch-Schönlein purpura, essential cryoglobulinemic vasculitis and cutaneous leukcytoclastic angiitis (Table 1). Prior to this the ACR classification criteria from 1990 were used (Table 2). In this chapter we will concentrate on the primary systemic vasculitic syndromes which have pulmonary involvement as a feature. Wegener's granulomatosis is excluded as it is discussed elsewhere in this book.

2. Giant cell arteritis

2.1. Prevalence and epidemiology

Giant cell arteritis is the most common of the systemic vasculitides. In Scandinavian countries the annual incidence rates are generally greater than 200 per million of the population aged 50 and older. In comparison, in southern Europe the incidence is less than 120 per million (Gonzalez-Gay and Garcia-Porrua, 2001). In both northern and southern Europe there has been a marked increase in the incidence of GCA in recent years (Petursdottir et al., 1999; Gonzalez-Gay et al., 2001). Giant cell arteritis affects older patients, the mean age being 70 years. The Chapel Hill consensus definition for GCA (Table 1) and the ACR classification criteria (Table 2) both stipulate that the patients should be over 50 years of age.

*Corresponding author.
Tel.: +44-207-928-9292; fax: +44-207-620-2658
E-mail address: david.d'cruz@kcl.ac.uk (D.P. D'Cruz)

DOI: 10.1016/S1571-5078(04)02005-7

Table 1
Chapel Hill consensus conference definitions

Large vessel vasculitis

Giant cell arteritis
Granulomatous arteritis of the aorta and its major branches with a predilection for the extracranial branches of the carotid artery
Often involves the temporal artery
Patients usually >50 years
May be associated with polymyalgia rheumatica

Takayasu's arteritis
Granulomatous inflammation of the aorta and its major branches
Patients usually >50 years

Medium vessel vasculitis

Polyarteritis nodosa
Necrotizing inflammation of medium-sized or small arteries without glomerulonephritis or vasculitis in the arterioles, capillaries or venules

Kawasaki disease
Arteritis of large, medium-sized and small arteries, associated with mucocutaneous lymph node syndrome

Small vessel vasculitis

Wegener's granulomatosis
Granulomatous inflammation involving the upper and lower respiratory tract, and necrotizing vasculitis affecting small to medium-sized vessels
Necrotizing glomerulonephritis is common

Microscopic polyangiitis
Necrotizing vasculitis, with few or no immune deposits, affecting small vessels
Necrotizing arteritis of small and medium-sized arteries may be present
Necrotizing glomerulonephritis is common
Pulmonary capillaritis often occurs

Churg–Strauss syndrome
Eosinophil-rich, granulomatous inflammation involving the respiratory tract, and necrotizing vasculitis affecting small to medium-sized vessels, associated with asthma and eosinophilia

Henoch-Schönlein purpura
Vasculitis with IgA-dominant immune deposits, affecting small vessels. Typically involves skin, gut and glomeruli. Associated with arthritis or arthralgia

Essential cryoglobulinaemic vasculitis
Vasculitis, with cryglobulin immune deposits, affecting small vessels and associated with cryoglobulins in serum
Skin and glomeruli are often involved

Cutaneous leukocytoclastic angitis
Isolated cutaneous leukocytoclastic angiitis without systemic vasculitis or glomerulonephritis

Table 2
ACR systemic vasculitis criteria, summarized from original papers

Large vessel vasculitis

Giant cell arteritis[a]
Age over 50 years at onset
New type of headache
Claudication of jaw or tongue
Scalp tenderness or nodules
Abnormal temporal artery on clinical examination
Temporal artery biopsy showing vasculitis, or item 4, can be used as a surrogate if biopsy not available

Takayasu's arteritis[b]
Age under 40 years at onset
Limb claudication
Diminished pulses
BP > 10 mm Hg difference between arms
Bruits
Abnormal arteriogram

Medium vessel vasculitis

Polyarteritis nodosa[c]
Weight loss
Livedo reticularis
Testicular pain or tenderness
Myalgias, myopathy or tenderness
Neuropathy
Hypertension
Renal impairment
Hepatitis B virus
Abnormal arteriography
Arterial biopsy showing PMN

Kawasaki disease
None available

Small vessel vasculitis

Wegener's granulomatosis[d]
Nasal or oral inflammation
Chest X-ray showing nodules, infiltrates (fixed) or cavities
Microscopic haematuria or red cell casts in urine
Granulomatous inflammation on biopsy

Microscopic polyangiitis
Not recognized

Churg–Strauss syndrome[e]
Asthma
Eosinophilia
Neuropathy
Pulmonary infiltrated (not fixed)
Sinusitis
Positive biopsy

Hypersensitivity vasculitis[f]
Age over 16 years at onset

Table 2 (*continued*)

Medications which may have precipitated onset
Palpable purpura
Rash
Positive biopsy
Henoch-Schönlein purpura[g]
Palpable purpura
Age at onset under 20 years
Bowel angina
Wall granulocytes on biopsy
Essential cryoglobulinemic vasculitis and cutaneous leukocytoclastic angiitis
Not recognized

Hunder et al. (1990) and Jeanette et al. (1994).

[a] Criteria classify GCA with 95.3% sensitivity and specificity 90.7%

[b] Three criteria classify TA with 90.55% sensitivity and 97.8% specificity.

[c] Three criteria classify PAN with 82.2% sensitivity and 86.6% specificity.

[d] Two criteria classify WG with 88.2% sensitivity and 92.0% specificity.

[e] Four criteria classify CSS with 85% sensitivity and 99.7% specificity.

[f] Three criteria classify HSV with 71% sensitivity and 83.9% specificity.

[g] Two criteria classify HSP with 87% sensitivity and 88% specificity.

Giant cell arteritis is more common in whites of Scandinavian extraction and uncommon in black, Asian and South American populations (Liu et al., 2001).

2.2. Aetiology/Pathogenesis

There is thought to be a genetic influence on the pathogenesis of GCA and there is an association with HLA-DRB1*04 alleles (Dababneh et al., 1998) in both susceptibility and severity. Unlike rheumatoid arthritis, however, there is no shared epitope homozygosity to predict severity of disease (Dababneh et al., 1998). In northwest Spain links between GCA and different tumour necrosis factor microsatellite polymorphisms have also been made (Mattey et al., 2000), but studies into links with adhesion molecule-1 have produced mixed results (Gonzalez-Gay and Garcia-Porrua, 2002). There are reports that cigarette smoking and history of vascular disease increase the risk of GCA (Gonzalez-Gay et al., 2001) and parvovirus B19 has recently been suggested as having a role in its pathogenesis (Gabriel et al., 1999). Giant cell arteritis and TA have a similar pathogenesis that distinguishes them from other vasculitides. Cellular immune responses involving T-cells, antigen-presenting cells, and macrophages are fundamental and there is no evidence of an autoantibody component (Weyand and Goronzy, 2003). Giant cell arteritis is a T-cell dependant disease (Weyand and Goronzy, 2002) and the CD4+ T-cell is the critical cell in organizing tissue injury in this vasculitic syndrome (Grunewald et al., 1972; Brack et al., 1997). The T-cell activation in the arterial wall requires the activation of specialized antigen-presenting cells and dendritic cells (Krupa et al., 2002). The antigen recognized by the CD4+ cells is unknown. Infectious agents, toxins, drugs, and autoantigens could all be possible and parvovirus, influenza virus, varicella virus and *Chlamydia pneumoniae* have all been suspected (Elling et al., 1996, 2000; Duhaut et al., 1999; Mitchell and Front, 2001). In GCA, T-cells leave the blood and enter the tissue via the vasa vasorum in the adventitia. Microvessels in the inflamed arteries produce a variety of adhesion molecules that regulate leukocyte transport (Wawryk et al., 1991; Lavignac et al., 1996; Cid et al., 2000). Activated dendritic cells produce the chemokines CCL19 and CCL21, which have a critical role in attracting T-cells and macrophages into the arterial wall (Krupa et al., 2002). Immature dendritic cells have a role in maintaining T-cell unresponsivness. In contrast to mature dendritic cells that induce T-cell responses, immature dendritic cells do not express the costimulatory molecules CD80 and CD86. Lesions in the temporal arteries from patients with GCA contain numerous dendritic cells in the adventitia and the inflamed wall. These dendritic cells are mature and activated (Krupa et al., 2002; Cid et al., 1989). The activation of endothelial cells and dendritic cells precedes T-cell recruitment to the tissue and the activation and differentiation of the dendritic cells are key events in the pathogenesis of GCA (Krupa et al., 2002).

2.3. Clinical manifestations

Giant cell arteritis was first described in 1932 by Horton et al. (1932). It is a granulomatous vasculitis of medium-sized and large arteries that affects older patients, with a mean age of 70 years. It has a predilection for the branches of the external carotid artery but is a systemic disease that can affect virtually any organ. Characteristic symptoms include temporal headaches and temporal artery tenderness, jaw claudication, polymyalgia rheumatica, fatigue, fever and visual disturbance including blindness. Although not characteristic, respiratory symptoms are not uncommon, but evidence of parenchymal lung disease is rare (Hunder, 1990; Larson et al., 1984). Parenchymal lung disease has, however, been reported in classical biopsy proven GCA patients. Cavitating and non-cavitating multiple large nodular opacities (Bradley et al., 1984; Kramer et al., 1987) and interstitial opacities (Kramer et al., 1987; Karam and Fulmer, 1982) have been demonstrated on both transbronchial and open lung biopsy (Bradley et al., 1984; Karam and Fulmer, 1982). Pulmonary artery involvement has been noted in GCA (Dennison et al., 1985; Glover et al., 1987) and pulmonary arteriole and venule involvement has also been noted in a patient 6 months before the diagnosis of GCA (biopsy proven) was made (Doyle et al., 1988). When the disease is untreated the prognosis is poor but treated early, the prognosis is good.

2.4. Investigations

2.4.1. Radiology

With the relatively rare involvement of the respiratory system in GCA radiological investigations of the chest are unusual. However, if parenchymal disease is suspected, conventional chest radiograph, CT or transbronchial or open lung biopsy would all undoubtedly be useful. If pulmonary artery involvement is suspected then pulmonary angiography would be the investigation of choice. With regards to the diagnosis of GCA, the gold standard is temporal artery biopsy which is discussed below.

However, promising techniques are high-resolution ultrasonography and colour duplex ultrasonography. Colour duplex ultrasonography may show a hypo-echoic halo around the perfused lumen in inflamed temporal arteries, which disappear with corticosteroid treatment (Schmidt et al., 1997). Ultrasonography is, however, dependent on blood flow abnormalities and it lacks the sensitivity to detect subtle inflammatory changes in the arterial wall (Schmidt, 2000). The extent of intimal hyperplasia and therefore luminal occlusion varies in patients with GCA and is modulated by the extent of platelet-derived growth factor production (Kaiser et al., 1998). Therefore patients with significant intimal hyperplasia and blood flow abnormalities could be diagnosed with ultrasonography, although those without significant intimal hyperplasia rely on biopsy to make the diagnosis.

2.4.2. Functional

Giant cell arteritis patients with proven interstitial patterns on chest radiograph have been shown to have restrictive patterns on pulmonary function testing (Kramer et al., 1987; Karam and Fulmer, 1982). In one study of 17 GCA patients without pulmonary symptoms or history of lung disease or tobacco use, three patients had restrictive patterns on pulmonary function tests, two had isolated reductions in transfer factor (DLCO) and one had obstructive physiology (Acritidis et al., 1988).

2.4.3. Positron emission tomography and nuclear medicine

Positron emission tomography (PET) scanning with radiolabelled glucose analogues enables in vivo measurement of glucose metabolism. It has the advantage over biopsy of being able to detect all active areas. Increased uptake in the large thoracic arteries is more common in GCA patients than controls with a 56% sensitivity and 98% specificity (Blockmans et al., 2000). This is due to the increased glycolysis in inactivated leukocytes and macrophages and is a characteristic feature of inflammation in GCA. Nuclear medicine scanning with gallium scintigraphy has been reported to localize inflammation in the aortic arch and pulmonary arteries in TA patients (Morita et al., 1993) and the temporal area in GCA patients. Both of these techniques are still largely only used for research purposes and their use in the clinical diagnosis of GCA has yet to be established.

2.4.4. Haematology and biochemistry

Typical features of chronic inflammation can been seen in any of the vasculitides: classically a normocytic, normochromic anaemia with a leucocytosis and thrombocytosis. Other inflammatory markers, in particular the erythrocyte sedimentation rate (ESR) and C-reactive protein (CRP), are often the only abnormal indices. They are, however, not always raised and up to 20% of GCA patients with positive biopsies have normal acute phase reactants (Mohan and Kerr, 2001).

2.4.5. *Tissue biopsy*

The gold standard for the diagnosis of GCA is a temporal artery biopsy. Skip lesions are characteristic so a biopsy of a minimum of 2–3 cm is required. If it is negative but clinical suspicion is still high, then biopsy of the opposite temporal artery may yield positive results in up to 15–20% of patients (Hall et al., 1983).

The findings are those of a panarteritis with mononuclear infiltrates penetrating all layers of the arterial wall. Typically, activated T-cells and macrophages are arranged in granulomas. Multinucleated giant cells, when present, are usually close to the fragmented internal elastic lumina. Often the intimal layer is hyperplastic, leading to concentric occlusion of the macrolumen. The classical granulomatous GCA is seen in about 50% of biopsies from symptomatic patients. The other 50% show a panarteritis with a mixed inflammatory infiltrate but with no giant cells. Patients biopsied prior to starting corticosteroids have the highest diagnostic yield of approximately 80%. After 1 week of treatment that yield deceases to 60% and then to 20% for patients on steroids for longer periods.

3. Takayasu's arteritis

3.1. *Prevalence and epidemiology*

The annual incidence of TA has been reported in Japan as 150 new cases per year from a population of 125 million (Koide, 1992). It is most common in Mexico and Far Eastern countries but, although no cases were reported in two European studies (Watts et al., 1995; Gonzalez-Gay and Garcia-Porrua, 1999), it is increasingly being recognized in the west. This disease is most common in young women during the childbearing years with the peak onset being in the third decade. Men are affected, however, and comprise between 10–30% of cases.

3.2. *Aetiology/Pathogenesis*

Takayasu's arteritis shares many histological abnormalities and pathogenic pathways with GCA and this distinguishes them from the other vasculitides. These are described in more detail above. Panarteritic inflammatory infiltrates cause marked thickening of the involved artery and subsequent luminal narrowing and occlusion, resulting in diffuse dilatation, aneurysms and thrombosis. Cellular immune responses involving T-cells, antigen-presenting cells and macrophages are fundamental elements in TA. However, in TA the T-cells may have additional effector functions, such as releasing the pore-forming protein perforin, which could directly contribute to the structural damage incurred by the aortic wall (Seko et al., 1994, 1996). The pathological findings when there is pulmonary artery involvement appear to be different from that in the systemic TA. Lie (1996) reviewed the pathology of five patients with TA and pulmonary involvement. Three types of vascular lesion were identified: the classic large vessel granulomatous GCA, a peculiar type of organized thrombus with prominent recanalization and neoangiogenesis, and plexogenic arteriopathy. Therefore the histological findings of pulmonary TA are distinct and differ from that of the systemic TA.

3.3. *Clinical manifestations*

Takayasu's arteritis is a form of large vessel granulomatous vasculitis. It predominantly affects the aorta and its main branches. The persistent inflammation often leads to stenosis, occlusion and aneurysm formation. Symptoms are predominately related to vascular insufficiency in the limbs, cerebral ischaemia and cardiac involvement. The gastrointestinal tract can also become symptomatic secondary to ischaemia. Systemic symptoms such as fatigue, weight loss, night sweats, fever and arthralgia are common. Characteristic clinical findings include absent or reduced pulses with vascular bruits and valvular disease, predominantly aortic regurgitation.

Myalgias, arthralgia, fatigue and fever are also common. At diagnosis, however, up to 20% of TA patients are asymptomatic and have been diagnosed coincidently. Pulmonary involvement in Takayasu's is almost exclusively secondary to vasculitis of the large or medium-sized pulmonary arteries. Pulmonary hypertension is a well-recognized finding (Lande and Bard, 1976; Moore et al., 1985; Chauvaud et al., 1987).

Takayasu's arteritis is a chronic relapsing disease—one study found that 45% of patients experienced relapse and another 23% never achieved remission (Kerr et al., 1994). Takayasu's arteritis is associated with significant morbidity and disease-related mortality is usually associated with congestive cardiac failure, cerebrovascular events, myocardial infarction, aneurysm rupture and renal failure (Kerr et al., 1994). Hypertension is also common. Koide (1992) reported hypertension as the major complaint on initial consultation in 45% of patients who were subsequently diagnosed with TA.

Five-year survival has been reported between 0 and 35% (Langford, 2001). One study, however, reported a survival of greater than 94% (Kerr et al., 1994).

3.4. Investigation

3.4.1. Radiology

Chest radiographs may be abnormal in up to 67% of patients with TA (Yamato et al., 1986). The common abnormalities are irregularities in the descending aorta, linear calcifications of the aortic wall, ectatic aortic arch and cardiomegaly. Decreased vascular markings secondary to pulmonary artery involvement are also seen, but less frequently. CT can demonstrate thickening and enhancement of the vascular wall in patients with active disease (Fig. 1). While magnetic resonance angiography is extremely useful in delineating gross vascular anatomy, most clinicians still regard invasive arterial angiography as the gold standard investigation. In terms of pulmonary disease, angiographic studies have estimated the frequency of pulmonary artery involvement in TA at between 70 and 86% (Yamato et al., 1986; Yamanda et al., 1992). Typical angiographic findings are stenosis, occlusion and aneurysm formation. A further angiographic study in patients with no respiratory symptoms showed that 50% had pulmonary arterial involvement (Lupi et al., 1975).

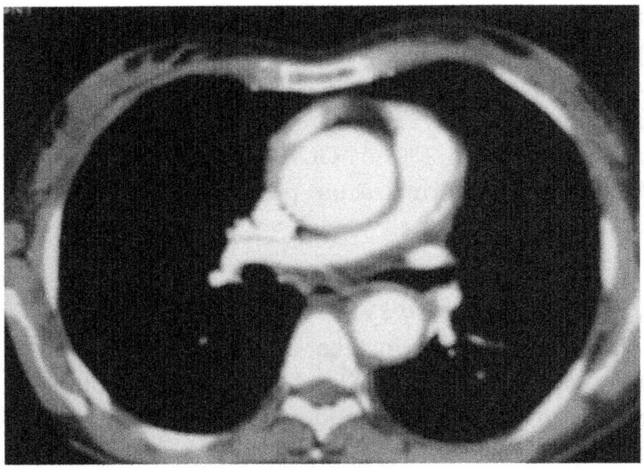

Figure 1. Takayasu's arteritis with pulmonary arteritis: CT scan with contrast showing thickening of pulmonary arterial wall and thickening of the aortic wall with dilatation of both the ascending and descending aorta.

Ventilation perfusion lung scans are often abnormal in TA (Umehara et al., 1991), which can result in an incorrect diagnosis of pulmonary embolism (Hayashi et al., 1986; Kerr et al., 1995). Fig. 2a and b shows a patient in whom the initial diagnosis was of pulmonary embolism, but the appearances were later ascribed to TA. It is also important to remember when considering this that thrombosis is, however, a complication of vasculitis, and has been seen in pulmonary arteritis (Kerr et al., 1995).

3.4.2. Functional

Nuclear medicine scanning with gallium scintigraphy has been reported to localize inflammation in the aortic arch and pulmonary arteries in TA patients (Morita et al., 1993), though the role of this has, however, yet to be established in the diagnosis of TA. It may be useful in following the response to treatment in some patients. There is also anecdotal unpublished evidence that FDG positron emission tomography may be useful in detecting arterial inflammation both at diagnosis and when following response to treatment.

3.4.3. Haematology and biochemistry

As for GCA, in TA an elevation of the acute phase reactants is expected. This is not always the case with

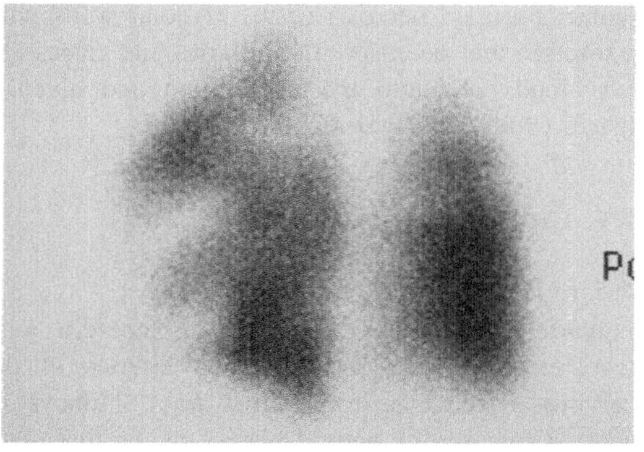

A

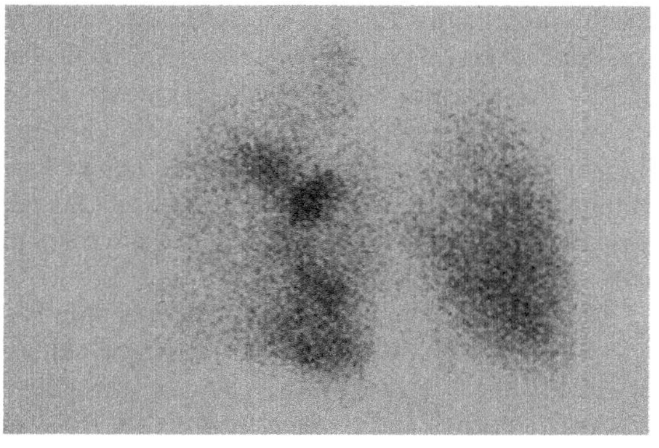

B

Figure 2. (a) Takayasu's arteritis with pulmonary arteritis: perfusion scan with multiple mismatched defects. (b) Takayasu's arteritis with pulmonary arteritis: normal ventilation scan of same patient.

up to 30% of angiogram proven TA patients having normal acute phase reactants. Interestingly up to 56% of TA patients who are otherwise in remission have a persistently raised ESR (Kerr et al., 1994; Wilke and Hoffman, 1995).

4. Microscopic polyangiitis and polyarteritis nodosa

4.1. Prevalence and epidemiology

The incidence and prevalence of microscopic polyangiitis and PAN have to be looked at carefully, since prior to the 1994 Chapel Hill consensus conference they were regarded as the same condition. In a prospective 6-year study from 1988 to 1994 of all systemic vasculitides in a community setting in Norwich, England, Watts et al. (1995) reported no cases of PAN meeting the Chapel Hill definition.

Subsequently, however, Watts et al. (2000 2001b) reported the annual incidence as 4.4 per million in Norway and 8.0 per million in the UK. There appears to be a geographical influence, with a higher incidence in southern compared to northern Europe, and in Kuwait the incidence has been reported as high as 16 per million (El-Reshaid et al., 1997).

Classical PAN affects men and women equally. Microscopic polyangiitis is more common in males. Neither have a racial predilection and the average age of onset for microscopic polyangiitis has been reported as 57 years in France (Guillevin et al., 1999), but both can occur in children and the elderly. Interestingly there is a geographical variation with an increased incidence of microscopic polyangiitis in Kuwait and Spain when compared to Norway (El-Reshaid et al., 1997; Gonzalez-Gay and Garcia-Porrua, 1999; Watts et al., 2001a).

4.2. Pathogenesis/Aetiology

4.2.1. Microscopic polyangiitis

Microscopic polyangiitis is a non-granulomatous small to medium-sized vessel vasculitis, characterized by pauci-immune necrotizing and cresentic glomerulonephritis. The absence of granulomas helps differentiate it from Wegener's granulomatosis. Diffuse alveolar haemorrhage, which is the main clinical manifestation of pulmonary involvement, is secondary to pulmonary capillaritis (see below). Microscopic polyangiitis is an antineutrophil cytoplasmic antibodies (ANCA) associated vasculitis with antibodies typically against myeloperoxidase. The role of ANCA in the pathogenesis of vasculitis, the different subgroups of ANCA, its antigenic targets, clinical associations and usefulness in diagnosis are discussed below.

Several mechanisms have been suggested as to how ANCA interacts with target antigens to cause necrotizing vasculitis. One hypothesis is that ANCA facilitate neutrophil adherence to vascular endothelial cells and indirectly mediates endothelial cell injury and transmigration of neutrophils into the perivascular space. Cytokines, IL-1, TGF-Beta and TNF prime neutrophils with ANCA antigens, making them accessible to ANCA, and also cause expression and up regulation of adhesion molecules on endothelial cells. Adherent neutrophils result in localized endothelial cell injury. These neutrophils may also pass between the injured endothelial cells into the perivascular space where they are characteristically seen histologically (Ewert et al., 1990; Falk et al., 1990; Savage et al., 1992; Cid, 1996). Interestingly, there are also links between ANCA and alpha$_1$-antitrypsin deficiency. Alpha$_1$-antitrypsin is a strong inhibitor of proteinase-3 and deficiency of alpha$_1$-antitrypsin is associated with systemic vasculitis. Myeloperoxidase can also inactivate alpha$_1$-antitrypsin and prolong the activity of proteinase-3 (Esnault et al., 1993; Savige et al., 1995).

4.3. Pulmonary capillaritis

The term pulmonary capillaritis is often used as a clinical diagnosis but is in fact a histopathological finding. It is seen in several diseases including (Sullivan and Hoffman, 1998):

(1) Churg–Strauss syndrome
(2) Wegener's granulomatosis
(3) Microscopic polyangiitis
(4) Henoch-Schönlein purpura
(5) Behçet's disease
(6) Systemic lupus erythematosus
(7) Rheumatoid arthritis
(8) Infection-related vasculitis
(9) Drug-related vasculitis
(10) Cryoglobulinemic vasculitis
(11) Malignancy-related vasculitis
(12) Polymyositis
(13) Sjögren's syndrome
(14) Antiphospholipid syndrome.

In many of these conditions there is an active glomerulonephritis with renal impairment, giving rise to the term pulmonary-renal syndrome.

Pulmonary capillaritis is a common histopathological finding in the clinical diffuse pulmonary haemorrhage (DPH) syndrome. The characteristic pathological features were described by Mark and Ramirez (1985). These include neutrophilic infiltration of the alveolar interstitium, fibrinous thrombi occluding capillaries and attaching to interalveolar septae, fibrinoid necrosis of the alveolar walls with disruption and necrosis of capillaries and release of red blood cells into the interstitium and alveolar spaces (Sullivan and Hoffman, 1998).

4.4. Clinical manifestations

4.4.1. Polyarteritis nodosa

Polyarteritis nodosa often presents acutely with involvement of the medium-sized arteries of the nervous system, gastrointestinal tract, kidneys or heart. Typically the natural history of the disease is for the presentation to be a severe illness, but if the patient recovers relapse is uncommon (Guillevin et al., 1996). Polyarteritis nodosa was first described by Kussmaul and Maier (1866) but since then it has gone though many changes in nomenclature. In the Chapel Hill consensus conference, patients with small vessel vasculitis were considered to be microscopic polyangiitis.

The presence of primary lung involvement in PAN is controversial. Early studies that indicated pulmonary involvement in 28–47% of cases can probably be ignored (Sweeney and Baggenstross, 1949; Rose and Spencer, 1957; Moskowitz et al., 1963) because these included microscopic polyangiitis. Following the Chapel Hill consensus conference pulmonary vasculitis and interstitial lung disease were then considered extremely rare in classical PAN (Hunninghake and Fauci, 1979; Kennedy and Fulmer, 1993). However, in a postmortem series ten patients with PAN were found to have bronchial vasculitis (Leavitt and Fauci, 1986) and a case report described medium-sized pulmonary artery vasculitis (Nick et al., 1996). Untreated PAN has a poor outcome with survival being as low as 13% (Frohnert and Sheps, 1967; Leib et al., 1979).

4.4.2. Microscopic polyangiitis

Microscopic polyangiitis is a small to medium-sized vessel vasculitis first distinguished from PAN by Wohlwill (1923) and then redefined by Davson et al. (1948) and described in detail by Savage et al. (1985). It is associated with severe pulmonary vasculitis and rapidly progressive glomerulonephritis. Although it is different from Wegener's granulomatosis in that it has no granulomatous inflammation, there are some similarities clinically and histologically.

4.4.3. *Diffuse pulmonary haemorrhage*

Diffuse pulmonary haemorrhage is a clinical syndrome commonly caused by necrotizing pulmonary capillaritis, most often associated with the primary vasculitides such as Wegener's granulomatosis, microscopic polyangiitis, Behçet's syndrome, mixed cryoglobulinaemia, SLE (Zamora et al., 1997) and Henoch-Schönlein purpura. Diffuse pulmonary haemorrhage is characterized by dyspnea, hypoxaemia, haemoptysis, anaemia, diffuse airspace shadowing on chest radiograph (Fig. 3) and raised transfer factor on pulmonary function tests. Many patients require ventilation and circulatory support on intensive care. It is important to always investigate for concomitant glomerulonephritis and to consider non-vasculitic causes when presented with this syndrome. Other diagnoses to consider would be chemical- or drug-related pneumonitis and idiopathic pulmonary haemosiderosis (Leatherman et al., 1984; Leatherman, 1987; Travis et al., 1990).

Unlike with Goodpasture's syndrome, there is no link between cigarette smoking and pulmonary vasculitis (Burns, 1998). Patients with pulmonary haemorrhage are more likely to have an IgM ANCA, whereas the most common ANCA is IgG (Jayne et al., 1989; Esnault et al., 1992).

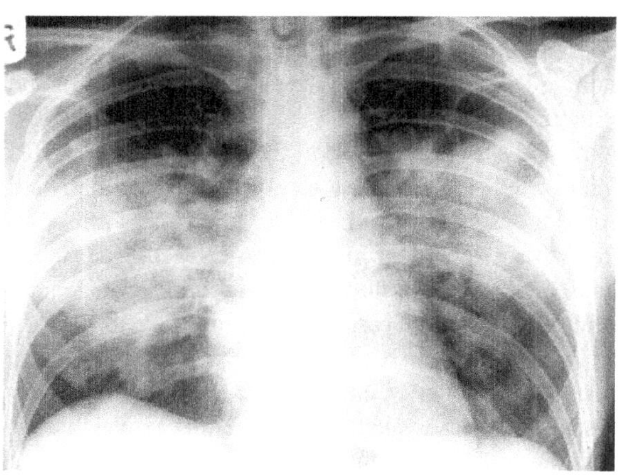

Figure 3. Microscopic polyangiitis with diffuse pulmonary haemorrhage: chest radiograph showing diffuse airspace midzone shadowing.

These patients with pulmonary haemorrhage have a worse prognosis and have high early mortality from respiratory failure or lung fibrosis (Haworth et al., 1985). Mortality may be as high as 50% despite expert care in centres of excellence (Haworth et al., 1985).

4.5. *Investigations*

4.5.1. *Classical polyarteritis nodosa*

4.5.1.1. Radiology. The investigation of choice is coeliac axis arteriography. The classical signs include a beaded appearance of the mesenteric or renal arteries, representing multiple microaneuysms. This was demonstrated by Bron et al. (1965), who showed that angiography could reveal microaneurysms and stenoses in medium-sized arteries. Although microaneurysms are not pathognomonic, they are commonly seen in PAN and rarely seen in other vasculitides. These lesions may disappear as the disease goes into remission (Darras-Joly et al., 1995). Approximately 70% of patients with a clinical diagnosis of PAN have positive angiographic findings.

4.5.1.2. Tissue biopsy. Biopsy can be invaluable when diagnosing PAN. A convenient tissue to biopsy in patients presenting with peripheral neuropathy, which is very common in PAN (affecting up to 80% of patients), is the sural nerve. The vascular lesions are characteristically focal and segmental. However, sural nerve biopsy sites often heal poorly and there is an increased risk of sepsis and ulceration, especially since the majority of these patients are subsequently immunosupressed with therapy. Although there is usually no evidence of myositis in PAN, a blind muscle biopsy may also reveal arteritis.

Necrotizing vasculitis with fibrinoid necrosis with the resultant formation of microaneurysms is typical. The unique histological feature of PAN is the coexistence of active necrotizing lesions and proliferative, fibrotic healing or healed lesions in different tissues or in different sections of the same tissue (Wilke and Hoffman, 1995).

4.5.1.3. Biochemistry, haematology and immunology. Evidence of inflammation is common with an ESR $>$ 60 mm per hour in 80–90% of patients, and elevated white cell count in 45–75%. Elevated CRP and a normocytic anaemia are also common and an eosinophilia is seen but not as often. Hepatitis B surface antigen should be sought but it is only seen in 7–36% of patients (Guillevin et al., 1989, 1995a,b). ANCA is rare in classical PAN, however, it has been reported and Hauschild et al. (1994) reported a frequency of 19.4% of ANCA in 36 patients with PAN.

4.5.2. *Microscopic polyangiitis*

4.5.2.1. Radiology. Findings consistent with DPH are the commonest radiological abnormality in microscopic polyangiitis occurring in up to 33% of patients. Other less common findings are pleural effusions and pulmonary oedema. Diffuse pulmonary haemorrhage does not occur in classical PAN.

The chest radiograph of DPH is characterized by diffuse or patchy air space shadowing with the periphery and apices typically being spared (Primack et al., 1995) (Fig. 3). The lesions are usually bilateral but may be asymmetrical. Air bronchograms are common 2–3 days after the acute episode. With repeat episodes of haemorrhage, the reticular pattern persists and progressive interstitial fibrosis develops. CT scanning shows bilateral consolidation or ground-glass shadowing in the acute stage (Fig. 4) and miliary 1–3 mm nodules in the subacute stage (Seo et al., 2000).

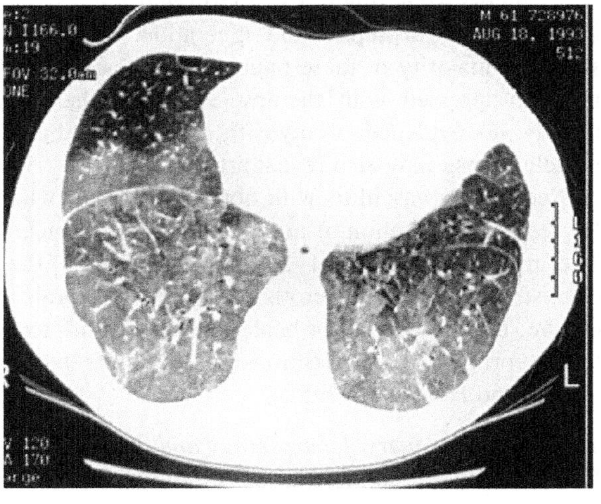

Figure 4. Microscopic polyangiitis with diffuse pulmonary haemorrhage: CT chest showing bilateral ground-glass shadowing indicating fluid in the alveolar spaces.

4.5.2.2. Functional. In patients with recurrent diffuse pulmonary haemorrhage, pulmonary fibrosis almost inevitably occurs and a restrictive pattern on lung function testing is found. This of course will occur in any condition where recurrent DPH is a feature. Much less common is severe airflow obstruction, but this has been reported (Brugiere et al., 1997).

4.5.3. *Biochemistry/Serology/Immunology*

Non-specific markers of inflammation are expected with a raised ESR, CRP, white cell and platelet count and a low albumin and a normocytic normochromic anaemia. Eosinophilia has been reported in up to 14% of patients (Adu et al., 1987). Complement C3 and C4 are normal or raised and rheumatoid factor and ANA have been reported in 39–50% and 21–33%, respectively.

Antineutrophil cytoplasmic antibodies were first described in 1982 in eight patients with glomerulonephritis, five of whom had pulmonary disease (Davies et al., 1982). They are directed against antigens in the cytoplasm of polymorphonuclear leucocytes and monocytes. They are divided into C (cytoplasmic), P (perinuclear) and A (atypical) on the basis of their indirect immunofluorescence staining patterns. Cytoplasmic antineutrophil cytoplasmic antibodies are usually directed against proteinase 3 (PR3) but have occasionally been reported to be directed against other proteins such as bactericidal permeability-increasing protein (BPI) (Zhao et al., 1996) and myeloperoxidase (Hoffman and Specks, 1998). The antigenic targets for p-ANCA are more varied and include the major antigen myeloperoxidase (Falk and Jennette, 1988), cathepsin (Yahya et al., 1997) and less commonly elastase, lactoferrin, cathepsin G, BPI (Zhao et al., 1996) and rarely PR3 (Hoffman and Specks, 1998). Antineutrophil cytoplasmic antibodies are associated with various systemic vasculitides of the small and medium-sized vessels, including Wegener's granulomatosis, microscopic polyangiitis and Churg–Strauss Syndrome (Hoffman and Specks, 1998). They have also been associated with numerous other non-vasculitic diseases such as inflammatory bowel disease (Stoffel et al., 1996), autoimmune hepatitis, sclerosing cholangitis (Stoffel et al., 1996), rheumatic autoimmune diseases (Hauschild et al., 1993), infections (Soto et al., 1994; Cho et al., 1995; Yahya et al., 1997) and malignancies (Edgar et al., 1993; Hoffman and Specks, 1998).

Antineutrophil cytoplasmic antibodies are useful in the diagnosis of the above conditions, although it has been debated in Wegener's granulomatosis whether they should be used as a disease marker to guide treatment. Some studies have supported this hypothesis (Cohen-Tervaert et al., 1989), however, other larger studies have suggested otherwise (Kerr et al., 1993). The use of ANCA in the diagnosis of Churg–Strauss syndrome is controversial. There have been no large studies performed. The frequency of positive ANCA, most often against myeloperoxidase (MPO), has reported at anywhere between 0–66% (Hauschild et al., 1993; Kerr et al., 1993; Cohen et al., 1995; Hagen et al., 1998).

5. Churg–Strauss syndrome

5.1. Prevalence and epidemiology

Churg–Strauss syndrome is extremely rare with an estimated annual incidence of approximately 3 per million (Reid et al., 1996). In Europe there have been two long-term prospective studies evaluating the incidence of primary systemic vasculitis, which included Wegener's granulomatosis, Churg–Strauss syndrome and PAN, as classified by the ACR criteria, and microscopic polyangiitis as defined by the Chapel Hill criteria. The incidence in Norwich, England and Lugo, Spain were 19.8 per million and 18.3 per million, respectively (Watts et al., 2001a). The prevalence of the same group of primary systemic vasculitis in Norwich was 144.5 per million (Watts et al., 2000). In both Norwich and Lugo there was a slight bias toward men. The mean age is approximately 30–45 years, but any age can be affected with no particular predilection to either sex.

5.2. Aetiology/Pathogenesis

The histological picture is distinct, being reported originally by Jacob Churg and Lotte Strauss in 1951, and consisted of necrotizing arteritis, eosinophilic infiltration of tissue and extravascular granulomas (Churg and Strauss, 1951). Pathological studies since have also revealed intravascular granulomas. The role of anti-neutrophil cytoplasmic antibodies in the pathogenesis of Churg–Strauss syndrome is controversial and has been discussed previously under the aetiology and pathogenesis of microscopic polyangiitis.

5.3. Clinical manifestations

This disease affects the small and medium-sized vessels. In Churg–Strauss syndrome asthma usually precedes evidence of vasculitis by months to years In as many as a fifth of cases they begin simultaneously. Along with asthma, eosinophilia, pulmonary infiltrates (Fig. 5) and allergic rhinitis are typical features. Allergic nasal and sinus disease in Churg–Strauss syndrome is not usually destructive, unlike in Wegener's granulomatosis. Several phases of the illness may be identified. The prodromal phase consists of allergic disease, asthma and allergic rhinitis, often with nasal polyps. The second phase is characterized by blood and tissue eosinophilia with clinical and radiographic evidence consistent with Loffler's syndrome or chronic eosinophilic pneumonia. A third phase of systemic vasculitis occurs but may be several years later (Lanham et al., 1984), and interestingly asthma often improves just prior to the development of the acute vasculitic phase.

In the lung pulmonary infiltrates are far more common (70–90%) than pulmonary nodules, which

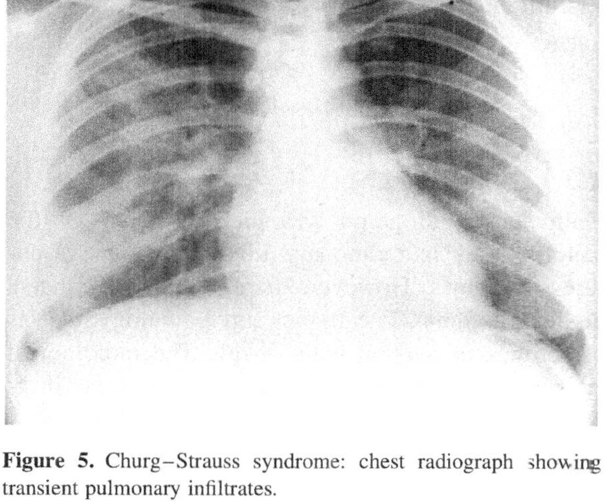

Figure 5. Churg–Strauss syndrome: chest radiograph showing transient pulmonary infiltrates.

are the most common pulmonary lesion in Wegener's granulomatosis. If lung nodules do occur they generally do not cavitate, as they often do in Wegener's granulomatosis (Hoffman and Kerr, 1994). Diffuse pulmonary infiltration and pleural disease rarely occur (Chumbley et al., 1977; Churg, 1983; Lanham et al., 1984). When compared to Wegener's granulomatosis, Churg–Strauss syndrome has a higher propensity for cardiac, neurological and gastrointestinal disease (Lane et al., 2003). In fact eosinophilic myocarditis occurs in approximately 50% of all Churg–Strauss syndrome patients (Lanham et al., 1984). Less often acute or chronic pericarditis, which can occasionally become restrictive, is seen (Lanham et al., 1984). Mild renal insufficiency is common in Churg–Strauss syndrome but renal failure is rare (Lanham et al., 1984). Cardiac disease resulting in congestive cardiac failure or myocardial infarction is the commonest cause of death (Lanham et al., 1984). Status asthmaticus or respiratory failure due to other causes only accounted for less than 10% of deaths (Lanham and Churg, 1991).

Churg–Strauss syndrome can either be a benign or aggressive illness (Chumbley et al., 1977; Churg 1983; Lanham et al., 1984). Patients with the worst 5-year survival are those with nervous system involvement, renal insufficiency, ischaemic gut disease and cardiomyopathy (Guillevin et al., 1995a,b). The mean survival time after the onset of signs and symptoms of vasculitis is 4.5 years (Chumbley et al., 1977), and patients with a short interval between the onset of asthma and onset of vasculitis have a poor prognosis.

5.4. Investigations

5.4.1. Radiology

Plain chest radiograph will pick up many of the abnormalities in pulmonary involvement in vasculitic syndromes. However, there is no doubt that a high-resolution CT can pick up pathology that is sometimes missed on plain X-ray. The radiological interpretation of these investigations can be difficult, and once immunosuppressive treatment has started it is made more difficult by the fact that nearly 50% of patients experience serious infectious complications related to treatment, with almost half of these being respiratory infections (Bradley et al. 1989; Sen, 1991). Radiological findings in the angiitis-granulomatosis group are nodular and patchy opacities, whereas the principal feature of those syndromes with pulmonary capillaritis is diffuse airspace shadowing.

Typical radiological findings in Churg–Strauss syndrome include non-segmental air space consolidation in a peripheral distribution similar to eosinophilic pneumonia, or multiple nodular lesions (Leavitt and Fauci, 1986; Weisbrod, 1989; Staples, 1991; Wilson, 1995). In contrast to Wegener's granulomatosis, cavitation of nodules is rare. Cardiomegaly and pericardial effusions are seen in patients with cardiac involvement.

5.4.2. Tissue biopsy

Although in some cases careful clinical history and examination along with radiological and laboratory investigations will give a diagnosis, often a tissue biopsy is required. Which tissue to biopsy is important to consider. In Wegener's granulomatosis and Churg–Strauss syndrome vasculitic skin lesions can be diagnostic, as can upper airway biopsy in Wegener's granulomatosis (Sams, 1980; Fulmer and Kaltreider, 1982; McCluskey and Fienberg, 1983; Fauci et al., 1983). It is important to note, however, that only a relative minority of patients have the classical histological findings on biopsy of upper airway tissues (D'Cruz et al., 1989). In syndromes with renal involvement such as Wegener's granulomatosis and microscopic polyangiitis percutaneous renal biopsy is the investigation of choice. If lung tissue is required then the decision is between transbronchial biopsy and open lung biopsy. Transbronchial biopsies are thought to be inferior to open lung biopsy but have a lower morbidity and mortality rate. Hoffman et al. (1992) performed a total of 82 open lung biopsies in patients with small vessel vasculitis, of which 89% showed evidence of combined vasculitis and necrosis. Granulomas and necrosis were found in 90%. Fifty-nine transbronchial biopsies were performed in 48 patients; in only four specimens was vasculitis identified and in only three of these were granulomas also seen.

6. Henoch-Schönlein purpura

6.1. Prevalence and epidemiology

Primarily a disease of children and the most common vasculitis in children, Henoch-Schönlein purpura is, however, well described in adults. The incidence rate has been reported as 13.5/100,000 in school-aged children (Robson and Leung, 1994), and 126.4 per million in Lugo, Spain (Calvino et al., 2001). The incidence in adults is, however, much less, reported as 14.3 per million and 13.0 per million in Lugo, Spain (Garcia-Porrua and Gonzalez-Gay, 1999) and Norwich, UK (Watts et al., 1998), respectively. Henoch-Schönlein purpura appears to be a seasonal disorder that occurs more commonly in the spring, autumn and winter, affecting males and females equally. In 50% of patients the disease onset is preceded by an upper respiratory tract infection. The median age of onset in children is 5.5 years in Northwest Spain (Calvino et al., 2001).

6.2. Aetiology/pathogenesis

Henoch-Schönlein purpura is known to follow Beta-haemolytic streptococcal infections (Kauffmann et al., 1980) and is a small vessel vasculitis characterized by immune complex deposits in small vessels and renal glomeruli where IgA is the pathogenic antibody. The aetiology of Henoch-Schönlein purpura has genetic associations with HLA-DRB1*01. Henoch-Schönlein purpura patients also have a decreased frequency of HLA-DRB1*07 (Amoli et al., 2001). Renal manifestations are associated with HLA-B*35 (Amoli et al., 2002a) and ILRN*2 (Amoli et al., 2002b) alleles.

6.3. Clinical manifestations

Henoch-Schönlein purpura is characterized by diffuse leukocytoclastic vasculitis involving the skin, joints, gastrointestinal tract and kidneys (Cream et al., 1970; Fauci, 1978; Kauffmann et al., 1980). It is primarily a disease of children although adult onset is well recognized. The clinical features typically include arthralgias, palpable purpura on the buttocks and lower limbs, abdominal pain and haematuria (Cream et al., 1970; Fauci, 1978). Pulmonary involvement is uncommon but can be fatal (Satinder et al., 1982). When the respiratory system is involved, symptoms range from cough to severe dyspnea (Fauci, 1978; Fulmer and Kaltreider, 1982). The disease is usually self-limiting but deaths from renal and respiratory failure have been reported.

6.4. Investigations

6.4.1. Radiology

Typically the chest radiograph only shows transient infiltrates or pneumonia, but occasionally a diffuse interstitial pattern has been observed.

6.4.2. Tissue biopsy

Typical biopsy appearances of either affected skin or kidneys are systemic necrotizing small-vessel vasculitis with neutrophils and neutrophil debris and deposits of pink amorphous fibrin within and around the small vessel walls. Abundant IgA deposition and C3 deposition are seen on immunofluorescence. If a skin biopsy is positive for Henoch-Schönlein purpura then the patient should always be investigated for coexisting renal disease.

6.4.3. Biochemistry, haematology and immunology

Routine lab tests are usually normal but the acute phase reactants may be raised. There are no diagnostic studies but a raised IgA in the appropriate clinical setting is suggestive of Henoch-Schönlein pupura. It is important to try and exclude other disorders and in particular serum clotted at 37°C should be sent for the presence of cryoglobulins.

7. Behçet's disease

7.1. Prevalence

The prevalence of Behçet's disease varies widely around the world. It is most common in eastern Mediterranean countries and the Far East. The worldwide prevalence varies from 1 in 10,000 to 1 in 300,000 (Michelson and Friedlaender, 1990; O'Duffy, 1990).

7.2. Epidemiology

The disease occurs mainly in young adults with the mean age of onset between 25 and 30 years old. (Zouboulis et al., 1997; Gurler et al., 1997; Davatchi, 1998). In Eastern countries the sex ratio is equal but in the West there is a female predilection.

In high prevalence areas Behçet's disease is associated with the HLA-B*5101 allele of HLA-B51 (Mizuki et al., 1997). In Western counties there is no strong association with HLA antigens (Gharibdoost et al., 1993). Eastern Behçet's disease is clinically more homogenous than it is in the west. Familial disease is noted but uncommon, and is not linked to any clear pattern of inheritance.

7.3. Aetiology/Pathogenesis

The histologic hallmark of Behçet's disease is a non-specific vasculitis of large and small arteries, veins, arterioles, venules and capillaries of both the systemic and the pulmonary circulations. Intrathoracic veins of all sizes may show perivascular infiltration with lymphocytes and mononuclear cells. The intima is swollen and the lumen is commonly thrombosed. Aortitis is manifested by a lymphocytic infiltration mixed with histocytes and eosinophils. Severe inflammation and destruction of the media weaken the aortic wall and set the stage for the formation of aneurysms.

Pulmonary arteries show periarterial or transmural lymphocytic, plasma cell and occasionally neutrophilic infiltration. There is mucoid degeneration of the media and intimal thickening of the larger elastic pulmonary arteries.

7.4. Clinical manifestations

Behçet's disease was first described by a Turkish dermatologist, Professor Hulusi Behçet. It is a systemic vasculitis characterized by recurrent oral and genital ulceration, ocular lesions (anterior or posterior uveitis or retinal vasculitis), skin lesions (erythema nodosum, pseudofolliculitis, papulopustular lesions) and pathergy. Other features include marked arthralgias occasionally with synovitis, a predilection to thrombosis and CNS involvement (headaches, meningoencephalitis, cranial nerve palsies and seizures). Arteries or veins of any size are involved, resulting in a wide spectrum of clinical symptoms and signs. A postmortem study of Behçet's patients showed arterial disease secondary to vasculitis in 36% of patients (O'Duffy, 1990). Pulmonary involvement in Behçet's disease is well recognized but rare, and the exact incidence is unknown (Raz et al., 1989). Haemoptysis is the most common clinical manifestation of pulmonary involvement (Grenier et al., 1981; Raz et al., 1989; Erkan and Cavdar, 1992), but fleeting infiltrates and pleuritis have also been reported (Cadman et al., 1976; Hunninghake and Fauci, 1979). Thoracic involvement includes aneurysms of the pulmonary artery, pulmonary infarction with haemorrhage and thrombosis of the superior vena cava (Ahn et al., 1995). Haemoptysis is secondary to either pulmonary artery-bronchial fistula, pulmonary capillaritis or pulmonary thromboembolism. It is extremely important to distinguish between patients with pulmonary embolism alone and patients with pulmonary-bronchial fistula, or a combination of the two, as catastrophic pulmonary haemorrhage can occur if the wrong patients are anticoagulated (Calamia and O'Duffy, 2001).

7.5. Investigation

Because of the lack of diagnostic tests in Behçet's disease it is often confused with other diseases. The presentation with mucosal ulcers and gastrointestinal involvement often leads to an initial diagnosis of Crohn's disease. Musculoskeletal involvement with arthralgias and synovitis can lead to mistaken diagnoses of rheumatoid or sometimes septic or crystal arthritis in the monoarticular presentation. Presentation with anterior uveitis and erythema nodosum may understandably lead to confusion with sarcoidosis.

7.5.1. Radiology

Typical radiological findings in Behçet's disease are widening of the mediastinum due to thrombosis of the superior vena cava (SVC), a lung mass due to pulmonary artery aneurysms and air space consolidation due to infarction or hemorrhage. CT scanning can demonstrate SVC thrombosis as well as air space consolidation and pulmonary artery aneurysms, if present. Stenosis of the pulmonary arteries can also occur and this is best visualized on pulmonary angiogram.

7.5.2. Biochemistry, haematology and immunology

Acute phase reactants can be normal in patients with active eye disease but are normally raised in those with large vessel vasculitis. Immune complexes may be raised but rheumatoid factor, cryoglobulins and complement levels are either normal or negative. HLA testing in patients from Eastern countries can be helpful but not so in patients from the West.

8. Relapsing polychondritis

8.1. Prevalence and epidemiology

Relapsing polychondritis is a rare condition that in 1992 had only been reported in 1000 patients worldwide (Irani et al., 1992). Michet (1990b) reported an incidence of 3.5 cases per million. Other than this there is a paucity of data regarding the epidemiology of the disease. Relapsing polychondritis may occur at any age, but the peak period is in the fifth decade with a mean age of 47 years Michet, 1990b). Caucasians are affected most commonly and it is rare in other ethnic groups; there is no sex predilection (Fig. 6).

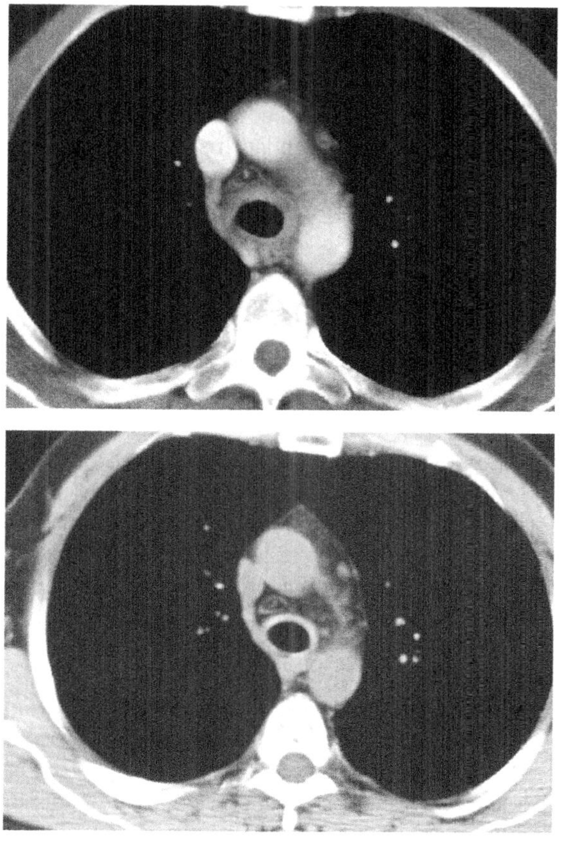

A B

Figure 6. (a) Relapsing polychondritis: CT scan showing inflammatory thickening of tracheal wall. (b) Relapsing polychondritis: CT scan of same patient after treatment showing marked improvement in tracheal inflammation.

8.2. Aetiology and pathogenesis

The aetiology of relapsing polychondritis is unknown. There are some genetic links. HLA-DR4 is increased in frequency in these patients (Luthra et al., 1981; Lang et al., 1993) and double transgenic mice for human HLA-DQ6 and HLA-DQ8 have developed chondritis and arthritis, which is similar to the human disease (Bradley et al., 1996). Cartilage destruction is mediated by release of degradative enzymes, including metalloproteinases and reactive oxygen metabolites from activated chondrocytes and inflammatory cells under the influence of immune-mediated cytokines such as interleukin 1 and tumor necrosis factor (Sridharan, 2001). Foidart et al. (1978) and Ebringer et al. (1981) have reported immune responses against type II collagen and Yang et al. (1993) detected antibodies to type II collagen and immune complexes in the serum of relapsing polychondritis patients. Titres of the anticollagen antibodies have been reported to correlate with the activity of the disease (Foidart et al., 1978).

Vasculitis is a common feature occurring in up to 56% of patients (McAdam et al., 1976). Various types of vasculitis have been reported, from cutaneous leukocytoclastic vasculitis to necrotizing vasculitis of the great vessels (McAdam et al., 1976; Michet, 1990a). Therefore it appears that relapsing polychondritis is a genetically influenced immune disease against type II collagen with vasculitis as a prominent pathological feature.

8.3. Clinical manifestations

The first case of relapsing polychondritis was first reported in 1923 by Jaksch-Wartenhorst (1923), but the term relapsing polychondritis was not used until 1960 when Pearson et al. (1960) reported two further cases. Three types of cartilage are characteristically involved: auricular cartilage, nasal cartilage and laryngotracheal cartilage. Uveitis, keratitis, scleritis, vestibular involvement, deafness and seronegative polyarthritis are part of the disease. McAdam's criteria (McAdam et al., 1976) are used as a guide to diagnosis (Table 3). Auricular chondritis is the initial manifestation in 40% of patients with 85% of patients eventually developing ear involvement. Hearing loss may occur from blockage of the Eustachian tube or the external auditory meatus. In up to 30% of patients inflammation of the internal auditory artery or its cochlear branch can cause deafness, tinnitus, ataxia, vertigo, nausea and vomiting (Cody and Sones, 1971; Moloney, 1978).

Nasal cartilage involvement can occur in up to 50% of patients and a seronegative non-deforming arthritis occurs in 33% of patients. This can be oligo- or poly-aticular and commonly involves central thoracic joints such as sternoclavicular, costochondral and sternomanubrial joints, which may lead to compromise of respiratory function in severe cases (McAdam et al., 1976).

Respiratory involvement in relapsing polychondritis is usually a result of laryngotracheal chondritis; medium-sized pulmonary vasculitis is recognized but is much rarer. Fifty percent of patients will eventually have laryngotracheal involvement resulting in hoarseness, non-productive cough, dyspnea, wheezing, inspiratory stridor, and tenderness over the larynx and proximal trachea (Eng and Sabanathan, 1991), and up to 26% result in laryngotracheal stricture (Sridharan, 2001). Stridor is caused by laryngeal cartilage inflammation and expiratory wheeze by bronchial cartilage destruction (Eng and Sabanathan, 1991). Mucosal oedema, strictures, and/or collapse of laryngeal or tracheal cartilage may cause life-threatening airway stenosis necessitating tracheostomy (Gilliland, 1999). Intubation for any reason may be difficult because the glottis may be narrowed due to oedema or cartilage destruction (Dunne and Sabanathan, 1994). Death may result from collapse of bronchial cartilage leading to pneumonia or respiratory insufficiency. Vasculitis is a common feature of relapsing polychondritis and it affects multiple systems and presents itself in many different ways. Cutaneous: leukocytoclastic vasculitis and subcutaneous nodules in 17–39% of patients; cardiovascular: aortitis, aortic aneurysms and aortic regurgitation in up to 10%; renal: segmental necrotizing cresentric glomerulonephritis in 22%; ocular: retinal vasculitis and chorioretinitis; and neurological: stroke, mononeuritis multiples, transverse myelitis and aseptic meningitis.

A series of 112 patients from the Mayo Clinic had a 5- and 10-year survival as 74 and 55%, respectively (Michet et al., 1986). The most frequent causes of death were infection, systemic vasculitis and malignancy. Only 10% were attributable to acute airway collapse.

Table 3
Diagnostic criteria for relapsing polychondritis

Recurrent chondritis of both auricles
Nonerosive inflammatory polyarthritis
Chondritis of nasal cartilage
Inflammation of ocular structures, including conjunctivitis, keratitis, scleritis/episleritis, and/or uvietis
Chondritis of the respiratory tract involving laryngeal and/or tracheal cartilages
Cochlear and/or vestibular damage manifest by meurosensory hearing loss, tinnitus, and/or vertigo

A definite diagnosis requires three or more clinical features to be present.

8.4. Investigations

8.4.1. Radiology

CT scanning of the trachea will usually show tracheal wall thickening secondary to oedema from inflammation and granulation tissue (Fig. 7a and b). Destruction of the tracheal cartilage may lead to softening and dynamic collapse of the airway, best shown on cine CT demonstrating flaccidity of the tracheal wall during inspiration. Direct visualization of the upper airways by fiberoptic endoscopy (Fig. 7) is necessary to fully characterize the extent of airway involvement (Eng and Sabanathan, 1991).

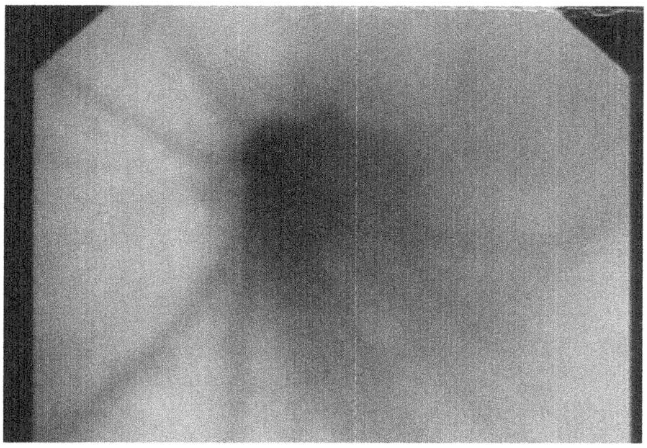

Figure 7. Relapsing polychondritis: fiberoptic bronchoscopy view showing floppy trachea collapsing on expiration.

Electrocardiogram (ECG) is recommended to detect early cardiac involvement and baseline echocardiography is advocated in screening for aortic valve disease, but no evidence supports its routine use (Buckley and Ades, 1992). Joint radiographs will typically show joint space narrowing without erosions (Booth et al., 1989).

8.4.2. Functional

Respiratory function testing would typically show extrathoracic airways obstruction with airway collapse on the inspiratory portion of the flow volume loop (Fig. 8). Because of the potential for serious airway involvement all patients, irrespective of symptoms, should undergo pulmonary function tests

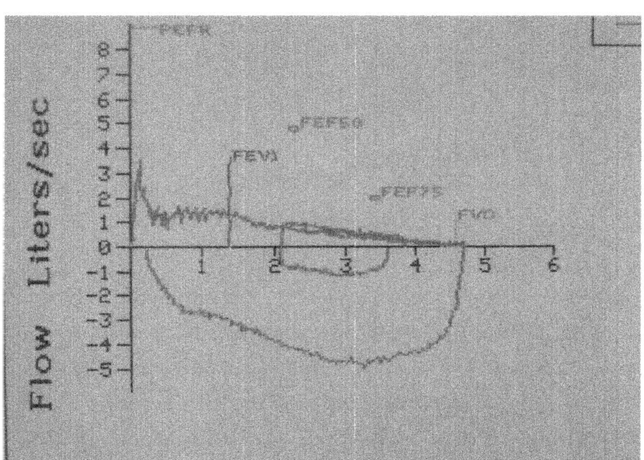

Figure 8. Relapsing polychondritis with severe tracheal involvement: flow volume loop showing expiratory tracheal collapse.

and as well direct visualiation of the upper airways by endoscopy.

8.4.3. Biochemistry, haematology and immunology

Mild leukocytosis and normochromic, normocytic anaemia occur in up to 50% of patients (Michet et al., 1986). Polyclonal hypergammaglobulinemia, elevated ESR and thrombocytosis are also seen. Antibodies to both native and denatured type II collagen are found in up to 50% of patients (Foidart et al., 1978; Ebringer et al., 1981; Yang et al., 1993). The sensitivity in one study was 33% with a specificity of 100%. This study also showed that during acute attacks the antibody titres were high, but they normalized with treatment with corticosteroid (Foidart et al., 1978).

9. Secondary vasculitis

9.1. Prevalence and epidemiology

Secondary vasculitis is most commonly observed in connective tissue diseases such as SLE and rheumatoid arthritis, or in relation to infections or solid or haematological malignancies (Gonzalez-Gay and Garcia-Porrua, 1999; Gonzalez-Gay et al., 2001). Rheumatoid vasculitis has a reported incidence of 12.5/million in Norwich, UK (Watts et al., 1995) and of 12.2/million in Lugo, Spain (Gonzalez-Gay and Garcia-Porrua, 1999).

In Norwich rheumatoid vasculitis was more common in men, and in Lugo most RA patients with vasculitis had the disease for more than 5 years, were rheumatoid factor positive and had other extra-articular features (Gonzalez-Gay and Garcia-Porrua, 1999).

In Lugo the incidence of vasculitis associated with SLE was 5.3 per million (Gonzalez-Gay and Garcia-Porrua, 1999). Of all the biopsy-proven secondary vasculitis recorded, severe bacterial infections and solid or haematological malignancies were responsible for 1.5 and 3%, respectively (Gonzalez-Gay and Garcia-Porrua, 1999; Gonzalez-Gay et al., 2001).

9.2. Clinical manifestations

Pulmonary vasculitis is seen, although not commonly, in SLE, rheumatoid vasculitis and systemic sclerosis (Hunninghake and Fauci, 1979). In SLE, pulmonary vasculitis secondary to leukocytoclastic vasculitis, granulomatous arteritis, necrotizing vasculitis and immune complex capillaritis have been described (Gross et al., 1972; Hunninghake and Fauci, 1979; Ingue et al., 1979; Armstrong and Steele, 1982; Leatherman et al., 1984). The most dramatic presentation is diffuse pulmonary haemorrhage and the clinical features are similar to those seen in microscopic polyangiitis (Zamora et al., 1997). In rheumatoid arthritis both necrotizing granulomatous vasculitis and diffuse pulmonary arteritis have been reported (Hunninghake and Fauci, 1979; Armstrong and Steele, 1982; Churg, 1983).

10. Leukocytoclastic vasculitis

Leukocytoclastic vasculitis is not recognized by the ACR classification criteria and in the Chapel Hill definition it is recognized only as a cutaneous vasculitis. There have, however, been reported cases of systemic leukocytoclastic vasculitis with pulmonary involvement. There is only limited data on its pathogenesis but they suggest that capillaritis and haemorrhagic alveolitis are the mechanisms involved. The aetiology of this vasculitis remains unclear but there are associations with drugs, chemicals, viral and bacterial infections and malignancy (Sams, 1980; Fulmer and Kaltreider, 1982).

10.1. Clinical manifestations

Leukocytoclastic vasculitis is most commonly isolated to cutaneous involvement, although it can become disseminated where the kidney, gastrointestinal tract and occasionally the lungs are involved (Winkelman and Ditto, 1964).Transient and diffuse infiltrates, pneumonia, pleural effusions and respiratory failure have been described (Winkelman and Ditto, 1964; Fulmer and Kaltreider, 1982). The prognosis is good if therapy is instituted early or if the causative agent is identified and removed, but only in 50–60% of patients is a cause found (Chandler and Fulmer, 1985).

11. Differential diagnosis

The vasculitides are a heterogeneous group of diseases that exhibit a wide range of clinical manifestations due to the often diffuse involvement of blood vessels. This has made this group of diseases historically very difficult to diagnose, especially considering their rarity. Due to the lack of pathognomonic tests, classification criteria have been based on the size of the vessel involved. These criteria are, however, classification and not diagnostic criteria which have been based, in the ACR criteria, on common features of a series of 1000 patients with vasculitis. They should therefore not be used for the differentiation of whether a patient does or does not have vasculitis. They are useful in the management of the patients who present with a classical clinical picture, as often GCA or Henoch-Schönlein purpura patients do, in terms of comparison of treatment and outcome, and are beneficial in understanding the natural history of the disease. They are also useful when studying groups of patients and for epidemiological studies. They are, however, not useful in diagnosing and managing individual patients, particularly when they have an atypical presentation. Therefore, as is often the case, if the patient does not present classically then all vasculitides should be considered as differentials. Patients in the early stages of the disease may not fulfil any of the criteria and often never will. Their diagnosis should be kept open and they should be carefully followed for development of any new classical features that may help confirm the exact diagnosis.

12. Treatment

12.1. General principles for treatment

Although the pulmonary vasculitides are quite a heterogeneous group of diseases their treatments are very similar. We will therefore discuss general principles of treatment but also highlight any specific treatments for each disease. Unfortunately the evidence base for these treatments is limited. Treatment for Wegener's granulomatosis is the most researched and we will briefly detail these findings. The lack of randomized controlled studies in other vasculitides means that this evidence is probably the best available in guiding treatment of the other vasculitides. When treating the vasculitides it is important for the physician and the patient to have clear and realistic goals. These disorders are not curable, however, a goal of inducing and maintaining prolonged remission and minimizing damage- or treatment-related morbidity should be the main aim.

The general principal for treating these vasculitides is to immunosuppress the patient with initially high doses of oral corticosteroid (some physicians will also use intial boluses of iv methylprednisolone 500–1000 mg iv for 3 days) and to consider cytotoxic agents, depending on each disease. Some diseases, such as GCA, often settle with corticosteroids alone, and others will require additional cytotoxics.

In Wegener's granulomatosis a standard regimen of cyclophosphamide and corticosteroids is initiated, which is followed by a gradual withdrawal of corticosteroids. The National Institute for Health (NIH) regimen is for oral cyclophosphamide 2 mg/kg/day with prednisolone 1 mg/kg/day (Talar–Williams et al., 1996). Assuming there is improvement after 1 month the prednisolone is slowly withdrawn over a period of 6–12 months. The cylophosphamide is recommended to continue for at least 1 year after complete remission. However, there have been many concerns over the side effects of long-term oral cyclophosphamide including haemorrhagic cystitis, bladder cancer, lymphoma and myelodysplasia. Infection is another concern: the mortality rate from infection related to over aggressive treatment is often higher than that from failure of the treatment to control the disease (Burns, 1998). However, the NIH regimen avoids leucopenia (aim for white cell count of 4 × 10 per dl) when using cyclophosphamide. Furthermore when corticosteroids are withdrawn after 3–4 months they are tapered to an alternate day schedule. Both these factors have resulted in a markedly lower rate of infection and mortality without loss of efficacy when compared to studies where daily tapering and leucopenia were a goal (Guillevin et al., 1997). Prophylaxis for infections is recommended. The routine use of anti-fungal suspensions and lozenges and prescription of Septrin (co-trimoxazole) prophylaxis for the prevention of Pneumocystis carinii infection is recommended. In Wegener's granulomatosis co-trimoxazole has the additional benefit of preventing relapses of upper airway involvement (DeRemee et al., 1985; Stegeman et al., 1996). These concerns over the side effects of long-term oral cyclophosphamide have led to other treatments being considered. The use of intermittent intravenous cyclophosphamide has been investigated in three prospective trials (Hoffman et al., 1990; Reinhold-Keller et al., 1994; Guillevin et al., 1997), and although they have shown some reasonable results the relapse rate was higher than in the NIH regimen. More encouragingly, in a recent trial which used corticosteroid and oral cyclophosphamide at the NIH dose for induction (average 3-months), the patients were then switched to weekly methotrexate with a similar remission rate and an improved incidence of side effects (Langford et al., 1999). Similar results were also reported in another study that used intermittent IV cyclophosphamide for induction in one of its treatment arms (De Groot et al., 1996). Most recently Jayne et al. (2003) completed a randomized trial of maintenance therapy in ANCA associated vasculitis. One hundred and fifty-five newly diagnosed generalized vasculitis patients were treated with oral cyclophosphamide 2 mg/kg and prednisolone 1 mg/kg tapering to 0.25 mg/kg by 12 weeks. Once remission was achieved, usually at 3 months, the patients were then randomly assigned to either oral cylophosphamide 1.5 mg/kg or azathioprine 2 mg/kg for the following 9 months. The primary end point was relapse and there was no significant difference in relapse between the two groups (cyclophosphamide: 13.7%; azathioprine 15.5%). The rate of severe adverse avents was high (10% induction, 11% azathioprine, 10% cyclophosphamide) but again there was no significant difference between the two maintenance groups. Cyclophosphamide is, however, generally regarded as a more toxic drug and more long-term side effects such as infertility and cancer, which would not have been identified in this study, have to be taken into account. This study is very encouraging for future management of ANCA-associated vasculitis but long-term relapse rate and the potential for repeated treatment courses are two unanswered questions.

There is evidence in randomized controlled trials for a beneficial effect of intravenous immunoglobulin (IVIG) treatment (Jayne et al., 1991), yet the ability of IVIG to remove circulating ANCA antibodies varies considerably depending on the batch of immunoglobulin used and on the manufacturer, which reflects the difficulty in quantifying ANCA specific anti-idiotype antibody levels in individual batches of donor serum. Plasma exchange has been shown in a randomized trial of vasculitis with renal involvement to benefit patients whose presenting creatinine level was above 500 μmol/l (Pusey et al., 1991).

12.2. GCA

A classic example of a vasculitis that responds dramatically to corticosteroids is GCA (Hunder, 1990). Corticosteroids are therefore the treatment of choice in GCA and not only do they produce a rapid improvement in localized and systemic symptoms but also they prevent visual complications (Aiello et al., 1993). Doses of 40–60 mg of prednisolne daily are traditionally used, based on studies in the 1950–1960s and 1970–1980s (Birkhead et al., 1957; Huston et al., 1978; Graham et al., 1981). Recently the use of Methotrexate as a adjuvant treatment in GCA was studied by Hoffman et al. (2002). They concluded that their study provided no evidence to support the use of methotrexate to control disease activity or to decrease the cumulative dose and toxicity of corticosteroids in patients with GCA. Therefore to date there is no evidence to support the use of cytotoxic therapy in GCA. Treatment evidence for pulmonary involvement in GCA is limited to a few case reports. In one paper on GCA patients with nodular opacities, treatment with corticosteroids led to marked improvement or complete resolution within months (Zeone et al., 1994). Two other papers report rapid resolution of clinical symptoms and clinical and radiographic signs with corticosteroids in two GCA patients, one with pulmonary nodules and the other with pleural effusions (Bradley et al., 1984; Romero et al., 1992).

12.3. Takayasu's arteritis

Establishing optimal treatment for TA has been difficult because there is no single parameter that can reliably assess the activity of the disease. A combination of clinical features, including systemic or ischaemic symptoms or signs and erythrocyte sedimentation rate with arteriographic changes, is typically used.

All 80% of symptomatic patients at diagnosis will require treatment, while the 20% who are asymptomatic can be educated to report symptoms immediately and carefully monitored. The treatment options in TA are corticosteroids alone, coticosteroids in combination with cytotoxics or surgery. Corticosteroids are regarded as the mainstay of treatment in TA though there is little conclusive evidence that they improve clinical features, radiographic appearances or overall outcome. The optimal doses and duration of treatment with corticosteroids remains unclear.

Cytotoxic therapy is generally used in patients with persistent disease activity despite coricosteroids or when corticosteroids can not be adequately tapered. Cytotoxic therapy has been researched by Kerr et al. (1994) and Hoffman et al. (1994). Kerr et al. found that 52% of Takayasu's patients required cytotoxic treatment with 40% of these going into remission. Hoffman et al. studied methotrexate in a glucocorticoid resistant population and found mixed results. A regimen of methotrexate (0.3 mg/kg/week) and corticosteroids (1 mg/kg/day) brought about remission in 81% of the patients with sustained remission of greater than a year in 25%, although relapse occurred in 54%. Cyclophosphamide may also be used but again the data to support its use is limited. In one paper seven patients treated with cyclophosphamide were all able to reduce their glucocorticoid dose and disease progression was halted in four (Shelhamer et al., 1985). Surgical modalities play an important role in treatment of TA.

Several factors need to be taken in to consideration. Although TA patients are young they have potential for suffering many medical problems including left ventricular hypertrophy, unrecognized hypertension, congestive cardiac failure and coronary artery disease secondary to the Takayasu's. Percutaneous angioplasty can be useful in correcting short stenoses of the aortic branches including the renal arteries (Tyagi et al., 1993). This is a difficult procedure, however. Unlike atherosclerosis, in TA all layers of the artery are affected and it is therefore rigid and non-compliant, so several attempts at angioplasty are often required and subsequent stenting provides the best results because of the risk of restenosis.

Surgical repair or bypass of grafting of fixed vascular lesions that are producing significant ischaemia have some reported success (Giodano et al., 1991). This includes repair or bypass grafting of stenotic pulmonary arteries (Moore et al., 1985; Chauvaud et al., 1987). The timing of these surgical procedures is controversial but there is a general consensus that surgery while the arteritis is still active is unwise. The anastomosis site is critical. It is best avoided in diseased arteries as Takayasu's affects all three layers of the artery and therefore makes anastamosis technically difficult. However, even though normal arteies are chosen carefully on arteriography for the anastamosis site, 44% of biopsies taken from arteries show microscopic evidence of active disease (Kerr et al., 1994) and this may have a impact on the integrity of the anastomosis site, especially in the long term.

12.4. Microscopic polyangiitis

There have been no prospective studies specifically studying treatment in microscopic polyangiitis so the evidence base for Wegener's granulomatosis is often followed. Therefore patients with microscopic polyangiitis with pulmonary haemorrhage and/or glomerulonephritis should be treated with cyclophosphamide and steroids as described above. In addition, plasma exchange is often used in patients with severe pulmonary–renal vasculitic syndromes where there is DPH and rapidly progressive glomerulonephritis.

12.5. Polyarteritis nodosa

There has been some controversy over the treatment of PAN and whether combined cyclophosphamide and corticosteroids are needed in all cases. This controversy has been compounded by the fact that many of the treatment studies have taken place before 1994 and have therefore included patients who would now be classified as microscopic polyangiitis. A study from France found the addition of cyclophosphamide and plasma exchange was beneficial in preventing relapse in PAN but did not significantly alter the 10-year survival rate which was 73% overall (Guillevin et al., 1991). The same French group led by Löic Guillevin studied survival from five separate trials and found no difference if cyclophosphamide was used in initial treatment (Guillevin et al., 1996). It should be pointed out that both of these studies included patients with Churg–Strauss syndrome and microscopic polyangiitis.

Poor prognostic factors in PAN are renal insufficiency, proteinuria > 1 g/day, gastrointestinal, neurological and central nervous system involvement. With none of the above the 5-year survival rate was 88% but when two factors were involved it dropped to just 56% (Guillevin et al., 1996). There have been some studies into the method of administration of cyclophosphamide but these have proved inconclusive (Genereau et al., 1994; Gayraud et al., 1997).

Therefore at present the optimal therapeutic approach to PAN is unclear. It would seem reasonable to conclude from the evidence available that a combination of corticosteroids and cyclophosphamide should be used in life-threatening multi-organ involvement, but in others initial therapy should be with corticosteroids only, with the addition of cytotoxics if the disease remains active or the corticosteroids cannot be tapered.

12.6. Behçet's disease

In cases of life-threatening Behçet's disease with pulmonary involvement, immunosuppression with cyclophosphamide and corticosteroids is recommended for induction treatment, to be switched to a less toxic immunosuppressant such as azathioprine or methotrexate for maintenance once remission is established, similar to the regimens described above. Life-threatening Behçet's is, however, quite a rarity and the more standard presentation would be with mucosal ulceration and arthralgias, which can be severe and disproportionate to the clinical findings. In these patients colchicine can be very useful, or pentoxifylline if colchicine is not tolerated, along with prednisolone, methotrexate or azathioprine if required.

12.7. Relapsing polychondritis

Because of the rarity of relapsing polychondritis the treatment regimens are empirical, and corticosteroids are regarded as the mainstay of treatment (0.5–1 mg/kg).

In milder cases with limited auricular, nasal and costochondritis, nonsteroidal anti-inflammatory drugs and colchicine are sometimes used.

In more severe cases with laryngotracheal involvement, systemic vasculitis, or necrotizing scleritis, if disease progresses despite adequate corticosteroid treatment then cytotoxic/immunosuppressive agents are used (Svenson et al., 1984; Hoang-Xuan et al., 1990; Anstey et al., 1991). In relapsing polychondritis with nephritis intravenous cyclophosphamide or oral cyclophosphamide plus corticosteroids have been successfully used (Ruhlen et al., 1981; Stewart and Mazanec, 1992). Acute flares of laryngotracheal disease can be treated with intravenous pulsed methylprednisolone (Lipnick and Fink, 1991) and local adrenaline injected into the inflamed tissues has been reported as being useful (Gaffney et al., 1992). However, this is only anecdotal and often tracheostomy is required. Larngeal stenting has mixed reports. They are recognized as having many complications including bleeding, ulceration and erosion of the tracheobronchial wall, migration of the stent, retention of secretions and granulation tissue formation (Nesbitt and Carrasco, 1996; Dasgupta et al., 1998). One report shows no increase in independence or survival (Dunne and Sabanathan, 1994) but a more recent study using self-expandible metallic stents (SEMs) was more promising (Bipin et al., 1999).

Key points

- Pulmonary vaculitis normally occurs as part of a systemic disease, but can occasionally occur in isolation.
- Pulmonary vasculitis is rare.
- The pathogenesis of pulmonary vasculitis is unclear but is thought to be due to immune complex deposition in connective tissue diseases such as SLE and HSP and alterations in cell mediated immunity in chronic granulomatous conditions.
- The pulmonary vasculitides are a heterogeneous group of diseases that can present in a number of different ways that are often atypical. Careful thought should be given to differential diagnosis and vasculitis should not be excluded early because of lack of classical features.
- A combination of radiological and immunological investigations is useful in diagnosing and monitoring disease. Wherever possible, appropriate tissue biopsy should be taken to help confirm the diagnosis.
- Treatment should be tailored to the individual patient and condition. In general corticosteroid treatment in combination with immunosupression with cyclophosphamide is required in the more severe cases. In some cases corticosteroids with a less toxic cytotoxic drug such as azathioprine or methotrexate, or corticosteroids alone, will suffice.
- Although mortality used to be high, with current treatment regimens, instigated early, the prognosis in general is good.

References

Acritidis, N.C., Andonopoulos, A.P., Gralanopoulou, V., et al. 1988. Pulmonary function of nonsmoking patients with giant cell arterits and/or polmyalgia rheumatica: a controlled study. Clin. Rheumatol. 7, 231–236.

Adu, D., Howie, A.J., Scott, D.G., Bacon, P.A., McGonigle, R.J., Micheal, J. 1987. Polyarteritis and the kidney. Q. J. Med. 62(239), 221–237.

Aiello, P.D., Trautmann, J.C., McPhee, T.J., et al. 1993. Visual prognosis in giant cell arteritis. Opthalmology 100, 550–555.

Ahn, J.M., Im, J.G., Ryoo, J.W., Kim, S.J., Do, Y.S., Choi, Y.W., et al. 1995. Thoracic manifestations of Behçet syndrome: radiographic and CT findings in nine patients. Radiology 194, 199–203.

Amoli, M.M., Thomson, W., Hajeer, A.H., et al. 2001. HLA-DRB1*01 association with Henoch-Schönlein purpura in patients from northwest Spain. J. Rheumatol. 28, 1266–1270.

Amoli, M.M., Thomson, W., Hajeer, A.H., et al. 2002a. HLA-B*35 association with nephritis in Henoch-Schönlein purpura. J. Rheumatol. 29, 948–949.

Amoli, M.M., Thomson, W., Hajeer, A.H., et al. 2002b. Interleukin-1 receptor antagonist gene polymorphism is associated with severe renal and renal sequelae in Henoch-Schönlein purpura. J. Rheumatol. 29 (7), 1404–1407.

Anstey, A., Mayou, S., Morgan, K., et al. 1991. Relapsing polychondritis: autoimmunity to type II collagen and treatment with cylosporin A. Br. J. Dermatol. 125, 588–591.

Armstrong, J.G., Steele, R.H. 1982. Localized pulmonary arteritis in rheumatoid disease. Thorax 37, 313–314.

Bipin, S., Dasgupta, A., Mehta, C. 1999. Management of airway manifestations of relapsing polychondritis: case reports and review of literature. Chest 116, 1669–1675.

Birkhead, N.C., Wagener, H.P., Shick, R.M. 1957. Treatment of temporal arteritis with adrenal Corticosteroids. JAMA 163, 821–827.

Blockmans, D., Stroobants, S., Maes, A., Mortelmans, L. 2000. Positron emission tomography in giant cell arteritis and polymyalgia rheumatica: evidence for inflammation of the aortic arch. Am. J. Med. 108 (3), 246–248.

Booth, A., Dieppe, P.A., Goddard, P.L., et al. 1989. The radiological manifestations of relapsing polychondritis. Clin. Radiol. 40, 147–149.

Brack, A., Geisler, A., Martinez-Taboada, V.M., Younge, B.R., Goronzy, J.J., Weyand, C.M. 1997. Giant cell vasculitis is a T cell- dependent disease. Mol. Med. 3, 530–543.

Bradley, J.D., Pinals, R.S., Blumenfeld, H.B., Poston, W.M. 1984. Giant cell arteritis with pulmonary nodules. Am. J. Med. 77, 135–140.

Bradley, J.D., Brandt, K.D., Katz, B.P. 1989. Infectious complications of cyclophosphamide treatment for vasculitis. Arthritis Rheum. 32, 45–53.

Bradley, D.S., Das, P., Griffiths, M.M., Luthra, H.S., David, C.S. 1996. Double transgenic HLA DQ6/8 mice provide a new model of polychondritis following type II collagen immunization. Arthrits Rheum. 39, S229.

Bron, K., Strott, C., Shapiro, A. 1965. The diagnostic value of angiographic observations in polyarteritis nodosa. A case of multiple aneurysms in the visceral organs. Arch. Intern. Med. 116, 454–459.

Brugiere, O., Raffy, O., Sleiman, C., Groussard, O., Rothchild, E., Mellot, F., Jebrak, G., Mal, H., Roue, C., Pariente, R., Fournier, M. 1997. Progressive obstructive lung disease associated with microscopic polyangiitis. Am. J. Respir. Crit. Care Med. 155, 739–742.

Buckley, L.M., Ades, P.A. 1992. Progressive aortic valve inflammation occurring despite apparent remission of relapsing polychondritis. Arthritis Rheum. 35, 812–814.

Burns, A. 1998. Pulmonary vasculitis. Thorax 53 (3), 220–227.

Cadman, E.C., Lundberg, W.B., Mitchell, M.S. 1976. Pulmonary manifestations in Behçet syndrome. Arch. Intern. Med. 136, 944–947.

Calamia, K.T., O'Duffy, J.D. 2001. Behçet's disease. In: G.S. Hoffman, C.M. Weyand (Eds.), Inflammatory Diseases of Blood Vessels. Marcel Dekker, New York, p. 473–490.

Calvino, M.C., Llorca, J., Garcia-Porrua, C., et al. 2001. Henoch-Schönlein purpura in children from northwestern Spain: a 20-year epidemiologic and clinical study. Medicine (Baltimore) 80, 279–290.

Chandler, D.B., Fulmer, J.D. 1985. Pulmonary vasculitis. Lung 163, 257–273.

Chauvaud, S., Mace, L., Brunewald, P., et al. 1987. Takayasu's arteritis with bilateral pulmonary artery stenosis: successful surgical correction. J. Thorac. Cardiovasc. Surg. 94, 246–250.

Cho, C., Asuncion, A., Tatum, A.H. 1995. False positive antineutrophil cytoplasmic antibody in aspergillosis with oxalosis. Arch. Pathol. Lab. Med. 119, 558–561.

Chumbley, L.E., Harrison, E.G., DeRemee, R.A. 1977. Allergic granulomatosis and angiitis (Churg–Strauss syndrome): report and analysis of 300 cases. Mayo Clin. Proc. 52, 477–484.

Churg, A. 1983. Pulmonary angiitis and granulomatosis revisted. Human Pathol. 14, 868–884.

Churg, J., Strauss, L. 1951. Allergic granulomatosis, allergic angiitis, and periarteritis nodosa. Am. J. Pathol. 27, 277–301.

Cid, M.C. 1996. New developments in the pathogenesis of systemic vasculitis. Curr. Opin. Rheumatol. 8, 1–11.

Cid, M.C., Campo, E., Ercilla, G., et al. 1989. Immunohistochemical analysis of lymphoid and macrophage cell subsets and their immunologic activation markers in temporal arteritis: influence of corticosteroid treatment. Arthrits Rheum. 32, 884–893.

Cid, M.C., Cebrian, M., Front, C., et al. 2000. Cell adhesion molecules in the development of inflammatory infiltrates in giant cell arteritis: inflammation-induced angiogenesis as the preferential site of leukocyte-endothelial cell interactions. Arthritis Rheum. 43, 184–194.

Cody, D.T.R., Sones, D.A. 1971. Relapsing polychondritis: audiovestibular manifestations. Laryngoscope 81, 1208–1222.

Cohen, P., Guillevin, L., Baril, L., et al. 1995. Persistence of antineutrophil cytoplasmic antibodies (ANCA) in asymptomatic patients with systemic polyarteritis nodosa or Churg-Stauss syndrome: follow-up of 53 patients. Clin. Exp. Rheumatol. 13, 193–198.

Cohen-Tervaert, J.W., Van-der-Woude, F.J., Fauci, A.S., et al. 1989. Association between active Wegener's granulomatosis and anticytoplasmic antibodies. Arch. Intern. Med. 149, 2461–2465.

Cream, J.J., Gumpel, J.M., Peachy, R.D.G. 1970. Schoenlein-Henoch purpura in the adult. Q. J. Med. 39, 461–484.

Dababneh, A., Gonzalez-Gay, M.A., Garcia-Porrua, C., et al. 1998. Giant cell arteritis and polymyalgia rheumatica can be differentiated by distinct patterns of HLA class II association. J. Rheumatol. 25, 2140–2145.

Darras-Joly, C., Lortholary, O., Cohen, P., Brauner, M., Guillevin, L. 1995. Regressing microaneurysms in 5 cases of hepatitis B virus related polyarteritis nodosa. J. Rheumatol. 22, 876–880.

Dasgupta, A., Dolmatch, B.L., Abi-Saleh, W.J., et al. 1998. Self-expandable metallic airway stent insertion employing flexible bronchoscopy: preliminary results. Chest 114, 106–109.

Davatchi, F. 1998. Epidemiology of Behçet's disease disease in Middle East and Asia. (A). Proceedings of the Eighth International Congress on Behçet's Disease, Reggio-Emilia, Italy, p. 36.

Davies, D.J., Moran, J.E., Naill, J.F., et al. 1982. Segmental necrotizing glomerulonephritis with antineutrophil antibody: possible arbovirus etiology. Br. Med. J. 285, 606.

Davson, J., Ball, J., Platt, R. 1948. The kidney in periarteritis nodosa. Q. J. Med. 17, 175–202.

D'Cruz, D.P., Baguley, E., Asherson, R.A., Hughes, G.R. 1989. Ear, nose and throat symptoms in subacute Wegener's granulomatosis. BMJ 299 (6696), 419–422.

De Groot, K., Reinhold-Keller, E., Tatsis, E., et al. 1996. Therapy for the maintenance of remission in sixty-five patients with generalized Wegener's granulomatosis. Methotrexate versus trimethoprin/sulfamethoxazole. Arthritis Rheum. 39, 2052–2061.

Dennison, A.R., Watkins, R.M., Gunning, A.J. 1985. Simultaneous aortic and pulmonary artery aneurysms due to Giant cell arteritis. Thorax 40, 156–157.

DeRemee, R.A., McDonald, T.J., Weiland, L.H. 1985. Wegener's granulomatosis: observations on the treatment with antimicrobial agents. Mayo Clin. Proc. 60, 27–32.

Doyle, L., McWilliam, L., Hasleton, P.S. 1988. Giant cell arteritis with pulmonary involvement. Br. J. Dis. Chest 82, 88–92.

Duhaut, P., Bosshard, S., Calvert, A., et al. 1999. Giant cell arteritis, polymyalgia rheumatica and viral hypotheses: a multicenter, prospective case-control study. J. Rheumatol. 26, 361–369.

Dunne, J.A., Sabanathan, S. 1994. Use of metallic stents in relapsing polychondritis. Chest 105, 864–867.

Ebringer, R., Rook, G., Swana, G.T., Bottazzo, G.F., Doniach, D. 1981. Autoantibodies to cartilage and type II collagen in relapsing polychondritis and other rheumatic diseases. Ann. Rheum. Dis. 40, 473–479.

Edgar, J.D.M., Rooney, D.P., McNamee, P., et al. 1993. An association between ANCA positive renal disease and malignancy. Clin. Nephrol. 40, 22–25.

Elling, P., Olsson, A.T., Elling, H. 1996. Synchronous variations of the incidence of temporal arteritis and polymyalgia rheumatica in different regions of Denmark: association with epidemics of *Mycoplasma pneumoniae* infection. J. Rheumatol. 23, 112–119.

Elling, H., Olsson, A.T., Elling, P. 2000. Human parvovirus and giant cell arteritis: a selective arteritic impact? Clin. Exp. Rheumatol. 18 (Suppl. 20), S12–S14.

El-Reshaid, K., Kapoor, M.M., El-Reshaid, W., et al. 1997. The spectrum of renal disease associated with microscopic polyangiitis and classic polyarteritis nodosa in Kuwait. Nephrol. Dial. Transplant 12, 1874–1882.

Eng, J., Sabanathan, S. 1991. Airway complications in relapsing polychondritis. Ann. Thorac. Surg. 91 (51), 686–692.

Erkan, F., Cavdar, T. 1992. Pulmonary vasculitis in Behçet's disease. Chest 146, 232–239.

Esnault, V.L., Soleimani, B., Keogan, M.T., et al. 1992. Associations of IgM with IgG ANCA in patients presenting with pulmonary haemorrhage. Kidney Int. 41, 1304–1310.

Esnault, V.L., Testa, A., Audrian, M. 1993. Alpha-1 antitrypsin genetic polymorphism in ANCA positive systemic vasculitis. Kidney Int. 43, 1329–1332.

Ewert, B.H., Jennette, J.C., Falk, R.J. 1990. Anti-myeloperoxidase antibodies stimulate neutrophils to damage human endothelia cells. Kidney Int. 41, 375–378.

Falk, R.J., Jennette, J.C. 1988. Anti-neutrophil cytolplasmic autoantibodies with specificity for myeloperoxidase in patients with systemic vasculitis and idiopathic necrotizing and cresentric glomerulonephritis. N. Engl. J. Med. 25, 1651–1657.

Falk, R.J., Terrell, R., Charles, L.A., et al. 1990. Anti-neutrophil cytoplasmic antibodies induce neutrophils to degranulatelate and produce oxygen radicals in vitro. Proc. Natl Acad. Sci. USA 87, 4115–4119.

Fauci, A.S. 1978. The spectrum of vasculitis-clinical, pathologic, immunologic, and therapeutic considerations. Ann. Intern. Med. 89, 660–676.

Fauci, A.S., Haynes, B.F., Katz, P., Wolff, S.M. 1983. Wegener's granulomatosis. Prospective clinical and therapeutic experience with 85 patients for 21 years. Ann. Intern. Med. 98, 76–85.

Foidart, J., Abe, S., Martin, G.R., Zizic, T.M., Barnett, E.V., Lawley, T.J., Katz, S.I. 1978. Autoantibodies to type II collagen in relapsing polychondritis. N. Engl. J. Med. 299, 1203–1207.

Frohnert, P.P., Sheps, S.G. 1967. Long-term follow-up study of polyarteritis nodosa. Am. J. Med. 43, 8–14.

Fulmer, J.D., Kaltreider, H.B. 1982. The pulmonary vasculitides. Chest 82, 615–624.

Gabriel, S.E., Espy, M., Erdman, D.D., et al. 1999. The role of parvovirus B19 in the pathogenesis of giant cell arteritis: a preliminary evaluation. Arthritis Rheum. 42, 1255–1258.

Gaffney, R.J., Harrison, M., Path, F.R.C., Blayney, A.W. 1992. Nebulized racemic ephedrine in the treatment of acute exacerbations of laryngeal relapsing polychondritis. J. Laryngol. Otol. 106, 63–64.

Garcia-Porrua, C., Gonzalez-Gay, M.A. 1999. Comparitive clinical and epidemiological study of hypersensitivity vasculitis versus Henoch-Schönlein purpura in adults. Semin. Arthritis Rheum. 28, 404–412.

Gayraud, M., Guillevin, L., Cohen, P., et al. 1997. Treatment of good-prognosis polyarteritis nodosa and Churg–Strauss syndrome: comparison of steroids and oral or pulse cyclophosphamide in 25 patients. Br. J. Rhematol. 36, 1290–1297.

Genereau, T., Lortholary, O., Leclerq, P., et al. 1994. Treatment of systemic vasculits with cyclophosphamide and steroids: daily oral low-dose cyclophosphamide administration after failure of a pulse intravenous high dose regimen in four patients. Br. J. Rheumatol. 33, 959–962.

Gharibdoost, F., Davatchi, F., Shahram, F., et al., 1993. Clinical manifestations of Behçet's diease in Iran: analysis of 2176 cases. In: P. Godeau, B. Wechsler (Eds.), Behçet's Disease. Elsevier, Paris, pp. 153–158.

Gilliland, B.C. 1999. Relapsing polychondritis and other Arthritides, 14th ed., Harrison's Principals of Internal Medicine, vol. 2. McGraw-Hall, New York, pp. 1951–1963.

Giodano, J.M., Leavitt, R.Y., Hoffman, G.S., Fauci, A.S. 1991. Experience with surgical treatment for Takayasu's disease. Surgery 109, 252–258.

Glover, M.U., Muniz, J., Bessone, L., et al. 1987. Pulmonary artery obstruction due to giant cell arteritis. Chest 91, 924–925.

Gonzalez-Gay, M.A., Garcia-Porrua, C. 1999. Systemic vasculitis in the adults in Northwestern Spain, 1988–1997. Clinical and epidemiological aspects. Medicine (Baltimore) 60, 170–172.

Gonzalez-Gay, M.A., Garcia-Porrua, C. 2001. Epidemiology of the vasculitides. Rheum. Dis. Clin. N. Am. 27, 729–749.

Gonzalez-Gay, M.A., Garcia-Porrua, C. 2002. Systemic vasculitides. Baillieres Best Pract. Res. Clin. Rheumatol. 16 (5), 833–845.

Gonzalez-Gay, M.A., Garcia-Porrua, C., Rivas, M.J., et al. 2001. Epidemiology of biopsy proven giant cell arteritis in northwestern Spain: trend over an 18 year period. Ann. Rheum. Dis. 60, 367–371.

Graham, E., Holland, A., Avery, A., Russell, R.W., et al. 1981. Prognosis in giant-cell arteritis. BMJ 282, 269–271.

Grenier, P., Bletry, O., Cornud, F., et al. 1981. Pulmonary involvement in Behçet's disease. Am. J. Roentgenol. 137, 565–569.

Gross, M., Eaterly, J.R., Earle, R.H. 1972. Pulmonary alterations in systemic lupus erythematosus. Am. Rev. Respir. Dis. 105, 572–577.

Grunewald, J., Andersson, R., Rydberg, L., et al. 1972. CD4+ and CD8+ T cell expansions using selected TCR V and J gene segments at the onset of giant cell arteritis. Arthritis Rheum. 37, 1221–1227.

Guilleveyin, L., Lahote, F., Cohen, P., et al. 1995. Corticosteroids plus pulse cyclophosphamide and plasma exchanges vs. corticosteroids plus pulse cyclophosphamide alone in the treatment of polyarteritis and Churg–Strauss syndrome patients with factors prediciting poor prognosis: a prospective, randomized trail of 62 patients. Arthritis Rheum. 38, 1638–1645.

Guillevin, L., Le, T., Gayraud, M. 1989. Systemic vasculitis of the polyarteritis nodosa group and infection with hepatitis B virus:a study in 98 patients. Eur. J. Int. Med. 1, 97–105.

Guillevin, L., Jarrousse, B., Lok, C., et al. 1991. Long term follow up after treatment of polyarteritis nodosa and Churg–Strauss angiitis with comparison of steroids, plasma exchange and cylophosphamide to steroids and plasma exchange. A prospective randomized trial of 71 patients. J. Rheumatol. 18, 567–574.

Guillevin, K.L., Lhote, F., Gallais, V., et al. 1995a. Gastrointestinal tract involvement in polyarteritis nodosa and Churg–Strauss syndrome. Ann. Med. Int. (Paris) 146, 260–267.

Guillevin, L., Lhote, F., Cohen, P., et al. 1995b. Polyarteritis nodosa related to hepatitis B virus. A prospective study with long-term observation of 41 patients. Medicine (Baltimore) 74, 238–253.

Guillevin, L., Lhorte, F., Gayraud, M., et al. 1996. Prognostic factors in polyarteritis nodosa and Churg–Strauss syndrome. A prospective study in 342 patients. Medicine (Baltimore) 75, 17–28.

Guillevin, L., Cordier, J.F., Lhorte, F., et al. 1997. A prospective, mulicenter, randomized trial comparing steroids and pulse cyclophosphamide versus steroids and oral cyclophosphamide in the treatment of generalized Wegener's granulomatosis. Arthritis Rheum. 40, 2187–2198.

Guillevin, L., Durand-Gasselin, B., Cevallos, R., et al. 1999. Microscopic polyangiitis: clinical and laboratory findings in eighty-five patients. Arthritis Rheum. 42, 421–430.

Gurler, A., Boyvat, A., Tursen, U. 1997. Clinical manifestations of Behçet's disease: an analysis of 2147 patients. Yonsei Med. J. 38, 423–427.

Hagen, E.C., Daha, M.R., Hermans, J., et al. 1998. Diagnostic value of standardized assays for antineutrophil cytoplasmic antibodies in idiopathic systemic vasculitis. Kidney Int. 53, 743–753.

Hall, S., Persellin, S., Lie, J.T., et al. 1983. The therapeutic impact of temporal artery biopsy. Lancet 2 (8361), 1217–1220.

Hauschild, S., Schmitt, W., Csernok, E., et al., 1993. ANCA in systemic vasculitides, collagen vascular diseases, rheumatic disorders and inflammatory bowel diease. In: W.L. Gross (Ed.), ANCA-Associated Vasculitides: Immunological and Clinical Aspects. Plenum Press, New York, pp. 245–251.

Hauschild, S., Csernok, E., Schmitt, W.H., Gross, W.L. 1994. Antineutrophil cytoplasmic antibodies in systemic polyarteritis nodosa with and without hepatitis B virus infection and Churg–Strauss syndrome—62 patients (Letter). J. Rheumatol. 21, 1173–1174.

Haworth, S.J., Savage, C.O.S., Carr, D., et al. 1985. Pulmonary haemorrhage complication Wegener's granulomatosis and microscopic polarteritis. BMJ 290, 1775–1778.

Hayashi, K., Nagasaki, M., Matsunaga, N., et al. 1986. Initial pulmonary artery involvement in Takayasu arteritis. Radiology 159, 401–403.

Hoang-Xuan, T., Foster, C.S., Rice, B.A. 1990. Scleritis in relapsing polychondritis. Response to therapy. Opthalmology 97, 892–898.

Hoffman, G.S., Kerr, G.S. 1994. Recognition of systemic vasculitis in the acutely ill patient. In: B.F. Mandell (Ed.), Acute Rheumatic and Immunologic Diseases. Marcel Dekker, New York, pp. 279–307.

Hoffman, G.S., Specks, U. 1998. Antineutrophil cytoplasmic antibodies (ANCA). Arthritis Rheum. 35, 1322–1329.

Hoffman, G.S., Leavitt, R.Y., Fleisher, T.A., et al. 1990 Treatment of Wegener's granulomatosis with intermittent high-dose intravenous cyclophosphamide. Am. J. Med. 89, 403–410.

Hoffman, G.S., Kerr, G.S., Leavitt, R.Y., et al. 1992. Wegener's granulomatosis: an analysis of 158 patients. Ann. Intern. Med. 116, 488–498.

Hoffman, G.S., Leavitt, R.Y., Kerr, G.S., et al. 1994. Treatment of glucocorticoid-resistant or relapsing Takayasu's arteritis with methotrexate. Arthrits Rheum. 37, 578–582.

Hoffman, G.S., Cid, M.C., Hellmann, D.B., et al. 2002. A multicenter, randomized, double-blind, placebo-controlled trial of adjuvant methotrexate treatment for giant cell arteritis. Arthritis Rheum. 46 (5), 1309–1318.

Horton, B.T., Magarth, T.B., Brown, G.E. 1932. An undescribed form of arteritis of the temporal vessels. Mayo Clin. Proc. 7, 700–706.

Hunder, G.C. 1990. Giant cell (temporal) arteritis. Rheum. Dis. Clin. N. Am. 16 (2), 399–409.

Hunder, G.G., Arend, W.P., Bloch, D.A., et al. 1990. The American College of Rheumatology criteria for the classification of vasculitis. Introduction. Arthritis Rheum. 33, 1065–1067.

Hunninghake, G.W., Fauci, A.S. 1979. Pulmonary involvement in the collagen vascular diseases. Am. Rev. Respir. Dis. 119, 471–503.

Huston, K.A., Hunder, G.G., Lie, J.T., et al. 1978. Temporal arteritis: a 25-year epidemiological, clinical, and pathologic study. Ann. Intern. Med. 88, 162–167.

Ingue, T., Kanayama, Y., Ohe, A., Kato, N., Horiguchi, T., Ishii, M., Jhiota, K. 1979. Immunopathological studies of pneumonitis in systemic lupus erythematosus. Ann. Intern. Med. 91, 30–34.

Irani, B.S., Martin Hirsch, D.P., Clark, D., et al. 1992. Relapsing polychondritis—a study of four cases. J. Laryngol. Otol. 106, 911–914.

Jaksch-Wartenhorst, R. 1923. Polychondropthia. Wien Arch. J. Intern. Med. 6, 93–100.

Jayne, D.R., Jones, S.J., Severn, A., et al. 1989. Severe pulmonary haemorrhage and systemic vasculitis in association with circulating anti-neutrophil cytoplasmic antibodies of IgM class only. Clin. Nephrol. 3, 101–106.

Jayne, D.R., Davies, D.J., Fox, C.J., et al. 1991. Treatment of systemic vasculitis with pooled intra-venous immunoglobulin. Lancet 337, 1137.

Jayne, D., Rasmussen, N., Andrassy, K., et al. 2003. A randomized trial of maintenance therapy for vasculitis associated with antineutrophil cytoplasmic autoantibodies. N. Engl. J. Med. 349, 36–44.

Jennette, J.C., Falk, R.J., Andrassy, K., et al. 1994. Nomencalture of systemic vasculitides: proposal of an international consensus conference. Arthritis Rheum. 37, 187–192.

Kaiser, M., Weyand, C.M., Bjornsson, J., Goronzy, J.J. 1998. Platelet-derived growth factor, intimal hyperplasia, and ischemic complications in giant cell arteritis. Arthritis Rheum. 41, 623–633.

Karam, G.H., Fulmer, J.D. 1982. Giant cell arteritis presenting as interstitial lung disease. Chest 82, 781–784.

Kauffmann, R.H., Herrmann, W.A., Meyer, C.J.L.M., Daha, M.R., Van Es, L.A. 1980. Circulating IgA-immune complexes in Henoch-Schoenlein purpura: a longitudinal study of their relationship to disease activity and vascular deposition of IgA. Am. J. Med. 69, 859–866.

Kennedy, J.I., Fulmer, J.D. 1993. Pulmonary vasculitides. In: M.I. Schwarz, T.E. King (Eds.), Interstitial Lung Disease, 2nd ed., Mosby-Year Book, St Louis, pp. 445–462.

Kerr, G.S., Fleisher, T.A., Hallahan, C.W., et al. 1993. Limited prognostic value of changes in antineutrophil cytoplasmic antibody titre in patients with Wegener's granulomatosis. Arthritis Rheum. 36, 365–371.

Kerr, G.S., Hallahan, C.W., Giordano, J., et al. 1994. Takayasu arthritis. Ann. Intern. Med. 120, 919–929.

Kerr, K.M., Auger, W.R., Fedullo, P.F., et al. 1995. Large vessel pulmonary arteritis mimicking chronic thromboembolic disease. Am. J. Respir. Crit. Care Med. 152, 367–373.

Koide, K. 1992. Takayasu's arteritis in Japan. Heart Vessels 7, 48–54.

Kramer, M.R., Melzer, E., Nesher, G., et al. 1987. Pulmonary manifestations of temporal arteritis. Eur. J. Respir. Dis. 71, 430–433.

Krupa, W.M., Dewan, M., Jeon, M.-S., et al. 2002. Trapping of misdirected dendritic cells in the granulomatous lesions of giant cell arteritis. Am. J. Pathol. 161, 1815–1823.

Kussmaul, A., Maier, K. 1866. Uber eine nicht bisher beschriebene eigenthumliche Arterienerkrankung (periarteritis nodosa), die mit Morbus Brightii und rapid fortschreitender allgemeiner Muskelahung einhergeht. Deutsche Archiv Klinische Medizin 1, 484–518.

Lande, A., Bard, R. 1976. Takayasu's arteritis: An unrecognized cause of pulmonary hypertension. Angiology 27, 114–121.

Lane, S.E., Watts, R.A., Scott, D.G.I. 2003. Wegener's Granulomatosis and Churg–Strauss syndrome: clinical features in a population-based cohort. Rheumatology 42 ((S)1), 134.

Lang, B., Rothenfuser, A., Lanchbury, J.S., et al. 1993. Susceptibility to relapsing polychondritis is associated with HLA-DR4. Arthritis Rheum. 36, 660–664.

Langford, C.A. 2001. Management of systemic vasculitis. Baillieres Best Pract. Res. Clin. Rheumatol. 15 (2), 281–297.

Langford, C.A., Talar-Williams, C., Barron, K.S., Sneller, M.C. 1999. A staged approach to the treatment of Wegener's granulomatosis: Induction of remission with glucocorticoids and daily cyclophosphamide switching to methotrexate for remission maintenance. Arthritis Rheum. 41, 2666–2673.

Lanham, J.G., Churg, J. 1991. Churg–Strauss syndrome. In: A. Churg, J. Churg (Eds.), Systemic Vasculitides. Igaku-Shoin, New York/Tokyo, pp. 101–120.

Lanham, J.G., Elkon, K.B., Pusey, C.D., Hughes, G.R. 1984. Systemic vasculitis with asthma and eosinophilia: a clinical approach to the Churg–Strauss syndrome. Medicine 63, 65–84.

Larson, T.S., Hall, S., Hepper, N.G.G., et al. 1984. Respiratory tract symptoms as a clue to giant cell arteritis. Ann. Intern. Med. 101, 594–597.

Lavignac, C., Jauberteau-Marchan, M.O., Liozon, E., Vidal, E., Catanzano, G., Liozon, F. 1996. Etude immunohistochimique des lesions d'arterite temporale de Horton avant et au cours de la corticotherapie. Rev. Med. Intern. 17, 814–820.

Leatherman, J.W. 1987. Immune alveolar haemorrhage. Chest 91, 891–897.

Leatherman, J.W., Davies, S.F., Hoidal, J.R. 1984. Alveolar haemorrhage syndromes: diffuse microvascular lung haemorrhage in immune and idiopathic disorders. Medicine 63, 343–361.

Leavitt, R.Y., Fauci, A.S. 1986. Pulmonary vasculitis. Am. Rev. Respir. Dis. 134, 149–166.

Leib, E.S., Restino, C., Paulus, H.E. 1979. Immunosuppressive and corticosteroid therapy of polyarteritis nodosa. Am. J. Med. 67, 941–947.

Lie, J.T. 1996. Isolated pulmonary Takayasu's arteritis: clinicopathologic characteristics. Mod. Pathol. 9 (5), 469–474.

Lipnick, R.N., Fink, C.W. 1991. Acute airway obstruction in relapsing polychondritis: treatment with pulse methylprednisolone. J. Rheumatol. 18, 98–99.

Liu, N.H., LaBree, L.D., Feldon, S.E., Rao, N.A. 2001. The epidemiology of giant cell arteritis: a 12-year retrospective study. Opthalmology 108, 1145–1149.

Lupi, E., Sanchez, G., Horwitz, S., et al. 1975. Pulmonary artery involvement in Takayasu's arteritis. Chest 67, 69–74.

Luthra, H.S., McKenna, C.H., Terasaki, P.I. 1981. Lack of association of HLA-A and B locus antigens with relapsing polychondritis. Tissue Antigens 17, 442–443.

Mark, E.J., Ramirez, J.F. 1985. Pulmonary capillaritis and hemorrhage in patients with systemic vasculitis. Arch. Pathol. Lab Med. 109, 413–418.

Mattey, D.L., Hajeer, A.H., Dababneh, et al. 2000. Association of giant cell arteritis and polymyalgia rheumatica with different tumour necrosis factor microsatellite polymorphisms. Arthritis Rheum. 43, 1749–1755.

McAdam, L.P., O'Hanlan, M.A., Bluestone, R., Pearson, C.M. 1976. Relapsing polychondritis: prospective study of 23 patients and a review of the literature. Medicine 55, 193–215.

McCluskey, R.T., Fienberg, R. 1983. Vasculitis in primary vasculitides, granulomatoses and connective tissue disease. Human Pathol. 14, 305–315.

Michelson, J.B., Friedlaender, M.H. 1990. Behçet's disease. Int. Opthalmol. Clin. 30, 271–278.

Mitchell, B.M., Front, R.L. 2001. Detection of varicella Zoster virus DNA in some patients with giant cell arteritis. Invest. Opthalmol. Vis. Sci. 42, 2572–2577.

Michet, C.J. 1990a. Vasculitis and relapsing polychondritis. Rheum. Dis. Clin. N. Am. 16, 441–444.

Michet, C.J. 1990b. Epidemiology of vasculitis. In: D.L. Conn (Ed.), Rheumatic Disease Clinics of North America. WB Saunders, Philadelphia, pp. 261–268, chapter 2.

Michet, C.J., McKenna, C.H., Luthra, H.S., O'Fallon, W.M. 1986. Relapsing polychondritis: survival and predictive role of early disease manifestations. Ann. Intern. Med. 104, 74–78.

Mizuki, N., Ota, M., Kimura, M., et al. 1997. Triplet repeat polymorphisms in the transmembrane region of the MICA gene: a strong association of six GCT repetitions with Behçet's disease. Proc. Natl Acad. Sci. USA 94, 1298–1303.

Mohan, N., Kerr, G.S. 2001. Diagnosis of vasculitis. Baillieres Best Pract. Res. Clin. Rheumatol. 15 (2), 203–223.

Moloney, J.R. 1978. Relapsing polychondritis: its otolaryngological manifestations. J. Laryngol. Otolaryngol. 92, 9–15.

Moore, J.W., Reardon, M.J., Cooley, D.A., et al. 1985. Severe Takayasu's arteritis of the pulmonary arteries: report of a case with successful surgical treatment. J. Am. Coll. Cardiol. 5, 369–373.

Morita, K., Saito, K., Miura, A.B., Ishikawa, H., Imai, H. 1993. The role of gallium scintigraphy, CT scan and MRI in the diagnosis of Takayasu's disease. J. Rheumatol. 20 (9), 1604.

Moskowitz, R.W., Baggenstross, A.H., Slocumb, C.H. 1963. Histopathologic classification or periarteritis nodosa: a study of 56 cases confirmed at necropsy. Mayo Clin. Proc. 38, 345–357.

Nesbitt, J.C., Carrasco, H. 1996. Expandable stents. Chest Surg. Clin. N. Am. 6, 305–328.

Nick, J., Tuder, R., May, R., Fisher, J. 1996. Am. J. Repir. Crit. Care Med. 153, 450–453.

O'Duffy, J. 1990. Vasculitis in Behçet's disease. Rheum. Dis. Clin. N. Am. 16, 423–431.

Pearson, C.M., Kline, H.M., Newcomer, V.D. 1960. Relapsing polychondritis. N. Engl. J. Med. 263, 51–58.

Petursdottir, V., Johansson, H., Nordborg, E., Nordborg, C. 1999. The epidemiology of biopsy-positive giant cell arteritis: special reference to cyclic fluctuations. Rheumatology 38, 1208–1212.

Primack, S.L., Miller, R.R., Muller, N.L. 1995. Diffuse pulmonary haemorrhage: clinical, pathological and imaging features. AJR 16, 295–300.

Pusey, C.D., Rees, A.J., Evans, D.J., et al. 1991. Plasma exchange in focal necrotizing glomerulonephritis without anti-GBM antibodies. Kidney Int. 40, 757–763.

Raz, I., Okon, E., Chajek-Shaul, T. 1989. Pulmonary manifestations in Behçet's syndrome. Chest 95, 585–589.

Reid, A.J.C., Scott, D.G.I., Watts, R.A., et al. 1996. Churg–Strauss syndrome in the United Kingdom: a 13 year experience. Sarcoidosis Vasc. Diffuse Lung Dis. 13, 271.

Reinhold-Keller, E., Kekow, J., Schnabel, A., et al. 1994. Influence of disease manifestation and antineutrophil cytoplasmic antibody titer on the response to pulse cyclophosphamide therapy in patients with Wegener's granulomatosis. Arthritis Rheum. 37, 919–924.

Robson, W.L.M., Leung, A.K.C. 1994. Henoch-Schönlein Purpura. Adv. Pediatr. 41, 163–194.

Romero, S., Vela, P., Padilla, I., Rosas, J., Martin, C., Aranda, I., et al. 1992. Pleural effusion as manifestation of temporal arteritis. Thorax 47, 398–399.

Rose, G.A., Spencer, H. 1957. Polyarteritis nodosa. Q. J. Med. 25, 43–81.

Ruhlen, J.L., Huston, K.A., Wood, W.G. 1981. Relapsing polychondritis with glomerulonephritis: improvement with prednisolone and cyclophosphamide. JAMA 245, 847–848.

Sams, W.M. 1980. Necrotizing vasculitis. J. Am. Acad. Dermatol. 3, 1–13.

Satinder, K., Cheifec, G. 1982. Fatal pulmonary Henoch-Schönlein syndrome. Chest 82(5) 654–656.

Savage, C.O., Winearls, C.G., Evans, D.J., Rees, A.J., Lockwood, C.M. 1985. Microscopic polyarteritis: presentation, pathology and prognosis. QJM 56 (220), 467–483.

Savage, C.O.S., Pottinger, B.E., Gaskin, G., et al. 1992. Autoantibodies developing to myeloperoxidase and proteinase-3 in systemic vasculitis stimulate neutrophil cytotoxicity towards cultured endothelial cells. Am. J. Pathol. 141, 335–342.

Savige, J.A., Chang, L., Cook, L., et al. 1995. Alpha-1 antitrypsin deficiency and anti-proteinase 3 antibodies in anti-neutrophil cytoplasmic antibody (ANCA) associated systemic vasculitis. Clin. Exp. Immunol. 100, 194–197.

Schmidt, W.A., Kraft, H.E., Vorpahl, K., Völker, L., Gromnica-Ihle, E.J. 1997. Colour duplex ultrasonography in the diagnosis of temporal arteritis. N. Eng. J. Med. 337 (19), 1336–1342.

Schmidt, W.A. 2000. Doppler ultrasonography in the diagnosis of giant cell arteritis. Clin. Exp. Rheumatol. 18 (4 Suppl. 20), S40–S42.

Seko, Y., Minota, S., Kawasaki, A., Shinkai, Y., Maeda, K., Yagita, H., Okumura, K., Sato, O., Takagi, A., Tada, Y., et al. 1994. Perforin-secreting killer cell infiltration and expression of a 65-kD heat-shock protein in aortic tissue of patients with Takayasu's arteritis. J. Clin. Invest. 93 (2) 750–758.

Seko, Y., Sato, O., Takagi, A., Tada, Y., Matsuo, H., Yagita, H., Okumura, K., Yazaki, Y. 1996. Restricted usage of T-cell receptor Valpha-Vbeta genes in infiltrating cells in aortic tissue of patients with Takayasu's arteritis. Circulation 93 (10) 1788–1790.

Sen, R.P. 1991. Pulmonary complications of combination therapy with cyclophophamide and prednisolone. Chest 99, 143–146.

Seo, J.B., Im, J.G., Chung, J.W., Song, J.W., Goo, J.W., Park, J.H., Yeon, K.M. 2000. Pulmonary vasculitis: the spectrum of radiological findings. Br. J. Radiol. 73 (875), 1224–1231.

Shelhamer, J.H., Volkman, D.J., Parillo, J.E., et al. 1985. Takayasu's arteritis and its therapy. Ann. Intern. Med. 103, 121–126.

Soto, A., Jorgensen, C., Oksman, F., et al. 1994. Endocarditis associated with ANCA. Clin. Exp. Rheumatol. 12, 203–204.

Sridharan, S.T. 2001. Relapsing polychondritis. In: G.S. Hoffman, C. Weyland (Eds.), Inflammatory Disease of the Blood Vessels. Marcel Dekker, New York, pp. 675–693.

Staples, C.A. 1991. Pulmonary angiitis and granulomatosis. Radiol. Clin. N. Am. 29, 973–982.

Stegeman, C.A., Cohen Tervaert, J.W., Yde Jong, P.E., et al. 1996. Trimethoprin-sulfamethoxazole (co-trimoxazole) for the prevention of relapses of Wegener's granulomatosis. N. Engl. J. Med. 335, 16–20.

Stewart, A.K., Mazanec, D.J. 1992. Pulse intravenous cyclophosphamide for kidney disease in relapsing polychondritis. J. Rheumatol. 19, 498–499.

Stoffel, M.P., Csernok, E., Herzberg, C., et al. 1996. Antineutrophil cytolplasmic antibodies (ANCA) directed against bactericidal/ permeability increasing protein (BPI): a new seromarker for inflammatory bowel disease and associated disorders. Clin. Exp. Immunol. 104, 54–59.

Sullivan, E.J., Hoffman, G.S. 1998. Pulmonary vasculitis. Clin. Chest Med. 19 (4), 759–776.

Svenson, K.L.G., Holmdahl, R., Klareskog, L., et al. 1984. Cyclosporin A treatment in a case of relapsing polychondritis. Scand. J. Rheumatol. 13, 329–333.

Sweeney, A.R., Baggenstross, A.H. 1949. Pulmonary lesions of periarteritis nodosa. Mayo Clin. Proc. 24, 35–43.

Talar-Williams, C., Hijazi, Y.M., Walther, M.M., et al. 1996. Cyclophosphamide induced cystitis and bladder cancer in patients with Wegener's granulomatosis. Ann. Intern. Med. 89, 403–410.

Travis, W.D., Colby, T.V., Lombard, C., et al. 1990. A clinicopathologic study of 34 cases of diffuse pulmonary haemorrhage with lung biopsy confirmation. Am. J. Surg. Pathol. 14, 1112–1125.

Tyagi, S., Singh, B., Kaul, U.A., et al. 1993. Balloon angioplasty for renovascular hypertension in Takayasu's arteritis. Am. Heart J. 125, 1386–1393.

Umehara, I., Shibuya, H., Nakagawa, T., et al. 1991. Comprehensive analysis of perfusion scintigraphy in Tayayasu's arteritis. Clin. Nucl. Med. 16, 352–357.

Watts, R.A., Carruthers, D.M., Scott, D.G.I. 1995. Epidemiology of systemic vasculitis: changing incidence or definition? Semin. Arthritis Rheum. 25, 28–34.

Watts, R.A., Jolliffe, V.A., Grattan, C.E., et al. 1998. Cutaneous vasculitis in a defined population-clinical and epidemiological associations. J. Rheumatol. 25, 920–924.

Watts, R.A., Lane, S.A., Bentham, G., Scott, D.G.I. 2000. Epidemiology of systemic vasculitis: a ten-year study in the United Kingdom. Arthritis Rheum. 43, 414–419.

Watts, R., Gonzalez-Gay, M.A., Lane, S.E., et al. 2001a. Geoepidemiology of systemic vasculitis- a comparison of the incidence in two regions of Europe. Ann. Rheum. Dis. 60, 170–172.

Watts, R.A., Lane, S.A., Scott, D.G.I., et al. 2001b. Epidemiology of vasculitis in Europe. Ann. Rheum. Dis. 60, 1156–1157.

Wawryk, S.O., Ayberk, H., Boyd, A.W., Rode, J. 1991. Analysis od adhesion molecules in the immunopathogenesis of giant cell arteritis. J. Clin. Pathol. 44, 497–501.

Weisbrod, G.L. 1989. Pulmonary angiitis and granulomatosis: a review. Can. Assoc. Radiol. J. 40, 127–134.

Weyand, C.M., Goronzy, J.J. 2002. Giant cell arthritis: pathogenesis. In: G.S. Hoffman, C.M. Weyand (Eds.), Inflammatory Diseases of Blood Vessels. Marcel Dekker, New York, pp. 413–423.

Weyand, C.M., Goronzy, J.J. 2003. Mechanisms of disease: medium- and large vessel vasculitis. N. Engl. J. Med. 349, 160–169.

Wilke, W.S., Hoffman, G.S. 1995. Treatment of glucocorticoid-resistant giant cell arteritis. Rheum. Dis. Clin. N. Am. 21 (1), 59–71.

Wilson, A.G. 1995. Immunologic diseases of the lungs. In: P. Armstrong, A.G. Wilson, P. Dee, D.M. Hansell (Eds.), Imaging of Diseases of the Chest, 2nd ed., Mosby-Year Book, St Louis, pp. 485–567.

Winkelman, R.K., Ditto, W.B. 1964. Cutaneous and visceral syndromes of necrotizing or allergic angiitis: a study of 38 cases. Medicine 69, 59–89.

Wohlwill, F. 1923. Uber die nur Mikroskopisch erkenbarre Form der Periarteritis nodosa. Virchows Archiv fur Pathologische Anatomie und Physiologie und fur Klinische Medizin 246, 377–411.

Yahya, T.M., Benedict, S., Shalabi, A., et al. 1997. Anti-neutrophil cytoplasmic antibody (ANCA) in malaria is directed against cathepsin G. Clin. Exp. Immunol. 110, 41–44.

Yamanda, M., Shibuya, H., Matsubara, O., et al. 1992. Pulmonary artery disease in Takayasu's arteritis: angiographic findings. Am. J. Radiol. 159, 263–269.

Yamato, M., Lecky, J.W., Hiramatsu, K., et al. 1986. Takayasu's arteritis: radiographic and angiographic findings in 59 patients. Radiology 161, 329–334.

Yang, C.L., Brinckmann, J., Rui, H.F., et al. 1993. Autoantibodies to cartilage collagens in relapsing polychondritis. Arch. Dermatol. Res. 285, 245–249.

Zamora, M.R., Warner, M.L., Tuder, R., Schwarz, M.I. 1997. Diffuse alveolar haemorrhage and systemic lupus erththematosus. Clinical presentation, histology, survival and outcome. Medicine (Baltimore) 76, 192–202.

Zeone, T., Souquet, P-J., Bohas, C., et al. 1994. Unusual manifestations of giant cell arteritis: pulmonary nodules, cough, conjunctivits and otitis with deafness. Eur. Respir. J. 7, 2252–2254.

Zhao, M.H., Jones, S.J., Lockwood, C.M. 1996. Bactericidal/ permeability increasing protein (BPI) is an important antigen for anti-neutrophil cytoplasm autoantibodies (ANCA) in vasculitis. Clin. Exp. Immunol. 99, 49–56.

Zouboulis, C.C., Kotter, I., Djawari, D., et al. 1997. Epidemiological features of Adamantiades-Behçet's disease in Germany and in Europe. Yonsei Med. J. 38, 411–422.

PART V

Pulmonary Involvement in Connective Tissue Disorders

Handbook of Systemic Autoimmune Diseases, Volume 2
Pulmonary Involvement in Systemic Autoimmune Diseases
A.U. Wells and C.P. Denton, editors

CHAPTER 6

Lung Disease in Lupus

Amy H. Kao[a], Janice M. Sabatine[a], Susan Manzi[b,*]

[a]*Division of Rheumatology and Clinical Immunology, University of Pittsburgh School of Medicine, Pittsburgh, PA, USA*

[b]*Division of Rheumatology and Clinical Immunology, University of Pittsburgh School of Medicine and University of Pittsburgh Graduate School of Public Health, S722 Biomedical Sciences Tower, 3500 Terrace Street, Pittsburgh, PA 15261, USA.*

1. Introduction

Systemic lupus erythematosus (SLE) is an autoimmune inflammatory disease that primarily affects women in the reproductive years, with various clinical presentations caused by the production of autoantibodies and the formation of complement-fixing immune complexes. Pulmonary complications, one of the predominant features of SLE, occur in more than half of the patients at some time during the course of their disease. In many cases, lung complications are not detected until autopsy, indicating that they are often not clinically evident. The general classification of pulmonary manifestations and their prevalence are summarized in Table 1. In this chapter we will review the epidemiology, clinical presentations, differential diagnosis, management, and outcome of the broad spectrum of pulmonary complications experienced by patients with SLE.

2. Pleural disease

2.1. Pleuritis with or without effusion

The most common pulmonary manifestation in patients with SLE is pleuritis with or without effusion, and it can occur concomitantly with pericarditis (Fig. 1) (Murin et al., 1998). In fact, pleuritis is more often encountered in SLE than in any other connective tissue disease. Symptoms usually include pleuritic chest pain, dyspnea, cough, and/or fever and are seen in approximately 45–60% of patients. Asymptomatic pleural involvement can be more prevalent. Autopsy series report pathologic changes consistent with pleuritis or pleural fibrosis in 50–93% of cases (Orens et al., 1994; Mochizuki et al., 1999). Asymptomatic pleural effusions have also been detected on chest radiographs and by other imaging techniques. Pleural effusions, seen in 16–50% of patients on plain chest radiographs, are usually small, and in about half of the cases are bilateral and equally distributed between the left and right hemithorax (Fig. 2) (Orens et al., 1994).

It can sometimes be difficult to definitely diagnose lupus pleuritis because several other conditions may present similarly (Table 2). Thoracentesis is appropriate for diagnosing pleuritis in patients with or without SLE presenting with pleural effusion. The characteristics of pleural fluid in SLE are listed in

*Corresponding author.
Tel.: +1-412-383-8734; fax: +1-412-383-8753
E-mail address: sxm6@pitt.edu (S. Manzi).

DOI: 10.1016/S1571-5078(04)02006-9

Table 1
Pulmonary manifestations of systemic lupus erythematosus

Organ involvement	Disease process	Prevalence of symptomatic disease
Pleura	Pleuritis with or without effusion	45–60%
	Pleural effusion	Unknown[a]
Parenchyma	Acute lupus pneumonitis with or without pulmonary hemorrhage	1–4%
	Diffuse alveolar hemorrhage	<2%
	Interstitial lung disease	3–8%
	Small airway disease	Few case reports
	Infectious pneumonia	44 & 76% in two autopsy series for bacterial bronchopneumonia
	Pulmonary edema	Unknown[a]
Pulmonary vasculature	Pulmonary arterial hypertension	5–14%
	Pulmonary embolism	35–42%[b]
	Acute reversible hypoxemia	Few case reports
Diaphragm	'Shrinking lung' syndrome	59 cases reported in literature

[a] Exact prevalence not known.
[b] Patients with SLE and antiphospholipid antibody.

Table 3 (Good et al., 1983). The diagnosis of exudative pleural effusion can be made based on pleural fluid LDH levels greater than 200 U/l, a fluid-to-serum LDH ratio greater than 0.6, or a fluid-to-serum total protein ratio greater than 0.5 based on the most commonly used Light's criteria (Light et al., 1972). Many studies also use different cutoff points of laboratory parameters (pleural LDH, pleural cholesterol, or protein ratio) to improve the differentiation of exudates from transudates (Paramothayan and Barron, 2002). Glucose levels are usually normal, in contrast to those in patients with rheumatoid arthritis, which are often less than 20 mg/dl. Pleural fluid sometimes contains anti-double-stranded DNA antibodies and lupus erythematosus (LE) cells. Although elevated ANA titers have been detected, they may not be specific for lupus pleuritis because nonlupus patients, particularly those with underlying malignancy or pleural or pericardial fluid, may have high ANA titers (Wang et al., 2000). Pleural biopsy with immunofluorescence staining is rarely performed in SLE because the histologic findings are nonspecific and include lymphocytic and plasma cell infiltration, fibrosis, and fibrinous pleuritis; however, it may be necessary for ruling out alternative etiologies such as tuberculosis.

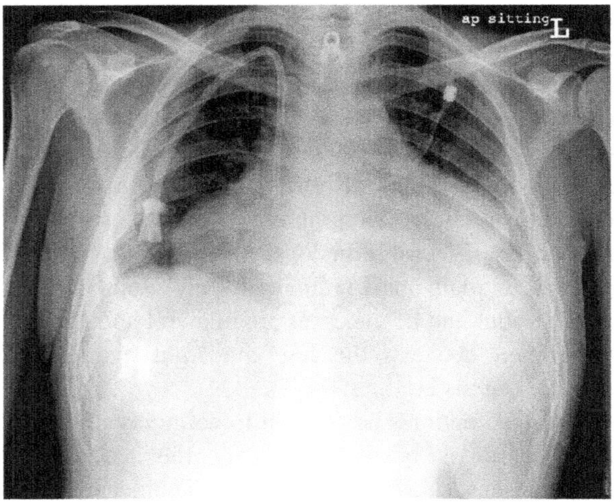

Figure 1. Chest radiograph (AP view) demonstrating small bilateral pleural effusions associated with a large pericardial effusion in a lupus patient presenting with pleuropericarditis.

Mild symptomatic cases of lupus pleuritis can be treated with nonsteroidal anti-inflammatory drugs (NSAIDs). However, in patients who do not improve or who have more severe symptoms, it may be necessary to use systemic corticosteroids (prednisone 10–40 mg daily). Pleuritis caused by drug-induced lupus usually resolves when the offending drug is discontinued. Most patients respond promptly to the above-mentioned regimen and their effusions usually resolve in a few days, although it may take several

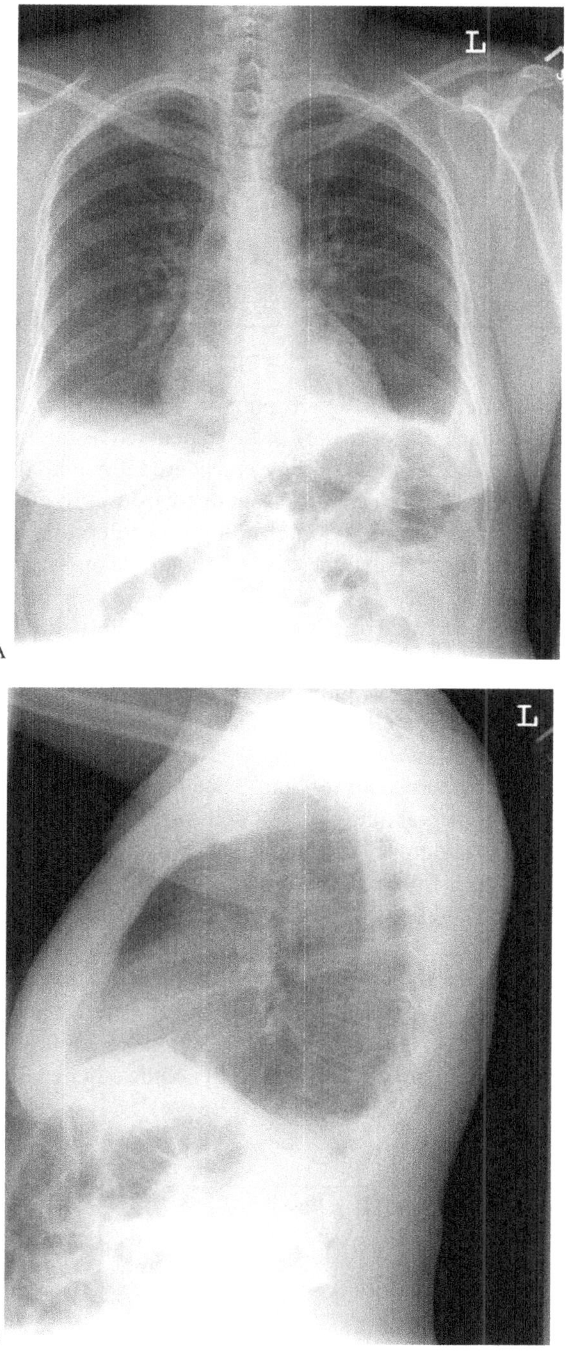

A

B

Figure 2. Chest radiograph (PA & lateral views) demonstrating asymptomatic bilateral pleural effusions with clear lung parenchyma.

weeks to see complete resolution radiographically. There is usually only minimal residual thickening after the effusion clears. Steroid-sparing agents such as hydroxychloroquine or azathioprine may be added when symptomatic pleuritis is slow to improve. In rare cases of refractory or chronic unremitting lupus pleuritis, it may be necessary to conduct pleurectomy or pleurodesis with a sclerosing agent such as talc or tetracycline (Glazer et al., 2000; Sharma et al., 2002).

2.2. Pleural effusion

Pleural effusions in patients with congestive heart failure or renal failure tend to be transudative as a result of volume overload and are characterized by a low cell and protein content. The most common cause of transudative effusion in patients with SLE is congestive heart failure, which occurs in 10% of lupus patients (Badui et al., 1985). Transudative pleural effusions can also develop in patients with SLE and nephrotic syndrome due to lupus nephritis because these patients commonly have hypoalbuminemia. Decreased serum albumin leads to low oncotic pressure, resulting in altered distribution of hydrostatic and oncotic pressure across the pleura. As a result, the rate of pleural fluid formation exceeds that of its reabsorption.

3. Parenchymal disease

3.1. Acute lupus pneumonitis/pulmonary hemorrhage

Acute lupus pneumonitis is part of a spectrum of pulmonary disease in SLE that results from acute injury to the alveolar-capillary component (Wiedemann and Matthay, 1989; Orens et al., 1994). Only 1–4% of patients with SLE manifest acute lupus pneumonitis (Orens et al., 1994), and it can be difficult to distinguish from infectious pneumonia. Typical presentations include fever, dyspnea, cough with scant sputum, and in some cases hemoptysis. Since coexisting pleuritis is common, patients may also experience pleuritic chest pain. Although rare (<2% of patients with SLE), diffuse alveolar

Table 2
Differential diagnosis of pleural effusion

Transudative effusion	Exudative effusion
Congestive heart failure	Infection
Renal disease (nephrotic syndrome)	Drugs[a] (e.g. procainamide, hydralazine, isoniazid, amiodarone or sulfasalazine)
Liver cirrhosis	Other connective tissue diseases (e.g. rheumatoid arthritis, systemic sclerosis, and adult Still's disease)
	Malignancy
	Pulmonary embolism

[a] Drugs that induce a lupus-like syndrome.

hemorrhage (DAH) is an often-lethal pulmonary complication of SLE with mortality rates exceeding 50% (Leatherman et al., 1984). DAH typically occurs in SLE as a pulmonary–renal syndrome (Liu et al., 1998; Chang et al., 2002). In one study, active nephritis was observed more frequently during episodes of alveolar hemorrhage (64%) than in the period prior to the first episode of DAH (28%) (Santos-Ocampo et al., 2000).

Patients with lupus pneumonitis are usually hypoxemic, tachypneic, and have diffuse or bibasilar rales on auscultation of the lungs. Infectious agents are usually not present in cultures of bronchoalveolar lavage unless infectious pneumonia is superimposed. If there is pulmonary hemorrhage, an acute decline in hemoglobin and an increase in diffusing capacity for carbon monoxide can occur. Basilar unilateral or bilateral alveolar or interstitial infiltrates, which can be patchy or diffuse, may be detected on bronchoscopy. High-resolution CT reveals scattered, bilateral ground-glass opacities or airspace consolidation (Fig. 3). Bronchoscopy may demonstrate bleeding and hemosiderin-laden macrophages (if the alveolar hemorrhage is not acute) in bronchoalveolar lavage. A lung biopsy should only be considered if potentially diagnostic tissue cannot be obtained from any other site. The pathologic findings in lupus pneumonitis are nonspecific and include alveolar wall inflammation (alveolitis), alveolar hemorrhage, edema, hyaline membranes, interstitial pneumonitis, capillary thrombosis, deposits of immunoglobulins and complement components (C3), and diffuse injury to the microvasculature (capillaritis) (Wiedemann and Matthay, 1989). It is rare to see gross vasculitis or necrosis. Electron microscopy of lung specimens shows subendothelial granular electron-dense deposits, characteristic of immune complexes, in the alveolar wall and in the walls of the arterioles (Churg et al., 1980). This funding suggests the possibility that the pathogenesis of lung and kidney disease in SLE is similar and involves microvascular injury due to immune-complex mediated processes (Hughson et al., 2001). Diagnosis of acute lupus pneumonitis requires a vigorous diagnostic evaluation to exclude other causes

Table 3
Characteristics of pleural fluid in SLE

Appearance	Serous or serosanguinous
Fluid type	Exudate
Protein	>3 g/dl
WBC	3000–5000 cells/ml (mononuclear or lymphocytic predominance)
Glucose	Equivalent to serum glucose level (>60 mg/dl)
Complement C3 and C4 levels	Decreased
Pleural fluid autoantibodies	Antinuclear antibody (also present in nonlupus patients with malignancy), anti-double-stranded DNA antibody
Cell sediment	LE cells

Permission granted to reproduce with modification from Kao, A.H., Manzi, S. 2002. How to manage patients with cardiopulmonary disease? Best Pract. Res. Clin. Rheumatol. 16, 211–227.

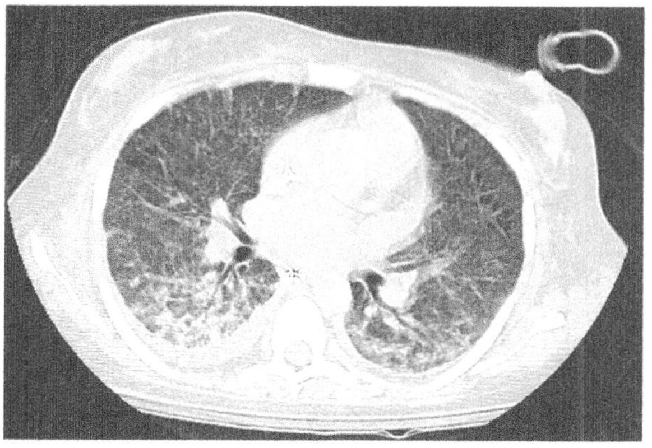

Figure 3. High-resolution chest CT scan demonstrating acute lupus pneumonitis with diffuse bilateral ground glass opacities, distended interlobular septa, and small bilateral pleural effusions.

of pulmonary infiltration (Specks, 2001), which are listed in Table 4. Differentiation among various etiologies is critical since patients with SLE frequently experience bacterial or opportunistic infections, particularly those patients on chronic immunosuppressive therapy.

It is crucial to start treatment of life-threatening hemorrhage promptly. The course of the disease is deteriorating, and patients often develop adult respiratory distress syndrome (ARDS) despite cytotoxic therapy. Owing to the lack of controlled studies to determine the efficacy of drug regimens in the treatment of acute lupus pneumonitis/DAH, current recommendations are based on case reports and clinical experience. Preferred treatment includes intravenous pulse methylprednisolone (1 g IV for 3 days) alone or in combination with pulse cyclophosphamide (0.5–1 g/m^2) or oral therapy (1–2 mg/kg/day) (Schwab et al., 1993). Other agents for treating steroid-resistant acute lupus pneumonitis include azathioprine, intravenous immunoglobulin, plasmapheresis, and immunoadsorption therapy, which have varying degrees of success (Isbister et al., 1981; Winder et al., 1993; Santiago et al., 1996; Graninger et al., 2002).

Table 4
Conditions with interstitial infiltrates that can mimic acute lupus pneumonitis ± alveolar hemorrhage

Infectious pneumonia
Coagulopathy
Uremia
Pulmonary embolism
Congestive heart failure
Wegener's granulomatosus
Microscopic polyangiitis
Goodpasture's syndrome
Behçet's disease
Pulmonary lymphangiomatosis
Pulmonary capillary hemangiomatosis
Idiopathic pulmonary hemosiderosis

3.2. Interstitial lung disease

The association of interstitial lung disease (ILD) with SLE was first described by Eisenberg et al. (1973). The prevalence of symptomatic ILD is approximately 3–8% of patients with SLE (Estes and Christian, 1971; Eisenberg et al., 1973; Jacobsen et al., 1998a,b; Kim et al., 2000).

In lupus patients, ILD may be a sequelae of acute lupus pneumonitis (Matthay et al., 1975) or it may be an insidious disease, at times accompanied by mild flares of pulmonary involvement. Patients typically present with dyspnea on exertion, occasional pleuritic chest pain, and nonproductive cough. Chest radiographs are recommended for symptomatic patients. The radiograph may be normal in the early course of disease or may show bilateral and basilar irregular linear opacities. Later in the disease, radiographs may reveal honeycombing and decreased lung volumes. Acute inflammatory changes may be distinguished from chronic scarring with high-resolution CT, an important distinction regarding anticipated response to treatment. Alveolar consolidation and ground glass opacities without significant honeycombing may identify patients with reversible disease. Pulmonary function tests typically reveal restrictive lung physiology with reduced vital capacity, total lung capacity, and diffusing capacity but with normal ratio of forced vital capacity in 1 s (FEV1) and forced vital capacity (FVC). Bronchoscopy with lavage or transbronchial biopsy, or laparoscopic or open lung biopsy, may eventually be necessary in many patients. Bronchial lavage often shows increased inflammatory cells, cytokines, and growth factors. Lung biopsies reveal interstitial fibrosis and lymphocytic infiltrates with peribronchial lymphoid hyperplasia. In more advanced ILD, extensive fibrosis of the alveolar wall with honeycomb changes is present. Immune complexes are deposited on the alveolar septae. These complexes have also been found in the lungs of lupus patients with acute lupus pneumonitis, pulmonary hemorrhage, and pulmonary hypertension.

Systemic steroids and immunosuppressive agents are routinely used to treat symptomatic ILD in SLE, although their effectiveness has not been established by controlled trials. In contrast to idiopathic ILD, which typically results in a rapid deterioration and severe restrictive lung disease, the clinical course of ILD in most lupus patients is slowly progressive and stabilizes over a period of time (Weinrib et al., 1990).

3.3. Small airway disease

Bronchiolitis obliterans, very uncommon in SLE, is airflow limiting caused by inflammation and fibrosis in the submucosal and peribronchiolar regions, typically in the absence of diffuse parenchymal inflammation. Findings on high-resolution CT are most commonly focal, sharply defined areas of decreased lung attenuation associated with reduced vessel sizes. These changes represent a combination of air trapping and oligemia (mosaic perfusion) in the absence of parenchymal consolidation. Both central and peripheral bronchiectasis may be present as well (Webb et al., 1996; Kim et al., 2000).

Cryptogenic organizing pneumonia (COP), previously known as bronchiolitis obliterans organizing pneumonia (BOOP), has been reported in a few cases (Fig. 4). It is a pathologic entity characterized by the formation of plugs of fibrous tissue in bronchioles and alveolar ducts (Gammon et al., 1992; Otsuka et al., 1996; Min et al., 1997). In this airway disease, cytotoxic therapy is typically reserved for patients who do not respond to corticosteroid treatment (Godeau et al., 1991; Min et al., 1997).

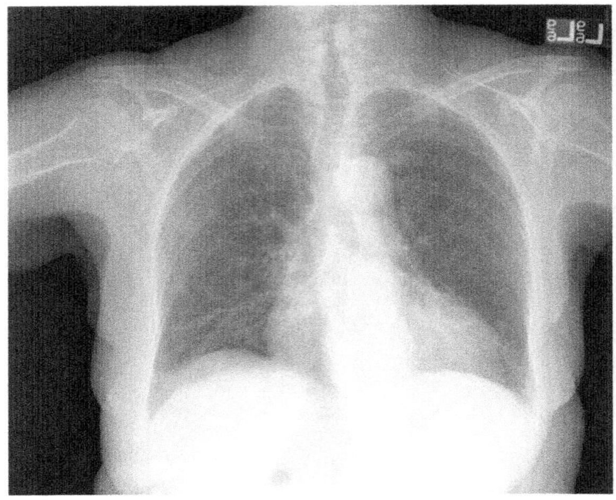

Figure 4. Chest radiograph demonstrating resolving cryptogenic organizing pneumonia (COP) with bibasilar interstitial thickening.

3.4. Infectious pneumonia

Infection is the most common cause of acute parenchymal disease in SLE and should be the primary consideration in the evaluation of new pulmonary infiltrates. Patients with SLE are susceptible to usual bacterial and opportunistic pathogens, and multiple pathogens may coexist. Bacterial bronchopneumonia was found in 44% of lupus patients in one autopsy series (Purnell et al., 1955) and in 76% of patients in another series (Haupt et al., 1981). It is important to recognize mycobacterial infections in patients with SLE, especially in areas where tuberculosis is endemic. The diagnosis of tuberculosis may be delayed since weight loss and fever may be mistakenly attributed to the underlying SLE. Miliary dissemination of tuberculosis and patchy consolidation are more common than cavitation on radiographs in patients with SLE (Kim et al., 1999). Similarly, because *Nocardia asteroids* targets the lungs and causes pulmonary infiltrates, pleural effusion, and central nervous system abnormalities, infection by this pathogen can be confused with the clinical manifestations of SLE. Physicians should suspect the presence of *Nocardia* species when chest wall extension is evident by CT scan. Although it is rare, this opportunistic infection is curable. The high mortality is usually caused by delay in diagnosis and treatment (Mok et al., 1997).

3.5. Pulmonary edema

When cardiac or renal failure leads to congestive heart failure, pulmonary edema can arise from volume overload by a process similar to that occurring during the development of pleural effusion. Whereas some cases of cardiac failure/cardiomyopathy are due to myocarditis, many are due to ischemic heart disease from accelerated atherosclerosis, hypertension, renal failure from lupus nephritis, valvular disease, or toxicity from medications.

4. Pulmonary vascular diseases

4.1. Pulmonary hypertension

SLE-associated pulmonary hypertension is more common than previously recognized, with prevalence ranging from 5 to 14% (Simonson et al., 1989; Li and Tam, 1999). Pulmonary artery pressures at rest and during exercise have been shown to be higher in unselected SLE patients than in normal subjects (Winslow et al., 1993). Therefore, it is likely that asymptomatic increases in pulmonary artery pressures are more common than symptomatic disease, particularly since pulmonary hypertension is more difficult to diagnose in early and mild cases. In a 5-year follow-up study of lupus patients, the prevalence of pulmonary hypertension increased from 14 to 43% even though systolic pulmonary artery pressures increased only modestly (23.4–27.5 mm Hg) (Winslow et al., 1995). Raynaud's phenomenon was also found to be more prevalent in patients with pulmonary hypertension (75 vs. 40%). Pulmonary hypertension is more common in younger lupus patients (18–49 years) and exhibits a striking female predominance (10:1, female:male). Symptoms include insidious onset of dyspnea on exertion, chest pain, and nonproductive cough. In cases of right heart failure or cor pulmonale, peripheral edema can be present. Physical examination may reveal a loud pulmonary heart sound (P2), a holosystolic murmur of tricuspid regurgitation, and signs of right ventricular enlargement. Enlargement of the pulmonary vasculature, cardiomegaly, and clear lung fields are typical findings on chest radiographs. Pulmonary pressure, right ventricular chamber size, and tricuspid insufficiency can be estimated with high sensitivity by echocardiography with Doppler. Increased right heart pressure in the setting of normal wedge pressure on cardiac catheterization confirms the diagnosis. In some cases, a pulmonary angiogram may be needed to rule out pulmonary embolism as the cause of increased right heart pressure.

The overall outcome of pulmonary hypertension in SLE is poor. Sudden cardiac death due to arrhythmia or cardiac failure accounts for the high mortality rates in patients with severe disease. Multiple factors are likely involved in the pathogenesis of pulmonary hypertension. Pulmonary arterial vasospasm may be a contributing factor in light of the frequent occurrence of Raynaud's phenomenon and its association with decreased survival in lupus patients with pulmonary hypertension (Simonson et al., 1989). Antiphospholipid antibodies may be important contributing factors since pulmonary vessel thrombosis has been noted in patients with antiphospholipid syndrome and pulmonary hypertension (De Clerck et al., 1991). Serum endothelin may also play a role since higher levels of this highly potent vasoconstrictor have been detected in lupus patients with pulmonary hypertension than in lupus patients without it (Shen et al., 1999). In addition, serum levels of endothelin strongly correlated with the severity of pulmonary artery pressure measured by Doppler. Although rare, pulmonary hypertension can also be a complication of long-standing interstitial lung disease. Since pulmonary artery vasculitis is uncommon, it is not a likely cause of pulmonary hypertension (Badui et al., 1985). However, partial improvement of hemodynamic abnormalities upon treatment with corticosteroids and cyclophosphamide suggest that vasculitis may have a contributory role. Prostacyclin and prostaglandin E1 have been tried successfully in SLE-associated pulmonary hypertension (Ignaszewski et al., 1993). In a multicenter, placebo-controlled trial, orally administered dual endothelin-receptor antagonist bosentan improved exercise capacity, indicated by the 6-min walking distance, in patients with pulmonary arterial hypertension (primary or associated with connective tissue diseases, such as systemic sclerosis and systemic lupus) (Rubin et al., 2002). In a subset of these patients, bosentan therapy resulted in improved right ventricular function and left ventricular early diastolic filling as detected by echocardiographic and doppler measures (Galie et al., 2003). Anticoagulation therapy should be considered in all lupus patients with pulmonary hypertension to prevent in situ thrombosis. Heart–lung transplantation may be an option for patients with severe pulmonary hypertension and otherwise quiescent disease.

4.2. Pulmonary embolism

Clinicians should suspect pulmonary embolism in any lupus patient having pleuritic chest pain and dyspnea, particularly if the patient has antiphospholipid antibodies or antiphospholipid syndrome. Approximately 35–42% of lupus patients with antiphospholipid antibodies experience thromboembolic events (Love and Santoro, 1990), the most common of which are deep vein thrombosis affecting the lower limbs and pulmonary embolism (Amigo and Khamashta, 2000).

Pulmonary angiography (Stein et al., 1992), spiral CT scans (Goodman et al., 1995; Remy-Jardin et al., 1996; van Rossum et al., 1996a,b; Mayo et al., 1997), and/or ventilation/perfusion scans (V/Q) (The PIOPED Investigators, 1990) can be used to document pulmonary embolism. Each of these imaging techniques has it own advantages and disadvantages. Although pulmonary angiography has been the 'gold standard' for confirming the presence of pulmonary emboli, it is an invasive procedure that causes major complications in 1–3% of patients and contributes to mortality in 0.3% (Stein et al., 1992). V/Q scans, which use radioisotopes, may be preferable to spiral CT and pulmonary angiography because these procedures use intravenous contrast material, which is contraindicated in patients with renal insufficiency. However, V/Q scans may be abnormal in conditions other than pulmonary embolism, such as pneumonia or emphysema. Spiral CT visualizes pulmonary emboli located in the central or segmental pulmonary arteries better than in the smaller peripheral arteries. It can also detect mediastinal tumors, bronchogenic carcinoma, aortic dissection, and hilar abnormalities.

4.3. Acute reversible hypoxemia syndrome

Abramson et al. (1991) first described a small group of acutely ill SLE patients with reversible 'unexplained' dyspnea with marked diffusion abnormalities but normal chest radiographs. Diffuse reversible injury to the lungs may result from aggregation of neutrophils following complement activation in active lupus. The patients described by Abramson responded to corticosteroid therapy within 72 h. It is possible that this syndrome is an early presentation of acute lupus pneumonitis that may be missed on routine chest radiographs (Susanto and Peters, 1997).

5. Diaphragm

5.1. 'Shrinking lung' syndrome

Hoffbrand and Beck (1965) first described a group of patients with unexplained dyspnea and restricted lung expansion with one or both hemidiaphragms elevated in chest radiographs, and thus coined the term 'shrinking lung syndrome'. This syndrome is a rare manifestation of SLE and is characterized by reduced lung volume, normal parenchyma, and a restrictive pulmonary function test with normal diffusion capacity. Weak respiratory muscles are evidenced by marked reduction of inspiratory transdiaphragmatic pressures (Martens et al., 1983). It has also been postulated that diaphragmatic dysfunction in SLE may result from a neuropathic process involving the phrenic nerve (Hardy et al., 2001). It is not entirely clear whether the muscle weakness is an isolated process affecting the diaphragm and respiratory muscles or is part of a generalized lupus-associated myopathy (Warrington et al., 2000; Hawkins et al., 2001). There are few pathologic studies. In one autopsy report, both hemidiaphragms of the patient were markedly thin with diffuse fibrotic changes (Rubin and Urowitz, 1983).

Shrinking lung syndrome has an insidious clinical course. The restrictive defect does not appear to be progressive. In a follow-up study over 38.5 patient-years (Martens et al., 1983), there was no relationship between functional pulmonary impairment and the extent of other organ involvement. The use of corticosteroid therapy for shrinking lung syndrome remains anecdotal because the etiology has not been established and defined therapy is lacking. Case reports of immunosuppressive agents such as methotrexate, azathioprine, and cyclophosphamide have shown varying results (Singh et al., 2002). In symptomatic patients, systemic corticosteroid therapy (prednisone 30–60 mg daily) may be beneficial (Walz-Leblanc et al., 1992). Lung function improves gradually over time in most patients (Bernstein et al., 1982). However, in patients who develop shrinking lung syndrome late in their disease and have no evidence of active lupus, the prognosis may not be as favorable (Mirinda et al., 2001).

6. Conclusion

There is a broad range of pulmonary manifestations associated with SLE. Although the most common is pleuritis, patients can also suffer from the insidious onset of ILD to the acute and potentially lethal DAH due to acute lupus pneumonitis. The severity of lung involvement ranges from clinically insignificant to life threatening in spite of aggressive treatment. Physicians should exclude infection as the cause of pulmonary involvement, since patients with SLE are susceptible to bacterial and opportunistic pathogens as a result of chronic immunosuppressive therapy. Randomized controlled clinical trials are needed to establish improved treatment regimens for pulmonary complications, and future research should be aimed at refining our knowledge of the pathogenesis of lung disease in SLE.

Acknowledgements

This work was supported by the Lupus Foundation of America, Western Pennsylvania Chapter; Arthritis Foundation, Western Pennsylvania Chapter/ACR Physician Scientist Development Award; NIH/MAC grant 1-P60-AR-44811 01; NIH R01 AR46588; and K24 AR02213.

Key points

- Pulmonary manifestations in SLE span a wide spectrum, the most common of which is pleuritis.
- Many cases of subclinical pulmonary disease such as pleurisy, pulmonary arterial hypertension, and ILD are being diagnosed with increasing frequency since the advent of improved noninvasive imaging techniques.
- Physicians should promptly consider infection, the most common cause of parenchymal disease in SLE, when evaluating patients with new pulmonary infiltrates. Acute lupus pneumonitis is an uncommon clinical manifestation of SLE.
- Pulmonary hemorrhage, although rare, is life threatening despite aggressive treatment with steroids and immunosuppressive therapies.
- Clinicians should suspect pulmonary embolism in any lupus patient having pleuritic chest pain and dyspnea, particularly if the patient has antiphospholipid antibodies or antiphospholipid syndrome.

References

Abramson, S.B., Dobro, J., Eberle, M.A., Benton, M., Reibman, J., Epstein, H., Rapoport, D.M., Belmont, H.M., Goldring, R.M. 1991. Acute reversible hypoxemia in systemic lupus erythematosus. Ann. Intern. Med. 114, 941–947.

Amigo, M.C., Khamashta, M.A. 2000. Antiphospholipid (Hughes) syndrome in systemic lupus erythematosus. Rheum. Dis. Clin. N. Am. 26, 331–348.

Badui, E., Garcia-Rubi, D., Robles, E., Jimenez, J., Juan, L., Deleze, M., Diaz, A., Mintz, G. 1985. Cardiovascular manifestations in systemic lupus erythematosus. Prospective study of 100 patients. Angiology 36, 431–441.

Bernstein, R.M., Ind, P.W., Elkon, K.B., Sewell, J.R., Gibson, G.J., Hughes, J.N.B., Hughes, G.R.V. 1982. Pulmonary function in SLE with a longitudinal study of shrinking lung syndrome. Arthritis Rheum. 25 (Suppl.), S7.

Chang, M.Y., Fang, J.T., Chen, Y.C., Huang, C.C. 2002. Diffuse alveolar hemorrhage in systemic lupus erythematosus: a single center retrospective study in Taiwan. Ren. Fail. 24, 791–802.

Churg, A., Franklin, W., Chan, K.L., Kopp, E., Carrington, C.B. 1980. Pulmonary hemorrhage and immune-complex deposition in the lung. Complications in a patient with systemic lupus erythematosus. Arch. Pathol. Lab. Med. 104, 388–391.

De Clerck, L.S., Michielsen, P.P., Ramael, M.R., Janssens, E., Van Maercke, Y.M., Van Marck, E.A., Stevens, W.J. 1991. Portal and pulmonary vessel thrombosis associated with systemic lupus erythematosus and anticardiolipin antibodies. J. Rheumatol. 18, 1919–1921.

Eisenberg, H., Dubois, E.L., Sherwin, R.P., Balchum, O.J. 1973. Diffuse interstitial lung disease in systemic lupus erythematosus. Ann. Intern. Med. 79, 37–45.

Estes, D., Christian, C. 1971. The natural history of systemic lupus erythematosus by prospective analysis. Medicine 50, 85–95.

Galie, N., Hinderliter, A.L., Torbicki, A., Fourme, T., Simmoneau, G., Pulido, T., Espinola-Zavaleta, N., Rocchi, G., Manes, A., Frantz, R., Kurzyna, M., Nagueh, S.F., Barst, R., Channick, R., Dujardin, K., Kronenberg, A., Leconte, I., Rainisio, M., Rubin, L. 2003. Effects of the oral endothelin-receptor antagonist bosentan on echocardiographic and doppler measures in patients with pulmonary arterial hypertension. J. Am. Coll. Cardiol. 41, 1380–1386.

Gammon, R.B., Bridges, T.A., al Nezir, H., Alexander, C.B., Kennedy, J.I. Jr. 1992. Bronchiolitis obliterans organizing pneumonia associated with systemic lupus erythematosus. Chest 102, 1171–1174.

Glazer, M., Berkman, N., Lafair, J.S., Kramer, M.R. 2000. Successful talc slurry pleurodesis in patients with nonmalignant pleural effusion. Chest 117, 1404–1409.

Godeau, B., Cormier, C., Menkes, C.J. 1991. Bronchiolitis obliterans in systemic lupus erythematosus: beneficial effect of intravenous cyclophosphamide. Ann. Rheum. Dis. 50, 956–958.

Good, J.T. Jr., King, T.E., Antony, V.B., Sahn, S.A. 1983. Lupus pleuritis. Clinical features and pleural fluid characteristics with special reference to pleural fluid antinuclear antibodies. Chest 84, 714–718.

Goodman, L.R., Curtin, J.J., Mewissen, M.W., Foley, W.D., Lipchik, R.J., Crain, M.R., Sagar, K.B., Collier, B.D. 1995. Detection of pulmonary embolism in patients with unresolved clinical and scintigraphic diagnosis: helical CT versus angiography. AJR Am. J. Roentgenol. 164, 1369–1374.

Graninger, M., Schmaldienst, S., Derfler, K., Graninger, W.B. 2002. Immunoadsorption therapy (therasorb) in patients with severe lupus erythematosus. Acta Med. Austriaca 29, 26–29.

Hardy, K., Herry, I., Attali, V., Cadranel, J., Similowski, T. 2001. Bilateral phrenic paralysis in a patient with systemic lupus erythematosus. Chest 119, 1274–1277.

Haupt, H.M., Moore, G.W., Hutchins, G.M. 1981. The lung in systemic lupus erythematosus. Analysis of the pathologic changes in 120 patients. Am. J. Med. 71, 791–798.

Hawkins, P., Davison, A.G., Dasgupta, B., Moxham, J. 2001. Diaphragm strength in acute systemic lupus erythematosus in a patient with paradoxical abdominal motion and reduced lung volumes. Thorax 56, 329–330.

Hoffbrand, B.I., Beck, E.R. 1965. Unexplained dyspnea and shrinking lung in SLE. Br. Med. J. 1, 1273–1277.

Hughson, M.D., He, Z., Henegar, J., McMurray, R. 2001. Alveolar hemorrhage and renal microangiopathy in systemic lupus erythematosus. Arch. Pathol. Lab. Med. 125, 475–483.

Ignaszewski, A.P., Percy, J.S., Humen, D.P. 1993. Successful treatment of pulmonary hypertension associated with systemic lupus erythematosus with prostaglandin I2 and prostaglandin E1. J. Rheumatol. 20, 595–596.

Isbister, J.P., Ralston, M., Hayes, J.M., Wright, R. 1981. Fulminant lupus pneumonitis with acute renal failure and RBC aplasia. Successful management with plasmapheresis and immunosuppression. Arch. Intern. Med. 141, 1081–1083.

Jacobsen, S., Petersen, J., Ullman, S., Junker, P., Voss, A., Rasmussen, J.M., Tarp, U., Poulsen, L.H., van Overeem Hansen, G., Skaarup, B., Hansen, T.M., Podenphant, J., Halberg, P. 1998a. A multicentre study of 513 Danish patients with systemic lupus erythematosus. I. Disease manifestations and analyses of clinical subsets. Clin. Rheumatol. 17, 468–477.

Jacobsen, S., Petersen, J., Ullman, S., Junker, P., Voss, A., Rasmussen, J.M., Tarp, U., Poulsen, L.H., van Overeem Hansen, G., Skaarup, B., Hansen, T.M., Podenphant, J., Halberg, P. 1998b. A multicentre study of 513 Danish patients with systemic lupus erythematosus. II. Disease mortality and clinical factors of prognostic value. Clin. Rheumatol. 17, 478–484.

Kim, H.Y., Im, J.G., Goo, J.M., Lee, J.K., Song, J.W., Kim, S.K. 1999. Pulmonary tuberculosis in patients with systematic lupus erythematosus. AJR Am. J. Roentgenol. 173, 1639–1642.

Kim, J.S., Lee, K.S., Koh, E.M., Kim, S.Y., Chung, M.P., Han, J. 2000. Thoracic involvement of systemic lupus erythematosus: clinical, pathologic, and radiologic findings. J. Comput. Assist. Tomogr. 24, 9–18.

Leatherman, J.W., Davies, S.F., Hoidal, J.R. 1984. Alveolar hemorrhage syndromes: diffuse microvascular lung hemorrhage in immune and idiopathic disorders. Medicine (Baltimore) 63, 343–361.

Li, E.K., Tam, L.S. 1999. Pulmonary hypertension in systemic lupus erythematosus: clinical association and survival in 18 patients. J. Rheumatol. 26, 1923–1929.

Light, R.W., Macgregor, M.I., Luchsinger, P.C., Ball, W.C. Jr. 1972. Pleural effusions: the diagnostic separation of transudates and exudates. Ann. Intern. Med. 77, 507–513.

Liu, M.F., Lee, J.H., Weng, T.H., Lee, Y.Y. 1998. Clinical experience of 13 cases with severe pulmonary hemorrhage in systemic lupus erythematosus with active nephritis. Scand. J. Rheumatol. 27, 291–295.

Love, P.E., Santoro, S.A. 1990. Antiphospholipid antibodies: anticardiolipin and the lupus anticoagulant in systemic lupus erythematosus (SLE) and in non-SLE disorders. Prevalence and clinical significance. Ann. Intern. Med. 112, 682–698.

Martens, J., Demedts, M., Vanmeenen, M.T., Dequeker, J. 1983. Respiratory muscle dysfunction in systemic lupus erythematosus. Chest 84, 170–175.

Matthay, R.A., Schwarz, M.I., Petty, T.L., Stanford, R.E., Gupta, R.C., Sahn, S.A., Steigerwald, J.C. 1975. Pulmonary manifestations of systemic lupus erythematosus: review of twelve cases of acute lupus pneumonitis. Medicine (Baltimore) 54, 397–409.

Mayo, J.R., Remy-Jardin, M., Muller, N.L., Remy, J., Worsley, D.F., Hossein-Foucher, C., Kwong, J.S., Brown, M.J. 1997. Pulmonary embolism: prospective comparison of spiral CT with ventilation–perfusion scintigraphy. Radiology 205, 447–452.

Min, J.K., Hong, Y.S., Park, S.H., Park, J.H., Lee, S.H., Lee, Y.S., Kim, H.H., Cho, C.S., Kim, H.Y. 1997. Bronchiolitis obliterans organizing pneumonia as an initial manifestation in patients with systemic lupus erythematosus. J. Rheumatol. 24, 2254–2257.

Mirinda, L., Karim, Y., Tench, C., Gordon, P., D'Cruz, D.P., Khamashta, M.A. 2001. Clinical features and outcome of the shrinking lung syndrome in systemic lupus erythematosus. Arthritis Rheum. 1688 (Suppl.), S334.

Mochizuki, T., Aotsuka, S., Satoh, T. 1999. Clinical and laboratory features of lupus patients with complicating pulmonary disease. Respir. Med. 93, 95–101.

Mok, C.C., Yuen, K.Y., Lau, C.S. 1997. Nocardiosis in systemic lupus erythematosus. Semin. Arthritis Rheum. 26, 675–683.

Murin, S., Wiedemann, H.P., Matthay, R.A. 1998. Pulmonary manifestations of systemic lupus erythematosus. Clin. Chest. Med. 19, 641–665.see also p. viii.

Orens, J.B., Martinez, F.J., Lynch, J.P. III 1994. Pleuropulmonary manifestations of systemic lupus erythematosus. Rheum. Dis. Clin. N. Am. 20, 159–193.

Otsuka, F., Amano, T., Hashimoto, N., Takahashi, M., Hayakawa, N., Makino, H., Ota, Z., Ogura, T. 1996. Bronchiolitis obliterans organizing pneumonia associated with systemic lupus erythematosus with antiphospholipid antibody. Intern. Med. 35, 341–344.

Paramothayan, N.S., Barron, J. 2002. New criteria for the differentiation between transudates and exudates. J. Clin. Pathol. 55, 69–71.

Purnell, D.C., Baggenstoss, A.H., Olsen, A.M. 1955. Pulmonary lesions in disseminated lupus erythematosus. Ann. Intern. Med. 42, 619–628.

Remy-Jardin, M., Remy, J., Deschildre, F., Artaud, D., Beregi, J.P., Hossein-Foucher, C., Marchandise, X., Duhamel, A. 1996. Diagnosis of pulmonary embolism with spiral CT: comparison with pulmonary angiography and scintigraphy. Radiology 200, 699–706.

Rubin, L.A., Urowitz, M.B. 1983. Shrinking lung syndrome in SLE—a clinical pathologic study. J. Rheumatol. 10, 973–976.

Rubin, L.J., Badesch, D.B., Barst, R.J., Galie, N., Black, C.M., Keogh, A., Pulido, T., Frost, A., Roux, S., Leconte, I., Landzberg, M., Simonneau, G. 2002. Bosentan therapy for pulmonary arterial hypertension. N. Engl. J. Med. 346, 896–903.

Santiago, K., Batuman, V., Meleg-Smith, S. 1996. A 31-year-old woman with lupus erythematosus and fatal multisystem complications. J. La State Med. Soc. 148, 379–384.

Santos-Ocampo, A.S., Mandell, B.F., Fessler, B.J. 2000. Alveolar hemorrhage in systemic lupus erythematosus: presentation and management. Chest 118, 1083–1090.

Schwab, E.P., Schumacher, H.R. Jr., Freundlich, B., Callegari, P.E. 1993. Pulmonary alveolar hemorrhage in systemic lupus erythematosus. Semin. Arthritis Rheum. 23, 8–15.

Sharma, S., Smith, R., Al Hameed, F. 2002. Fibrothorax and severe lung restriction secondary to lupus pleuritis and its successful treatment by pleurectomy. Can. Respir. J. 9, 335–337.

Shen, J.Y., Chen, S.L., Wu, Y.X., Tao, R.Q., Gu, Y.Y., Bao, C.D., Wang, Q. 1999. Pulmonary hypertension in systemic lupus erythematosus. Rheumatol. Int. 18, 147–151.

Simonson, J.S., Schiller, N.B., Petri, M., Hellmann, D.B. 1989. Pulmonary hypertension in systemic lupus erythematosus. J. Rheumatol. 16, 918–925.

Singh, R., Huang, W., Menon, Y., Espinoza, L.R. 2002. Shrinking lung syndrome in systemic lupus erythematosus and Sjogren's syndrome. J. Clin. Rheumatol. 8, 340–345.

Specks, U. 2001. Diffuse alveolar hemorrhage syndromes. Curr. Opin. Rheumatol. 13, 12–17.

Stein, P.D., Athanasoulis, C., Alavi, A., Greenspan, R.H., Hales, C.A., Saltzman, H.A., Vreim, C.E., Terrin, M.L., Weg, J.G. 1992. Complications and validity of pulmonary angiography in acute pulmonary embolism. Circulation 85, 462–468.

Susanto, I., Peters, J.I. 1997. Acute lupus pneumonitis with normal chest radiograph. Chest 111, 1781–1783.

The PIOPED Investigators, 1990. Value of the ventilation/perfusion scan in acute pulmonary embolism. Results of the prospective investigation of pulmonary embolism diagnosis (PIOPED). JAMA 263, 2753–2759.

van Rossum, A.B., Pattynama, P.M., Ton, E.R., Treurniet, F.E., Arndt, J.W., van Eck, B., Kieft, G.J. 1996a. Pulmonary embolism: validation of spiral CT angiography in 149 patients. Radiology 201, 467–470.

van Rossum, A.B., Treurniet, F.E., Kieft, G.J., Smith, S.J., Schepers-Bok, R. 1996b. Role of spiral volumetric computed tomographic scanning in the assessment of patients with clinical suspicion of pulmonary embolism and an abnormal ventilation/perfusion lung scan. Thorax 51, 23–28.

Walz-Leblanc, B.A., Urowitz, M.B., Gladman, D.D., Hanly, P.J. 1992. The 'shrinking lungs syndrome' in systemic lupus erythematosus–improvement with corticosteroid therapy. J. Rheumatol. 19, 1970–1972.

Wang, D.Y., Yang, P.C., Yu, W.L., Kuo, S.H., Hsu, N.Y. 2000. Serial antinuclear antibodies titre in pleural and pericardial fluid. Eur. Respir. J. 15, 1106–1110.

Warrington, K.J., Moder, K.G., Brutinel, W.M. 2000. The shrinking lungs syndrome in systemic lupus erythematosus. Mayo Clin. Proc. 75, 467–472.

Webb, W.R., Muller, N.L., Naidich, D.P. 1996. Disease characterized primarily by linear and reticular opacities. In: W.R. Webb, N.L. Muller, D.P. Naidich (Eds.), High Resolution CT of the Lung, 2nd ed, Lippincott-Raven, Philadelphia, p. 109–148.

Weinrib, L., Sharma, O.P., Quismorio, F.P. Jr. 1990. A long-term study of interstitial lung disease in systemic lupus erythematosus. Semin. Arthritis Rheum. 20, 48–56.

Wiedemann, H.P., Matthay, R.A. 1989. Pulmonary manifestations of the collagen vascular diseases. Clin. Chest. Med. 10, 677–722.

Winder, A., Molad, Y., Ostfeld, I., Kenet, G., Pinkhas, J., Sidi, Y. 1993. Treatment of systemic lupus erythematosus by prolonged administration of high dose intravenous immunoglobulin: report of 2 cases. J. Rheumatol. 20, 495–498.

Winslow, T.M., Ossipov, M., Redberg, R.F., Fazio, G.P., Schiller, N.B. 1993. Exercise capacity and hemodynamics in systemic lupus erythematosus: a Doppler echocardiographic exercise study. Am. Heart. J. 126, 410–414.

Winslow, T.M., Ossipov, M.A., Fazio, G.P., Simonson, J.S., Redberg, R.F., Schiller, N.B. 1995. Five-year follow-up study of the prevalence and progression of pulmonary hypertension in systemic lupus erythematosus. Am. Heart. J. 129, 510–515.

Handbook of Systemic Autoimmune Diseases, Volume 2
Pulmonary Involvement in Systemic Autoimmune Diseases
A.U. Wells and C.P. Denton, editors

CHAPTER 7

Pulmonary Involvement in the Antiphospholipid Syndrome

Gerard Espinosa[a], Ricard Cervera[a,*], Mario García-Carrasco[a], Josep Font[a], Ronald A. Asherson[b]

[a]*Department of Autoimmune Diseases, Hospital Clínic, Barcelona, Catalonia, Spain*
[b]*Rheumatic Diseases Unit, Department of Medicine, University of Cape Town Health Sciences Centre, Groote Schuur Hospital, Cape Town, South Africa*

1. Introduction

The antiphospholipid syndrome (APS) is a systemic autoimmune disorder characterized by a combination of arterial and/or venous thrombosis, recurrent fetal loss, often accompanied by a mild-to-moderate thrombocytopenia, and elevated titers of antiphospholipid antibodies (aPL), namely, the lupus anticoagulant (LA) and/or anticardiolipin antibodies (aCL) and/or antibodies to β2 Glycoprotein 1 (Greaves et al., 2000). The APS may be divided into two categories. 'Primary' APS occurs in patients without clinical evidence of any major autoimmune disease (Asherson et al., 1989), whereas 'secondary' APS occurs in association with autoimmune diseases, mainly systemic lupus erythematosus (SLE) but also with other conditions e.g. other 'autoimmune' conditions, carcinomas, vasculitic syndromes and drug administration (Font et al., 1989; Levine et al., 2003). A recent consensus statement provides simplified criteria for the diagnosis of the antiphospholipid syndrome (Wilson et al., 1999)

Pulmonary manifestations which may be associated with this syndrome in both the primary and secondary forms include pulmonary embolism and infarction (Espinosa et al., 2002), pulmonary hypertension (Piette and Hunt, 2000; Luchi et al., 1992), adult respiratory distress syndrome (ARDS) (Ghosh et al., 1993), intraalveolar hemorrhage (Howe et al., 1988) and primary thrombosis of lung vessels, both large (Cucurull et al., 1996) and small (Maggiorini et al., 1997), as well as pulmonary capillaritis (Gertner and Lie, 1993). Less frequently, a postpartum syndrome (Branch et al., 1986) and fibrosing alveolitis (Savin et al., 1994) associated with the APS have been documented. Many of these manifestations are interrelated and have been reported as occuring simultaneously in the same patient (Hillerdal, 1997).

*Corresponding author.
Tel./fax: +34-93-227-5774.
E-mail address: rcervera@clinic.ub.es (R. Cervera).

DOI: 10.1016/S1571-5078(04)02007-0

2. Pulmonary manifestations in the APS

2.1. Pulmonary embolism and infarction

The first major pulmonary complication to be documented was pulmonary thromboembolic disease. This does not differ clinically from 'ordinary' embolic disease in aPL negative patients. It constitutes the most frequent pulmonary manifestation of the APS and may be the first manifestation of the disease (Espinosa et al., 2002). In the study of the Euro-Phospholipid Project Group performed on 1000 patients with APS, pulmonary embolism was the presenting manifestation in 9% of patients and appeared *during* the evolution of disease in 14% (Cervera et al., 2002). Pulmonary embolism most commonly originates from the deep veins of the lower extremities, but may also arise from many other sites, including the inferior vena cava and other large vessels (Mintz et al., 1984), tricuspid valve vegetations (Brucato et al., 1994) or right-sided intracardiac thrombosis (Day et al., 1995; O'Hickey et al., 1993). The last site underlines the need to systematically perform an echocardiographic investigation in all patients with APS and pulmonary embolism. Recurrent pulmonary emboli may give rise to *pulmonary hypertension* (Brucato et al., 1994) which may, unusually and in severe cases, be accompanied by isolated tricuspid valve insufficiency (Cucurull et al., 1996; Turjanski et al., 1998). Pulmonary embolism can also evolve to *infarction* occurring in 10–15% of cases and cavitation has been reported in up to 7% of patients with pulmonary infarction (Libby et al., 1985). Recently, Bertoli et al. (2002) described the case of a female patient with a diagnosis of primary APS, pulmonary thromboembolism and infarction followed by lung *cavitation*.

The management of the acute thrombotic event is no different in APS patients to that in a general population. Patients are required to be anticoagulated with heparin followed by warfarin. Long term (possibly life-long) oral anticoagulation is the optimum prophylactic treatment for recurrent thrombosis and appears to be more effective than antiaggregants (Khamashta et al., 1995; Muñoz-Rodríguez et al., 1999). Nevertheless, the recommended therapeutic International Normalized Ratio (INR) remains controversial. Because increasing the target INR from a range of 2.0–3.0 to a range of 3.1–4.0 is likely to be associated with a doubling of the risk of major hemorrhage, it is important to know whether the higher intensity treatment is more effective. Retrospective studies suggest that patients with antiphospholipid antibodies have a high risk of recurrent thrombosis while receiving moderate intensity warfarin (INR 2.0 to 3.0) and that this risk is lower with a higher intensity of anticoagulant therapy (target INR, 3.1 to 4.5) (Khamashta et al., 1995; Krnic-Barrie et al., 1997; Rosove and Brewer, 1992). However, these results must be interpreted with caution, because the studies were retrospective, recurrent thrombosis was not confirmed by independent adjudication, and the INR at the time of the thrombotic events was uncertain.

Recently, a Canadian consortium reported the results of a prospective, randomized, controlled study of the use of two doses of warfarin for prevention of thrombosis in patients with the APS who had previous thrombosis (Crowther et al., 2003). A total of 114 patients were treated with either moderate-intensity warfarin (target INR, 2.0 to 3.0) or high-intensity warfarin (target INR, 3.1 to 4.0). In both treatment groups, the rate of recurrent thrombosis was low, and the lower dose of warfarin was as effective as the higher dose. Adverse effects were similar among patients in the two groups. These results balance those of a previous report of treatment with higher doses of anticoagulant agents (Ruiz-Irastorza et al., 2002). In that study, 66 patients with APS and previous thrombosis were included. All received oral anticoagulation to a target international normalized ratio of 3.5. The authors concluded that the risk of intracranial and fatal bleeding in patients with definite APS and previous thrombosis treated with oral anticoagulation to a target INR of 3.5 was similar to that in groups of patients treated to lower target ratios.

Multicenter prospective trials are needed to determine the optimal range of anticoagulation which is not associated with an increased risk of bleeding. While awaiting these results, we recommend that the INR be maintained between 2.5 and 3.5 (Muñoz-Rodríguez et al., 1999).

2.2. Pulmonary hypertension

The prevalence of pulmonary hypertension in APS associated to SLE and the primary APS has been estimated to be between 1.8 and 3.5%, respectively (Vianna et al., 1994). In the Indiana cohort of primary APS patients, 3% had symptomatic pulmonary hypertension (McCarty, 2000). In the study performed by the Euro-Phospholipid Project Group including patients with APS (primary and secondary), the prevalence of pulmonary hypertension was 2.2% (Cervera et al., 2002).

The development of pulmonary hypertension in APS may result from various causes. Recurrent pulmonary embolism is the leading cause of pulmonary hypertension in APS (Piette and Hunt, 2000). The prevalence of the aPL in patients with chronic thromboembolic pulmonary hypertension varies between 10% (Moser et al., 1990; Jamieson et al., 1993) and 20% (Sandoval et al., 1996). It is likely that chronic thromboembolic pulmonary hypertension following pulmonary thromboembolism develops more frequently in the presence of aPL. In a study of 24 consecutive medical patients with chronic thromboembolic pulmonary hypertension, 12 had aPL, and 75% had at least one abnormality associated with hypercoagulability (Colorio et al., 2001). The association of pulmonary hypertension with aPL was first documented in 1983 (Asherson et al., 1983). Since this original communication, there have been many other reports describing this association, not only with SLE (Tam and Li, 1998; Asherson et al., 1986; Mackworth-Young et al., 1984; Anderson and Ali, 1984; Asherson et al., 1986) but also in the primary APS (Asherson et al., 1989; Font et al., 1991; Jeffrey et al., 1989; Alarcón-Segovia et al., 1989; Nagai et al., 1997). In a prospective analysis of 500 patients with SLE, a statistically significant association between pulmonary hypertension and the presence of IgA aCL above 2 SD has been described (Alarcón-Segovia et al., 1989). An extended study performed on 667 patients with SLE confirmed the association of pulmonary hypertension with aPL, but the criteria used were not precisely defined (Alarcón-Segovia et al., 1989). On the other hand, there are several studies which have failed to demonstrate any association with pulmonary hypertension and the presence of aPL (Petri et al., 1987; Miyata et al., 1993). Several cases of 'primary' (non-thromboembolic) pulmonary hypertension complicating primary APS have been described (Asherson et al., 1989; Luchi et al., 1992; Nagai et al., 1997; De la Mata et al., 1994; Rana et al., 2001). Luchi et al. (1992) interpreted their case as the coexistence of pulmonary thrombosis with primary pulmonary hypertension, which would explain the plexogenic lesions found on lung biopsy. However, plexogenic lesions are also known to occur in chronic thromboembolic pulmonary hypertension. Rana et al. (2001) described a case of 55-year-old male with APS who developed pulmonary hypertension induced by in situ thrombosis in pulmonary microvasculature.

The role of aPL in the pathophysiology of 'idiopathic' primary pulmonary hypertension is unclear at this time. In a group of 30 patients with idiopathic (non-SLE) primary pulmonary hypertension, four had aPL (LA in two and low IgG aCL in three) (Asherson et al., 1990). Karmochkine et al. (1996) determined the prevalence of aPL in 38 patients with primary and secondary (heart failure, congenital heart defect and various lung diseases) pulmonary hypertension. Eleven patients (29%) had aPL without differences between primary and secondary pulmonary hypertension. Positive aPL were detected only in patients with precapillary pulmonary hypertension. The authors concluded that aPL might play a role in the initiation and/or progression of in situ thromboses frequently observed in precapillary pulmonary hypertension. Conversely, a recent study described a higher prevalence of aPL in thromboembolic pulmonary hypertension compared to primary pulmonary hypertension (Wolf et al., 2000). Keeping in mind that all forms of severe pulmonary hypertension may be complicated by superimposed in situ thrombosis (Rana et al., 2001; Chaouat et al., 1996), there is a risk in categorizing some patients with pulmonary hypertension as suffering from a definite APS (Wilson et al., 1999). Other possible explanations include a role for activated platelets, an interaction between aPL and endothelial cells on the pulmonary vasculature leading to vascular remodeling, and the implication of endothelin-1, a peptide that induces vasoconstriction and stimulates the proliferation of vascular muscle cells. High levels of endothelin-1 have been found in both plasma and lung tissue of patients with primary pulmonary hypertension (Cacoub et al., 1997), as well as in plasmas of APS patients with arterial thrombosis (Atsumi et al., 1998). Portal hypertension (Bayraktar et al., 2001) or pulmonary veno-occlusive disease (Hussein et al., 1999) associated with pulmonary hypertension may also occasionally be encountered with aPL positivity.

Regarding management of these cases, chronic anticoagulation is required in all cases in order to prevent new thrombotic events (Haworth, 1998) and this seems particularly true for patients with APS (Khamashta et al., 1995). If pulmonary hypertension is secondary to recurrent thromboembolism, an inferior vena cava filter may be recommended (Auger et al., 1995). In some patients with very severe disease, successful thromboendarterectomy has been performed (Cucurull et al., 1996; Sandoval et al., 1996; Ando et al., 1998). Other modalities of treatment are those used in 'idiopathic' or connective tissue disease-associated primary pulmonary hypertension. It is recommended that patients be given vasodilators such as calcium channel blockers; unfortunately, only one-third of patients respond to this vasodilator therapy (Tam and Li, 1998; Rich et al., 1992). Furthermore, in severe cases, continuous intravenous prostacyclin infusion with a pump may be useful (Humbert et al., 1998) and bosentan — the new anti-endothelin 1 agent — is a promising drug. Cyclophosphamide has also appeared to be beneficial in connective tissue disease-associated primary pulmonary hypertension, but there is no experience of this therapy in APS-associated primary pulmonary hypertension (Tam and Li, 1998). Finally, diverse surgical procedures (atrial septectomy and double lung, single lung or heart–lung transplantation) in patients refractory to medical regimens are documented. The mortality remains high and, in general, the outcome in patients with pulmonary hypertension and APS is usually fatal (Luchi et al., 1992; Anderson and Ali, 1984; Asherson et al., 1990), although a patient with primary APS and primary pulmonary hypertension has been described with a survival from the time of diagnosis of more than 20 years (Nagai et al., 1997).

2.3. Pulmonary arterial thrombosis

In some patients, the thrombotic obstruction occurs at the level of the large, elastic pulmonary arteries. Six such patients with APS and major pulmonary arterial thromboses have been described up to the present time (Luchi et al., 1992; Cucurull et al., 1996; Sandoval et al., 1996; Nakagawa et al., 1992). Five were treated with thromboendarterectomy, the procedure being successful in four. A fatal outcome in the remaining patients was, in fact, expected because of the severe clinical and hemodynamic abnormalities which were present. Despite good results with surgical intervention, maintenance of long-term oral anticoagulation is considered prudent.

2.4. Pulmonary microthrombosis

A minority of APS patients have presented with widespread thrombotic occlusions involving the small pulmonary arteries or alveolar capillary lumens (Ghosh et al., 1993; Maggiorini et al., 1997; Gertner and Lie, 1993; Brucato et al., 1994; Kerr et al., 1997). Three of these six patients showed isolated microthromboses on lung biopsy without evidence of pulmonary capillaritis or alveolar hemorrhage (Maggiorini et al., 1997; Gertner and Lie, 1993; Brucato et al., 1994). These three patients had been diagnosed previously as primary APS. Clinically, the first presented with fever, cough, mild haemoptysis and shortness of breath at rest and at minimal exercise. Chest radiography showed bilateral patchy infiltrates. With pulse methylprednisolone followed by 50 mg prednisone daily and heparin the patient's condition improved dramatically within days. The second patient presented with fever and pain in her left chest, showing a consolidation of the left lingula and a pleural effusion on chest radiography. Unfortunately, the treatment and evolution of this patient was not reported. The third patient presented with dyspnea and pulmonary hypertension with involvement of tricuspid and mitral valves. His clinical course deteriorated progressively in spite of high doses steroids and continuous intravenous heparin, and he died of intractable cardiac failure. The remaining cases demonstrated alveolar hemorrhage and pulmonary capillaritis on the lung biopsies, presenting with the clinical picture of ARDS. Two of these patients died, one of them despite high dose steroids, heparin, aspirin and azathioprine. The remaining patient improved gradually with the administration of i.v. pulses of methylprednisolone.

2.5. Adult respiratory distress syndrome

The adult respiratory distress syndrome (ARDS) is an uncommon, devastating clinical syndrome of acute lung injury with non-cardiac pulmonary edema, characterized by an acute onset with arterial hypoxemia refractory to treatment with supplemental oxygen. Radiographically, there are bilateral infiltrates which may be patchy or asymmetric and there may be accompanying pleural effusions (Ware and Matthay, 2000). To date, 61 patients with ARDS and the APS have been reported (Ghosh et al., 1993; Hillerdal et al., 1991; Ingram et al., 1987; Argento and DiBenedetto, 1998; Asherson et al., 1998, 2001). Fifty-five of them were suffering from catastrophic APS (Asherson et al., 1998, 2001) with a mortality of 54%, despite treatment with full anticoagulation, high-dose steroids and immunosupression. Histologic examination of lung specimens revealed extensive small vessel thromboses, intraalveolar hemorrhage, and hyaline membrane formation with or without pulmonary capillaritis. The mechanism of ARDS in APS is unclear. Antiphospholipid antibodies were detected in the bronchoalveolar lavage of patients with ARDS, suggesting involvement of autoimmune mechanisms in the pathogenesis of ARDS (Nakos et al., 2001; Wiedermann et al., 2003). In the absence of inflammatory changes, an acute increase in hydrostatic pressure by an occluding embolus may cause exudation of fluid from blood vessels into the lung parenchyma (Ingram et al., 1987). Pulmonary microembolism may cause vascular injury in the pulmonary circulation and increase the transport of proteins through the pulmonary microvascular barrier into the parenchyma (Ghosh et al., 1993). The management consists of, in addition to anticoagulation, high-dose steroids, and occasionally pulse cyclophosphamide and plasma exchange.

2.6. Intraalveolar pulmonary hemorrhage

Diffuse alveolar hemorrhage is always a potentially life-threatening situation and may be the initial manifestation of APS (Gertner, 1999). Patients are usually middle-aged with a male predominance and may present with symptoms of cough, dyspnea, and fever, with or without hemoptysis, progressing to acute respiratory failure (Specks, 2001). The main laboratory features encountered are hypoxemia and anemia and chest radiography shows rapidly changing and extensive alveolar infiltrates. The diagnosis is one of exclusion and, as with other systemic autoimmune disease, other causes of diffuse alveolar hemorrhage such as uremia, coagulopathy, pulmonary embolus or infection need to be excluded. Bronchioalveolar lavage may be useful showing hemosiderin-laden macrophages. Lung biopsy should only be considered if potentially diagnostic tissue cannot be obtained from any other site (Crausman et al., 1995). Histopathologically, alveolar hemorrhage and microvascular thrombosis with or without pulmonary capillaritis are the main findings (Gertner and Lie, 1993; Hillerdal et al., 1991; Asherson et al., 2001). Almost all patients who were treated with corticosteroids have improved, regardless of additional treatment with cyclophosphamide. Therefore, the treatment of diffuse alveolar hemorrhage in APS should commence with corticosteroids (usually with high dose intravenous, e.g. 1 g methylprednisolone daily for 3–5 days) if the patient presents with severe respiratory distress. Two patients who did not respond to intravenous hydrocortisone and pulse methylprednisolone improved with plasma exchange (Howe et al., 1988; Waterer et al., 1999), and one patient improved upon institution of intravenous immunoglobulin therapy (Gertner, 1999). With respect to anticoagulation, if there is active bleeding it may be necessary to withhold it, but with a view to the reinstitution of therapy as soon as the pulmonary status improves. Another point of importance is the potential for relapse without immunosupressive therapy. This occurred in three patients (Gertner, 1999; Aronoff and Callen, 1997). Thus, a subset of patients may require long-term immunosupression, as is the case in other types of pulmonary capillaritis.

2.7. Other pulmonary manifestations

2.7.1. Postpartum syndrome

Branch et al. (1986) described, in several patients, a clinical picture consisting of spiking fevers, pleuritic chest pain and dyspnea with chest radiographs showing pleural effusions and patchy infiltrates. Cardiac conduction defects were present in one patient. Another case with similar characteristics was described in 1994 by Kupferminc et al. (1994). A woman developed fever, pulmonary infiltrates, cardiac conduction defects, and renal insufficiency following severe preeclampsia in the postpartum period.. She tested positive for LA and aCL, and responded to steroid therapy and plasmapheresis. These cases may, in fact, be examples of microangiopathy and possible catastrophic APS.

2.7.2. Fibrosing alveolitis

Only three case reports to date have documented the association of fibrosing alveolitis and APS (Savin et al., 1994; Kelion et al., 1995; Magro et al., 2001). The first was a male with primary APS who developed insidious diffuse pulmonary infiltrates. Histopathologic examination of the lung showed alveolitis and fibrosis. The second was a patient with cryptogenic fibrosing alveolitis who developed pulmonary embolism and myocardial infarction with APS. The third was a 28-year-old man who underwent a single lung transplantation for rapidly progressive interstitial pneumonitis. Following transplantation, primary APS was diagnosed following a thromboembolic event and continued dyspnea. Review of his native lung and allograft tissue showed diffuse hemorrhage secondary to capillary injury, probably reflecting aPL effects on endothelium. It is possible that this rare association might simply reflect the concurrence of two entities in the same patient without a causal relationship between aPL and this condition.

3. Final remarks

In conclusion, patients with APS may develop a broad spectrum of pulmonary involvement, pulmonary thromboembolism and pulmonary hypertension being the most frequent complications described. In addition to these manifestations, patients with microvascular pulmonary thrombosis, pulmonary capillaritis and alveolar hemorrhage have also been documented. Clinicians should seriously consider these types of vascular injury when evaluating patients with APS who present with dyspnea, fever and infiltrates on chest radiography. These conditions might occur as separate entities or may, in fact, form part of ARDS. Therefore, in the presence of these clinical features, clinicians must consider searching and testing for aPL when no other etiology can be determined. There is a high frequency of ARDS in patients with catastrophic APS.

As regards treatment, long-term anticoagulation is essential in all cases, in order to prevent the occurrence of new thrombotic events. There is insufficient experience with immunosupression in APS-associated pulmonary hypertension. High-dose steroids may be useful in cases of non-inflammatory vasculopathy (ARDS, pulmonary microthrombosis and alveolar hemorrhage). The role of cyclophosphamide and other therapeutic modalities such as plasma exchange or the administration of immunoglobulins has not, as yet, been well researched. The clinical setting will usually dictate whether additional treatments are required in these cases.

Key points

- Pulmonary embolism constitutes the most frequent pulmonary manifestation of the APS. Recurrent pulmonary embolism is the leading cause of pulmonary hypertension in the APS. The mortality of pulmonary hypertension in APS patients remains high. There is a high frequency of ARDS in patients with catastrophic APS with a high mortality. Diffuse alveolar hemorrhage is always a potentially life-threatening situation and may be the initial manifestation of APS.
- Long-term anticoagulation is essential in all cases, in order to prevent the occurrence of new thrombotic events. Patients are required to be anticoagulated with heparin followed by warfarin. Nevertheless, the recommended therapeutic INR remains controversial. High-dose steroids may be useful in cases of non-inflammatory vasculopathy (ARDS, pulmonary microthrombosis and alveolar hemorrhage).

References

Alarcón-Segovia, D., Sánchez-Guerrero, J. 1989. Primary antiphospholipid syndrome. J. Rheumatol. 16, 482–488.

Alarcón-Segovia, D., Deleze, M., Oria, C.V., Sánchez-Guerrero, J., Gómez-Pacheco, L., Cabiedes, J., et al. 1989. Antiphospholipid antibodies and the antiphospholipid syndrome in systemic lupus erythematosus. A prospective analysis of 500 consecutive patients. Medicine (Baltimore) 68, 353–365.

Alarcón-Segovia, D., Pérez-Vázquez, M.E., Villa, A.R., Drenkard, C., Cabiedes, J. 1992. Preliminary classifcation criteria for the antiphospholipid syndrome within systemic lupus erythematosus. J. Rheumatol. 21, 275–286.

Anderson, E.N., Ali, M.R. 1984. The lupus anticoagulant, pulmonary thromboembolism and fatal pulmonary hypertension. Ann. Rheum. Dis. 43, 760–763.

Ando, M., Takamoto, S., Okita, Y., Matsukawa, R., Nakanishi, N., Kyotani, S., et al. 1998. Operation for chronic pulmonary thromboembolism accompanied by thrombophilia in 8 patients. Ann. Thorac. Surg. 66, 1919–1924.

Argento, A., DiBenedetto, R.J. 1998. ARDS and adrenal insufficiency associated with the antiphospholipid antibody syndrome. Chest 113, 1136–1138.

Aronoff, D.M., Callen, J.P. 1997. Necrosing livedo reticularis in a patient with recurrent pulmonary hemorrhage. J. Am. Acad. Dermatol. 37, 300–302.

Asherson, R.A., Mackworth-Young, C.G., Boey, M.L., Hull, R.G., Saunders, A., Gharavi, A.E., et al. 1983. Pulmonary hypertension in systemic lupus erythematosus. Br. Med. J. 287, 1024–1025.

Asherson, R.A., Hackett, D., Gharavi, A.E., Harris, E.N., Kennedy, H.G., Hughes, G.R.V. 1986. Pulmonary hypertension in systemic lupus erythematosus. A report of three cases. J. Rheumatol. 12, 416–420.

Asherson, R.A., Khamashta, M.A., Ordi-Ros, J., Derksen, R.H.W.M., Machin, S.J., Path, F.R.C., et al. 1989. The 'primary' antiphospholipid syndrome: major clinical and serological features. Medicine (Baltimore) 68, 366–374.

Asherson, R.A., Higenbottam, T.W., Dinh Xuan, A.T., Khamashta, M.A., Hughes, G.R.V. 1990. Pulmonary hypertension in a lupus clinic: experience with twenty-four patients. J. Rheumatol. 17, 1292–1298.

Asherson, R.A., Cervera, R., Piette, J.C., Font, J., Lie, J.T., Burcoglu, A., et al. 1998. Catastrophic antiphospholipid syndrome. Clinical and laboratory features of 50 patients. Medicine (Baltimore) 77, 195–207.

Asherson, R.A., Cervera, R., Piette, J.C., Shoenfeld, Y., Espinosa, G., Petri, M.A., et al. 2001. Catastrophic Antiphospholipid Syndrome. Clues to the Pathogenesis from a Series of 80 Patients. Medicine (Baltimore) 80, 355–377.

These 2 studies describe the prevalence of clinical and immunologic features and the outcome of the first 130 patients with catastrophic APS.

Atsumi, T., Khamashta, M.A., Haworth, R.S., Brooks, G., Amengual, O., Ichikawa, K., et al. 1998. Arterial disease and thrombosis in the antiphospholipid syndrome: a pathogenic role of endothelin-1. Arthritis Rheum. 41, 800–807.

This study shows high levels of endothelin-1 in plasmas of APS patients with arterial thrombosis.

Auger, W.R., Permpikul, P., Moser, K.M. 1995. Lupus anticoagulant, heparin use, and thrombocytopenia in patients with chronic thromboembolic pulmonary hypertension: a preliminary report. Am. J. Med. 99, 392–396.

Bayraktar, Y., Tanaci, N., Egesel, T., Gokoz, A., Balkanci, F. 2001. Antiphospholipid syndrome presenting as portopulmonary hypertension. J. Clin. Gastroenterol. 32, 359–361.

Bertoli, A.M., Tabares, A.H., Casas, J.P., Saurit, V., Caeiro, F., Alvarellos, A. 2002. Lung cavitation in primary antiphospholipid syndrome. Lupus 11, 57–59.

Branch, D.W., Kochenour, N.K., Rok, N.S., Scott, J.R. 1986. A new postpsrtum syndrome associated with antiphospholipid antibodies. Proceedings of the Second International Symposium on Antiphospholipid Antibodies, 3–10.

Brucato, A., Baudo, F., Barberis, M., Redaelli, R., Casadei, G., Allegri, F., et al. 1994. Pulmonary hypertension secondary to thrombosis of the pulmonary vessels in a patient with the primary antiphospholipid syndrome. J. Rheumatol. 21, 942–944.

Cacoub, P., Dorent, R., Nataf, P., Carayon, A., Riquet, M., Noe, E., et al. 1997. Endothelin-1 in the lungs of patients with pulmonary hypertension. Cardiovasc. Res. 33, 196–200.

Cervera, R., Piette, J.C., Font, J., Khamashta, M.A., Shoenfeld, Y., Camps, M.T. 2002. Antiphospholipid Syndrome. Clinical and immunologic manifestations and patterns of disease expression in a cohort of 1,000 Patients. Arthritis Rheum. 46, 1019–1027.

This multicenter study describes the prevalence of the main clinical and immunologic features of 1000 APS patients at disease onset and during the evolution.

Chaouat, A., Weitzenblum, E., Higenbottam, T. 1996. The role of thrombosis in severe pulmonary hypertension. Eur. Respir. J. 9, 356–363.

Colorio, C.C., Martinuzzo, M.E., Forastiero, R.R., Pombo, G., Adamczuk, Y., Carreras, L.O. 2001. Thrombophilic factors in chronic thromboembolic pulmonary hypertension. Blood Coagul. Fibrinol. 12, 427–432.

Crausman, R.S., Achenbach, G.A., Pluss, W.T., O'Brien, R.F., Jennings, C.A. 1995. Pulmonary capillaritis and alveolar hemorrhage associated with the antiphospholipid antibody syndrome. J. Rheumatol. 22, 554–556.

Crowther, M.A., Ginsberg, J.S., Julian, J., Math, J.M., Denburg, J., Hirsh, J., et al. 2003. A Comparison of two intensities of warfarin for the prevention of recurrent thrombosis in patients with the antiphospholipid antibody syndrome. N. Engl. J Med. 349, 1133–1138.

Cucurull, E., Ordi-Ros, J., Murtra, M., Mellibovsky, L., Orriols, R., Vilardell, M. 1996. Pulmonary thromboendarterectomy in a patient with primary antiphospholipid syndrome. Med. Clin. (Barc.) 106, 498–500.

Day, S.M., Rosenzweig, B.P., Kronzon, I. 1995. Transesophageal echocardiographic diagnosis of right atrial thrombi associated with the antiphospholipid syndrome. J. Am. Soc. Echocardiogr. 8, 937–940.

De la Mata, J., Gomez-Sanchez, M.A., Aranzana, M., Gomez-Reino, J.J. 1994. Long-term iloprost infusion therapy for severe pulmonary hypertension in patients with connective tissue diseases. Arthritis Rheum. 37, 1528–1533.

Espinosa, G., Cervera, R., Font, J., Asherson, R.A. 2002. The lung in the antiphospholipid syndrome. Ann. Rheum. Dis. 61, 195–198.

Font, J., Cervera, R., López-Soto, A., Pallarés, L., Bosch, X., Ampurdanés, S., et al. 1989. Anticardiolipin antibodies in patients with autoimmune diseases: isotype distribution and clinical associations. Clin. Rheumatol. 8, 475–483.

Font, J., López-Soto, A., Cervera, R., Balasch, J., Pallarés, L., Navarro, M., et al. 1991. The 'primary' antiphospholipid syndrome: antiphospholipid antibody pattern and clinical features of a series of 23 patients. Autoimmunity 9, 69–75.

Gertner, E. 1999. Diffuse alveolar hemorrhage in the antiphospholipid syndrome: spectrum of the disease and treatment. J. Rheumatol. 26, 805–807.

This study describes the clinical manifestations, laboratory findings, and treatment of 5 patients with the APS who develop diffuse alveolar hemorrhage.

Gertner, E., Lie, J.T. 1993. Pulmonary capillaritis, alveolar haemorrhage, and recurrent microvascular thrombosis in primary antiphospholipid syndrome. J. Rheumatol. 20, 1224–1228.

Ghosh, S., Walters, H.D., Joist, J.H., Osborn, T.G., Moore, T.L. 1993. Adult respiratory distress syndrome associated with antiphospholipid antibody syndrome. J. Rheumatol. 20, 1406–1408.

Greaves, M., Cohen, H., Machin, S.J., Mackie, I. 2000. Guidelines on the investigation and management of the antiphospholipid syndrome. Br. J. Hematol. 109, 704–715.

Haworth, S.G. 1998. Primary pulmonary hypertension. J. R. Coll. Physicians Lond. 32, 187–190.

Hillerdal, G. 1997. The lung physician and the antiphospholipid syndrome. Eur. Respir. J. 10, 511–512.

Hillerdal, G., Hagg, A., Licke, G., Wegenius, G., Scheibenpflug, L. 1991. Intra-alveolar hemorrhage in the anticardiolipin antibody syndrome. Scand. J. Rheumatol. 20, 58–62.

Howe, H.S., Boey, M.L., Fong, K.Y., Feng, P.H. 1988. Pulmonary hemorrhage, pulmonary infarction, and the lupus anticoagulant. Ann. Rheum. Dis. 47, 869–872.

Humbert, M., Sanchez, O., Fartoukh, M., Jagot, J.L., Sitbon, O., Simmonneau, G. 1998. Treatment of severe pulmonary hypertension secondary to connective tissue diseases with continuous IV epoprostenol (prostacyclin). Chest 114 (Suppl. 1), 80–82.

Hussein, A., Trowitzsch, E., Brockmann, M. 1999. Pulmonary veno-occlusive disease, antiphospholipid antibody and pulmonary hypertension in an adolescent. Klin. Padiatr. 211, 92–95.

Ingram, S.B., Goodnight, S.H., Bennett, R.M. 1987. An unusual syndrome of a devastating non-inflammatory vasculopathy associated with anticardiolipin antibodies. Arthritis Rheum. 30, 37–42.

Jamieson, S.W., Auger, W.R., Fedullo, P.F., Channick, R.N., Kriett, J.M., Tarazi, R.Y., et al. 1993. Experience and results with 150 pulmonary thromboendarterectomy operations over a 29-month period. J. Thorac. Cardiovasc. Surg. 106, 116–127.

Jeffrey, P., Asherson, R.A., Rees, P.J. 1989. Recurrent deep venous thrombosis and thromboembolic pulmonary hypertension in the 'primary' antiphospholipid syndrome. Clin. Exp. Rheumatol. 7, 567–569.

Karmochkine, M., Cacoub, P., Dorent, R., Laroche, P., Nataf, P., Piette, J.C., et al. 1996. High prevalence of antiphospholipid antibodies in precapillary pulmonary hypertension. J. Rheumatol. 23, 286–290.

Kelion, A.D., Cockcroft, J.R., Ritter, J.M. 1995. Antiphospholipid syndrome in a patient with rapidly progressive fibrosing alveolitis. Postgrad. Med. J. 71, 233–235.

Kerr, J.E., Poe, R., Kramer, Z. 1997. Antiphospholipid antibody syndrome presenting as a refractory noninflammatory pulmonary vasculopathy. Chest 112, 1707–1710.

Khamashta, M.A., Cuadrado, M.J., Mujic, F., Taub, N.A., Hunt, B.J., Hughes, G.R.V. 1995. The management of thrombosis in the antiphospholipid-antibody syndrome. N. Engl. J. Med. 332, 993–997.

Krnic-Barrie, S., O'Connor, C.R., Looney, S.W., Pierangeli, S.S., Harris, E.N. 1997. A retrospective review of 61 patients with antiphospholipid syndrome: analysis of factors influencing recurrent thrombosis. Arch. Intern. Med. 157, 2101–2108.

These two studies suggest that oral anticoagulant treatment in APS patients with venous thromboembolism should be carried on longer than in aPL-negative patients with DVT or PE.

Kupferminc, M.J., Lee, M.J., Green, D., Peaceman, A.M. 1994. Severe postpartum pulmonary, cardiac, and renal syndrome associated with antiphospholipid antibodies. Obstet. Gynecol. 83, 806–807.

Levine, J.S., Branch, W., Rauch, J. 2003. The antiphospholipid syndrome. N. Engl. J. Med. 346, 752–763.

This is an extensive review of the various clinical manifestations and management of APS.

Libby, L., King, T., Laforce, F.M., Schwarz, M.I. 1985. Pulmonary cavitation following pulmonary infarction. Medicine 64, 342–348.

Luchi, M.E., Asherson, R.A., Lahita, R.G. 1992. Primary idiopathic pulmonary hypertension complicated by pulmonary arterial thrombosis. Association with antiphospholipid antibodies. Arthritis Rheum. 35, 700–705.

Mackworth-Young, C.G., Gharavi, A.E., Boey, M.L., Hughes, G.R.V. 1984. Portal and pulmonary hypertension in a case of systemic lupus erythematosus: possible relationship with clotting abnormalities. Eur. J. Rheumatol. Inflamm. 7, 71–74.

Maggiorini, M., Knoblauch, A., Schneider, J., Russi, E.W. 1997. Diffuse microvascular pulmonary thrombosis associated with primary antiphospholipid antibody syndrome. Eur. Respir. J. 10, 727–730.

Magro, C.M., Pope-Harman, A., Moh, P., Ross, P. Jr. 2001. Primary antiphospholipid antibody syndrome caused by isolated anti-phosphatidylethanolamine antibodies presenting as cryptogenic fibrosing alveolitis with recurrent pulmonary hemorrhage after single-lung transplantation. J. Heart Lung Transplant 21, 1232–1236.

McCarty, G.A. 2000. Vascular pathology of the antiphospholipid antibody syndrome. In: M.A. Khamashta (Ed.), Hughes Syndrome. The Antiphospholipid Syndrome. Springer, London, pp. 263–280.

Mintz, G., Acevedo-Vazquez, E., Gutierrez-Espinosa, G., Avelar-Garnica, F. 1984. Renal vein thrombosis and inferior vena cava thrombosis in systemic lupus erythematosus. Arthritis Rheum. 27, 539–544.

Miyata, M., Suzuki, K., Sakuma, F., Watanabe, H., Kaise, S., Nishimaki, T., et al. 1993. Anticardiolipin antibodies are associated with pulmonary hypertension in patients with mixed connective tissue disease or systemic lupus erythematosus. Int. Arch. Allergy Immunol. 100, 351–354.

Moser, K.M., Auger, W.R., Fedullo, P.F. 1990. Chronic major-vessel thromboembolic pulmonary hypertension. Circulation 81, 1735–1743.

Muñoz-Rodríguez, F.J., Font, J., Cervera, R., Reverter, J.C., Tàssies, D., Espinosa, G., et al. 1999. Clinical study and follow-up of 100 patients with the antiphospholipid syndrome. Semin. Arthritis Rheum. 29, 182–190.

Nagai, H., Yasuma, K., Katsuki, T., Shimakura, A., Usuda, K., Nakamura, Y., et al. 1997. Primary antiphospholipid syndrome and pulmonary hypertension with prolonged survival. A case report. Angiology 48, 183–187.

Nakagawa, Y., Masuda, M., Shiihara, H., Tsuruta, Y., Abe, H., Miura, M., et al. 1992. Succesful pulmonary thromboendarterectomy for chronic thromboembolic pulmonary hypertension associated with anticardiolipin antibodies: report of a case. Surg. Today 22, 548–552.

Nakos, G., Kitsiouli, E., Maneta-Peyret, L., Cassagne, C., Tsianos, E., Lekka, M. 2001. The characteristics of bronchoalveolar lavage from a patient with antiphospholipid syndrome who developed acute respiratory distress syndrome. Clin. Rheumatol. 20, 91–97.

O'Hickey, S., Skinner, C., Beattie, J. 1993. Life-threatening right ventricular thrombosis in association with phospholipid antibodies. Br. Heart. J. 70, 279–281.

Petri, M., Rheinschmidt, M., Whiting-O'Keefe, Q., Hellmann, D., Corash, L. 1987. The frequency of lupus anticoagulant in systemic lupus erythematosus. A study of sixty consecutive patients by activated partial thromboplastin time, Russell viper venom time, and anticardiolipin antibody level. Ann. Intern. Med. 106, 524–531.

Piette, J.C., Hunt, B.J. 2000. Pulmonary hypertension and antiphospholipid antibodies. In: M.A. Khamashta (Ed.), Hughes Syndrome. The Antiphospholipid Syndrome. Springer, London, pp. 96–104.
The authors review the expanding knowledge of the pathogenic disease pathways of pulmonary hypertension in APS.

Rana, M., Endo, H., Watabe, H., Tanaka, S., Kondo, H. 2001. A case of primary antiphospholipid syndrome complicated with pulmonary hypertension. Ryumachi 41, 869–874.

Rich, S., Kaufmann, E., Levy, P.S. 1992. The effect of high doses of calcium-channel blockers on survival in primary pulmonary hypertension. N. Engl. J. Med. 327, 76–81.

Rosove, M.H., Brewer, P.M. 1992. Antiphospholipid thrombosis: clinical course after the first thrombotic event in 70 patients. Ann. Intern. Med. 117, 303–308.

Ruiz-Irastorza, G., Khamashta, M.A., Hunt, B.J., Escudero, A., Cuadrado, M.J., Hughes, G.R. 2002. Bleeding and recurrent thrombosis in definite antiphospholipid syndrome: analysis of a series of 66 patients treated with oral anticoagulation to a target international normalized ratio of 3.5. Arch. Intern. Med. 162, 1164–1169.

Sandoval, J., Amigo, M.C., Barragan, R., Izaguirre, R., Reyes, P.A., Martínez-Guerra, M.L., et al. 1996. Primary antiphospholipid syndrome presenting as chronic thromboembolic hypertension. Treatment with thromboendarterectomy. J. Rheumatol. 23, 772–775.

Savin, H., Hoberman, M., Kott, E., Lishner, M., Kitai, Y., Kidron, D., et al. 1994. Fibrosing alveolitis associated with primary antiphospholipid antibodies. J. Rheumatol. 33, 977–980.

Specks, U. 2001. Diffuse alveolar hemorrhage syndromes. Curr. Opin. Rheumatol. 13, 12–17.

Tam, L.-S., Li, E.K. 1998. Succesful treatment with immunosupression, anticoagulation and vasodilator therapy of pulmonary hypertension in SLE associated with secondary antiphospholipid syndrome. Lupus 7, 495–497.

Turjanski, A.A., Finkielman, J.D., Vazquez-Blanco, M. 1998. Isolated tricuspid valve disease in antiphospholipid syndrome. Lupus 8, 474–476.

Vianna, J.L., Khamashta, M.A., Ordi-Ros, J., Font, J., Cervera, R., López-Soto, A., et al. 1994. Comparison of the primary and secondary antiphospholipid syndrome: a European multicenter study of 114 patients. Am. J. Med. 96, 3–9.

Ware, L.B., Matthay, M.A. 2000. The acute respiratory distress syndrome. N. Engl. J. Med. 342, 1334–1349.

Waterer, G.W., Latham, B., Waring, J.A., Gabbay, E. 1999. Pulmonary capillaritis associated with the antiphospholipid antibody syndrome and rapid response to plasmapheresis. Respirology 4, 405–408.

Wiedermann, F.J., Lederer, W., Mayr, A.J., Sepp, N., Herold, M., Schobersberger, W. 2003. Prospective observational study of antiphospholipid antibodies in acute lung injury and acute respiratory distress syndrome: comparison with catastrophic antiphospholipid syndrome. Lupus 12, 462–467.

Wilson, W.A., Gharavi, A.E., Koike, T., Lockshin, M.D., Branch, D.W., Piette, J.-C., et al. 1999. International consensus statement on preliminary classification criteria for definite antiphospholipid syndrome: report of an international workshop. Arthritis Rheum. 42, 1309–1311.

Wolf, M., Boyer-Neumann, C., Parent, F., Eschwege, V., Jaillet, H., Meyer, D., et al. 2000. Thrombotic risk factors in pulmonary hypertension. Eur. Respir. J. 15, 395–399.

Handbook of Systemic Autoimmune Diseases, Volume 2
Pulmonary Involvement in Systemic Autoimmune Diseases
A.U. Wells and C.P. Denton, editors

CHAPTER 8

Rheumatoid Arthritis and the Lung

Joel David*, Sally Edmonds
Department of Rheumatology, Nuffield Orthopaedic Centre, Oxford OX3 7LD, UK.

1. Introduction

Rheumatoid arthritis (RA) is the most common inflammatory disease (Tanoue, 1998), the hallmark of which is a small and large joint inflammatory erosive arthritis. The cause of the disease remains unknown; however, a large number of observed immunological phenomena are recognised, many of which are utilised in targeted therapy. Pulmonary complications of rheumatoid are common. Autopsy studies suggest pulmonary involvement in up to 50% of patients (Hunninghake and Fauci, 1979; King, 1998). However, with more sensitive diagnostic tools such as high resolution CT (HRCT), up to 70% of patients will be found to have some pulmonary abnormality. The identification of systemic disease is important as it is associated with a greater mortality, especially in patients less than 50 years of age (Gordon et al., 1973).

Drugs used to treat RA may cause pulmonary side-effects that may be indistinguishable from pulmonary manifestations of the RA itself. HRCT, brocho-alveolar lavage and even biopsy may be required in the diagnosis.

Smoking confers a worse prognosis on RA and also increases susceptibility to methotrexate-related pulmonary injury. The treatment of RA-related lung disease remains challenging.

*Corresponding author.
Tel.: +44-1865-227724; fax: +44-1865-227938
E-mail address: joeldavid@noc.anglox.nhs.uk (J. David).

DOI: 10.1016/S1571-5078(04)02008-2

2. Epidemiology

RA occurs worldwide in about 1% of the adult population (Lawrence et al., 1989), although its regional and temporal prevalence is variable. There is a suggestion of a decline in the incidence of RA over the last 40 years (Doran et al., 2002). RA affects women more commonly than men (2:1 to 3:1), although some of the extra-articular manifestations, including rheumatoid nodules and lung disease, are more common in men (Weyand et al., 1998). These differences could also result from associated factors such as smoking, rather than genetic factors or hormonal differences between the genders (Saag et al., 1997). The peak age of onset of RA is in the fifth decade (Yukioka et al., 1998), but it may occur as early as the second. It also appears that new onset RA is occurring in much older individuals than was previously the case (Imanaka et al., 1997).

RA is a multi-factorial disease and, given its increased prevalence in women, it seems likely that hormones have an important, if not completely elucidated, influence. In most women, the disease remits during pregnancy, only to return, often more severely than before, in the post partum period (Nicholas and Panayi, 1988). There are conflicting data on the relationship between both oral contraceptives and hormone replacement therapy and RA (Vandenbroucke et al., 1986; Carette et al., 1989; Brennan et al., 1997).

Family studies indicate a genetic predisposition to RA. Monozygotic twins are at least four times more likely to be concordant for RA than dizygotic twins (Aho et al., 1986). One of the major genetic factors in the aetiology of RA is the class II major histocompatability complex (MHC) gene product HLA-DR4 (Walport et al., 1992). Up to 70% of patients with classic or definite RA express HLA-DR4, compared with 28% of control individuals. In some ethnic groups, there is an association between RA and HLA-DR1 and HLA-Dw16. These observations form the basis for the suggestion that shared epitopes determine susceptibility to RA (Gregersen et al., 1987).

Other characteristics, in addition to the genetic, gender and age-related factors mentioned above, almost certainly predispose to the development of RA. These include socio-economic status (Berkanovic et al., 1996), educational level (Callahan and Pincus, 1988), and stress (Persson et al., 1999). Smoking not only appears to predispose to the development of RA, but may also influence the severity and predispose to the development of some of the extra-articular manifestations (Doyle et al., 2000).

The prevalence and incidence of many of the extra-articular features of RA, including lung disease, is not accurately known. There is a striking tendency for patients to develop more than one extra-articular feature. For example, nodules, vasculitis and pulmonary involvement frequently coexist (Scott et al., 1981a,b). Pleuropulmonary disease is clinically apparent in about 10% of patients with RA, but is detected in over half of patients with early disease when detailed investigations are used (Gabbay et al., 1997). The natural history of both RA and associated pulmonary disease is changing with the increased use of immunosuppressive drugs such as methotrexate and, more recently, the biologics. Refractory pleural effusions and obstructive airways disease such as bronchiolitis obliterans are becoming less common. There is an emergence of pulmonary tuberculosis and other infections associated with the use of the biologics (Keane et al., 2001). For most expressions of rheumatoid-related lung disease, male sex, rheumatoid factor (RF) positivity and the presence of subcutaneous rheumatoid nodules remain the main risk factors. The course of extra-articular manifestations of rheumatoid does not always parallel joint disease and may even dominate clinical expression. Intra-thoracic complications of rheumatoid may precede the onset of joint disease in up to 20% (King, 1998).

3. Clinical manifestations

The spectrum of rheumatoid-associated lung disease is broad (Table 1).

3.1. Serositis and effusions

Pleural disease is common in RA, and in post-mortem series the incidence has been between 38 and 73% (King, 1998). Involvement of the pleura may be silent clinically or may result in pleurisy or a pleural effusion, or both. As is true of most of the other pulmonary manifestations of RA, serositis and effusions are more common in men than in women. Pleural effusions occur in approximately 5% of patients with RA (Shannon and Gale, 1992). They may resolve spontaneously or become chronic or recurrent. Rheumatoid effusions are usually unilateral (Light, 1990) and small to moderate in size. They may cause symptoms such as chest pain, dyspnoea and fever and about one third of patients will have

Table 1
Pulmonary manifestations of rheumatoid arthritis

Pleural disease
Pleuritis
Effusion
Pneumothorax
Bronchpleural fistula
Empyema
Nodulosis
Rheumatoid nodulosis
Caplan's syndrome
Airway disease
Crico-arytenoid arthritis
Upper airway involvement
Sjogren's syndrome
Airway obstruction
Bronchiectasis
Bronchiolitis obliterans with organising pneumonia
Bronchiolitis obliterans
Interstitial lung disease
Pulmonary vascular disease
Vasculitis
Primary pulmonary hypertension
Secondary pulmonary hypertension
Drug related disease
Pulmonary infection
Other
Fibrobullous disease
Amyloidosis

concurrent interstitial lung disease (ILD) or pulmonary rheumatoid nodules (Light, 1990).

Rheumatoid pleural effusions are exudates, with high protein and lactate dehydrogenase levels (Lillington et al., 1971; Light, 1990). There is a low glucose concentration (Carr and Power, 1960) which is thought to be caused by impaired glucose transport from blood to pleural fluid (Dodson and Hollingsworth, 1966), in contrast to empyema and malignant effusions, where the low glucose content is probably secondary to increased consumption of glucose by cells within the effusion. Rheumatoid effusions usually have a low pH (<7.2) and leukocyte counts within them are generally less than 10,000/ml, with a lymphocytic or polymorphonuclear predominance (Light, 1990; Shannon and Gale, 1992). Other findings include reduced pleural fluid C3, C4 and CH50 levels and increased RF levels (Light, 1990; King, 1998), although these do not help to distinguish rheumatoid effusions from other causes of effusion such as SLE, tuberculosis, bacterial empyema and malignancy. Cytology may reveal granular leukocytes with cytoplasmic inclusion bodies known as RA cells (Feagler et al., 1971; Light, 1990), but these may occur in other conditions and are, therefore, non-specific (Joseph and Sahn, 1993). Hyaluronan levels have also been shown to be high in rheumatoid pleural fluid, perhaps secondary to the local production of pro-inflammatory cytokines (Söderblom et al., 1999).

3.2. Nodules

Rheumatoid pulmonary nodules have the same histology as those found in subcutaneous tissue and seem to be more common in patients with extra pulmonary nodules (Maini and Zvaifler, 1998). Pulmonary rheumatoid nodules are thought to be the only specific pleuropulmonary manifestation of RA (King, 1998), and are strongly associated with seropositivity, rarely occurring in patients who are negative for RF (Maini and Zvaifler, 1998). The prevalence of pulmonary nodules varies, depending on whether they are identified by plain chest X-ray (CXR), CT of the chest or by post-mortem or lung biopsy. In one large series of 516 patients, only two nodules were identified by plain CXR (Walker and Wright, 1968). In a series of 77 patients who underwent HRCT of the chest, 17 (22%) were found to have nodular densities (Cortet et al., 1995). In another series of 40 patients who underwent open lung biopsy, microscopic nodules were identified in 13 (32%) (Yousem et al., 1985). The significance of such micro nodular disease is unclear, particularly because such findings are often seen in normal people without connective tissue disease. Nodules are usually asymptomatic, but if they are close to the pleural surface, may result in pleural effusion, pneumothorax, pyopneumothorax and bronchopulmonary fistula (Shannon and Gale, 1992; King, 1998). Cavitation of nodules within the parenchyma may also rarely lead to haemoptysis and infection (Dieppe, 1975; King, 1998). Of all the pulmonary manifestations of RA, nodules are associated with the most favourable prognosis (Yousem et al., 1985). Nodules, whether pulmonary or subcutaneous, may antedate clinical arthritis. If they occur in the context of RA, other causes of nodulosis must be excluded: in particular, malignancy and infection. More widespread nodulosis may also occur, particularly in men with RA, so-called 'rheumatoid nodulosis' (Wisnieski and Askari, 1981). This is a distinct entity from Caplan's syndrome, which was first described in 1953 in Welsh coal miners with RA, who had multiple pulmonary nodules, probably related to silica deposition in the lung (Caplan, 1953).

3.3. Interstitial lung disease

ILD is the most common symptomatic pulmonary manifestation of RA. It is seen more often in men than women, especially in the context of a high RF titre and severe articular disease. Radiographically, ILD associated with RA is indistinguishable from idiopathic pulmonary fibrosis (IPF) and ILD associated with other connective tissue diseases. The most common finding is of asymmetrical bilateral basal interstitial abnormalities (Walker and Wright, 1968; Remy-Jardin et al., 1994). HRCT is the most sensitive method of detecting ILD; the prevalence using this technique is reported as being up to 47% (Fujii et al., 1993; Remy-Jardin et al., 1994). However, a recent study using HRCT has shown evidence of ILD in 19% of hospital outpatients with RA (Dawson et al., 2001).

As with any fibrosing lung disease, ILD in RA is associated with a reduction in lung volumes and pulmonary compliance and abnormalities in diffusing capacity for carbon monoxide (DLCO) (Shannon and Gale, 1992; King, 1998). RA patients with ILD tend to demonstrate a neutrophilic alveolitis and an increase in the absolute number of macrophages, as assessed by bronchoalveolar lavage (BAL) (Gilligen et al., 1990; King, 1998). A recent prospective study correlated HRCT, lung function tests (PFT) and BAL cytology in patients with ILD associated with RA (Biederer et al., 2003). HRCT appeared to be the most appropriate investigation for the detection and follow up of ILD, and PFT and BAL only partially correlated with lesion profusion or grading on HRCT, but they provided valuable information about dynamic lung function and differential diagnoses.

The symptoms of ILD usually occur after the onset of arthritis, but in approximately one fifth of patients, lung disease predates articular disease (King, 1998). Patients may be asymptomatic, but the commonest complaints are dyspnoea and cough (Roschmann and Rothenberg, 1987). As with other causes of lung fibrosis, finger clubbing is common and may be seen in up to 75% of cases (King, 1998), although probably not as frequently as in idiopathic lung fibrosis (Rajasekaran et al., 2001). In general, ILD associated with RA tends to follow a more benign course than the idiopathic form of the disease, but patients may develop end stage respiratory failure (Dixon et al., 1957). It does appear, however, that RA patients with ILD carry a worse prognosis than RA patients with other lung diseases such as pulmonary nodules or BOOP (Hakala, 1988). It is important, therefore, that ILD is diagnosed as early as possible and monitored so that the appropriate therapy may be initiated.

3.4. Bronchiectasis

The prevalence of bronchiectasis may be as high as 40% (Despaux et al., 1998) but changes on HRCT can be seen in up to 70% (Perez et al., 1998). Bronchiectasis in RA is often asymptomatic; the prevalence of *symptomatic* disease is probably much lower, around 3% in one study (Allain et al., 1997). The predilection for bronchiectasis in RA may be related to an increased susceptibility to airway infection (Bamji and Cooke, 1983). There may also be a genetic susceptibility in some patients (Hillarby et al., 1993). More recently, it has been suggested that a mutation on the cystic fibrosis transmembrane conductance regulator gene may predispose to the development and severity of bronchiectasis in RA patients (Puechal et al., 1999). The co-existence of RA and bronchiectasis confers a worse prognosis, with a reduced five-year survival when compared to RA alone (Swinson et al., 1997).

3.5. Bronchiolitis obliterans with organising pneumonia

Bronchiolitis obliterans with organising pneumonia (BOOP) may be associated with RA, other connective tissue diseases, infection and drug toxicity. It is characterised pathologically by the presence of granulation tissue in the lumen of the bronchioles and alveolar ducts (Muller and Miller, 1995). Organising pneumonia usually occurs distal to this process.

Patients with BOOP present with non-specific symptoms, which include productive cough, dyspnoea, weight loss and fever (Rees et al., 1991). Crackles are usually heard on auscultation. The CXR typically shows patchy bilateral infiltrates and the CT scan may show consolidation in these areas (Cohen et al., 1994). BOOP tends to show a restrictive, rather than an obstructive, picture on lung function testing (Muller and Miller, 1995). The diagnosis of BOOP may be confirmed by either surgical or transbronchial biopsy. In a series of 40 patients with RA undergoing lung biopsy, BOOP was the second most common histological abnormality (Yousem et al., 1985). On the whole, the prognosis for BOOP is better than for either ILD or obliterative bronchiolitis (OB). Patients may, however, progress to end stage respiratory failure and death, and it may be that BOOP associated with connective tissue disease has a worse prognosis than other types of BOOP (Epler et al., 1985). In the more severe cases, it is possible that BOOP either coexists with or predates the development of fibrotic lung disease (Cohen et al., 1994).

3.6. Obliterative bronchiolitis

The association of OB with RA was first noted in 1977 (Geddes et al., 1977). Unlike the other pulmonary manifestations of RA, OB seems to be more common in women. The cause of OB remains unclear, but usually occurs in patients who are RF positive and have well-established joint disease. Patients most often present with dyspnoea and a non-productive cough, which usually worsen rapidly—in contrast to the other types of lung disease associated with RA. The CXR is usually normal, but may show signs of hyperinflation.

OB is less common than BOOP, and is characterised pathologically by the presence of submucosal and peribronchiolar fibrosis resulting in extrinsic narrowing and obliteration of the bronchiolar lumen (Muller and Miller, 1995). Small bronchi and bronchioles are primarily involved. Histologically, the typical finding is of fibrosis with little active inflammation (Muller and Miller, 1995). The diagnosis of OB should be considered in any RA patient who has rapidly progressive air flow obstruction accompanied by dyspnoea and cough. The outlook for these patients is poor.

3.7. Rheumatoid drugs and the lung

3.7.1. Nonsteroidal anti-inflammatory drugs

Nonsteroidal anti-inflammatory drugs (NSAIDs) may be associated with hypersensitivity and bronchospasm in susceptible individuals (Zilnik, 1997). Patients will experience cough, fever, dyspnoea and skin rash, usually accompanied by peripheral eosinophilia. The CXR may show bilateral interstitial infiltrates and the BAL fluid shows marked eosinophilia. Symptoms resolve on cessation of the NSAID (Tanoue, 1998). The newer cyclooxygenase II inhibitor (COX II) drugs are associated with fluid retention and non-cardiogenic pulmonary oedema may rarely occur (author's experience).

3.7.2. Gold

Gold-induced pulmonary disease may be difficult to diagnose, particularly when interstitial pneumonia appears in the course of therapy. Tomioka and King (1997) defined the clinical features and prognosis in order to differentiate it from that secondary to the rheumatoid process itself. They identified 140 cases of gold-induced pulmonary disease. Interestingly, the development of pulmonary disease most often followed improvement in systemic disease, presumably induced by gold. Features that distinguish gold-induced disease from rheumatoid lung include female sex, the presence of fever and rash, eosinophilia, raised IgE levels, proteinuria, thrombocytopenia, post injection reactions to gold (Scott et al., 1981a,b) and the absence of subcutaneous nodules or clubbing. Lymphocytosis on BAL and more recently CT scan findings (Sinha et al., 2001) have been useful in making a diagnosis. Alveolar opacities occur along the broncho-vascular bundles on CT scanning. Gold-induced pulmonary disease may be considered a distinct entity distinguishable from rheumatoid lung. It usually improves with cessation of therapy or treatment with corticosteroids.

Chakravarty and Webley (1992) treated 62 RA patients with gold, penicillamine and azathioprine and monitored their lung function over a two-year period. They found 46% of patients treated with gold and 21% treated with penicillamine, developed a restrictive defect after two years and there was a significant reduction in vital capacity and gas transfer ($p < 0.001$) in both groups. A significant improvement in pulmonary function occurred in the gold treated patients ($p < 0.05$) a year after treatment was discontinued. Alveolar macrophages obtained at BAL demonstrate that gold is retained for prolonged periods in pulmonary tissue following treatment. This does not, however, demonstrate in itself any relationship between gold and chronic lung disease (Garcia et al., 1987).

3.7.3. D-Penicillamine

D-Penicillamine is rarely used nowadays for RA. There are three forms of pulmonary disease with which it has been associated: OB, ILD and a pulmonary-renal syndrome with alveolar haemorrhage (Stein et al., 1980; Zitnik and Cooper, 1990)

3.7.4. Sulphasalazine

Pulmonary toxicity is a rare side effect of sulphasalazine. Parry et al. (2002) described 50 cases.

The typical presentation was of new onset dyspnoea and infiltrates on CXR. Commonly the patients presented with cough and fever. Eosinophilia was noted in half the cases. Sputum production, allergy history, rash, chest pain and weight loss were inconsistent findings. The commonest pulmonary pathology was that of an eosinophilic pneumonia with interstitial infiltrate with or without fibrosis. Fatal reports were infrequent. Most patients were managed by drug withdrawal although 40% required corticosteroids.

3.7.5. Methotrexate

Methotrexate is the most commonly used second-line agent for RA in the western world. It is a folic acid antagonist. Pulmonary toxicity is described in 0.5–12% although most papers suggest about 3% (Zisman et al., 2001). Perhaps the most accurate estimate of prevalence, based on the largest prospective series to date, is 1% (Cannon and Finck, 2000). The most frequent symptom is that of sub-acute progression over several weeks of a dry cough, dyspnoea, fever and bi-basal crackles. Peripheral eosinophilia occurs in about a third of cases. The CXR maybe normal, but more commonly reveals bilateral interstitial or mixed interstitial and alveolar infiltrates with a predilection for the bases. HRCT scanning may demonstrate diffuse ground glass opacification, reticular opacities, centrilobular nodules, septal lines or widespread consolidation (Arakawa et al., 2003). Pulmonary function studies may reveal a restrictive ventilatory defect and/or impaired gas exchange. Histological findings in methotrexate induced pulmonary disease show cellular interstitial infiltrates, granulomas, fibrosis and atypical epithelial cells. There is most often diffuse alveolar damage. Once methotrexate-induced lung disease is suspected, the drug should be withdrawn. Corticosteroids may accelerate resolution. The prognosis is usually favourable but occasionally the outcome may be fatal.

There is no evidence that methotrexate is associated with chronic lung disease (Dawson et al., 2003).

Alarcon et al. (1997) examined patients for potential risk factors for the development of methotrexate-induced lung injury. They and other workers (Ohosone et al., 1997) found that older age groups, diabetes, existing rheumatoid pleuropulmonary involvement and previous reactions to disease modifying drugs (DMARDs) all increase the chances of developing methotrexate-induced lung disease. Surfactant proteins have been used to detect and monitor methotrexate-associated lung injury (Miyata et al., 2002).

Methotrexate-induced pneumonitis appears to be more common in patients with RA than in those where the methotrexate is used for psoriatic arthritis (Salaffi et al., 1997). This may be because pre-existing lung disease is more common in RA; there may also be a disease susceptibility gene for this.

BAL cell profile in methotrexate induced pneumonitis suggests a lymphocytic alveolitis with a preferential increase in CD4+ cells (Schnabel et al., 1997). This pattern differs from that of ILD due to RA and may, therefore, also assist in making an earlier diagnosis.

Some patients may complain of a persistent isolated dry cough on methotrexate therapy and all their pulmonary investigations are normal including HRCT and BAL cytology. This may occur as a result of an irritant effect of methotrexate on the airways (Schnabel et al., 1996).

Opportunistic infection such as pneumocystis carinii is important to exclude when pulmonary symptoms occur in a rheumatoid patient treated with methotrexate. This infection is particularly likely to occur with concurrent corticosteroid therapy, when NSAIDs are used or when there is renal impairment (Krebs and Gibbons, 1996).

There have been a few recent reports of a pneumonitis that has occurred in RA patients treated with methotrexate and biologics. This suggests that anti-TNF therapy may have a permissive or synergistic role in the expression of methotrexate pneumonitis (Courtney et al., 2003).

3.7.6. Biologics

Anti-TNF drugs such as infliximab, etanercept and adalimumab are increasingly used for aggressive RA either at onset, or in those patients who have already received numerous DMARDs. These patients may have pre-existing pulmonary disease. Gomez-Reino et al. (2003) reviewed infliximab and etanercept safety. They reported the results of 71 participating centres, which comprised 1578 treatments with infliximab (86%) or etanercept (14%) in 1540 patients.

There were 17 cases of tuberculosis (TB) treated with infliximab. The estimated incidence of TB associated with infliximab in the rheumatoid population was significantly greater than background rates prior to 2001 (Keane et al., 2001; Mayordomo et al., 2002).

Delayed hypersensitivity reactions and acute respiratory distress syndrome following infliximab infusions have been described (Riegert-Johnson et al., 2002). In these cases an eosinophilic pneumonia occurs, responsive to corticosteroid therapy. Etanercept, too, has been linked with lung injury in the form of non-caseating pulmonary granulomas. Withdrawal of the drug achieved clinical stabilisation (Peno-Green et al., 2002).

3.8. Smoking and rheumatoid arthritis

Studies looking for a causal relationship between cigarette smoking and RA have been inconsistent, although overall, smoking probably does have a small contributory role to play, particularly in men. A prospective population study in Finland suggested that exposure to tobacco smoke, or some factor or cluster of factors associated with smoking, may trigger the production of RF, and this, in men, may subsequently contribute to the development of RA (Heliövaara et al., 1993). Other studies have also shown a link between smoking and RF production or the development of sero-positive arthritis (Tuomi et al., 1990; Symmons et al., 1997). In a nationwide study of disease-discordant twins, Silman et al. (1996) showed clear evidence of an association between smoking and disease, in spite of the fact that the majority of the twin pairs were concordant for cigarette smoking. This latter study was true for both sexes, and whilst men seem to be at most risk of developing RA in association with smoking, one study has shown that the duration, although not the intensity, of cigarette smoking is associated with a modest increased risk of RA in women as well (Karlson et al., 1999). Further studies have shown a positive relationship between the number of cigarettes smoked and the development of RA (Hutchinson et al., 2001; Reckner Olsson et al., 2001). Interestingly, smoking in RA patients without a family history of RA was more prevalent than in RA patients with a positive family history of RA; this is true for the number of pack years smoked, for smoking at the time of disease onset and even in those with a simple history of having previously smoked. A recent study has attempted to quantify the influence of cigarette smoking on the risk of developing RA (Stolt et al., 2003). This case-control study over four years found that current smokers, ex-smokers, and ever-smokers of both sexes had an increased risk for sero-positive RA, but not for sero-negative RA. The increased risk was only apparent among subjects who had smoked for 20 years or more, was evident at an intensity of smoking of 6–9 cigarettes a day and remained for up to 10–19 years after smoking cessation. The risk increased with increasing cumulative dose of smoking.

Smoking also has an effect on RA disease activity and severity. In a study of 336 patients with RA, Saag et al. (1997) showed that smokers with more than 25 pack years were 3.1 times more likely to be RF positive (IgM and IgA) and 2.4 times more likely to show radiographic erosions than never smokers. In another study of 63 women with advanced RA, Másdóttir et al. (2000) found that the patients who were heavy smokers (more than 20 pack years) develop more severe RA than those who smoked less or not at all. Wolfe (2000) confirmed the relationship of smoking, disease severity and RF positivity but did not demonstrate alterations in day-to-day disease activity measures. The mechanism by which smoking influences RA susceptibility/severity is still unclear. Mattey et al. (2002) postulated that genes associated with detoxification or activation of chemicals in tobacco smoke could be important. This group had already found that increased severity in RA is associated with a null polymorphism at the glutathione S-transferase (GST) M1 locus (Mattey et al., 1999). The GSTM1 enzyme detoxifies known or suspected carcinogens found in tobacco smoke. Their data suggest firstly that disease outcome in female RA patients with a history of smoking is significantly worse than those who have never smoked. Secondly, the data provide evidence that the risk of developing severe disease in women with RA is increased in those who have the GSTM1-null polymorphism and who have also smoked. The authors suggest that this association may be due in part to a relationship between the GSTM1 polymorphism and RF production in smokers.

Smoking appears to be one of the main predictors for the development of some of the extra-articular manifestations of RA including pericarditis, pleuritis, cutaneous vasculitis, Felty's syndrome, neuropathy, ophthalmological manifestations, glomerulonephritis and other types of vasculitis (Turesson et al., 2003). This association was independent of RF, and the authors suggest that smoking in some way drives the rheumatoid process towards extra-articular involvement and that this is perhaps because of the effect that smoking has on blood vessels. Vascular abnormalities are clearly pivotal in rheumatoid vasculitis, but may also be important in other extra-articular manifestations such as pericarditis and rheumatoid nodules. In addition, smoking is a well-known predictor of cardiovascular disease, and it is now well documented that patients with RA have increased cardiovascular morbidity (McEntegart et al., 2001). Smoking may also exert its deleterious effects by altering nitric oxide pathways (Farrell and Blake, 1996).

There is evidence of a downward trend in the incidence of extra-articular manifestations of RA, especially rheumatoid vasculitis, observed with a decrease in worldwide tobacco use and overall improved mortality in RA (Albano et al., 2001). This having been said, it is interesting to note that the commonest cause of respiratory symptoms in RA patients is chronic airways obstruction related to smoking (Banks et al., 1992).

4. Morbidity and mortality of rheumatoid lung disease—comparison with other autoimmune lung diseases

The excess mortality associated with RA arises largely from its extra-articular involvement (Leigh and Fries, 1991), including increased frequency of infections and cardiovascular, renal, and pulmonary diseases (Wolfe, 1996). Overall, infection is the leading cause of death in RA, and even where there is underlying lung disease, such as pulmonary fibrosis, superimposed infection poses a greater risk than the fibrosis itself (Hakala, 1988). Like RA, systemic lupus erythematosus (SLE) may affect all the components of the respiratory system. Infection rates are also increased in SLE, particularly patients treated with glucocorticoids, and are an important cause of morbidity and mortality (Nived et al., 1985). BOOP in both RA and SLE carries a good prognosis and is steroid responsive. In both diseases, 'pure' OB carries a much worse prognosis than BOOP and is generally not treatment responsive. A rare complication of SLE, not seen in RA, is the 'shrinking lung syndrome'. The long-term prognosis of this condition is reasonable and may respond to immunosuppressive therapy (Karim et al., 2002). Two other conditions associated with lupus and not usually with RA, are acute lupus pneumonitis and pulmonary haemorrhage, both of which carry a poor prognosis (Wiedemann and Matthay, 1992). Whilst ILD is common in RA, it is not as prevalent as in systemic sclerosis (SSc), in which it is said to occur in some form in most patients (White, 2003). In addition, the prognosis is much worse in SSc with some 15% of patients progressing to severe restrictive lung disease. Pulmonary fibrosis remains a major cause of death in patients with SSc. Primary pulmonary hypertension (PAH) occurs in RA (Dawson et al., 2000), but is usually milder than in SSc (Denton and Black, 2003) or dermatomyositis and polymyositis (in which pulmonary hypertension is usually associated with pulmonary fibrosis) (Yazici and Kagan, 2002). Similarly, ILD tends to be less progressive than in patients with anti-Jo-1 antibody positive myositis, who may develop a rapidly progressive, diffuse alveolitis, which may decompensate into adult respiratory distress syndrome, with a poor prognosis and an often fatal outcome (Clawson and Oddis, 1995).

Thus, whilst pulmonary manifestations are common in patients with RA, they tend to be more benign than those associated with the other connective tissue diseases.

5. Treatment of rheumatoid lung disease

The treatment of rheumatoid lung disease is largely anecdotal as there are no good randomised controlled trials. Progressive ILD due to RA is difficult to treat. Traditionally high doses of oral corticosteroids with the addition of cyclophosphamide or chlorambucil have been used (Nanki et al., 2002).

Pneumonitis, when it occurs in RA, may be due to low dose oral methotrexate, infection or the rheumatoid process itself, and these processes may be difficult to distinguish. Methotrexate lung injury is treated by withdrawing the drug, oxygen therapy, and, rarely, steroids are needed. In one case report (Suwa et al., 1999), where infection had been excluded, there had been no response to the withdrawal of methotrexate and treatment with corticosteroids. It was only when intravenous cyclophosphamide was initiated that rapid physiological and radiographic improvement occurred.

There have been several anecdotal reports of azathioprine and D-penicillamine being useful for rheumatoid ILD (Chang et al., 2002). Cyclosporin-A in conjunction with cyclophosphamide has also been used with good effect in some cases (Puttick et al., 1995).

Rheumatoid effusions do not generally require specific treatment, although if they are large and causing significant breathlessness, they may need draining. They usually respond to the DMARDs used to treat the articular disease.

BOOP is generally steroid responsive. This contrasts with OB alone, which is not treatment responsive and consequently carries a worse prognosis.

There have been recent reports of clinical response of RA associated pulmonary fibrosis to the use of biological agents. Vassallo et al., 2003 describes a patient who had sustained improvement in dyspnoea, cough and exercise tolerance following TNF Alpha inhibition therapy, with stabilisation of pulmonary function.

When rheumatoid lung disease is associated with drug toxicity (NSAIDs, sulphasalazine and gold), resolution usually occurs with cessation of the drug. In approximately 40%, corticosteroids will aid in this resolution.

Key points

- HRCT suggests that approximately 70% of patients with RA will have pulmonary disease.
- RA is associated with pleural disease, pulmonary nodulosis, airways and ILD.
- Pulmonary fibrosis in RA is milder that that seen in cryptogenic fibrosis or that associated with other inflammatory connective tissue diseases. It is also less commonly associated with clubbing.
- Methotrexate is the most commonly used DMARD for RA: it is associated with a 3% incidence of non-chronic pulmonary toxicity.
- Immunosuppressive drugs and the biologics are changing the natural history of RA and associated pulmonary disease.
- There is emergence of pulmonary TB and other infections with the use of the biologics.
- Smoking has a negative effect on the activity and severity of RA.
- The treatment of the pulmonary disease associated with RA remains largely anecdotal.

References

Alarcon, G.S., Kremer, J.M., Macaluso, M., Weinblatt, M.E., Cannon, G.W. 1997. Risk factors for methotrexate-induced lung injury in patients with rheumatoid arthritis. A multicenter case-control study. Methotrexate-Lung Study Group. Ann. Intern. Med. 127, 356.

Aho, K., Koskenvuo, M., Tuominen, J., Kaprio, J. 1986. Occurrence of rheumatoid arthritis in a nationwide series of twins. J. Rheumatol. 13, 899.

Albano, S.A., Santana-Sahagun, E., Weisman, M.H. 2001. Cigarette smoking and rheumatoid arthritis. Semin. Arthritis Rheum. 31, 146.

Allain, J., Saraux, A., Guedes, C., Valls, I., Devauchelle, V., Le Goff, P. 1997. Prevalence of symptomatic bronchiectasis in patients with rheumatoid arthritis. Revue du Rhumatisme (Engl. Ed.) 64, 531.

Arakawa, H., Yamasaki, M., Kurihara, Y., Yamada, H., Nakajima, Y. 2003. Methotrexate-induced pulmonary injury: septal CT findings. J. Thorac. Imag. 18, 231.

Bamji, A., Cooke, N. 1983. Rheumatoid arthritis and chronic bronchial suppuration. Scand. J. Rheumatol. 14, 15.

Banks, J., Banks, C., Cheong, B. 1992. An epidemiological and clinical investigation of pulmonary function and respiratory symptoms in patients with rheumatoid arthritis. Q. J. Med. 85, 795.

Berkanovic, E., Oster, P., Wong, W.K. 1996. The relationship between socio-economic status and recently diagnosed rheumatoid arthritis. Arthritis Care Res. 9, 257.

Biederer, J., Schnabel, A., Muhle, C., Gross, W.L., Heller, M., Reuter, M. 2003. Correlation between HRCT findings, pulmonary function tests and bronchoalveolar lavage cytology in interstitial lung disease associated with rheumatoid arthritis. Eur. Radiol. October 14 [Epub ahead of print].

Brennan, P., Bankhead, C., Silman, A., Symmons, D.P.M. 1997. Oral contraceptives and rheumatoid arthritis: results from a primary care-based incident case-control study. Semin. Arthritis Rheum. 26, 817.

Callahan, L.F., Pincus, T. 1988. Formal education level as a significant marker of clinical status in rheumatoid arthritis. Arthritis Rheum. 31, 1346.

and the Embrel ERA Investigators Group, Simpson, K.M., and the Leflunomide Investigators Group, Strand V., Cannon, G.W., Finck, B.K. 2000. Methotrexate-induced pulmonary Disease during treatment of rheumatoid arthritis in large clinical trials. Arthritis Rheum. 43, 341.

Caplan, A. 1953. Certain unusual radiologic appearances in the chest of coal miners suffering from rheumatoid arthritis. Thorax 8, 29.

Carette, S., Marcoux, S., Gingras, S. 1989. Postmenopausal hormones and the incidence of rheumatoid arthritis. J. Rheumatol. 16, 911.

Carr, D.T., Power, M.H. 1960. Pleural fluid glucose with special reference to its concentration in rheumatoid pleurisy with effusion. Dis. Chest 37, 321.

Chakravarty, K., Webley, M. 1992. A longitudinal study of pulmonary function in patients with rheumatoid arthritis treated with gold and D-penicillamine. Br. J. Rheumatol. 31, 829.

Chang, H.K., Park, W., Ryu, D.S. 2002. Successful treatment of progressive rheumatoid interstitial lung disease with cyclosporine: a case report. J. Kor. Med. Sci. 17, 270.

Clawson, K., Oddis, C.V. 1995. Adult respiratory distress syndrome in polymyositis patients with the anti-Jo-1 antibody. Arthritis Rheum. 35, 1519.

Cohen, A.J., King, T.E., Downey, G.P. 1994. Rapidly progressive bronchiolitis obliterans with organising pneumonia. Am. J. Respir. Crit. Care Med. 149, 1670.

Cortet, B., Flipo, R.M., Remy-Jardin, M., Coquerelle, P., Duquesnoy, B., Remy, J., Delcambre, B.D. 1995. Use of high resolution computed tomography of the lungs in patients with rheumatoid arthritis. Ann. Rheum. Dis. 54, 815.

Courtney, P.A., Alderdice, J., Whitehead, E.M. 2003. Comment on methotrexate pneumonitis after initiation of infliximab therapy for rheumatoid arthritis. Arthritis Rheum. 49, 617.

Dawson, J.K., Goodson, N.G., Graham, D.R., Lynch, M.P. 2000. Raised pulmonary artery pressures with Doppler echocardiography in rheumatoid arthritis patients. Rheumatology 39, 1320.

Dawson, J.K., Graham, D.R., Desmond, J., Fewins, H.E., Lynch, M.P. 2003. Investigation of the chronic pulmonary effects of low-dose oral methotrexate in patients with rheumatoid arthritis: a prospective study incorporating HRCT scanning and pulmonary function tests. Rheumatology 42, 802.

Dawson, J.K., Fewins, H.E., Desmond, J., Lynch, M.P., Graham, D.R. 2001. Fibrosing alveolitis in patients with rheumatoid arthritis as assessed by high resolution computed tomography, chest radiography, and pulmonary function tests. Thorax 56, 622.

Denton, C.P., Black, C.M. 2003. Pulmonary hypertension in systemic sclerosis. Rheum. Dis. Clin. N. Am. 29, 335.

Despaux, J., Manzoni, P., Toussirot, E., Auge, B., Cedoz, J.P., Wendling, D. 1998. Prospective study of the prevalence of bronchiectasis in rheumatoid arthritis using high-resolution computed tomography. Revue du Rhumatisme (Engl. Ed.) 65, 453.

Dieppe, P.A. 1975. Empyema in rheumatoid arthritis. Ann. Rheum. Dis. 34, 181.

Dixon, A.S., Dixon, J., Ball, J. 1957. Honeycomb lung and chronic rheumatoid arthritis. Ann. Rheum. Dis. 16, 241.

Dodson, W.H., Hollingsworth, J.W. 1966. Pleural effusion in rheumatoid arthritis. Impaired transport of glucose. N. Engl. J. Med. 276, 1337.

Doran, M.F., Pond, G.R., Crowson, C.S., O'Fallon, W.M., Gabriel, S.E. 2002. Trends in incidence and mortality in rheumatoid arthritis in Rochester, Minnesota, over a forty-year period. Arthritis Rheum. 46, 625.

Doyle, J.J., Eliasson, A.H., Argyros, G.J., Dennis, G.J., Finger, D.R., Hurwitz, K.M., Phillips, Y.Y. 2000. Prevalence of pulmonary disorders in patients with newly diagnosed rheumatoid arthritis. Clin. Rheumatol. 19, 217.

Epler, G.R., Colby, T.V., McCloud, T.C., Carrington, C.B., Gaensler, E.A. 1985. Bronchiolitis obliterans organising pneumonia. N. Engl. J. Med. 312, 152.

Farrell, A.J., Blake, D.R. 1996. Nitric oxide. Ann. Rheum. Dis. 55, 7.

Feagler, J.R., Sorenson, G.D., Rosenfeld, M.G., Osterland, C.K. 1971. Rheumatoid pleural effusion. Arch. Pathol. 92, 257.

Fujii, M., Adachi, S., Shimizu, T., Hirota, S., Sako, M., Kono, M. 1993. Interstitial lung disease in rheumatoid arthritis: assessment with high resolution computed tomography. J. Thoracic Imag. 8, 54.

Gabbay, E., Tarala, R., Will, R., Carroll, G., Adler, B., Cameron, D., Lake, F.R. 1997. Interstitial lung disease in recent onset rheumatoid arthritis. Am. J. Crit. Care Med. 156, 528.

Garcia, J.G., Munim, A., Nugent, K.M., Bishop, M., Hoie-Garcia, P., Parhami, N., Keogh, B.A. 1987. Alveolar macrophage gold retention in rheumatoid arthritis. J. Rheumatol. 14, 435.

Geddes, D.M., Corrin, B., Brewerton, D.A., Davies, R.J., Turner-Warwick, M. 1977. Progressive airway obliteration in adults and its association with rheumatoid disease. Q. J. Med. 184, 427.

Gilligen, D.M., O'Connor, C.M., Ward, K. 1990. Bronchoalveolar lavage in patients with mild and severe rheumatoid lung disease. Thorax 45, 591.

Gregersen, P.K., Silver, J., Winchester, R.J. 1987. The shared epitope hypothesis. An approach to understanding the molecular genetics of susceptibility to rheumatoid arthritis. Arthritis Rheum. 30, 1205.

Gomez-Reino, J.J., Carmona, L., Valverde, V.R., Mola, E.M., Montero, M.D. 2003. Treatment of rheumatoid arthritis with tumour necrosis factor inhibitors may predispose to significant increase in tuberculosis risk: a multicenter active-suveillance report. Arthritis Rheum. 48, 2122.

Gordon, D.A., Stein, J.L., Broder, I. 1973. The extra-articular features of rheumatoid arthritis. A systematic analysis of 127 cases. Am. J. Med. 54, 445.

Hakala, M. 1988. Poor prognosis in patients with rheumatoid arthritis hospitalised for interstitial lung fibrosis. Chest 93, 114.

Heliövaara, M., Aho, K., Aromma, A., Knekt, P., Reunanen, A. 1993. Smoking and risk of rheumatoid arthritis. J. Rheumatol. 20, 1830.

Hillarby, M.C., McMahon, M.J., Grennan, D.M., Cooper R.G., Clarkson, R.W., Davies, E.J., Sanders, P.A., Chattopadhyay, C., Swinson, D. 1993. HLA associations in subjects with rheumatoid arthritis and bronchiectasis but not with other pulmonary complications of rheumatoid disease. Br. J. Rheumatol. 32, 794.

Hunninghake, G.W., Fauci, A.S. 1979. Pulmonary involvement in collagen vascular disesases. Am. Rev. Respir. Dis. 119, 471.

Hutchinson, D., Shepstone, L., Moots, R., Lear, J.T., Lynch, M.P. 2001. Heavy cigarette smoking is strongly associated with rheumatoid arthritis (RA), particularly in patients without a family history of RA. Ann. Rheum. Dis. 60, 223.

Imanaka, T., Shichikawa, K., Inoue, K., Shimaoka, Y., Takenaka, Y. 1997. Increase in age at onset of rheumatoid arthritis in Japan over a 30 year period. Ann. Rheum. Dis. 56, 313.

Joseph, J., Sahn, S.A. 1993. Connective tissue disease and the pleura. Chest 1904, 262.

Karim, M.Y., Miranda, L.C., Tench, C.M., Gordon, P.A., D'Cruz, D.P., Khamashata, M.A., Hughes, G.R. 2002. Presentation and prognosis of the shrinking lung syndrome in systemic lupus erythematosus. Sem. Arthritis Rheum. 31, 289.

Karlson, E.W., Lee, I.-Min., Cook, N.R., Manson, J.E., Buring, J.E., Hennekens, C.H. 1999. A retrospective cohort study of cigarette smoking and risk of rheumatoid arthritis in female health professionals. Arthritis Rheum. 42, 910.

Keane, J., Gershon, S., Wise, R.P., Mirabile-Levens, E., Kasznica, J., Schwieterman, W.D., Siegel, J.N., Braun, M.M. 2001. Tuberculosis associated with Infliximab, a tumour necrosis factor alpha-neutralizing agent. N. Engl. J. Med. 345, 1098.

King, T.E. Jr. 1998. Interstitial lung diesease. In: M.I. Schwarz, T.E. King, Jr. (Eds.), Connective tissue disease, 3rd edn., BC Decker, Hamilton, Ont., Canada, p. 451.

Krebs, S., Gibbons, R.B. 1996. Low-dose methotrexate as a risk factor for *Pneumocystis carinii* pneumonia. Mil. Med. 161, 58.

Lawrence, R.C., Hochberg, M.C., Kelsey, J.L., McDuffie, F.C., Medsger, T.A. Jr., Felts, W.R., Shulman, L.E. 1989. Estimates of the prevalence of selected arthritic and musculoskeletal diseases in the United States. J. Rheumatol. 16, 427.

Leigh, J.P., Fries, J.F. 1991. Mortality predictors among 263 patients with rheumatoid arthritis. J. Rheumatol. 18, 1307.

Light, R. 1990. Pleural disease due to collagen vascular disease, 2nd edn., Pleural Diseases, Lea & Febiger, Philadelphia.

Lillington, G.A., Carr, D.T., Mayne, J.G. 1971. Rheumatoid pleurisy with effusion. Arch. Int. Med. 128, 764.

Maini, R.V., Zvaifler, N.J. 1998. Rheumatoid arthritis and other synovial disorders. In: J.H. Klippel, P.A. Dieppe (Eds.), Rheumatology, 2nd edn., Mosby, London.

Másdóttir, B., Jónsson, T., Manfreðsdóttir, V., Víkingsson, A., Brekkan, Á., Valdimarsson, H. 2000. Smoking, rheumatoid factor isotypes and severity of rheumatoid arthritis. Rheumatology 39, 1202.

Mattey, D.L., Hassell, A.B., Plant, M., Dawes, P.T., Ollier, W.R., Jones, P.W., Fryer, A.A., Alldersea, J.E., Strange, R.C. 1999. Association of polymorphism in glutathione S-transferase loci with susceptibility and outcome in rheumatoid arthritis: comparison with shared epitope. Ann. Rheum. Dis. 57, 164.

Mattey, D.L., Hutchinson, D., Dawes, P.T., Nixon, N.B., Clarke, S., Fisher, J., Brownfield, A., Alldersea, J., Fryer, A.A., Strange, R.C. 2002. Smoking and disease severity in rheumatoid arthritis. Arthritis Rheum. 46, 640.

Mayordomo, L., Marenco, J.L., Gomez-Mateos, J., Rejon, E. 2002. Pulmonary military tuberculosis in a patient with anti-TNF-alpha treatment. Scand. J. Rheumatol. 31, 44.

McEntegart, A., Capell, H.A., Creran, D., Rumsley, A., Woodward, M., Lowe, G.D.O. 2001. Cardiovascular risk factors, including thrombotic variables, in a population with rheumatoid arthritis. Rheumatology 40, 640.

Miyata, M., Sakuma, F., Fukayam, E., Kobayashi, H., Rai, T., Saito, H., Kasukawa, R., Suzuki, S. 2002. Detection and monitoring of methotrexate-associated lung injury using serum markers KL-6 and SP-D in rheumatoid arthritis. Intern. Med. 41, 467.

Muller, N.L., Miller, R.R. 1995. Diseases of the bronchioles: CT and histopathologic findings. Radiology 196, 3.

Nanki, N., Fujita, J., Yamaji, Y., Maeda, H., Kurose, T., Kaji M. 2002. Nonspecific interstitial pneumonia/fibrosis completely recovered by adding cyclophosphamide to corticosteroids. Intern. Med. 41, 867.

Nicholas, N.S., Panayi, G.S. 1988. RA and pregnancy. Clin. Exp. Rheumatol. 6, 179.

Nived, O., Sturfelt, G., Wollheim, F. 1985. Systemic lupus erythematosus and infection: a controlled and prospective study including an epidemiological group. Q. J. Med. 55, 271.

Ohosone, Y., Okano, Y., Kameda, H., Fujii, T., Hama, N. Hirakata, M., Mimori, T. 1997. Clinical characteristics of patients with rheumatoid arthritis and methotrexate induced pneumonitis. J. Rheumatol. 24, 2299.

Parry, S.D., Barbatzas, C., Peel, E.T., Barton, J.R. 2002. Sulphasalazine and lung toxicity. Eur. Respir. J. 19, 756.

Peno-Green, L., Lluberas, G., Kingsley, T., Brantley, S. 2002. Lung injury linked to etanercept therapy. Chest 122, 1858.

Perez, T., Remy-Jardin, M., Cortet, B. 1998. Airways involvement in rheumatoid arthritis: clinical, functional, and HRCT findings. Am. J. Respir. Crit. Care Med. 157, 1658.

Persson, L.O., Berglund, K., Sahlberg, D. 1999. Psychological factors in chronic rheumatic diseases—a review. The case of rheumatoid arthritis, current research and some problems. Scand. J. Rheumatol. 28, 137.

Puechal, X., Fajac, I., Bienvenu, T., Desmazes-Dufeu, N., Hubert, D., Kaplan, J.C., Menkes, C.J., Dusser, D.J. 1999. Increased frequency of cystic fibrosis deltaF508 mutation in bronchiectasis associated with rheumatoid arthritis. Eur. Respir. J. 13, 1281.

Puttick, M.P., Klinkhoff, A.V., Chalmers, A., Ostrow, D.N. 1995. Treatment of progressive rheumatoid interstitial lung disease with cyclosporine. J. Rheumatol. 22, 2163.

Rajasekaran, B.A., Shovlin, D., Lord, P., Kelly, C.A. 2001. Interstitial lung disease in patients with rheumatoid arthritis: a comparison with cryptogenic fibrosing alveolitis. Rheumatology 40, 1022.

Reckner Olsson, Å., Skogh, T., Wingren, G. 2001. Comorbidity and lifestyle, reproductive factors, and environmental exposures associated with rheumatoid arthritis. Ann. Rheum. Dis. 60, 934.

Rees, J.H., Woodhead, M.A., Sheppard, M.N., du Boiss, R.M., Remy-Jardin, M. 1991. Rheumatoid arthritis and cryptogenic organising pneumonitis. Respir. Med. 85, 243.

Remy-Jardin, M., Remy, J., Cortet, B., Mauri, F., Delcambre, M. 1994. Lung changes in rheumatoid arthritis: CT findings. Radiology 193, 375.

Riegert-Johnson, D.L., Godfrey, J.A., Myers, J.L., Hubmayr, R.D., Sandborn, W.J., Loftus, E.V. Jr. 2002. Delayed hypersensitivity reaction and acute respiratory distress syndrome following infliximab infusion. Inflamm. Bowel Dis. 8, 186.

Roschmann, R.A., Rothenberg, R.J. 1987. Pulmonary fibrosis in rheumatoid arthritis: a review of clinical features and therapy. Semin. Arthritis Rheum. 16, 174.

Saag, K.G., Cerhan, J.R., Kolluri, S., Ohashi, K., Hunninghake, G.W., Schwartz, D.A. 1997. Cigarette smoking and rheumatoid arthritis severity. Ann. Rheum. Dis. 56, 463.

Salaffi, F., Manganelli, P., Carotti, M., Lamanna, G., Cervini, C. 1997. Methotrexate-induced pneumonitis in patients with rheumatoid arthritis and psoriatic arthritis: report of five cases and review of the literature. Clin. Rheumatol. 16, 296.

Schnabel, A., Dalhoff, K., Bauerfeind, S., Barth, J., Gross, W.L. 1996. Sustained cough in methotrexate therapy for rheumatoid arthritis. Clin. Rheumatol. 15, 277.

Schnabel, A., Richter, C., Bauerfeind, S., Gross, W.L. 1997. Bronchoalveolar lavage cell profile in methotrexate induced pneumonitis. Thorax 52, 377.

Scott, D.G.I., Bacon, P.A., Tribe, C.R. 1981. Systemic rheumatoid vasculitis: a clinical and laboratory study of 50 cases. Medicine (Baltimore) 60, 288.

Scott, D.L., Brady, G.V., Aitman, T.J., Zaphiropoulos, G.C., Hawkins, C.F. 1981. Relationship of gold and penicillamine therapy to diffuse interstitial lung disease. Ann. Rheum. Dis. 40, 136.

Shannon, T.M., Gale, M.E. 1992. Noncardiac manifestations of rheumatoid arthritis in the thorax. J. Thoracic Imag. 7, 19.

Silman, A.J., Newman, J., MacGregor, A.J. 1996. Cigarette smoking increases the risk of rheumatoid arthritis. Arthritis Rheum. 39, 732.

Sinha, A., Silverstone, E.J., O'Sullivan, M.M. 2001. Gold-induced pneumonitis: computed tomography findings in a patient with rheumatoid arthritis. Rheumatology 40, 7.

Söderblom, T., Pettersson, T., Nyberg, P., Teppo, A.M., Linko, L., Riska, H. 1999. High pleural fluid hyaluronan concentrations in rheumatoid arthritis. Eur. Respir. J. 13, 519.

Stein, H.B., Patterson, A.C., Offer, R.C. 1980. Adverse effects of D-penicillamine in rheumatoid arthritis. Ann. Intern. Med. 92, 24.

Stolt, P., Bengtsson, C., Nordmark, B., Lindblad, S., Lundberg, I., Klareskog, L., Alfredsson, L. and the other members of the EIRA study group 2003. Quantification of the influence of cigarette smoking on rheumatoid arthritis: results from a population based case-control study using incident cases. Ann. Rheum. Dis. 62, 835.

Suwa, A., Hirakata, M., Satoh, S., Mimori, T., Utsumi, K., Inada, S. 1999. Rheumatoid arthritis associated with methotrexate-induced pneumonitis: improvement with IV cyclophosphamide therapy. Clin. Exp. Rheumatol. 17, 355.

Swinson, D.R., Symmons, D., Suresh, U., Jones, M., Booth, J. 1997. Decreased survival in patients with co-existent rheumatoid arthritis and bronchiectasis. Br. J. Rheumatol. 36, 689.

Symmons, D.P.M., Bankhead, C.R., Harrison, B.J., Brennan, P., Barrett, E.M., Scott, D.G.I., Silman, A.J. 1997. Blood transfusion, smoking, and obesity as risk factors for the development of rheumatoid arthritis. Arthritis Rheum. 40, 1955.

Tanoue, L. 1998. Pulmonary Manifestations of Rheumatoid Arthritis. Clin. Chest Med. 19, 667.

Tomioka, R., King, T.E. Jr. 1997. Gold-induced pulmonary disease: clinical features, outcome and differentiation from rheumatoid lung disease. Am. J. Respir. Crit. Care 153, 1011.

Tuomi, T., Heliövarra, M., Palosuo, T., Aho, K. 1990. Smoking, lung function, and rheumatoid factors. Ann. Rheum. Dis. 49, 753.

Turesson, C., O'Fallon, W.M., Crowson, C.S., Gabriel, S.E., Matteson, E.L. 2003. Extra-articular disease manifestations in rheumatoid arthritis: incidence trends and risk factors over 46 years. Ann. Rheum. Dis. 62, 722.

Vandenbroucke, J.P., Witteman, J.C., Valkenburg, H.A., Boersma, J.W., Cats, A., Festen, J.J., Hartman, A.P., Huber-Bruning, O., Rasker, J.J., Weber, J. 1986. Noncontraceptive hormones and rheumatoid arthritis in perimenopausal and postmenopausal women. JAMA 255, 1299.

Vassallo, R., Matteson, E., Thomas, C.F. Jr. 2003. Clinical response of rheumatoid arthritis-associated fibrosis to tumour necrosis factor-alpha inhibition. Chest 122, 1093.

Walker, W.C., Wright, V. 1968. Pulmonary lesions and rheumatoid arthritis. Medicine 47, 501.

Walport, M.J., Ollier, W.E.R., Silman, A.J. 1992. Immunogenetics of rheumatoid arthritis and the Arthritis and Rheumatism Council's National Repository. Br. J. Rheumatol. 31, 701.

Weyand, C.M., Schmidt, D., Wager, U., Goronzy, J.J. 1998. The influence of sex on the phenotype of rheumatoid arthritis. Arthritis Rheum. 41, 817.

White, B. 2003. Interstitial lung disease in scleroderma. Rheum. Dis. Clin. N. Am. 29, 371.

Wiedemann, H.P., Matthay, R.A. 1992. Pulmonary manifestations of systemic lupus erythematosus. J. Thorac. Imag. 7, 1.

Wisnieski, J.J., Askari, A.D. 1981. Rheumatoid nodulosis. A relatively benign rheumatoid variant. Arch. Intern. Med. 141, 615.

Wolfe, F. 1996. The natural history of rheumatoid arthritis. J. Rheumatol. 23 (Suppl. 44), 13.

Wolfe, F. 2000. The effect of smoking on clinical, laboratory and radiographic status in rheumatoid arthritis. Arthritis Rheum. 27, 630.

Yazici, Y., Kagan, L.J. 2002. Clinical presentation of the idiopathic inflammatory myopathies. Rheum. Dis. Clin. N. Am. 28, 823.

Yousem, S.A., Colby, T.V., Carrington, C.B. 1985. Lung biopsy in rheumatoid arthritis. Am. Rev. Respir. Dis. 131, 770.

Yukioka, M., Wakitani, S., Murata, N., Toda, Y., Ogawa, R., Kaneshige, T., Ochi, T. 1998. Elderly onset rheumatoid arthritis and its association with HLA-DRB1 alleles in Japanese. Br. J. Rheumatol. 37, 98.

Zitnik, R.J., Cooper, J.A.D. 1990. Pulmonary disease due to antirheumatic agents. Clin. Chest Med. 111, 139.

Zilnik, R.J. 1997. Drug induced lung disease due to nonchemotherapeutic agents. In: A.P. Fishman (Ed.), Pulmonary Diseases and Disorders. McGraw Hill, New York, p. 1017.

Zisman, D.A., McCune, W.J., Tino, G., Lynch, J.P. 3rd 2001. Drug-induced pneumonitis: the role of methotrexate. Sarcoidosis Vasc. Diffuse Lung Dis. 18, 243.

Handbook of Systemic Autoimmune Diseases, Volume 2
Pulmonary Involvement in Systemic Autoimmune Diseases
A.U. Wells and C.P. Denton, editors

CHAPTER 9

Sjögren's Syndrome and the Lung

Spyros A. Papiris[a,1], Haralampos M. Moutsopoulos[b,*]

[a]*Department of Critical Care and Pulmonary Services, 45–47 Ipsilantou Str., "Evangelismos Hospital", School of Medicine, National and Kapodistrian University of Athens, GR 10675, Athens, Greece*

[b]*Department of Pathophysiology, "Laiko Hospital", School of Medicine, National and Kapodistrian University of Athens, 76 M. Asias Str., Goudi, GR 11527, Athens, Greece.*

1. Introduction

Sjögren's syndrome, an autoimmune epithelitis, is a chronic, slowly progressive inflammatory autoimmune disease, characterized by lymphocytic infiltration of the exocrine glands and epithelia in multiple sites, leading to diminished or absent glandular secretions and to a more or less generalized, mucosal dryness (Moutsopoulos et al., 1980; Talal et al., 1987; Moutsopoulos, 1994; Moutsopoulos, 2001). Sjögren's syndrome presents with a wide spectrum: from lacrimal and salivary exocrinopathy to systemic disease (lungs, liver, kidneys, and other organs or tissues), and, later in the illness and in a small number of patients (≈5%), an associated B-cell lymphoid malignancy (Bunim and Talal, 1963; Kassan et al., 1978; Royer et al., 1997; Voulgarelis et al., 1999). Sjögren's syndrome can occur alone (primary Sjögren's syndrome) or in association with almost all of the other rheumatic autoimmune disorders (secondary Sjögren's syndrome) (Moutsopoulos et al., 1980). The co-existing rheumatic disease may be already present at the time of diagnosis of Sjögren's syndrome, or may later become apparent. Pulmonary manifestations have been reported in both the primary and the secondary forms of the syndrome (Alarcón-Segovia et al., 1965; Kelly et al., 1991; Cairns et al., 1992). In the latter case the co-existing rheumatic disorder influences the pattern of pulmonary expression (Papiris et al., 1999a).

Pulmonary involvement was first recognized 60 years ago, by Henrik Sjögren (1933), who described similar histopathological changes in the exocrine glands of the bronchi to those commonly observed in the salivary glands. Since then, pulmonary involvement in primary Sjögren's syndrome has been the subject of various studies and several pulmonary manifestations have been described, including bronchial and bronchiolar disease, interstitial pneumonia, and a spectrum of lymphoproliferative diseases (Table 1). However, pulmonary manifestations, though frequent and pleomorphic, are rarely clinically severe (Hunninghake and Fauci, 1979; Segal et al., 1981; Constantopoulos et al., 1985; Papathanasiou et al., 1986; Gardiner, 1993; Papiris et al., 1999a; Cain et al., 1998; Davidson et al., 2000).

In primary Sjögren's syndrome, some discrepancy in the available literature still exists concerning the frequency, the pattern of abnormalities, and the clinical significance of the respiratory involvement. This may be attributed to the fact that previous studies

[1]Tel.: +30-2107201952; fax: + 30-2107293470
E-mail address: papiris@otenet.gr (S.A. Papiris)

*Corresponding author.
Tel.: +30-2107771095/89480; fax: +30-2107462664
E-mail address: hmoutsop@med.uoa.gr (H.M. Moutsopoulos).

DOI: 10.1016/S1571-5078(04)02009-4

Table 1
Respiratory manifestations in Sjögren's syndrome

Upper airways disease
Nasal mucosa infiltration and dryness ('rhina sicca')
Epistaxis
Sinusitis
Oral cavity major and minor salivary glands involvement (xerostomia)
Lymphocytic infiltration of the tracheobronchial submucosal glands (xerotrachea)
Subepithelial bronchial and bronchiolar lymphocytic infiltration (lymphocytic bronchitis/bronchiolitis)
Bronchial hyperresponsiveness
Lymphoproliferative disorders
Diffuse lymphoid hyperplasia of the lungs
Peribronchiolar (reactive lymphoid hyperplasia/follicular bronchiolitis)
Diffuse alveolar interstitial, (lymphoid interstitial pneumonia, LIP)
Pseudolymphoma
Lymphomatoid granulomatosis.
Malignant B-cell non-Hodgkin's lymphoma
Other diffuse interstitial pneumonias
Pulmonary fibrosis, usual interstitial pneumonia (UIP) type
Non-specific interstitial pneumonia (NSIP)
Cryptogenic organizing pneumonia (COP)
Diffuse panbronchiolitis
Multiple lung cysts or bullae
Vasculitis and primary pulmonary hypertension
Pulmonary amyloidosis
Pleural disease (mainly in the secondary Sjögren's syndrome)

have focused on a single abnormality, included exclusively symptomatic patients, or have failed to distinguish between primary and secondary disease (Gardiner, 1993; Cain et al., 1998; Papiris et al., 1999a).

2. Prevalence

The prevalence of primary Sjögren's syndrome is approximately 0.5–1% in the general population, and 10–30% in patients with other rheumatic autoimmune disorders. The prevalence of respiratory involvement in Sjögren's syndrome can be estimated from a number of manifestations, such as symptoms (cough, dyspnea) (Constantopoulos et al., 1985; Mialon et al., 1997), functional (Kelly et al., 1991) or radiological abnormalities (Franquet et al., 1997; Uffmann et al., 2001), and bronchoalveolar lavage findings (Hatron et al., 1987; Dalavanga et al., 1991). Therefore, any statement of prevalence is influenced by methodology and also by the referral values used. In one of the largest series to date, Kelly et al. (1991), performing standard spirometry and measurement of diffusing capacity, and using standardized residuals to control values, reported abnormal pulmonary function in 24 of 100 unselected patients with primary Sjögren's syndrome.

3. Epidemiology

Sjögren's syndrome affects predominantly middle-aged women (female-to-male ratio 9:1) although it occurs in all ages, including childhood. Accordingly, respiratory manifestations are present, almost exclusively, in middle-aged women.

4. Etiology/Pathogenesis

This generalized exocrinopathy is associated with dense lymphocytic infiltrates of glandular tissues and a marked B lymphocytic cell hyperreactivity which is manifested by various serum autoantibodies directed against non-organ specific antigens such as immunoglobulins (rheumatoid factor) or extractable nuclear and cytoplasmic antigens (Ro/SSA, La/SSB). The majority of tissues infiltrating lymphocytes, including those of the airways (Papiris et al., 1997), are CD4 T-cells (Adamson et al., 1983) that bear the α/β T-cell receptor (TCR) and express various markers of activation, including class II major histocompatibility complex (MHC) HLA-DR proteins, adhesion molecules, and the cytokines interleukin-2 (IL-2) and interferon-γ (IFN-γ) (Fox et al., 1985; Moutsopoulos et al., 1986; Brookes et al., 1995).

Several lines of evidence indicate that epithelial cells may have a critical role in the induction and perpetuation of the immune responses in the inflamed tissues. The glandular epithelial cells of patients with Sjögren's syndrome display an activated phenotype. They inappropriately express the oncogenes c-myc and p53 (Skopouli et al., 1992; Tapinos et al., 1999), whereas the expression of nuclear autoantigenic proteins (La/SSB) is translocated to the cell-surface (Yannopoulos et al., 1992; De Wilde et al., 1996;

Haneji et al., 1997). Furthermore, in patients with Sjögren's syndrome, the glandular epithelial cells express molecules implicated in the lymphoid recruitment and in the expansion of the inflammation, such as the lymphoattractant chemokines BCA-1, ELC, STCP-1/MDC, SLC and TARC (Xanthou et al., 2001), ICAM-1 adhesion molecules (Kapsogeorgou et al., 2001), and the proinflammatory cytokines IL-1, IL-6 and tumor necrosis factor-α (TNFα) (Boumpa et al., 1995). Most importantly, glandular epithelial cells of Sjögren's syndrome patients appear suitably equipped for the presentation of antigenic peptides and the transmittance of activation signals to T-cells. They express MHC class I and class II molecules (Moutsopoulos et al., 1986; Lindahl et al., 1985; Fox et al., 1986), functional B7 costimulatory molecules (Manoussakis et al., 1999; Kapsogeorgou et al., 2001), and CD40 molecules (Dimitriou et al., 2002). These phenomena support the capacity of the epithelial cells of the exocrine glands to act as non-classic antigen-presenting cells and most likely indicate that they are actively involved in the regulation of the local immune responses and the pathogenesis of Sjögren's syndrome.

Programmed cell death, or apoptosis, is considered to be an important pathogenetic mechanism in various autoimmune disorders, by which intracellular auto-antigens are presented to the immune system. In Sjögren's syndrome, apoptotic processes are thought to play a major role in the destruction of the salivary epithelia. Increased apoptosis is detected in the salivary gland tissues obtained from Sjögren's syndrome patients by DNA fragmentation and TUNEL assay (Polichronis et al., 1998). The increased expression of Fas (Apo1/CD95) protein and its ligand (FasL/CD95L) among the epithelial cells of patients suggest their intervention in the apoptotic mechanisms that operate in epithelial cells (Kong et al., 1997; Polichronis et al., 1998; Matsumura et al., 1998; Fujihara et al., 1999; HumphreysBeher et al., 1999; Abu-Helu et al., 2001). The expression of anti-apoptotic Bcl-2 molecules (Polichronis et al., 1998), as well as apoptosis-inducing enzymes (perforin, granzymes) (Xanthou et al., 1999) by the infiltrating lymphocytes most likely indicates their role in the induction of epithelial destruction. Moreover, recent data from studies on cultured salivary gland epithelial cells attest the injurious role of T-cell derived cytokines, which are produced in the inflammatory glandular lesions of Sjögren's syndrome patients and particularly that of IFNγ, in the survival of epithelial tissues (Abu-Helu et al., 2001). Such noxious effects were demonstrated to occur through the induction of Fas-mediated programmed cell death and anoikia only if IFNγ is present (Abu-Helu et al., 2001).

5. Clinical manifestations

5.1. Upper airways involvement

'Rhina sicca', dryness and crusting of the nasal mucosa, is not an uncommon complaint of patients with Sjögren's syndrome. Epistaxis and sinusitis may occasionally occur, and are considered complications of nasal dryness and crusting (Case records of the Massachusetts General Hospital, 2001). Xerostomia, due to involvement of the major and minor salivary glands of the oral cavity, is one of the most classic manifestations of Sjögren's syndrome. Dryness also extends to the pharynx. However, upper airways involvement does not appear to have any significant respiratory implications.

5.2. Lower airways involvement

5.2.1. Large airways involvement

The lower airways appear to be a frequent respiratory target in well-classified patients with primary Sjögren's syndrome. Indeed, the most common clinical manifestation of airways involvement in primary Sjögren's syndrome is a dry cough of variable intensity, which may be observed in up to 50% of patients (Mialon et al., 1997). A 'sicca' cough is usually considered the result of the desiccation of the tracheobronchial tree ('xero-trachea' from the Greek ξηρός = dry) due to the involvement of the bronchial glands by the inflammatory process (Ellman and Parkes Weber, 1949; Ellman et al., 1951; Constantopoulos et al., 1984). Inflammatory cell infiltration of the submucosal glands of the large airways (bronchial inflammatory exocrinopathy) was first described 60 years ago by Sjögren (1933). However, very few studies have since attempted to characterize systematically the histopathological changes and/or the pattern of the cellular infiltrate at glandular or extraglandular sites of the large airways. Andoh et al. (1993) in a study of six autopsied patients with Sjögren's syndrome (two with primary and four with secondary Sjögren's syndrome) reported hyperplasia of airway secretory cells and submucosal glands, suggesting that airways exocrine gland destruction may not be invariably present (or at least may not be present at all phases of the course of disease), and that factors other than exocrine gland destruction may be related to the presence of a cough in at least some of these patients. Furthermore, Papiris et al. (1997) performed endobronchial biopsies and studied the extraglandular cellular infiltrate of large bronchi of patients with Sjögren's syndrome (six with the primary and four with the secondary form of the syndrome) using histochemistry and immunohistochemistry. The pathology showed an increased number of CD4 positive T lymphocytes in the lamina propria (defined as the 100μ beneath the subepithelial basement membrane) of the bronchial mucosa of the large airways, outside of the bronchial submucosal glands, suggesting that in Sjögren's syndrome in the large airways the same infiltrate that is observed in the major salivary glands may also involve the subepithelial extraglandular tissues (lymphocytic bronchitis). However, further studies are necessary to characterize better the pattern and significance of the involvement of large airways in Sjögren's syndrome.

5.2.2. Small airways involvement

All patterns of functional abnormalities (obstructive, restrictive, and mixed) in patients with primary Sjögren's syndrome have been described in the available literature (Gardiner, 1993; Cain et al., 1998). This might reflect, in part, the pleomorphy of lung involvement (airways and/or parenchymal disease) as well as failure to distinguish between the primary and the secondary forms of the disease. In our experience and in that of others, probably the most frequent functional abnormality in well-selected patients with primary Sjögren's syndrome is small airways obstruction, which is usually mild. Constantopoulos et al. (1985) reported, in eight out of 36 patients with primary Sjögren's syndrome, isolated small airways obstruction with significantly diminished maximal expiratory flows at 25% of vital capacity (MEF_{25}) and suggestive flow-volume curves. Segal et al. (1981) found obstructive abnormalities in nine out of 13 patients with primary Sjögren's syndrome. Newball and Brahim (1977) reported airways obstruction in six out of 13 patients with primary Sjögren's syndrome. Papiris et al. (1999b), in a controlled study, found a high prevalence of mild obstructive abnormalities in a large population of 61 non-smoking patients with primary Sjögren's syndrome, using the MEF_{50}, and the MEF_{25} as sensitive indices to detect minor degrees of small airways obstruction. Lahdensuo et al. (1995) detected, in half of their patients with primary Sjögren's syndrome, pulmonary hyperinflation as defined by a higher residual volume to total lung capacity ratio (RV/TLC), in association with diminished peripheral flows. Mialon et al. (1997) reported reduced MEF_{25} in 72% of patients, also suggesting peripheral airways obstruction. Small airways obstruction in patients with primary Sjögren's syndrome is probably the result of a chronic mononuclear cell infiltration (lymphocytic bronchiolitis) around the small bronchioles with or without hyperplasia of the bronchus-associated lymphoid tissue (BALT) (Ellman et al., 1951; Newball and Brahim, 1977; Sutinen et al., 1977; Constantopoulos et al., 1985; Cairns et al., 1992; Gardiner et al., 1993; Yousem et al., 1985; Colby, 1998). However, as a result of the indolent course of the disease in the majority, relatively few patients have been studied histologically and there is a lack of sufficient data in the literature regarding the morphological status of both small and large airways in patients with primary Sjögren's syndrome. Bronchial hyperresponsiveness of uncertain clinical and pathogenetic significance has also been described in Sjögren's syndrome patients (Potena et al., 1990; Gudbjörnsson et al., 1991).

5.2.3. Clinical implications and pathogenetic considerations of lower airways involvement

Lymphocytic bronchitis/bronchiolitis in primary Sjögren's syndrome, though frequent, is rarely clinically important and does not seem to predispose to infective exacerbations. Mialon et al. (1997) describe a low prevalence of recurrent respiratory infection. The diagnosis of Sjögren's related bronchitis/bronchiolitis may be difficult since the small airways represent the 'silent zone' of the lung, and large airways involvement does not seem to significantly influence lung volumes and flows. Abnormalities may also be absent on conventional chest radiograms and diffuse or focal signs of hyperinflation and air trapping are only observed in the most severe cases, which is uncommon in primary Sjögren's syndrome. High-resolution computerized tomography (HRCT) lung scanning with additional expiratory images is more sensitive, and suggestive diagnostic findings of bronchiolar involvement include bronchiolar wall thickening with a 'tree-in-bud' appearance, peribronchial nodules, bronchiolectasis/bronchiectasis, mosaic perfusion, air trapping, and cystic lesions. Simple spirometry is usually normal and more sophisticated physiologic maneuvers such as expiratory airflow at low lung volumes, closing volumes, and dynamic compliance may be necessary to detect small airways involvement. Histologic confirmation by transbronchial or preferably by video-assisted lung biopsy is required for confident diagnosis only when the coexistence of other lung complications, such as follicular bronchiolitis and/or any form of interstitial pneumonia, or lymphoma development is suspected (Papiris et al., 1999a).

The pathogenetic significance of lymphocytic bronchitis/bronchiolitis in primary Sjögren's syndrome remains obscure. Lymphocytic infiltrates outside the salivary and lacrimal glands have been also described in other tissues such as the liver and kidneys. Renal biopsies of patients with Sjögren's syndrome show focal lymphocytic infiltrates around tubules that extend and occupy the interstitium, resulting clinically in a tubular defect with or without acidosis (Siamopoulos et al., 1986). Skopouli et al. (1994) reported that the main histopathological finding in the liver biopsies of patients with Sjögren's syndrome and circulating antimitochondrial antibodies and/or elevated liver enzymes is a lymphocytic infiltration around cholangial ducts similar to that found in stage I biliary cirrhosis.

5.2.4. Current theory

Moutsopoulos (1994) proposed that Sjögren's syndrome should be referred to as 'Autoimmune Epithelitis' and advanced the hypothesis that the extraglandular manifestations in Sjögren's syndrome might be related to the attraction by immune effector cells to epithelia, such as those of renal tubules, bronchi and cholangial ducts, that maintain an exocrine function or, at least, have common ion transporting properties. These epithelia might share common antigens with the exocrine glands that appear to attract the 'attention' of the immune system, which mounts a cellular and humoral immune response against these molecules, leading to dysfunction and disease. According to this concept, at least some of the extraglandular manifestations of the disease (lung, kidney, and liver involvement) might not represent a strictly extraglandular localization of the disease, but might be part of the generalized exocrine dysfunction observed in the syndrome. Carbonic anhydrase II, a basic metalloenzyme important for the regulation of acid–base status (Spicer et al., 1984; Okazaki et al., 1989; Inagaki et al., 1991; Nishimori et al., 1993, 1994, 1995) and alpha-fodrin, an actin-binding protein found at the periphery of chromaffin cells involved in secretion (Haneji et al., 1997), are among the candidate autoantigens in Sjögren's syndrome. Although this hypothesis is very intriguing, further studies are necessary to clarify the detailed pathogenetic mechanisms of the extraglandular manifestations in Sjögren's syndrome, and to determine the relationship between the respiratory tract and other sites of involvement.

5.3. Lymphoproliferative diseases

Sjögren's syndrome is at the crossroads of autoimmune disease and lymphoid malignancy since it may express a spectrum of lymphoproliferative diseases. Infiltrative lung lesions in which the lymphocytes are the main cellular component, as in Sjögren's syndrome, include a divergent group of disorders spanning a spectrum from inflammatory lesions to malignant neoplasms (Colby and Carrington, 1983). Minor lymphocytic proliferation in the lung is thought to derive from BALT. In Sjögren's syndrome, lung lymphoproliferative diseases range from benign to malignant lymphomatous infiltration, including diffuse lymphoid hyperplasia of the lungs, which may be peribronchiolar (reactive lymphoid hyperplasia/follicular bronchiolitis) and/or alveolar interstitial (lymphocytic interstitial pneumonia, LIP), pseudolymphoma, lymphomatoid granulomatosis, and malignant (usually B-cell non-Hodgkin's) lymphoma (Bunim and Talal, 1963; Kassan et al., 1978; Zulman et al., 1978; Yousem et al., 1985; Anderson and Talal, 1972; Bonner et al., 1973; Liebow and Carrington, 1973; Fortul et al., 1985; Katzenstein, 1997; Royer et al., 1997; Kobayashi et al., 1988; Voulgarelis et al., 1999; Mariette, 1999). The evolution from benign lymphocytic infiltration to malignant non-Hodgkin's lymphoma is probably a multistep process, the underlying molecular events of which are still unknown.

Small, usually inconspicuous aggregates of lymphoid tissue occur along the bronchial tree, especially at division points and adjacent to distal respiratory bronchioles, and are known as BALT or 'pulmonary microtonsills'. BALT in association with the analogous tissue in the gastrointestinal tract, the gut-associated lymphoid tissue (GALT), comprise the so-called mucosal-associated lymphoid tissue (MALT). This system in the lung is thought to play an essential role in the prevention of infection of inhaled microorganisms, by serving as the pulmonary site for secondary lymphoid differentiation, where the naïve lymphocytes initially contact an inhaled antigen to become antigen specific memory or immune effector cells. Once primed by the antigen, memory cells circulate throughout the BALT compartment and the remaining lung parenchyma awaiting exposure to the same provoking antigen (Agostini et al., 1993). BALT can be the source of various pathologic lesions, ranging from various forms of hyperplasia to malignant neoplasms (Katzenstein, 1997).

Follicular bronchiolitis may present idiopathically as a separate syndrome but is most commonly observed in rheumatoid arthritis (with or without Sjögren's syndrome), HIV infection, or as a sequel to viral infections (Yousem et al., 1985). In patients with primary Sjögren's syndrome, follicular bronchiolitis usually coexists with lymphocytic bronchitis/bronchiolitis, reactive lymphoid hyperplasia and/or LIP. Histopathologically, it is characterized by lymphoid hyperplasia surrounding terminal bronchioles, with protrusion into their lumen (BALT hyperplasia associated with small airways obstruction). Small germinal centers are usually present in the lymphoid tissue. Intraluminal inflammation or fibrosis and mural scarring are absent. In rare cases, follicular bronchiolitis may be associated with destruction of the alveolar walls and cyst or bullae formation (Kobayashi et al., 1988). The clinical and radiologic manifestations may 'paradoxically' mimic interstitial lung disease with reticular and reticulo-nodular infiltrates on the chest radiogram, while physiologic tests may disclose restriction or obstruction (Wells and du Bois, 1993). A tree-in-bud pattern seen on HRCT in a patient with Sjögren's syndrome is highly suggestive of follicular bronchiolitis, provided that infection is excluded. Transbronchial, video-assisted or open lung biopsy is necessary to obtain histologic confirmation. In symptomatic patients, glucocorticosteroids may be administered with a favorable response.

Lymphoid interstitial pneumonia is a diffuse infiltrative lung disorder first described by Carrington and Liebow (1966). It is a classic but uncommon component of primary Sjögren's syndrome ($\approx 5\%$ of patients, accounting for more than 25% of all LIPs), but occurs also in HIV infection, other infections (e.g. Epstein-Barr virus, Legionella pneumophila), allogeneic bone marrow transplantation, common variable immunodeficiency, chronic liver disease and a few other conditions (Swigris et al., 2002). Histologically, it is characterized by an interstitial infiltrate of mature lymphocytes, plasma cells, and other lymphoreticular elements, which expand the interstitial septa and fill the alveolar spaces (Katzenstein, 1997). Interstitial lymphoid nodules with germinal centers may be visible in some areas. Frequently, it coexists with lesions typical of follicular bronchiolitis (it is hypothesized that the pulmonary lesions may have originated in the bronchial wall at sites of BALT hyperplasia) (Swigris et al., 2002) and the overlapping list of causes of the two conditions suggests a close relation. In addition both follicular bronchiolitis and LIP may evolve into malignant lymphoma. Clinically patients with LIP present with cough and progressive dyspnea. Systemic symptoms such as fever, night sweats, and weight loss are less common. Lung auscultation often reveals bibasilar crackles. Clubbing is absent. The chest radiograph shows a diffuse reticular or reticulonodular pattern with lower lobe predominance. HRCT is the radiographic procedure of choice to better define pulmonary opacities in LIP. Thickened bronchovascular bundles, nodules of varying sizes, and ground glass opacities are common. Pulmonary function studies may document restriction with low diffusing capacity. Transbronchial or, preferably, thoracoscopic or open lung biopsy is necessary for diagnosis. Lymphoid interstitial pneumonia may have a favorable course.

Pseudolymphoma, or inflammatory pseudotumor, of the lung is histologically similar to LIP but differs radiographically, in that it causes isolated mass-like densities rather than diffuse infiltrates (Saltzstein, 1963; Katzenstein, 1997). Pseudolymphomas may be solitary or multiple and occasionally bilateral. Pulmonary pseudolymphomas may occasionally evolve to malignant lymphomas or be lymphomas from the beginning, and their differentiation from the well-differentiated lymphocytic lymphoma (WDLL) is difficult. Polyclonality characterizes the inflammatory infiltrate in both LIP and pseudolymphoma.

Lymphomatoid granulomatosis (LYG) is a rare, angiocentric and angiodestructive lymphoreticular proliferative and granulomatous disease involving predominantly the lungs, skin, and nervous system that shares overlapping features between Wegener's granulomatosis and malignant lymphoma (Liebow et al., 1972; Katzenstein et al., 1979). According to Katzenstein (1997), LYG is not related pathogenetically to Wegener's granulomatosis or the other angiitides and granulomatoses. There is enough evidence to consider LYG a form of T-cell lymphoma and to justify a subclassification of LYG into categories of 'LYG lymphoma' and 'pure LYG', when diagnostic lymphomatous areas are absent or, more probably, have not been sampled. Histologically, LYG is characterized by a combination of a dense mononuclear infiltrate, which consists of a mixture of small lymphocytes, plasma cells, histiocytes, immunoblasts, and atypical lymphoid cells, in association with marked transmural infiltration of arteries and veins and extensive parenchymal necrosis. Video-assisted thoracoscopic or open lung biopsy is required for its diagnosis. A few cases have been associated with primary Sjögren's syndrome (Liebow et al., 1972; Weisbrot, 1976).

The spectrum of malignant lymphoproliferation in Sjögren's syndrome extends from an increased frequency of mixed monoclonal cryoglobulinemia, and increased levels of circulating CD5-positive B-cells, circulating monoclonal immunoglobulins and free light chains, to malignant non-Hodgkin's lymphomas. The occurrence of non-Hodgkin's lymphomas is the most serious complication of Sjögren's syndrome (Bunim and Talal, 1963; Kassan et al., 1978; Zulman et al., 1978; Royer et al., 1997; Voulgarelis et al., 1999; Mariette, 1999; Voulgarelis and Moutsopoulos, 2001). In these patients, 20% of deaths are attributable to lymphoma (Ioannidis et al., 2002). Bunim and Talal (1963) first reported an increased incidence of non-Hodgkin's lymphomas in patients with Sjögren's syndrome and suggested that the chronic antigenic stimulation triggered a malignant transformation event. This finding was followed by several cases reporting an association between Sjögren's syndrome and lymphomas. Kassan et al. (1978) found that the relative risk of lymphoma in Sjögren's syndrome is 44 times higher than in an age, sex and race matched control population. Subsequently, Zulman et al. (1978) showed that these lymphomas are primarily of B-cell origin, containing exclusively IgMk immunoglobulin in their cytoplasm. B-cell lymphomas are considered to be the result of a monoclonal expansion of a malignant B-cell clone. Recently, Royer et al. (1997) described 16 non-Hodgkin's lymphomas occurring in patients with underlying Sjögren's syndrome. These lymphomas arose not only in salivary glands (seven cases) but also in other mucosal extranodal sites, including the stomach (four cases), the lung (three cases), the skin (three cases), the buccal mucosa (one case), the thymus (one case) and in nodal sites (eight cases). Low-grade marginal zone lymphomas were diagnosed in 12 of the 16 patients, nine of MALT type in mucosal sites and three exclusively nodal. The term 'low-grade marginal zone lymphoma' has been proposed to encompass both the monocytoid B-cell lymphomas, which appear as the nodal counterpart of MALT lymphomas, and the MALT lymphomas. The four other patients presented with a high-grade B-cell lymphoma that was probably a histological transformation of an underlying low-grade marginal zone lymphoma, involving, in three cases, skin, stomach, and parotid. In this series, lymphomas were not associated with viruses known to be present in other types of lymphoma. Voulgarelis et al. (1999) described the disease characteristics, the clinical course, and the evolution in 33 patients with Sjögren's syndrome and malignant lymphomas followed up in nine European medical centers. Lymphomas in this study were primarily situated in the marginal zone (49%), with the manifestations mostly extranodal (79%) and most often identified in the salivary glands. The lungs were involved by lymphoma in two patients (6%). Other lung manifestations were observed in ten patients (31%). Lymphadenopathy (66%), skin vasculitis (33%), peripheral nerve involvement (24%), low-grade fever (25%), anemia (48%), and lymphopenia (79%) were observed significantly more frequently in patients with lymphomas than in the general Sjögren's syndrome population. Patients with high-to-intermediate grade lymphoma had a worse prognosis. The presence of symptoms such as fever, night sweats, and weight loss, as well as tumor bulk (>7 cm), were additional independent risk factors for death. Finally, in a recent study, Ioannidis et al. (2002) sought to determine the incidence and predictors of adverse long-term outcomes by studying 723 consecutive patients with primary Sjögren's syndrome followed over a 20-year-period. During this period they recorded 39 deaths (seven due to lymphoma) and 38 diagnoses of lymphoproliferative disease, and found that the presence of palpable purpura and low C4 levels at the first visit may distinguish high-risk patients (type I primary Sjögren's syndrome) from patients with an uncomplicated disease course (type II, low-risk primary Sjögren's syndrome).

Primary lung lymphomas in Sjögren's syndrome are uncommon. Strimlan et al. (1976) reported that a review of 343 patients with Sjögren's syndrome revealed three patients with malignant pulmonary lymphoma. The rare occurrence of primary malignant tracheal lymphoma has also been described (Kamholz et al., 1987). Radiographically, pulmonary lymphomas may present as solitary or multiple opacities, or diffuse interstitial infiltrates, and in some cases may simulate other benign lymphoproliferative lesions (Fig. 1). Lung cysts are more suggestive of follicular bronchiolitis with associated lymphoid interstitial pneumonia and may help in the differential diagnosis (Honda et al., 1999). However, the patchy and bronchocentric distribution, the presence of hilar or mediastinal lymphadenopathy, and the involvement of the pleural space are characteristics of high-grade lymphoma. Thoracoscopic or open lung biopsy is usually necessary to obtain adequate tissue. Histological elements in favor of lymphoma include a patchy distribution, lymphangitic spread, and the demonstration by immunocytochemical stains of a monoclonal cell line as opposed to the polyclonality observed in the diffuse lymphoid hyperplasia of the lungs and the pseudolymphomas.

5.4. Other forms of interstitial pneumonias

Recently, an international Consensus Statement defining the clinical manifestations, pathology, and radiologic features of patients with idiopathic interstitial pneumonias has been produced and published as a collaborative effort by the American Thoracic Society and the European Respiratory Society (2002). The new classification comprises the following clinicopathologic entities with their relative histological patterns in order of relative frequency: (1) idiopathic pulmonary fibrosis (IPF), usual interstitial pneumonia pattern, (2) non-specific interstitial pneumonia (NSIP), non-specific interstitial pneumonia pattern, (3) cryptogenic organizing pneumonia (COP), formerly called bronchiolitis obliterans organizing pneumonia (BOOP), organizing pneumonia pattern, (4) acute interstitial pneumonia, diffuse alveolar damage pattern, (5) respiratory bronchiolitis-associated interstitial lung disease (RB-ILD), respiratory bronchiolitis pattern, (6) desquamative interstitial pneumonia (DIP), desquamative interstitial pneumonia pattern, and (7) lymphoid interstitial pneumonia (LIP), lymphoid interstitial pneumonia pattern. Several of the above-described clinicopathological entities may also be secondary to different conditions such as rheumatic autoimmune disorders, drugs-related pulmonary toxicity or lung damage related to the inhalation of inorganic or organic dusts. Furthermore, several of the above, in addition to the classic LIP previously described, have been reported (though infrequently) in Sjögren's syndrome patients.

Interstitial pulmonary fibrosis in the form of the usual interstitial pneumonia pattern is rather uncommon in patients with Sjögren's syndrome. In the series of 343 patients studied by Strimlan et al. (1976), pulmonary fibrosis was histopathologically diagnosed in only two patients. In this series, however, there was

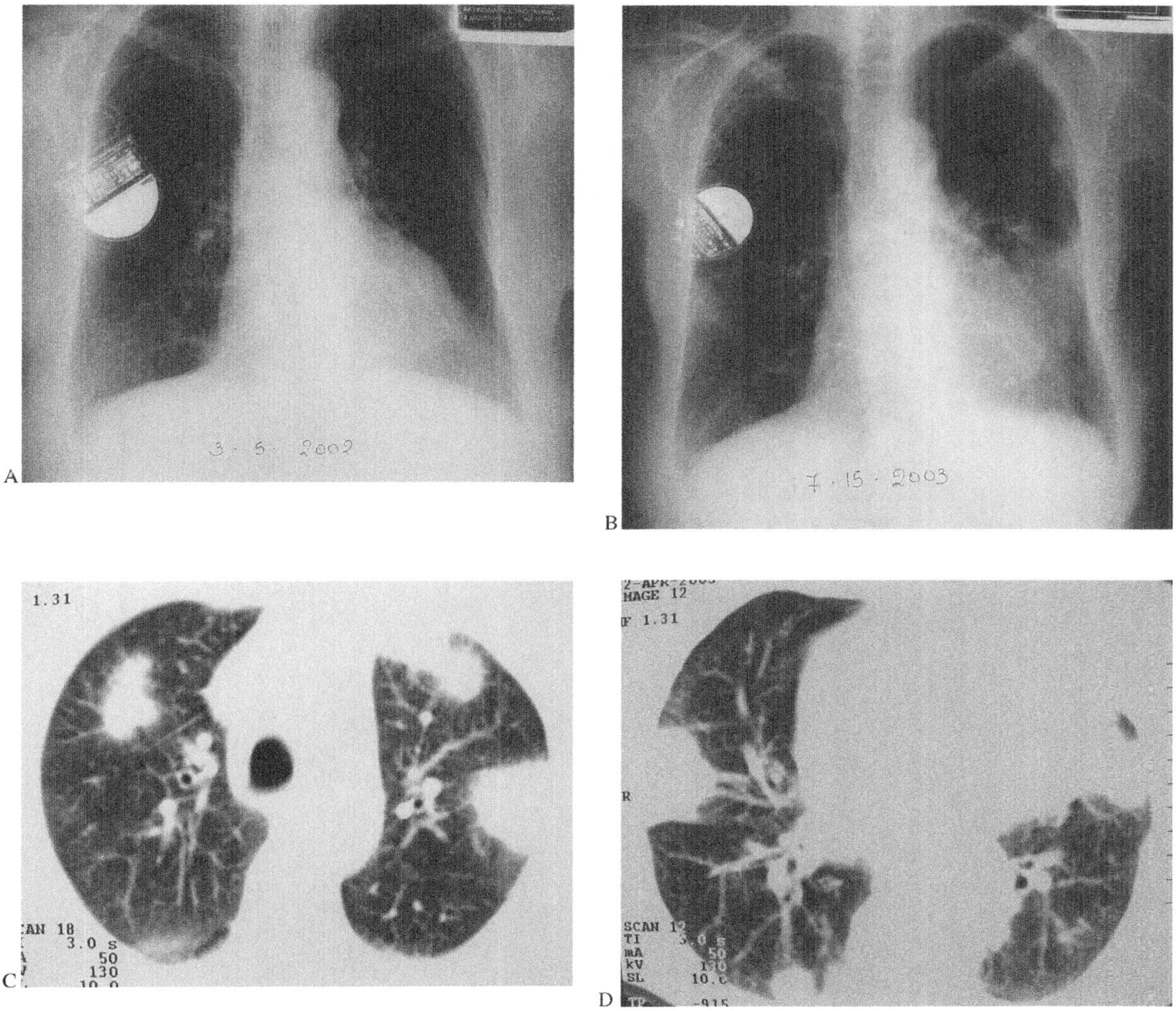

Figure 1. This 73-year-old woman was presented with keratoconjounctivitis sicca, xerostomia and recurrent swelling of the parotid glands 12 years before. A posteroanterior chest radiograph (A) performed during a routine visit on March 2002 shows clear lung fields. A few months later the patient gradually developed progressive dyspnea on exertion, fatigue, and weight loss. A new posteroanterior chest radiograph (B) performed on July 2003 revealed multiple wedge-shaped peripheral-based opacities on both lungs. The computerized tomography of the chest (C and D) performed soon after disclosed multiple peripheral nodular or wedge-shaped opacities in both lungs. Video-assisted lung biopsy permitted the identification of an extranodal pulmonary marginal zone B-cell lymphoma. In (E) the parenchymal consolidation due to lymphocytic infiltration and hyalinosis of the stroma is evident (hematoxylin and eosin, original magnification: 20 × magnification). In (F) small B lymphocytes with lymphoplasmocytoid features (immunophenotype: CD20 + ve, CD5 − ve, CD23 − ve, CD10 − ve, cyclin D1 − ve, IgMk) infiltrate the bronchial epithelium–lymphoepithelial lesion (hematoxylin and eosin, original magnification: 200 × magnification). (Histopathology slides are courtesy of Dr D. Rontogianni.)

no distinction between the primary and secondary form of Sjögren's syndrome. Since then, most reports of interstitial pulmonary fibrosis in patients with Sjögren's syndrome have been found in patients with the secondary form of the syndrome (Gardiner, 1993). Pulmonary fibrosis has also been described in patients with primary Sjögren's syndrome, although the histopathologic changes have been poorly documented and the diagnosis was usually based on radiological and functional data alone (Gardiner et al., 1993).

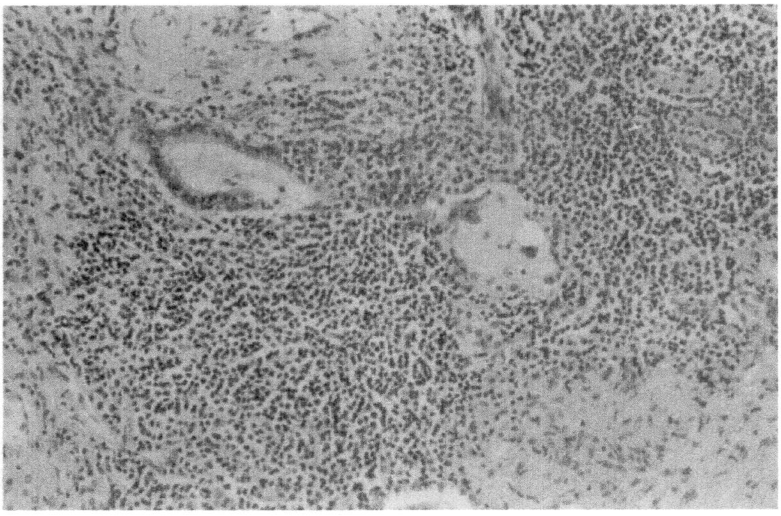

E

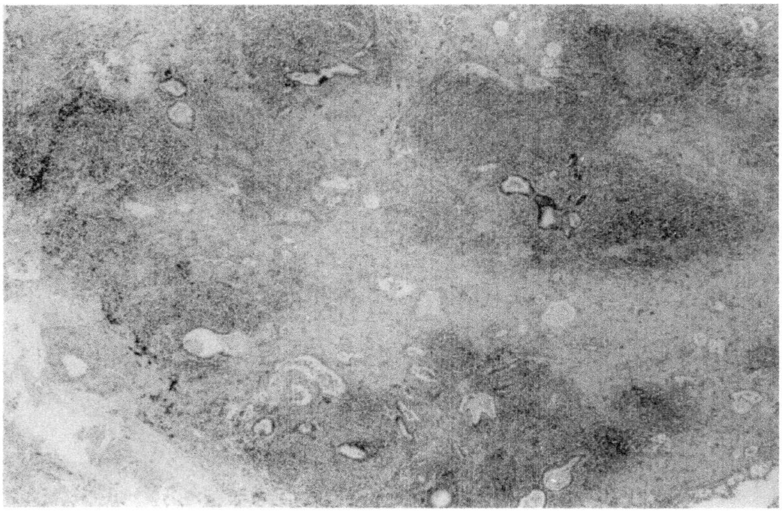

F

Figure 1. *(continued)*

Deheinzelin et al. (1996) performed open lung biopsy in 12 patients with primary Sjögren's syndrome and found a spectrum of interstitial lung disease, from follicular bronchiolitis to LIP to fibrosis with honeycombing. Azathioprine, either alone or in combination with corticosteroids, obtained a favorable response in pulmonary function. Recently, Yamadori et al. (2002) performed surgical biopsies in nine patients with primary Sjögren's syndrome and found six patients with UIP histology and three with NSIP. Non-specific interstitial pneumonia is a form of idiopathic interstitial pneumonia with similar clinical features to those of idiopathic pulmonary fibrosis, UIP type, but with a better prognosis. It appears to be more common than UIP in some autoimmune rheumatic disorders, in particular in scleroderma and polymyositis/dermatomyositis.

Cryptogenic organizing pneumonia (COP), formerly called bronchiolitis obliterans organizing pneumonia (BOOP), is defined pathologically by the presence of granulation tissue plugs, composed of fibroblasts and a connective tissue matrix within the lumens of the distal airspaces (bronchioles, alveolar ducts and alveoli) (Epler et al., 1985). The clinical picture is usually that of a non-resolving pneumonia. COP represents a non-specific reaction to acute lung injury and can been seen in a variety of circumstances including several of the autoimmune rheumatic disorders (Wright et al., 1992). A few cases have been reported in primary Sjögren's syndrome (Matteson and Ike, 1990; Usui et al., 1992). Most cases of COP are steroid-responsive, but some cases may progress rapidly to respiratory insufficiency and death (Usui et al., 1992; Cohen et al., 1994).

5.5. Diffuse panbronchiolitis

Diffuse panbronchiolitis is a unique form of chronic obstructive lung disease of unknown etiology, associated with sinusitis, and largely restricted to Japan (Homma et al., 1983). Histologically, it is characterized by a transmural infiltrate of lymphocytes and plasma cells around the respiratory bronchioles. Foamy macrophages fill the adjacent alveoli and mucus and neutrophils fill the lumen of the affected bronchioles. The natural history of the disease is slowly progressive (several years) and death may occur due to respiratory failure. The clinical course may improve with the introduction of prolonged treatment with macrolide antibiotics. Two cases have been reported in association with Sjögren's syndrome (Okano et al., 1991; Ubucata et al., 1991).

5.6. Multiple lung cystic lesions or bullae

Bulla formation is a rare but well-described pulmonary manifestation in Sjögren's syndrome and usually accompanies other lung lesions such as follicular bronchiolitis, and lymphoid interstitial pneumonia (Bonner et al., 1973; Kobayashi et al., 1988; Inase et al., 1990; Case records of the Massachusetts General Hospital, 2001; Meyer et al., 1997; Sakamoto et al., 2002; Hubscher et al., 2002). On CT scanning Honda et al. (1999) found that lung cysts were the most helpful finding in distinguishing lymphoid interstitial pneumonia from malignant lymphoma. Cyst formation is believed to be related to bronchiolar obstruction and distal overinflation due to a check-valve mechanism (Bonner et al., 1973).

5.7. Vasculitis and primary pulmonary hypertension

Pulmonary hypertension is another very rare complication of primary Sjögren's syndrome due to the primary involvement of lung circulation, and very few cases have been reported in the literature thus far (Case records of the Massachusetts General Hospital, 1975).

5.8. Pulmonary amyloidosis

Amyloidosis is the extracellular deposition of the fibrous protein amyloid in one or more sites of the body. The secondary or reactive form of the disease, usually associated with chronic infectious or inflammatory diseases, is the form described in Sjögren's syndrome, though primary amyloidosis has also been described associated with MALT lymphoma (Kobayashi et al., 1988; Bonner et al., 1973; Sugai, 2002).

5.9. Pleural disease

Pleural effusions appear to be an extremely rare manifestation of Sjögren's syndrome and, when present, are largely confined to the secondary form of the disease. In the series published by Bloch et al. (1965) none of the 62 patients with Sjögren's syndrome presented with a pleural effusion. However, in the series of Strimlan et al. (1976) that included 349 patients, five had pleural effusion (<1%). Of these five patients, three had rheumatoid arthritis, or systemic lupus erythematosus, but two had no other autoimmune rheumatic disorder associated. Pleural fluid characteristics have been described in two patients and were lymphocyte-predominant exudates with normal pH and glucose levels and low adenosine deaminase levels (Alvarez-Sala et al., 1989; Ogihara et al., 1995).

6. Diagnostic investigations

Recently a joint American–European Consensus group proposed a modified classification criteria set, new rules for correctly classifying patients with primary and secondary Sjögren's syndrome, and a list of exclusion criteria (Vitali et al., 2002). The classification criteria set includes:

I. Ocular symptoms: a positive response to at least one of the following questions:
   1. Have you had daily, persistent, troublesome dry eyes for more than three months?
   2. Do you have a recurrent sensation of sand or gravel in the eyes?
   3. Do you use tear substitutes more than three times a day?
II. Oral symptoms: a positive response to at least one of the following questions:
   1. Have you had a daily feeling of dry mouth for more than three months?
   2. Have you had recurrently or persistently swollen salivary glands as an adult?
   3. Do you frequently drink liquids to aid in swallowing dry food?
III. Ocular signs: that is, objective evidence of ocular involvement defined as a positive result of at least one of the following two tests:
   1. Schirmer's test, performed without anaesthesia (≤ 5 mm in 5 min)
   2. Rose bengal score or other ocular dye score (≥ 4 according to van Bijsterveld's scoring system)
IV. Histopathology: focal lymphocytic sialoadenitis in minor salivary glands (obtained through normal-appearing mucosa), evaluated by an expert histopathologist, with a focus score ≥ 1, defined as a number of lymphocytic foci (which are adjacent to normal-appearing mucous acini and contain more than 50 lymphocytes) per 4 mm^2 of glandular tissue.
V. Salivary gland involvement: defined by a positive result for at least one of the following diagnostic tests:
   1. Unstimulated whole salivary flow (≤ 1.5 ml in 15 min)
   2. Parotid sialography showing the presence of diffuse sialectasias (punctate, cavitary or destructive pattern), without evidence of obstruction in the major ducts
   3. Salivary scintigraphy showing delayed uptake, reduced concentration and/or delayed excretion of tracer
VI. Autoantibodies to Ro(SSA) or La(SSB) antigens, or both.

   Accordingly, in patients without any potentially associated disease, primary Sjögren's syndrome may be defined as follows:
   A. The presence of any four of the six items is indicative of primary Sjögren's syndrome, as long as either item IV (Histopathology) or VI (Serology) is positive
   B. The presence of any three of the four objective criteria items (that is, items III, IV, V, VI)
   C. The classification tree procedure represents a valid alternative method for classification, although it should be more properly used in clinical–epidemiological survey.

Otherwise, in patients with a potentially associated disease (for instance, another well-defined connective tissue disease), the presence of item I or item II plus any two from among items III, IV, and V may be considered as indicative of secondary Sjögren's syndrome.

Exclusion criteria include: past head and neck radiation treatment, hepatitis C infection, acquired immunodeficiency syndrome, pre-existing lymphoma, sarcoidosis, graft-versus-host disease and, finally, use of anticholinergic drugs.

6.1. Radiological

The frequency of abnormalities on the chest radiograph varies considerably in different series from 1.7 to 33% (Silbiger and Peterson, 1967; Whaley et al., 1973; Strimlan et al., 1976). A reticulonodular pattern of basal predominance is most frequently observed. Lung biopsy performed in a small number of patients has shown that this pattern may be caused by different histological abnormalities such as follicular bronchiolitis, lymphoid interstitial pneumonia, interstitial fibrosis or even frank lymphoma (Fig. 1). HRCT lung scanning is more sensitive than plain films. Uffmann et al. (2001) examined by HRCT 37 consecutive, asymptomatic patients with primary Sjögren's syndrome and normal chest radiographs and found abnormalities, such as interlobular septal thickening, micronodules, ground glass attenuation, and parenchymal cysts, in a large proportion of cases (65%). Intralobular opacities, honey-combing, bronchial wall thickening, bronchiectasis, and pleural irregularities were less commonly observed (Uffmann et al., 2001). Overall, HRCT abnormalities are reported in 4–65% of patients with Sjögren's syndrome, and specific findings of airway involvement such as bronchial wall thickening, bronchiolectasis, and patchy or diffuse air-trapping are observed in 22–50% (Meyer et al., 1997; Franquet et al., 1997, 1999; Uffmann et al., 2001; Taouli et al., 2002) (Fig. 2). Franquet et al. (1999) evaluated with expiratory HRCT 34 patients with primary Sjögren's syndrome and disclosed a mosaic pattern of lung attenuation, a sign of bronchiolar disease, in 50%. In this study the extent of air trapping did not correlate with functional indices, which according to the authors might suggest the existence of a subclinical bronchiolar inflammatory process that may precede detectable abnormalities in lung function studies. Furthermore, Franquet et al. (1997) evaluated with HRCT 50 non-smoking patients with primary Sjogren's syndrome and found that interstitial fibrosing alveolitis and small airways disease represented the majority of the abnormalities. In their series, bronchiolar abnormalities and linear opacities were seen in 65% of the patients, ground glass opacities in 41%, rounded opacities in 29%, honeycombing in 24% and patchy areas of airspace consolidation in 6%. Bronchiolar abnormalities alone were found in 23% of patients (Franquet et al., 1997). In the series of Taouli et al. (2002), 54% of patients with primary Sjögren's syndrome had HRCT signs of airway disease, 20% had interstitial fibrosis and 14% had a pattern suggestive of LIP. In the same study, a good correlation with pulmonary function tests was shown. Cystic changes of 5–30 mm in diameter with air trapping may be ascribable to bronchiolar obstruction and development of a valve mechanism on the basis of lymphocytic wall infiltration (Meyer et al., 1997). In the series of Johkoh et al. (1999), including 22 patients with LIP, 10 of whom had Sjogren's syndrome, cystic lesions were reported in 68%. HRCT findings in the context of diffuse interstitial pneumonia include patchy, predominantly peripheral, subpleural, bibasal reticular abnormalities in UIP, a more or less extensive ground glass pattern in LIP, a variable combination of both the above patterns in NSIP, and focal infiltrates in organizing pneumonia.

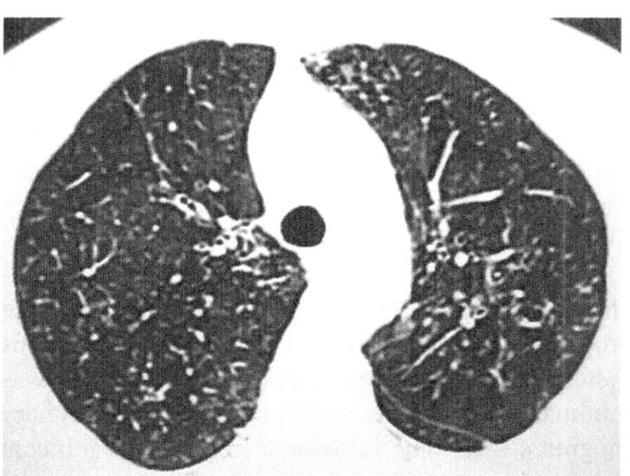

Figure 2. Asymptomatic 55-year-old woman with primary Sjögren's syndrome. High resolution CT scan obtained at the level of the lower lobes shows, in the periphery of the lung, focal areas of bronchial wall thickening, with characteristic tree-in-bud appearance and sparse peribronchial nodules (courtesy of Dr K. Malagari).

6.2. Functional

Pulmonary function tests in Sjögren's syndrome are more valuable in the estimation of severity, following the course of disease, and monitoring responses to therapy than for diagnosis since, as previously discussed, all patterns of physiological abnormalities (obstructive, restrictive, and mixed) have been described. Among the various pulmonary function indices, the most precise and reproducible index is the vital capacity (VC), although in early and mild disease it may be normal. Vital capacity and diffusing capacity for carbon monoxide (DLCO) are of particular value in cases of diffuse interstitial involvement. Expiratory flows at low lung volumes, MEF_{50}, and the MEF_{25}, are appropriate indices with which to detect early airways involvement. Gas exchange abnormalities and respiratory insufficiency are uncommon in these patients and may be observed only in rare cases with advanced stage diffuse interstitial involvement, from the UIP, NSIP, LIP, or COP patterns of disease.

6.3. Biochemistry/Serology/Immunology

B-cell hyperreactivity is a key immunological feature of Sjögren's syndrome and manifests with hypergammaglobulinemia, circulating immune complexes, and multiple autoantibodies directed against both organ and non-organ specific autoantigens (Harley, 1987). Although not specific for Sjögren's syndrome, rheumatoid factors, antinuclear antibodies, antihistone and anti-ds-stranded DNA antibodies are found in high levels and quite frequently ($\approx$70% of patients). The analysis of the antigenic specificity of serum antinuclear antibodies most often reveals the presence of autoantibodies against two distinct ribonucleoproteins termed Ro (or SSA) and La (or SSB). Anti-Ro (SSA) and anti-La (SSB) antibodies are found in 40–60% and 25–40%, respectively, of primary Sjögren's syndrome patients, and their detection constitutes a diagnostic criterion (Vitali et al., 2002). Their detection in serum of Sjögren's syndrome patients is associated with high-intensity inflammatory infiltration of the minor salivary glands, earlier onset and longer disease duration, recurrent parotid gland enlargement, splenomegaly, lymphadenopathy and vasculitis (Manoussakis et al., 1986). Furthermore, Davidson et al. (2000) found that pulmonary disease occurs predominantly in anti-Ro (SSA) antibody positive patients and presents early in the course of the disease. However, the cause and role of anti-Ro (SSA) and anti-La (SSB) autoantibodies remain unclear. Finally, anti-Ro (SSA) and anti-La (SSB) antibodies are not entirely specific for primary Sjögren's syndrome and may also be found in several other rheumatic autoimmune disorders (including systemic lupus erythematosus, subacute cutaneous lupus, rheumatoid arthritis and polymyositis), whether associated with secondary Sjögren's syndrome or not. In agreement with the increased prevalence of B-cell lymphomas among Sjögren's syndrome patients, evidence of oligoclonal B-cell expansion is found quite early in the disease course. Monoclonal light chains or immunoglobulins can be found in the serum and urine of 80–100% of patients with evidence of systemic involvement, compared to approximately 25–40% of patients with only glandular disease. In addition, approximately 30% of patients with primary Sjögren's syndrome exhibit high serum levels of mixed polyclonal–monoclonal cryoglobulins, which usually contain an IgMk-monoclonal rheumatoid factor. Cryoglobulinaemia is associated with systemic disease, antibodies to Ro (SSA), and a higher risk of developing lymphoma (Tzioufas et al., 1996).

7. Differential diagnosis

The differential diagnosis of Sjögren's syndrome includes adverse effects of drugs, sarcoidosis, lipoproteinemias (types II, IV, and V) age-related atrophy, chronic graft-versus-host disease, lymphomas, amyloidosis, and infection by human immunodeficiency virus or hepatitis C virus (Manoussakis and Moutsopoulos, 2000). The identification of serum autoantibodies to Ro(SSA) or La(SSB) proteins is a strong indication of primary Sjögren's syndrome. Therefore, the correct diagnosis of Sjögren's syndrome requires complete clinical, pathological and serological evaluation of patients, as well as the application of the recently described international criteria (Vitali et al., 2002).

8. Prognosis and treatment

Skopouli et al. (2000) studied the evolution of the clinical picture and laboratory profiles of primary Sjögren's syndrome, the incidence and predictors for systemic sequelae, and the impact of primary Sjögren's syndrome on overall survival in a prospective cohort study of 261 patients with the disease. They found that the initial presentation of primary Sjögren's syndrome determines subsequent outcome. The presence of palpable purpura, low levels of C4, and mixed monoclonal cryoglobulins are adverse prognostic factors. The risk of developing serious systemic sequelae in the absence of these factors was minimal. Furthermore, they documented that primary Sjögren's syndrome is associated with a significant increase in mortality compared with the general population. However, in the absence of any risk factors, most patients have a mortality rate equal to that of the general population.

Currently, there is no consensus treatment for Sjögren's syndrome, which remains fundamentally an incurable disease (Manoussakis and Moutsopoulos, 2001). The treatment is generally aimed at alleviating the dryness symptoms and related morbidities. More recent approaches to therapy for Sjögren's syndrome have included therapies that increase glandular excretion using muscarinic (M3) receptor agonists. Systemic manifestations are treated with steroids, non-steroidal anti-inflammatory drugs, hydroxychlorochine, or cytotoxic agents, but in general these therapies are marginally effective and have potentially serious side effects.

The pleomorphy of the respiratory manifestations and their variability in clinical severity, which may range from mild to severe and occasionally life-threatening disease, require special therapeutic measures. Oily applications and lubricants are not advised to alleviate symptoms in patients with 'rhina sicca' since their aspiration to the lungs may pose serious problems (lipoid pneumonia). Sinusitis should be treated adequately with antibiotics and, if indicated, with surgical drainage. For severe dry cough due to 'xerotrachea', normal saline nebulizations and high doses of bromexine or analogous expectorants might be tried (although efficacy is unproven). Muscarinic (M3) receptor antagonists such as pilocarpine hydrochloride, and sivimeline, should not be advised since bronchial hyper-responsiveness has been described in these patients and there may be an unacceptable risk of airways obstruction. Corticosteroids are the most widely used treatment for follicular bronchiolitis and LIP, and are thought to arrest or improve symptoms in a large proportion of patients. Corticosteroids are also effective in patients with COP and NSIP. In patients with UIP, low-dose corticosteroids and azathioprine are usually recommended.

Combined chemotherapy is recommended in patients with low-grade lymphoma transforming to high grade and for those with high-grade lymphoma. A regimen of proven efficacy is cyclophosphamide, doxorubicin, vincristine and prednisone (CHOP). Rituximab, a chimeric murine–human anti-CD20 monoclonal antibody that targets B lymphocytes, has been approved by the Food and Drug Administration for treatment of relapsed and/or refractory low grade B-cell non-Hodgkin's lymphomas (Brown et al., 1989; Somer et al., 2003). This monoclonal antibody binds to an epitope of the transmembrane CD20 protein that is expressed on most mature B lymphocytes, as well as B-cell lymphoma cells, and causes cell death by induction of apoptosis, complement-mediated cell lysis, and antibody-dependent cell-mediated cytotoxicity (Shan et al., 1998). Improvement in Sjögren's syndrome general manifestations following therapy with Rituximab for marginal zone lymphoma has been recently described (Somer et al., 2003) and opens new roads for exploration.

Acknowledgements

The authors wish to thank Dr Efstathia Capsogeorgou for revision of the part related to the etiology/pathogenesis, Dr Katerina Malagari for revision of all the radiological parts and for providing Fig. 2, and Dr Dimitra Rontogianni for providing diagnosis and the histopathological slides of the case reported in Fig. 1(E and F).

Key points

- Sjögren's syndrome, an autoimmune epithelitis, is characterized by: (a) a lymphocytic infiltration of the exocrine glands and epithelia in multiple sites, including those of the upper and lower airways, leading to diminished or absent glandular secretions and to a more or less generalized, mucosal dryness, and (b) a marked B lymphocytic cell hyperreactivity manifested by various serum autoantibodies, such as those directed against the Ro(SSA) and La(SSB) ribonucleoproteins, or immunoglobulins (rheumatoid factor).
- Pulmonary involvement in primary Sjögren's syndrome includes: (a) upper and lower, large and small airways disease (common, but mild in severity), (b) different patterns of diffuse interstitial pneumonia, such as chronic organizing pneumonia (COP), non-specific interstitial pneumonia (NSIP), and usual interstitial pneumonia (UIP) (uncommon, but of variable severity), and (c) a spectrum of lymphoproliferative diseases, extending from follicular bronchiolitis to lymphocytic interstitial pneumonia (LIP) and, finally, to

malignant B-cell non-Hodgkin's lymphoma (in a small but significant number of patients and of variable severity).

- Currently, there is no consensus treatment for Sjögren's syndrome which remains fundamentally an incurable disease. The treatment is generally aimed at alleviating the dryness symptoms and related morbidities. The pleomorphy of the respiratory manifestations and their variability in clinical severity that may range from mild to severe and occasionally life-threatening disease require special therapeutic measures.

References

Abu-Helu, R.F., Dimitriou, I.D., Kapsogeorgou, E.K., Moutsopoulos, H.M., Manoussakis, M.N. 2001. Induction of salivary gland epithelial cell injury in Sjögren's syndrome: in vitro assessment of T cell-derived cytokines and Fas protein expression. J. Autoimmun. 17, 141.

Adamson, T.C., Fox, R.I., Frisman, D.M., Howell, F.V. 1983. Immunohistologic analysis of lymphoid infiltrates in primary Sjögren's syndrome using monoclonal antibodies. J. Immunol. 130, 203.

The first characterization of the T lymphocytic subpopulations involved in the inflammatory infiltrate in Sjögren's syndrome.

Agostini, C., Chilosi, M., Zambello, R., Trentin, L., Semenzato, G. 1993. Pulmonary immune cells in health and disease: lymphocytes. Eur. Respir. J. 6, 1378.

This important article encompasses all the aspects of the role of lymphocytes in health and disease in the lungs.

Alarcón-Segovia, D., Divertie, M.B., Brown, A.L. 1965. Pleuropulmonary manifestations associated with Sjögren's syndrome. Arthritis Rheum. 8, 427.

One of the first articles that tried to characterize lung involvement in Sjögren's syndrome but without distinction between primary and secondary disease.

Alvarez-Sala, R., Sanchez-Toril, F., Garcia-Martinez, J., Zaera, A., Maza, J.F. 1989. Primary Sjögren's syndrome and pleural effusion. Chest 96, 1440.

American Thoracic Society/European Respiratory Society, 2002. International multidisciplinary consensus classification of the idiopathic interstitial pneumonias. Am. J. Respir. Crit. Care Med. 165, 277.

The ultimate consensus classification on idiopathic interstitial pneumonias.

Anderson, L.G., Talal, T.L. 1972. The spectrum of benign to malignant lymphoproliferation in Sjögren's syndrome. Clin. Exp. Immunol. 10, 199.

Andoh, Y., Shimura, S., Sawai, T., Sasaki, H., Takishima, T., Shirato, K. 1993. Morphometric analysis of airways in Sjögren's syndrome. Am. Rev. Respir. Dis. 148, 1358.

Bloch, K.J., Buchanan, W.W., Wohl, M.J. 1965. Sjögren's syndrome. Medicine 44, 187.

Bonner, H., Ennis, R.S., Geelhoed, G.W., Tarpley, T.M. 1973. Lymphoid infiltration and amyloidosis of lung in Sjögren's syndrome. Arch. Pathol. 95, 42.

Boumpa, D., Skopouli, F.N., Moutsopoulos, H.M. 1995. Cytokine mRNA expression in the labial salivary glands tissues from patients with primary Sjögren's syndrome. Br. J. Rheumatol. 34, 326.

Brookes, S.M., Price, E.J., Venables, P.J.W., Maini, R.N. 1995. Interferon-gamma and epithelial cell activation in Sjögren's syndrome. Br. J. Rheumatol. 34, 226.

Brown, S.L., Miller, R.A., Horning, S.J., Czerwinski, D., Hart, S.M., McElderry, R., Basham, T., Warnke, R.A., Merigan, T.C., Lery, R. 1989. Treatment of B-cell lymphomas with anti-idiotype antibodies alone and in combination with alpha interferon. Blood 73, 651.

Bunim, J.J., Talal, N. 1963. The association of malignant lymphoma with Sjögren's syndrome. Trans. Assoc. Am. Physicians 76, 45.

The first recognition of malignancy insurgence in Sjögren's syndrome.

Cain, H.C., Noble, P.W., Matthay, R.A. 1998. Pulmonary manifestations of Sjögren's syndrome. Clin. Chest Med. 19 (4), 687.

Cairns, D., Shelley, L., Burke, W.M.J., Bryant, D.H., Yeates, M., Penny, R., Breit, S.N. 1992. The differing patterns of interstitial lung involvement in connective tissue diseases. J. Rheumatol. 19, 1089.

Carrington, B.C., Liebow, A.A. 1966. Lymphocytic interstitial pneumonitis. Am. J. Pathol. 48, 36.

The first attempt to classify idiopathic interstitial pneumonias. Largely, still valid.

Case records of the Massachusetts General Hospital, 1975. Case 28-1975. N. Engl. J. Med. 193, 136.

Case records of the Massachusetts General Hospital, 2001. Case 17-2001. N. Engl. J. Med. 344, 1701.

Cohen, A., King, T.A., Downey, G. 1994. Rapidly progressive bronchiolitis obliterans with organizing pneumonia. Am. J. Respir. Crit. Care Med. 149, 1670.

Colby, T.V. 1998. Pulmonary pathology in patients with systemic autoimmune diseases. Clin. Chest Med. 19 (4), 587.

Colby, T.V., Carrington, C. 1983. Lymphoreticular tumors and infiltrates of the lung. Pathol. Ann. 18, 27.

Constantopoulos, S.H., Drosos, A.A., Maddison, P.J., Moutsopoulos, H.M. 1984. Xerotrachea and interstitial lung disease in primary Sjögren's syndrome. Respiration 46, 310.

Constantopoulos, S.H., Papadimitriou, C.S., Moutsopoulos, H.M. 1985. Respiratory manifestations in primary Sjögren's syndrome: a clinical, functional and histologic study. Chest 88, 226.

Dalavanga, Y.A., Constantopoulos, S.H., Galanopoulou, V., Zerva, L., Moutsopoulos, H.M. 1991. Alveolitis correlates with clinical pulmonary involvement in primary Sjögren's syndrome. Chest 99, 1384.

Davidson, B.K., Kelly, C.A., Griffiths, I.D. 2000. Ten year follow up of pulmonary function in patients with primary Sjögren's syndrome. Ann. Rheum. Dis. 59 (9), 709.

Deheinzelin, D., Capelozzi, V.L., Kairala, R.A., Barbas, J.V., Saldiva, P.H.N., de Carvalho, C.R.R. 1996. Interstitial lung disease in primary Sjögren's: clinical pathological evaluation and response to treatment. Am. J. Respir. Crit. Care Med. 154, 794.

De Wilde, P.C.M., Kater, I., Bodeutsch, C., van den Hoogen, F.H.J., van de Putte, L.B.A., van Venrooij, W.J. 1996. Aberrant expression pattern of SS-B/La antigen in the labial salivary glands of patients with Sjögren's syndrome. Arthritis Rheum. 39, 783.

Dimitriou, I.D., Kapseogergou, E.K., Moutsopoulos, H.M., Manoussakis, M.N. 2002. CD40 on salivary gland epithelial cells: high constitutive expression by cultured cells from Sjögren's syndrome patients indicating their intrinsic activation. Clin. Exp. Immunol. 127, 386.

Ellman, P., Parkes Weber, F. 1949. Sjögren's disease with dryness of the bronchial mucosa and uncertain lung lesion. Br. Med. J. 1, 304.

Ellman, P., Parkes Weber, F., Goddier, T.E.W. 1951. A contribution to the pathology of Sjögren's syndrome. Q. J. Med. 77, 33.

Epler, G.R., Colby, T.V., McLoud, T.C., Carrington, C.B., Gaensler, E.A. 1985. Bronchiolitis obliterans organizing pneumonia. Chest 312, 152.

The first classic and systematic description of bronchiolitis obliterans organizing pneumonia (BOOP).

Fortul, T.I., Cano-Valle, F., Oliva, E., Barrios, R. 1985. Follicular bronchiolitis in association with connective tissue diseases. Lung 163, 305.

Fox, R.I., Theophilopoulos, A.N., Altman, A. 1985. Production of interleukin 2 (IL 2) by salivary gland lymphocytes in Sjögren's syndrome: detection of reactive cells by using antibody directed to synthetic peptides of IL 2. J. Immunol. 135, 3109.

Fox, R.I., Bumol, T., Fantozzi, R., Bone, R., Schreiber, R. 1986. Expression of histocompatibility antigen HLA-DR by salivary gland epithelial cells in Sjögren's syndrome. Arthritis Rheum. 29, 1105.

Franquet, T., Gimenez, A., Monill, J.M., Diaz, C., Geli, C. 1997. Primary Sjogren's syndrome and associated lung disease: CT findings in 50 patients. AJR Am. J. Roentgenol. 169, 655.

Franquet, T., Diaz, C., Domingo, P., Gimenez, A., Geli, C. 1999. Air-trapping in primary Sjogren's syndrome: correlation of expiratory CT with pulmonary function tests. J. Comput. Assist. Tomogr. 23, 169.

Fujihara, T., Fujita, H., Tsubota, K., Saito, K., Tsuzaka, K., Abe, T., Takeutsi, T. 1999. Preferential localization of CD8 + $\alpha E\beta 7$ + T cells around acinar epithelial cells with apoptosis in patients with primary Sjögren's syndrome. J. Immunol. 163, 2226.

Gardiner, P. 1993. Primary Sjögren's syndrome. Bailliere's Clin. Rheumatol. 7, 59.

An excellent review.

Gardiner, P., Ward, C., Allison, A., Ashcroft, T., Simpson, W., Walters, H., Kelly, C. 1993. Pleuropulmonary abnormalities in primary Sjögren's syndrome. J. Rheumatol. 20, 831.

Gudbjörnsson, B., Hedenström, H., Stålenheim, G., Hällgren, R. 1991. Bronchial hyperresponsiveness to methacoline in patients with primary Sjögren's syndrome. Ann. Rheum. Dis. 50, 36.

Haneji, N., Nakamori, T., Takio, K., Yanagi, K., Higashiyama, H., Saito, I., Noji, S., Sugino, H., Hayashi, Y. 1997. Identification of alpha-fodrin as a candidate autoantigen in primary Sjögren's syndrome. Science 276, 604.

Harley, J.B. 1987. Autoantibodies in Sjögren's syndrome. In: N. Talal, H.M. Moutsopoulos, S.S. Kassan (Eds.), Sjögren's Syndrome. Clinical and Immunological Aspects. Springer-Verlag, Berlin, p. 218.

Hatron, P.-Y., Wallaert, B., Gosset, D., Tonnel, A.-B., Gosselin, B., Voisin, C., Devulder, B. 1987. Subclinical lung inflammation in primary Sjögren's syndrome. Arthritis Rheum. 30, 1226.

Homma, H.A., Yamanaka, S., Tanimoto, N., Tamura, M., Chijimatsu, Y., Kira, S., Izumi, T. 1983. Diffuse panbronchiolitis: a disease of the transitional zone of the lung. Chest 83, 63.

Honda, J.H., Johkoh, T., Ichikado, K., Tomiyama, N., Maeda, M., Mihara, N., Higashi, M., Hamada, S., Naito, H., Yamamoto, S., Nakamura, H. 1999. Differential diagnosis of lymphocytic interstitial pneumonia and malignant lymphoma on high resolution CT. AJR Am. J. Roentgenol. 173, 71.

Hubscher, O., Re, R., Iotti, R. 2002. Cystic lung disease in Sjögren's syndrome. J. Rheumatol. 29, 2235.

Humphreys-Beher, M.G., Peck, A.B., Dang, H., Talal, N. 1999. The role of apoptosis in the initiation of autoimmune response in Sjögren's syndrome. Clin. Exp. Immunol. 116, 383.

Hunnighake, G.W., Fauci, A.S. 1979. Pulmonary involvement in the collagen vascular diseases. Am. Rev. Respir. Dis. 199, 279.

An excellent review.

Inagaki, Y., Jinno-Yoshida, Y., Hamasaki, Y., Ueki, H. 1991. A novel autoantibody reactive with carbonic anhydrase in sera from patients with systemic lupus erythematosus and Sjögren's syndrome. J. Dermatol. Sci. 2 (3), 147.

Inase, N., Usui, Y., Tachi, H., Takayama, S., Nakyama, M., Orenaga, M., Miura, H., Kimula, Y. 1990. Sjögren's syndrome with bronchial gland involvement and multiple bullae. Respiration 57, 286.

Ioannidis, J.P.A., Vassiliou, V.A., Moutsopoulos, H.M. 2002. Long-term risk of mortality and lymphoproliferative disease and predictive classification of primary Sjögren's Syndrome. Arthritis Rheum. 46, 741.

Johkoh, T., Müller, N.L., Pickford, H.A., Hartman, T.E., Ichikado, K., Akira, M., Honda, O., Nakamura, M. 1999. Lymphocytic interstitial pneumonia: thin-section CT findings in 22 patients. Radiology 212, 567.

Kamholz, S., Sher, A., Barland, P., Rosen, N., Rakoff, S., Becker, N. 1987. Sjögren's syndrome: Severe upper airways obstruction due to primary malignant tracheal lymphoma developing during successful treatment of lymphocytic interstitial pneumonitis. J. Rheumatol. 14, 588.

Kapseogergou, E.K., Moutsopoulos, H.M., Manoussakis, M.N. 2001a. Functional expression of a costimulatory B7.2 (CD86) protein on human salivary gland epithelial cells that interacts with the CD28 receptor, but has reduced binding to CTLA4. J. Immunol. 166, 3107.

In this article it is shown for the first time that epithelial cells like antigen presenting cells can provide the second signal for T-cell activation.

Kapseogergou, E.K., Dimitriou, I.D., Abu-Helu, R.F., Moutsopoulos, H.M., Manoussakis, M.N. 2001b. Activation of epithelial and myoepithelial cells in the salivary glands of patients with Sjögren's syndrome: high expression of intercellular adhesion molecule-1 (ICAM.1) in biopsy specimens and cultured cells. Clin. Exp. Immunol. 124, 126.

Kassan, S.S., Thomas, T.L., Moutsopoulos, H.M., Hoover, R., Kimberly, R.P., Budman, D.R., Costa, J., Decker, J.L., Chused, T.M. 1978. Increased risk of lymphoma in sicca syndrome. Ann. Intern. Med. 89, 888.

It is the classic paper that estimated the increased risk for lymphoma development in Sjögren's syndrome.

Katzenstein A.-L. (Ed.) 1997. Primary lymphoid lung lesions. Katzestein and Askin's Surgical Pathology of Non Neoplastic Lung Disorders, 3rd ed, Saunders, Philadelphia, p. 223.

Katzenstein, A.-L.A., Carrington, B.C., Liebow, A.A. 1979. Lymphomatoid granulomatosis: a clinicopathological study of 152 cases. Cancer 43, 360.

A classic paper on LYG.

Kelly, C., Gardiner, P., Pal, B., Griffiths, I. 1991. Lung function in primary Sjögren's syndrome: a cross sectional and longitudinal study. Thorax 46, 180.

Kobayashi, H., Matsuoka, R., Kitamura, S., Tsunoda, N., Saito, K. 1988. Sjögren's syndrome with multiple bullae and pulmonary nodular amyloidosis. Chest 94, 438.

Kong, L., Ogawa, N., Nakabayashi, T., Liu, G.T., D'souza, E., McGuff, H.S., Guerrero, D., Talal, N., Dang, H. 1997. Fas and fas ligand expression in the salivary glands of patients with primary Sjögren's syndrome. Arthritis Rheum. 40, 87.

Lahdensuo, A., Korpela, M. 1995. Pulmonary findings in patients with primary Sjogren's syndrome. Chest 108, 316.

Liebow, A.A., Carrington, C.B. 1973. Diffuse pulmonary lymphoreticular infiltrates associated with dysproteinaemia. Med. Clin. N Am. 57, 809.

Liebow, A.A., Carrington, B.C., Friedman, P.J. 1972. Lymphomatoid granulomatosis. Human Pathol. 3, 457.

The classic paper on LYG.

Lindahl, G., Hedfords, E., Klareskog, L., Forsum, U. 1985. Epithelial HLA-DR expression in T lymphocyte subsets in salivary glands in Sjögren's syndrome. Clin. Exp. Immunol. 61, 475.

Manoussakis, M.N., Moutsopoulos, H.M. 2000. Sjögren's syndrome: autoimmune epithelitis. Bailliere's Clin. Rheumatol. 14, 73.

Manoussakis, M.N., Moutsopoulos, H.M. 2001. Sjogren's syndrome: current concepts. Adv. Intern. Med. 47, 191.

Manoussakis, M.N., Tziuofas, A.G., Pange, P.J.E., Moutsopoulos, H.M. 1986. Serological profiles in subgroups of patients with Sjögren's syndrome. Scand. J. Rheumatol. 61, 89.

Manoussakis, M.N., Dimitriou, I.D., Kapseogeorgou, E.K., Xanthou, G., Paikos, S., Polichronis, M., Moutsopoulos, H.M. 1999. Expression of B7 costimulatory molecules in patients with Sjögren's syndrome. Arthritis Rheum. 41, 229.

Mariette, X. 1999. Lymphomas in patients with Sjögren's syndrome: review of the literature and physiopathologic hypothesis. Leukemia Lymphoma 33, 93.

Matsumura, T., Umemiya, K., Kagami, M., Tomoika, H., Tanabe, E., Sugiyama, T., Sueishi, M., Nakajima, A., Azuma, M., Okumura, K., Sumida, T. 1998. Glandular and extraglandular expression of the Fas–Fas ligand and apoptosis in patients with Sjögren's syndrome. Clin Exp. Rheumatol. 16, 561.

Matteson, E.L., Ike, R.W. 1990. Bronchiolitis obliterans organizing pneumonia and Sjögren's syndrome. J. Rheumatol. 17, 676.

Meyer, C.A., Pina, J.S., Taillon, D., Goodwin, J.D. 1997. Inspiratory and expiratory high-resolution CT findings in the patient with Sjogren's syndrome and cystic lung disease. AJR Am. J. Roentgenol. 168, 101.

Mialon, P., Barthelemy, L., Sebert, P., Le Henaff, C., Sami, D., Pennec, Y.L., Le Goff, P., Youinou, P. 1997. A longitudinal study of lung impairment in patients with primary Sjögren's syndrome. Clin. Exp. Rheumatol. 15, 349.

Moutsopoulos, H.M. 1994. Sjögren's syndrome: autoimmune epithelitis. Clin. Immunol. Immunopathol. 72, 162.

A new intriguing proposal on Sjögren's syndrome pathogenesis.

Moutsopoulos, H.M. 2001. Sjögren's syndrome. In: E. Braunwald, A.S. Fauci, D.L. Kasper, S.L. Hauser, D.L. Longo, J.L. Jameson (Eds.), Harrison's Principles of Internal Medicine. McGraw-Hill, New York, p. 1947.

Moutsopoulos, H.M., Chused, T.M., Mann, D.L., Klippel, J.H., Fauci, A.S., Frank, M.M., Lawley, T.J., Hamburger, M.I. 1980. Sjögren's syndrome (sicca syndrome): current issues. Ann. Intern. Med. 92 (Part 1), 212.

The classic article on the different aspects of Sjögren's syndrome.

Moutsopoulos, H.M., Hooks, J.J., Chan, C.C., Dalavanga, Y.A., Skopouli, F.N., Detrick, B. 1986. HLA-DR expression by labial minor salivary gland tissues in Sjögren's syndrome. Ann. Rheum. Dis. 45, 677.

Newball, H.H., Brahim, S.A. 1977. Chronic obstructive airway disease in patients with Sjögren's syndrome. Am. Rev. Respir. Dis. 115, 295.

Nishimori, I., Okazaki, K., Yamamoto, Y., Morita, M., Tamura, S., Yamamoto, Y. 1993. Specific cellular immune responses to pancreatic antigen in chronic pancreatitis and Sjögren's syndrome. J. Clin. Immunol. 13 (4), 265.

Nishimori, I., Yamamoto, Y., Okazaki, K., Morita, M., Onodera, M., Kino, Y., Tamura, S., Yamamoto, Y. 1994. Identification of autoantibodies to a pancreatic antigen in patients with idiopathic chronic pancreatits and Sjögren's syndrome. Pancreas 9 (3), 374.

Nishimori, I., Bratanova, T., Toshkov, I., Caffrey, T., Mogaki, M., Shibata, Y., Hollingsworth, M.A. 1995. Induction of experimental autoimmune sialoadenitis by immunization of PL/J mice with carbonic anhydrase II. J. Immunol. 154, 4865.

Ogihara, T., Nakatani, A., Ito, H., Irokawa, M., Ban, S., Takahashi, A., Nishinarita, M., Oka, Y. 1995. Sjögren's syndrome with pleural effusion. Intern. Med. 34, 811.

Okano, A., Sato, A., Suda, T., Suda, I., Yasuda, K., Iwata, M., Chida, K. 1991. A case of diffuse panbronchiolitis complicated by malignant thymoma and Sjögren's syndrome. Jpn. J. Thorac. Dis. 29, 262. (in Japanese; abstract in English).

Okazaki, K., Tamura, S., Morita, M., Nishimori, I., Yamamoto, Y., Yamamoto, Y. 1989. Interspecies crossreactive antigen of the pancreatic duct cell prepared by monoclonal antibody. Int. J. Pancreatol. 5, 359.

Papathanasiou, M.P., Constantopoulos, S.H., Tsampoulas, C. 1986. Reappraisal of respiratory abnormalities in primary and secondary Sjögren's syndrome. A controlled study. Chest 90, 370.

Papiris, S.A., Saetta, M., Turato, G., La Corte, R., Trevisani, L., Mapp, C.E., Maestrelli, P., Fabbri, L., Potena, A. 1997. CD_4 positive T-lymphocytes infiltrate the bronchial mucosa in patients with Sjögren's syndrome. Am. J. Respir. Crit. Care Med. 156, 637.

Papiris, S.A., Kassan, S.S., Moutsopoulos, H.M. 1999a. Lung involvement in primary Sjögren's syndrome. Sem. Respir. Crit. Care Med. 20 (2), 179.

Papiris, S.A., Maniati, M., Constantopoulos, S.H., Roussos, C., Moutsopoulos, H.M., Skopouli, F.N. 1999b. Lung involvement in primary Sjögren's syndrome is mainly related to the small airway disease. Ann. Rheum. Dis. 58, 61.

Polichronis, M., Tapinos, N.I., Theocharis, S.E., Economou, A., Kittas, C., Moutsopoulos, H.M. 1998. Modes of epithelial cell death and repair in Sjögren's syndrome (SS). Clin. Exp. Immunol. 114, 485.

Potena, A., La Corte, R., Fabbri, L.M., Papi, A., Trotta, F., Ciaccia, A. 1990. Increased bronchial responsiveness in primary and secondary Sjögren's syndrome. Eur. Respir. J. 3, 548.

Royer, B., Cazals-Hatem, D., Sibilia, J., Agbalika, F., Cayuela, J.-M., Soussi, T., Maloisel, F., Clauvel, J.-P., Brouet, J.-C., Mariette, X. 1997. Lymphomas in patients with Sjögren's syndrome are marginal zone B-cell neoplasm, arise in diverse extranodal and nodal sites, and are not associated with viruses. Blood 90, 766.

Sakamoto, O., Saita, N., Ando, M., Kohrogi, H., Suga, M., Ando, M. 2002. Two cases of Sjögren's syndrome with multiple bullae. Intern. Med. 41, 124.

Saltzstein, S.L. 1963. Pulmonary malignant lymphomas and pseudolymphomas: classification, therapy and prognosis. Cancer 16, 928.

A classic article on lung lymphomas.

Segal, I., Fink, G., Machtey, I., Gura, V., Spitzer, S.A. 1981. Pulmonary function abnormalities in Sjögren's syndrome and the sicca complex. Thorax 36, 286.

Shan, D., Ledbetter, J.A., Press, O.W. 1998. Apoptosis of malignant human B-cells by ligation of CD20 with monoclonal antibodies. Blood 91, 1644.

Siamopoulos, K.C., Mavridis, A.K., Elisaf, M., Drosos, A.A., Moutsopoulos, H.M. 1986. Kidney involvement in primary Sjögren's syndrome. Scand. J. Rheumatol. 61 (s), 156.

Silbiger, M.L., Peterson, C.C. 1967. Sjögren's syndrome: its roentgenological features. Am. J. Roentgenol. 100, 554.

Sjögren, H. 1933. Zur Kenntnis der Keratoconjunctivitis sicca (Keratitis filiformis bei Hypofunction der Tranendrusen). Acta Ophthamologica (SII), 1.

The first systematic description of a new syndrome.

Skopouli, F.N., Kousvelari, E.E., Mertz, P., Jaffe, E.S., Fox, P.C., Moutsopoulos, H.M. 1992. C-myc mRNA expression in minor salivary glands of patients with Sjögren's syndrome. J. Rheumatol. 19, 693.

Skopouli, F.N., Barbatis, C., Moutsopoulos, H.M. 1994. Liver involvement in primary Sjögren's syndrome. Br. J Rheumatol. 33, 745.

Skopouli, F.N., Dafni, U., Ioannidis, J.P.A., Moutsopoulos, H.M. 2000. Clinical evolution, and morbidity and mortality of primary Sjogren's syndrome. Semin. Arthritis Rheum. 29, 296.

Somer, B.G., Tsai, D.E., Downs, L., Weinstein, B., Schuster, S.J. 2003. Improvement in Sjögren's syndrome following therapy with rituximab for marginal zone lymphoma. Arthritis Rheum. 49, 394.

Spicer, S.S., Sens, M.A., Hennigar, R.A., Stoward, P.J. 1984. Implications of the immunohistochemical localization of the carbonic anhydrase isozymes for their function in normal and pathologic cells. Ann. NY Acad. Sci. 429, 382.

Strimlan, C.V., Rosenow, E.C. III, Divertie, M.B., Harrison, E.G. 1976. Pulmonary manifestations in Sjögren's syndrome. Chest 70, 354.

Sugai, S. 2002. Mucosa-associated lymphoid tissue (MALT) lymphoma and primary amyloidosis in the lung in Sjögren's syndrome. Intern. Med. 41, 251.

Sutinen, S., Sutinen, S., Huhti, E. 1977. Ultrastructure of lymphoid interstitial pneumonia. Am. J. Clin. Pathol. 67, 328.

Swigris, J.J., Berry, G.J., Raffin, T.A., Kuschner, W.G. 2002. Lymphoid interstitial pneumonia. A narrative review. Chest 122, 2150.

An excellent review.

Talal, N., Moutsopoulos, H.M., Kassan, S.S. 1987. Sjögren's Syndrome: Clinical and Immunological Aspects. Springer, Heidelberg.

The classic text on Sjögren's syndrome.

Taouli, B., Brauner, M.W., Mourey, I., Lemouchi, D., Grenier, P.A. 2002. Thin-section chest CT findings of primary Sjögren's syndrome: correlation with pulmonary function. Eur. Radiol. 12, 1504.

Tapinos, N.I., Polihronis, M., Moutsopoulos, H.M. 1999. Lymphoma development in Sjogren's syndrome: novel p53 mutations. Arthritis Rheum. 42 (7), 1466.

Tzioufas, A.G., Boumba, D.A., Skopouli, F.N., Moutsopoulos, H.M. 1996. Mixed monoclonal cryoglobulinemia and monoclonal rheumatoid factor cross-reactive idiotypes as predictive factors for development of lymphoma in primary Sjögren's syndrome. Arthritis Rheum. 39, 767.

Ubucata, M., Sugiyama, S., Ohno, S., Sugama, Y., Kitamura, S. 1991. A case of Sjögren's syndrome with a clinical course similar to diffuse panbronchiolitis. Jpn. J. Thorac. Dis. 29, 387. (in Japanese; abstract in English).

Uffmann, M., Kiener, H.P., Bankier, A.A., Baldt, M.M., Zontsich, T., Herold, C.J. 2001. Lung manifestation in asymptomatic patients with primary Sjögren's syndrome: assessment with high resolution CT and pulmonary function tests. J. Thorac. Imaging 16 (4), 282.

Usui, Y., Kimula, Y., Miura, H., Kodaira, Y., Takayama, S., Nakayama, M., Kataoka, N. 1992. Bronchiolitis obliterans organizing pneumonia associated with primary Sjögren's syndrome who died of superimposed diffuse alveolar damage. Respiration 59, 122.

Vitali, C., Bombardieri, S., Jonsson, R., Moutsopoulos, H.M., Alexander, E.L., Carsons, S.E., Daniels, T.E., Fox, P.C., Fox, R.I., Kassan, S.S., Pillemer, S.R., Talal, N., Weisman, M.H., The European study group on classification criteria for Sjögren's syndrome 2002. Classification criteria for Sjögren's syndrome: a revised version of the European criteria proposed by the American–European consensus group. Ann. Rheum. Dis. 61, 554.
The ultimate consensus criteria.

Voulgarelis, M., Moutsopoulos, H.M. 2001. Malignant lymphoma in Sjögren's syndrome. IMAJ 3, 761.

Voulgarelis, M., Dafni, U.G., Isenberg, D.A., Moutsopoulos, H.M., The members of the European concerted action on Sjögren's syndrome 1999. Arthritis Rheum. 42, 1765.

Weisbrot, I.M. 1976. Lymphomatoid granulomatosis of the lung, associated with a long history of benign lymphoepithelial lesions of the salivary glands and lymphoid interstitial pneumonitis. Am. J. Clin. Pathol. 66, 792.

Wells, A.U., du Bois, R.M. 1993. Bronchiolitis in association with connective tissue disorders. Clin. Chest. Med. 14 (4), 655.

Whaley, K., Webb, J., McAvoy, B.A., Hughes, G.R., Lee, P., MacSween, R.N., Buchanan, W.W. 1973. Sjögren's syndrome: clinical associations and immunological phenomena. Q. J. Med. 42, 513.

Wright, J.L., Cagle, P., Churg, A., Colby, T.V., Myers, J. 1992. Diseases of the small airways. Am. Rev. Respir. Dis. 1146, 240.

Xanthou, G., Tapinos, N.I., Polihronis, M., Nezis, I.P., Margaritis, L.H., Moutsopoulos, H.M. 1999. CD4 cytotoxic and dendritic cells in the immunopathologic lesion of Sjögren's syndrome. Clin. Exp. Immunol. 118, 154.

Xanthou, G., Polihronis, M., Tzioufas, A.G., Paikos, S., Sideras, P., Moutsopoulos, H.M. 2001. 'Lymphoid' chemokine messenger RNA expression by epithelial cells in the chronic inflammatory lesion of the salivary glands of Sjogren's syndrome patients: possible participation in lymphoid structure formation. Arthritis Rheum. 44 (2), 408.

Yamadori, I., Fujita, J., Banoh, S., Tokuda, M., Tanimoto, Y., Kataoka, M., Yamasaki, Y., Yoshinuchi, T., Ohtsuki, Y., Ishida, T. 2002. Nonspecific interstitial pneumonia as pulmonary involvement in Sjögren's syndrome. Rheumatol. Int. 22 (3), 89.

Yannopoulos, D.J., Roncin, S., Lamour, A., Pennec, Y.L., Moutsopoulos, H.M., Youinou, P. 1992. Conjunctival epithelial cells from patients with Sjögren's syndrome inappropriately express major histocompatibility complex molecules, La(SSB) antigen, and heat-shock proteins. J. Clin. Immunol. 12, 259.

Yousem, S.A., Colby, T.V., Carrington, C.B. 1985. Follicular bronchitis/bronchiolitis. Human Pathol., 700.

Zulman, J., Jaffe, R., Talal, N. 1978. Evidence that the malignant lymphoma of Sjögren's syndrome is a monoclonal B-cell neoplasm. N. Engl. J. Med. 299, 1215.
The first characterization of the type of lymphomas arising in Sjögren's syndrome.

Handbook of Systemic Autoimmune Diseases, Volume 2
Pulmonary Involvement in Systemic Autoimmune Diseases
A.U. Wells and C.P. Denton, editors

CHAPTER 10

Interstitial Disease in Systemic Sclerosis

Nicole S. Goh, Roland M. du Bois*

Interstitial Lung Disease Unit, Royal Brompton Hospital, Sydney Street, London SW3 6NP, UK

1. Introduction

The term 'scleroderma' is used to encompass a heterogenous group of conditions linked by the presence of varying degrees of skin sclerosis (Black, 1993). The simplest division of the scleroderma-related disorders is into localised and systemic forms. The term 'systemic sclerosis' (SSc) is used for the latter form and is a reflection of the frequent involvement of internal organs.

SSc is further subdivided into limited (lcSSc) and diffuse cutaneous subsets (dcSSc), which are principally distinguished by the extent of skin fibrosis and the forms of organ involvement. Patients with lcSSc typically have skin sclerosis limited to the hands, and to a lesser extent, the face and neck. Vascular manifestations are prominent and they classically suffer from the CREST syndrome (calcinosis, Raynaud's phenomenon, oesophageal dysmotility, sclerodactyly and telangiectasia).

Patients with dcSSc, in contrast, have extensive skin involvement, extending proximally, often to the chest and abdominal wall. They are also at greater risk for developing renal, lung and cardiac complications.

SSc is, therefore, a connective tissue disease characterised clinically by varying degrees of skin fibrosis and visceral organ involvement (Leroy et al., 1988; Medsger, 1997). Pulmonary involvement is common in SSc and includes a variety of manifestations (see Table 1.), pulmonary interstitial fibrosis (PIF) and pulmonary vascular disease being the most common.

Since the advent of ACE inhibitors and effective gastrointestinal drugs, pulmonary involvement has become the most common cause of scleroderma-related death. The early detection and treatment of lung disease is, therefore, important to halt progression and, in certain cases, reverse disease. The course of disease, however, is highly variable, ranging from indolent to rapidly progressive. Treatments available are potentially toxic, carrying their own risk of morbidity and mortality. A vigilant surveillance of disease detection, assessment of disease prognosis and timing of treatment is, therefore, imperative in the management of patients.

The most common interstitial lung disease (ILD) in SSc is diffuse interstitial fibrosis (PIF/SSc) and unless otherwise stated, the rest of the chapter will focus on this manifestation of SSc.

2. Prevalence

Interstitial fibrosis is the most common pulmonary manifestation in SSc, occurring in roughly 80% of patients (Arroliga et al., 1992). The definition of prevalence is, however, not entirely straightforward and depends on the criteria used. Respiratory symptoms, present in well over 50% of patients, are an unreliable marker. They do not discriminate between PIF and pulmonary vascular disease and can be confounded by musculoskeletal disease or general debility. On the other hand, some patients

*Corresponding author.
Tel.: +44-20-7351-8327; fax: +44-20-7351-8336
E-mail address: r.dubois@rbh.nthames.nhs.uk (R.M. du Bois).

DOI: 10.1016/S1571-5078(04)02010-0

Table 1
Pulmonary manifestations of SSc

Pulmonary interstitial fibrosis[a]
Pulmonary vascular disease[a]
Pleural disease
Aspiration pneumonia
Organising pneumonia[b]
Diffuse alveolar damage[b]
Cuirasse[b]
Alveolar haemorrhage[b]
Drug-associated pneumonitis

[a] Most common.
[b] Rare.

present late due to the same confounders. Chest radiography abnormalities have been reported in 25–65% of patients (Minai et al., 1998) and computed tomography (CT) further detects limited disease in a proportion of patients with normal chest radiography (Harrison et al., 1989). Autopsy series have reported a prevalence of up to 75% of patients (D'Angelo et al., 1969; Wiedemann and Matthay, 1989) and lung function abnormalities have been seen in up to 90%. In addition, PIF is one of the American Rheumatism Association's (ARA) preliminary diagnostic criteria for the disease (Masi et al., 1980), and can precede the systemic disease, sometimes by years, and thus can impact on true prevalence figures.

3. Epidemiology

The epidemiology of SSc is not fully defined due to the relative rarity of the disease, the difficulty in diagnosis and its extreme clinical variability. SSc is predominantly a disease of women, with a female to male ratio ranging from 3:1 to 8:1 (Steen et al., 1997). The peak incidence is between 45 and 64 years of age (Medsger, 1997) and there appears to be an increased incidence in blacks, with an earlier onset than in whites (Laing et al., 1997). Black patients have also been reported to have more diffuse disease, associated with worse survival (Laing et al., 1997). Although women are affected more frequently than men, the factors responsible for this are not apparent.

An excess of female cases compared with male cases has been observed to be more marked in the child-bearing years than in older age groups (Steen et al., 1997). In a study comparing female patients with SSc and controls (Beebe et al., 1997), no significant associations were seen with age at menarche, ever being pregnant, or oral contraceptive use, although oestrogen replacement therapy was associated with a small but significant increased risk of developing SSc. In contrast, a reduced risk of SSc among parous women compared with nulliparous women has been reported (Pisa et al., 2002).

In a retrospective study on the issue of parity on disease progression, it was observed that nulliparous women had an earlier onset of disease, more diffuse disease, more severe lung involvement, and a higher SSc related mortality (Artlett et al., 2002b). In contrast, it has also been reported that women with PIF had more children than those without PIF (Launay et al., 2001). In addition, nulliparous women were no more likely to have diffuse disease than those with one or more children.

4. Aetiology/Pathogenesis

4.1. Aetiology

The aetiology of SSc is unknown. It is, however, generally accepted that the disease results from complex interactions between environmental factors in a genetically susceptible hosts, leading to variable disease expression.

4.1.1. Genetic factors

Strong evidence for genetic factors in SSc is supported by (1) the observation of familial clustering and the increased prevalence in twin studies; (2) the increased prevalence of autoantibody positivity and other autoimmune diseases in the relatives of patients with SSc; (3) differences in SSc prevalence and clinical manifestations among different ethnic groups; (4) HLA associations with the disease and more strongly, with specific autoantibodies; (5) the potential influences of various genetic polymorphisms on the severity and progression of disease (Johnson et al., 2002).

SSc has been shown to cluster in families, although at a low frequency of about 1.5% (Englert et al., 1999; Arnett et al., 2001). In the first large population-based study in SSc from Sydney, Australia, a population prevalence rate of roughly 1.4 per million was observed in 715 SSc patients (710 families) (Englert et al., 1999). Given the low prevalence of the disease, estimated to be between 0.021 and 0.024% (Chandran et al., 1995; Mayes et al., 2003), the occurrence of disease seen in family members of patients with SSc confers the highest relative risk for the disease. Although the concordance of SSc among identical twins is only 5.9%, this lends further support to the role of genetic factors in the pathogenesis of SSc (Feghali and Wright, 1995).

The familial occurrence of SSc with other autoimmune diseases, such as systemic lupus erythematosus (SLE), has been well reported (Hagberg et al., 1961; du Bois et al., 1971; Flores et al., 1984; Arnett et al., 1984; Maddison et al., 1993). In a study of 63 family members of patients with SSc, multiple cases of SSc were seen in one family with similar disease expressions. Other connective tissue diseases were found in nine families, and other non-specific features of connective tissue diseases such as Raynaud's phenomenon and arthritis occurred commonly, especially in female relatives. ANA have also been detected more frequently in relatives than in controls (Maddison et al., 1993; McHugh et al., 1994; Whyte et al., 1994); relatives with anti-Scl-70 (Whyte et al., 1994) and anti-centromere antibodies (McHugh et al., 1994) also had SSc in these studies.

A high prevalence of SSc has been found in Choctaw-Native Americans in the state of Oklahoma (Arnett et al., 1996a). The prevalence of SSc in this population was at least 20 times greater than in the general population and appeared to be associated with differences in MHC allele expressions when compared to other ethnic groups. Disease expression also appears to be different among ethnic groups. African American patients are more likely to have anti-Scl-70 antibodies, and more systemic involvement with a higher occurrence of PIF. In contrast, Caucasian patients are more likely to have anti-centromere antibodies with more limited disease and less systemic manifestations (Johnson et al., 2002).

Certain HLA haplotypes have been associated with SSc. These include HLA-DR5 (DRB1*1101 and 1104, DQA1*0501, DQB1*0301) and DR3 (DRB1*0301, DQA1*0501, DQB1*0201) haplotypes in American and European white populations (Gladman et al., 1981; Arnett et al., 1990), and HLA-DR2 (DRB1*1502, DQB1*0601) (Kuwana et al., 1993b) in Japanese. In particular relation to the lungs, Briggs et al. (1991) found that the presence of DR3/DRw52a or anti-Scl-70 antibodies gave a relative risk of 16.7 for the development of PIF. More recently, Gilchrist et al. (2001) found strong associations between clinical phenotypes and autoantibody status. In a study of over 200 patients, the presence of Scl-70 was associated with PIF, and Scl-70 was in turn found to be associated with HLA-DPB1*1301 and HLA-DRB1*11. The presence of anticentromere autoantibody on the other hand was linked to HLA-DRB1*04 and HLA-DRB1*08. Table 2 outlines genetic associations with other autoantibody subsets.

The potential influence of various genetic polymorphisms on the severity and progression of the fibrotic process by promoting increased collagen gene expression have been studied in SSc. Two different single nucleotide polymorphisms in the gene for transforming growth factor β (TGFβ 1), a potent profibrotic cytokine, have been reported to be present in higher frequency in patients with SSc than in normal individuals (Crilly et al., 2002), although other studies have not confirmed this.

Fibrillin-1 is an important structural protein expressed in many tissues, including skin, and is a major component of elastic microfibrils found in the extracellular matrix (ECM). A genetically determined mutant fibrillin protein is responsible for the type I tight skin (Tsk) mouse model of scleroderma (Jimenez and Gershwin, 1996; Falkner et al., 1998). By analogy, certain single nucleotide polymorphism in the non-coding region of the fibrillin-1 gene has been found to be associated with development of SSc in Choctaw and Japanese populations (Tan et al., 2001).

Type I collagen is produced in excess in patients with SSc. The presence of certain nucleotide repeats associated with higher expression of COL1A2 (gene for type I collagen) were found more frequently in SSc cases (Hata et al., 2000).

Table 2
Human leucocyte antigens associations with autoantibodies seen in patients with SSc

Autoantibody	HLA associations	Ethnic group	References
ACA	DR1 (DRB1*0101: DQB1*0501) DRB1*0104	Choctaw, White, African, Japanese, Hispanics Whites, Hispanics	Reveille et al. (1992b, 2001), Morel et al. (1995)
Anti Scl-70	DR5/11 (DRB1*1101, 1104) DQB1*0301; DPB1*1301 DR2 (DRB1*1502; DQB1*0601; DPB1*0901) DR2 (DRB1*1602; DQB1*0301; DPB1*1301)	White African Japanese, Choctaw	Reveille et al. (1992a, 2001), Kuwana et al. (1993b), Tan et al. (1999)
Anti-PM-Scl	DR3 (DRB1*0301, DQB1*0201)	White	Marguerie et al. (1992)
Anti-Th/To	DR5/11 (DRB1*1104, DQB1*0301)		Falkner et al. (1998)
Anti-RNAP	? DQB1*0201		Fanning et al. (1998), Falkner et al. (2000)
Anti-U3-RNP/ antifibrillarin	DR6/13 (DRB1*1302: DQB1*0604)	White and Africans	Arnett et al. (1996b)

4.1.2. Environmental factors

4.1.2.1. Infectious agents. Infectious agents have been considered to play a possible causative role in SSc. This hypothesis is based on observations that production of specific autoantibodies in SSc may be due to an antigen-driven response triggered by 'molecular mimicry' between self-antigens sharing structural similarities to a foreign protein of viral or bacterial origin. The two most recently implicated viruses are the parvovirus and the human cytomegalovirus (HCMV). Ferri et al., (1999) detected parvovirus B19 infection in the bone marrow of 12 out of 21 SSc patients and it was also observed that SSc patients with bone marrow B19 infection showed a shorter mean disease duration to presentation or death than B19-negative patients. Autoantibodies against cell surface antigens have been considered pathogenic by inducing endothelial cell damage. A higher prevalence of IgG-anti HMCV antibodies capable of binding the HCMV late protein UL-94 and inducing apoptosis in human endothelial cells has been observed (Lunardi et al., 2000).

4.1.2.2. Chemicals. A number of chemicals have been implicated in the aetiology of SSc, based on either case reports or epidemiology studies. One of the earliest associations was seen with silica dust (Bramwell, 1914), although more recent evidence has not supported this (Silman and Jones, 1992). Vinyl chloride polymers (Veltman et al., 1975), and organic solvents such as benzene, xylene and trichloroethylene (Nietert et al., 1998; Nietert et al., 1999), have all been implicated. In addition, an association between solvent-associated hobbies and the development of SSc with anti-Scl-70 antibodies has also been observed (Nietert et al., 1999). Associations between silicone breast implants and the development of SSc have been previously reported (van Nunen et al., 1982; Kumagai et al., 1984). However, further evidence has not supported a causative relationship (Hochberg and Perlmutter, 1996; Edworthy et al., 1998; Janowsky et al., 2000). 'Epidemics' caused by the ingestion of contaminated rapeseed oil (toxic oil syndrome) (Tabuenca, 1981) and L-tryptophan (Silver et al., 1990a; Kamb et al., 1992) lend further support to the notion that toxic exposures could play a role in the development of SSc, at least in some patients, perhaps those with a genetic predisposition.

4.2. Microchimerism

The exchange of cells between the mother and the foetus in both directions has been recognised during normal human pregnancy (Hall et al., 1995; Lo et al., 1996). Perhaps more surprising is the observation that the exchange can persist both in the foetus (Maloney et al., 1999) and the mother (Bianchi et al., 1996) for a prolonged period of time; well into adulthood for the foetus and decades after the completion of pregnancy for the mother. It has been recently proposed that an allogeneic foeto-maternal reaction, possibly a manifestation of an intergenerational HLA incompatibility, may be involved in the pathogenesis of SSc (Nelson et al., 1998; Artlett et al., 1998). These engrafted cells have been postulated to become activated by an environmental trigger and subsequently mount a graft-vs.-host reaction towards the mother or the offspring, which may result in the development of SSc. A higher concentration of male DNA in both peripheral blood (Nelson et al., 1998; Artlett et al., 1998) and skin (Artlett et al., 1998) was detected in SSc females who had given birth to sons compared to control females. Microchimerism of maternal origin in blood and tissues of the offspring has also been observed and might explain the occurrence of SSc in nulliparous women and in men (Maloney et al., 1999).

This hypothesis is still controversial as several studies have shown that foetal Y chromosome DNA is present in normal controls. Other studies have, however, suggested that it may be the quantity and not the mere presence of foetal cells that may be the crucial contributory factor in the pathogenesis of SSc (Ohtsuka et al., 2001; Artlett et al., 2002a).

4.3. Pathogenesis

Although the pathogenesis of SSc is complex and incompletely understood, dysregulation of cellular and humoral immunity, vascular injury and widespread tissue fibrosis are important in the development of the disease. Cell–cell, cell–cytokine, and cell–matrix interactions are involved. It is generally accepted that early immunological events and vascular changes result in the generation of a population of activated fibrogenic fibroblasts, which is generally considered to be the effector cell in the disease.

The earliest structural features of ILD in SSc include pulmonary capillary endothelial and epithelial injury, interstitial oedema and inflammatory cell infiltration. It is likely that endothelial and/or epithelial injury precede inflammation and fibrosis although the initiating factor is not known (Harrison et al., 1991b).

Although the mechanisms which lead to the deposition of excess collagen and other ECM in the lungs are not well understood, it is thought that mediators released after lung injury play a crucial role in the activation of fibroblasts. There are many potential sources of fibroblast growth factors in the lung. These include alveolar macrophages (Rom et al., 1988; Wallaert et al., 1988; Kinsella et al., 1989), injured or regenerating endothelial and epithelial cells (Gibbons and Dzau, 1990), inflammatory cells such as lymphocytes and mast cells (Agelli and Wahl, 1986; Reiser and Last, 1986), and mesenchymal cells such as interstitial fibroblasts, myofibroblasts and smooth muscle cells. Mediators may also enter the lung interstitium from the circulation as a result of endothelial cell injury and capillary leakage (Harrison et al., 1990).

The ECM most relevant to fibrosis are the collagens, proteoglycans, fibronectin, fibrillin, tenascin, and SPARC (secreted protein, acidic and rich in cysteine; osteonectin; BM-40). Adhesive receptors (integrins) on fibroblasts and other connective tissue cells that are specific for ECM macromolecules also play important roles in fibrosis. Avila et al. (1999) found a strong association between fibronectin polymorphisms and interstitial fibrosis. Fibronectin, released by alveolar macrophages, has been found to be overexpressed in the respiratory tract of scleroderma patients with interstitial fibrosis. This may contribute to the recruitment and attachment of the fibroblasts in scleroderma lung disease (Silver et al., 1990b).

Many cytokines and growth factors have been implicated in the pathogenesis of fibrosis (see Table 3).

Transforming growth factor-beta (TGF-β) is considered one of the key molecules involved in the pathogenesis of SSc (Smith and Leroy, 1990). It is secreted in a latent form and has to be activated in order to exert its profibrotic action. Sources of TGF-β include macrophages, lymphocytes, platelets, fibroblasts, epithelial and endothelial cells.

One of the important effects of TGF-β is the stimulation of ECM synthesis (Varga et al., 1987; Kissin et al., 2002). TGF-β also decreases the synthesis of collagen-degrading metalloproteinases and stimulates the production of protease inhibitors such as the tissue inhibitor of metalloproteinase-1 (TIMP-1). Increased TGF-β signalling appears to

Table 3
Cytokines and growth factors implicated in the pathogenesis of fibrosis

Growth factor/cytokine	Potential cellular sources in fibrosis	References
Transforming growth factor-beta (TGF-β)	Macrophages/monocytes, lymphocytes, platelets, fibroblasts, endothelial cells, epithelial cells	Fine and Goldstein (1987), Raghu et al. (1989), Smith and Leroy (1990), Deguchi and Kishimoto (1991), Corrin et al. (1994), Coker et al. (2001)
Connective tissue growth factor (CTGF)	Fibroblasts	Sato et al. (2000b), Leask et al. (2002)
Platelet derived growth factor (PDGF)	Macrophages, platelets, fibroblasts, endothelial cells	Ohba et al. (1994), Ludwicka et al. (1995), Shimizu et al. (2000)
Tumour necrosis factor (TNF)	Monocytes/macrophages, fibroblasts	Postlethwaite and Seyer (1990), Bolster et al. (1997), Hasegawa et al. (1997b), Sime et al. (1998), Pantelidis et al. (2001), Young et al. (2002)
Insulin growth factor (IGF)	Macrophages, fibroblasts, endothelial cells	Rom et al. (1988), Harrison et al. (1994)
Basic fibroblast growth factor (bFGF)	Macrophages, mast cells, neutrophils, eosinophils	Vaillant et al. (1996), Denton et al. (1997)
Endothelin	Endothelial cells	Cambrey et al. (1994), Vancheeswaran et al. (1994), Abraham et al. (1997)
Oncostatin M	T lymphocytes, macrophages	Ihn et al. (1997), Ihn and Tamaki (2000), Luzina et al. (2002)
Interleukin-1 (IL1)	Macrophages, fibroblasts, endothelial cells	Postlethwaite et al. (1984), Shahar et al. (1996), Luzina et al. (2002)
Interleukin-4 (IL4)	Th2 lymphocytes	Postlethwaite and Seyer (1991), Postlethwaite et al. (1992), Atamas and White (1999), Sakkas et al. (1999)
Interleukin-6 (IL6)	Macrophages, fibroblasts, Th2 lymphocytes, endothelial cells	Duncan and Berman (1991), Fries et al. (1994), Shahar et al. (1996), Hasegawa et al. (1999)
Interleukin-8 (IL8)	Endothelial cells, Th2 lymphocytes	Southcott et al. (1995), Pantelidis et al., (1997), Kadono et al., (1998), Furuse et al. (2003)
Interleukin-13 (IL13)	Th2 lymphocytes	Hasegawa et al. (1997a), Oriente et al. (2000), Fallon et al. (2000)
Tissue inhibitor metalloproteinase-1 (TIMP-1)	Fibroblasts	Kirk et al. (1995), Kikuchi et al. (1997), Susol et al. (2000), Young-Min et al. (2001)
Monocyte-chemotactic protein (MCP-1)	Macrophages, fibroblasts	Zhang et al. (1994), Suga et al. (1999), Hasegawa et al. (1999), Yamamoto et al. (2001), Moore et al. (2001), Galindo et al. (2001), Luzina et al. (2002)
Pulmonary and activation-regulated chemokine (PARC)	Macrophages, epithelial cells	Hieshima et al. (1997), Pardo et al. (2001), Luzina et al. (2002), Atamas et al. (2003)

result from a number of pathways. TGF-β can act in an autocrine loop to sensitise fibroblasts and maintain them in a persistently activated state. Activated monocytes can also secrete TGF-β, and it appears that the SSc fibroblasts might also express increased numbers of TGF-β receptors.

Collagen gene activation via TGF-β is an intricate process (Massague, 2000) and involves the Smad family of proteins (Wrana and Attisano, 2000). Bioactive TGF-β binds to the cell surface TGF-β receptor in target cells and becomes activated via phosphorylation. Signalling from the phosphorylated receptor to the nucleus occurs through Smad 2, 3 and 4. Smad 7 is an inhibitory Smad that can bind to the TGF-β receptor complex and prevent the action of Smad 2 and 3. It has been recently suggested that reduced levels of Smad 7 may play an important role in the pathogenesis of SSc (Dong et al., 2002), although more recent data point to Smad7 overexpression in SSc (Asano et al., 2004). The role of Smad-independnet signaling is unclear but may be central to maintaining a persistent profibrotic fibroblast phenotype.

Increased levels of TGF-β mRNA and protein have been demonstrated in the lungs of SSc patients with PIF (Deguchi and Kishimoto, 1991; Corrin et al., 1994; Ludwicka et al., 1995; Coker et al., 2001). Bronchoalveolar mononuclear cells were found to have more than a 10-fold enhancement in TGF-β gene transcription compared to controls (Deguchi and Kishimoto, 1991). Immunohistochemistry on lung biopsies of patients with PF/SSc demonstrated the presence of intracellular TGF-β in alveolar macrophages, bronchial epithelium and hyperplastic type II pneumocytes, and the presence of extracellular TGF-β in fibrous tissue immediately beneath the bronchial and hyperplastic alveolar epithelium. In contrast, the alveolar epithelium and interstitium were negative for both forms in a normal lung (Corrin et al., 1994). TGF-β has been shown to stimulate the synthesis of procollagen, fibronectin and glycosaminoglycans by lung fibroblast cell lines (Fine and Goldstein, 1987; Raghu et al., 1989; Dubaybo and Thet, 1990; McAnulty et al., 1991). In vitro, TGF-β has also been found to stimulate procollagen production in fibroblasts derived from the lungs of patients with SSc (Raghu et al., 1989; Harrison et al., 1991a).

Connective tissue growth factor (CTGF) is a TGFb-induced protein strongly implicated as an inducer of tissue fibrosis (Leask et al., 2002). CTGF is synthesised by fibroblasts and endothelial cells under the influence of TGF-β. Elevated serum CTGF levels found in patients with SSc were found to correlate with the extent and severity of skin sclerosis and the severity of pulmonary fibrosis (Sato et al., 2000b).

Increased levels of platelet growth factor (PDGF) have been found in bronchoalveolar lavage fluid (BAL) from patients with SSc (Ohba et al., 1994; Ludwicka et al., 1995). This increase may reflect activation of the coagulation cascade. Thrombin, found to be significantly increased in the lungs of SSc patients compared to controls, increased the expression of PDFG and upregulated PDGF receptors to modulate fibroblast proliferation (Ohba et al., 1994; Shimizu et al., 2000).

The SSc fibroblast (both lung and skin) has been shown to be different from normal fibroblasts. It produces more ECM, including collagens I, III, V, VI and VII, tenascin, proteoglycans, fibronectin, laminin and fibrillin-1 (Varga and Bashey, 1995; Shi-Wen et al., 1997). In addition, it proliferates faster, is more resistant to apoptosis (Jelaska and Korn, 2000; Santiago et al., 2001) and shows exaggerated responses to subsequent cytokine stimulation (Yamakage et al., 1992; Denton et al., 1997; Yamamoto et al., 2001). The proportion of alpha-smooth muscle actin (a-SMA)-positive cells is elevated in cultures of SSc fibroblasts (Jelaska and Korn, 2000). As these fibroblast-derived cells display morphological and biochemical features of both fibroblasts and contractile muscle cells, they are called myofibroblasts. Myofibroblasts appear to play a role in matrix synthesis and they have been shown to synthesise increased amounts of collagens, TIMP and other ECM components in vitro (Kirk et al., 1995). In addition, myofibroblasts appear to be a major source of TGF-β and chemokines in various tissues during the fibrotic process (Zhang et al., 1995). TGF-β is a potent inducer of a-SMA synthesis and myofibroblast transdifferentiation (Desmoulière et al., 1993; Vaughan et al., 2000). During physiological processes of matrix remodelling, myofibroblasts undergo apoptosis. TGF-β not only induces the generation of myofibroblasts, but also suppresses their apoptosis (Zhang and Phan, 1999). Hence, TGF-β appears to play an important role in the persistence of myofibroblasts in tissues during pathological fibrosis.

5. Clinical manifestations

An insidious onset of breathlessness on exertion, a dry cough and fatigue are the most common symptoms in patients with PIF/SSc. A substantial proportion of patients, however, may not present till late in the disease due to other co-morbidities. Chest pain is uncommon and haemoptysis rare; if present, another cause should be looked for. The earliest examination findings consist of bibasilar, fine inspiratory crackles. As the disease progresses, these crackles may become coarser, continue into the expiratory phase and extend upwards to involve the upper zones. Although often accompanied by other systemic signs, the pulmonary findings of SSc may precede the other signs. Digital clubbing is rare.

6. Diagnostic investigations

6.1. Radiological

6.1.1. Chest radiography

The classical abnormality of PIF/SSc on chest radiography consists of a reticulonodular pattern in the bases and periphery. As the disease progresses, there is loss of lung volume associated with more extensive changes. In early disease, however, the chest radiograph is not a sensitive tool and should be used as an initial screen only in conjunction with other investigations.

6.1.2. Computed tomography

CT scanning has revolutionised the approach to ILD in SSc. Not only is it highly sensitive for the detection (Harrison et al., 1989), quantification of severity and characterisation of PIF/SSc, but also its role in prognosis is becoming more apparent.

CT is highly sensitive for the detection of abnormality and is able to identify limited disease in patients with normal chest radiographs (Harrison et al., 1989). The characteristic CT findings in PIF/SSc consist of bilateral reticular shadowing, in a peripheral, subpleural distribution, most predominant posteriorly at the bases but becoming more anterior as the disease progresses. This probably represents a combination of fine intralobular fibrosis and inflammation. It is often difficult to determine which of these predominates but the co-existence of traction of the small airways confirms that at least some of the change is due to fibrosis (Wells et al., 1992). In the majority of patients with SSc and diffuse lung disease, the CT pattern resembles that seen in idiopathic non-specific interstitial pneumonia (NSIP).

CT has been used to distinguish variations in diffuse lung disease pattern that suggest different histopathological subtypes. Although most CT studies have concentrated on idiopathic pulmonary fibrosis (IPF), a disease that has a much worse prognosis than PIF/SSc, the principles of CT interpretation are likely to be the same in rheumatological diseases.

Diagnosis of IPF requires the presence of a histopathological pattern of usual interstitial pneumonia (UIP) (consensus statement 2002). Until relatively recently, the diagnostic label 'IPF' included patients whose biopsies comprised a mixture of histopathologic patterns including UIP, NSIP, desquamative interstitial pneumonia and diffuse alveolar damage (DAD). It has now become clear that idiopathic NSIP has a better prognosis than idiopathic UIP (clinically IPF by the new definition) (Daniil et al., 1999; Nicholson et al., 2000). There is increasing evidence that CT appearances are highly predictive of the histopathologic pattern in IPF (Flaherty et al., 2002, 2003b). In a study exploring the relationships between CT and histopathological patterns on survival in patients with NSIP and UIP, Flaherty et al. (2003b) found that patients with a histopathological pattern of UIP, with a CT interpretation that was not that of probable or definite UIP, fared better than patients with histopathological UIP and a CT pattern that was indicative of definite or probable UIP (i.e. pathology and CT concordant) and worse than those with a histopathological diagnosis of NSIP. The role of CT in discriminating between different histopathologic patterns in idiopathic interstitial pneumonias is becoming increasingly clear, and this has important implications for the assessment of prognosis. These prognostic statements cannot yet be extrapolated to patients with PIF/SSc or other rheumatological diseases, as will be discussed subsequently.

CT is, nonetheless, a reliable tool for quantifying severity of disease in patients with PIF/SSc. It has been shown to be a sensitive and reproducible method of determining the morphological extent of disease (Schurawitzki et al., 1990; Collins et al., 1994).

6.2. Functional

6.2.1. Lung function testing

A restrictive ventilatory defect together with a reduction in gas transfer is typically seen in patients with PIF. Hypoxia is common but hypercapnia is generally a late sign.

A reduced gas transfer, which is often minor, is present in the majority of patients (Owens et al., 1983). A greater reduction, however, can be a reflection of either interstitial fibrosis or pulmonary vascular disease. If there is no loss of volume, then lone pulmonary vascular disease is the most likely explanation. The pattern of likely lung disease can often be predicted from the autoantibody profile. In the presence of a positive anti-Scl 70, a reduced gas transfer (DL_{CO}) is likely to indicate interstitial fibrosis. In the absence of pulmonary vascular disease, DL_{CO} is a reliable functional marker of morphological severity of interstitial fibrosis. In a large cohort of patients with PIF, DL_{CO} correlated better than other lung function indices with the total morphological extent of disease on CT (Wells et al., 1997b).

In a study of patients with severe interstitial fibrosis, Steen et al. (1994a) observed that despite being asymptomatic early in the course of the disease, the greatest reduction in forced vital capacity (FVC) was seen in the first 4 years of the disease.

Arterial blood gas (ABG) estimation commonly reveals a reduced P_aO_2 with a normal or low P_aCO_2. Hypoxia is usually not marked until late in the disease process. Hypercapnia, if present, is often a preterminal event. Exercise increases both ventilation–perfusion mismatching and diffusion abnormalities. This results in increasing hypoxia, widening of the alveolar-arterial oxygen gradient and increasing dead space ventilation (a rise in dead space volume; increased V_D/V_T ratio).

6.2.2. ^{99m}Tc-DTPA clearance

The clearance of inhaled ^{99m}Tc-DTPA (technetium labelled diethylene-triamine-penta-acetate) from the lung is a measure of epithelial barrier integrity. An increased clearance ($t_{1/2} < 40$ min) is considered abnormal and has been described in a variety of ILDs, including PIF/SSc (Harrison et al., 1989; Wells et al., 1993a) and IPF (Wells et al., 1993a; Mogulkoc et al., 2001). The rapidity of ^{99m}Tc-DTPA clearance has been shown to have prognostic value. Normal clearance predicts subsequent disease stability defined by lung function tests. A persistently abnormal test puts the patient in a group that includes those individuals who are more likely to have a subsequent decline in lung function.

6.2.3. Bronchoalveolar lavage

Although the cell constituents of BAL are not specific for the diagnosis of PIF/SSc, the value of BAL is in excluding complicating infections, drug reactions, coexisting disease and malignancy. In PIF/SSc, the most common abnormality is an increase in neutrophil numbers but in some patients eosinophils ± lymphocyte numbers may also be increased in various combinations. An increased cellularity has been reported in subclinical disease (Wallaert et al., 1986; Wallaert, 1990). The significance of subclinical alveolitis, however, remains uncertain. Bronchoalveolar lavage is viewed as an index of prognosis in some centres.

6.3. Biochemistry/Serology/Immunology

No features of routine full blood count and biochemistry profile are specific for scleroderma. Anaemia of chronic disease may be present. Abnormalities due to disease elsewhere, such as renal dysfunction, may be identified. Abnormal liver function, thyroid function, and muscle enzymes may identify a co-existing autoimmune disease.

Antinuclear antibodies (ANAs) and, more specifically, extractable nuclear antigens are serologic hallmarks of patients with systemic autoimmune disease (Hahn, 1998) that may allow subclassification of patients with an established diagnosis of an autoimmune or connective tissue disease (Phan et al., 2002). A positive ANA is seen in more than 95% of patients with scleroderma (Bunn et al.).

ANAs produce a wide range of patterns and reflect the presence of antibodies to one or a combination of nuclear antigens. The nuclear staining pattern, however, has a relatively low sensitivity and specificity for different autoimmune diseases. The different patterns include homogenous or diffuse, peripheral or rim, speckled, nucleolar and centromeric. In the context of scleroderma, a speckled pattern (suggesting the presence of anti-Scl-70 (antitopoisomerase I)), a nucleolar pattern (suggesting the presence of proteins of the small nucleolar RNP complex (anti-fibrillarin, Mpp10 and hU3-55K), and anti Th/To antibodies), or a centromeric pattern (suggesting the presence of anti-centromere antibodies) are useful. Anti-RNApolymerase and anti-topoisomerase reactivities may also give anti-nucleolar staining.

The autoantibodies classically associated with subsets of SSc are anti-centromere antibodies (ACA) and anti-Scl-70 (otherwise known as anti-topoisomerase I). When a patient presents with their lung disease before the more systemic features, ACA and anti-Scl-70 antibodies are very useful in distinguishing patients with SSc from otherwise healthy individuals with Raynaud's syndrome, from patients with other connective tissue disease, and from unaffected family members. In general, the sensitivity is between 20 and 35% with a specificity of >95% (Reveille et al., 2003). Whereas ACA is predictive of limited skin involvement, anti-Scl-70 is more often associated with diffuse skin involvement and the development of pulmonary fibrosis and other internal organ involvement. The presence of ACA and anti-Scl70 are almost mutually exclusive, with rare exceptions reported in the literature (Dick et al., 2002).

ACA has been reported in 20–30% of patients with SSc, depending on the ethnicity of the patient. In a study of 230 patients, individuals with ACA were more likely to have abnormal DL_{CO} but a normal chest radiograph and FVC, indicating the presence of pulmonary vascular disease (Jacobsen et al., 1998). ACA has been associated with a lower frequency of radiographic IPF and a lesser severity of disease (Steen et al., 1988; Kuwana et al., 1994; Kane et al., 1996).

Anti-topoisomerase-1 antibodies are found in 15–20% of patients with SSc and are independent of ethnicity; they are found in about 40% of patients with dcSSc and less than 10% of patients with lcSSc (Spencer-Green et al., 1997; Reveille et al., 2003). Reactivity is associated with both the presence (Reveille et al., 2003) and severity of radiographic PIF (Steen et al., 1988; Jacobsen et al., 1998).

Other antinucleolar reactivities (ANoA) (Reimer et al., 1988) in SSc include anti-PM-Scl (Oddis et al., 1992), anti-U3-RNP/antifibrillarin (Blaszczyk et al., 1990), anti-Th/To (Reddy et al., 1983), and the anti-RNA polymerase family (RNAP), including anti-RNA polymerase I (Reimer et al., 1987), II (Kuwana et al., 1993a) and III (Okano et al., 1993). ANoA have been reported in 15–40% of patients with SSc (Bernstein et al., 1982; Steen et al., 1988). Anti-PM-Scl (Kuwana et al., 1994; Harvey et al., 1997) and Anti-Th/To (Harvey et al., 1997; Jacobsen et al., 1998; Kuwana et al., 2002) antibodies are predictive of limited skin involvement, whereas Anti-RNA polymerase (Okano et al., 1993; Kuwana et al., 1994; Chang et al., 1998; Harvey et al., 1999) and anti U3-RNP (Reimer et al., 1988; Kuwana et al., 1994; Arnett et al., 1996b; Jacobsen et al., 1998; Tormey et al., 2001) antibodies are predictive of diffuse cutaneous involvement.

6.4. Investigational assays

Lung epithelium-specific proteins, in particular Krebs von den Lungen 6 (KL-6), surface protein A (SP-A) and surface protein D (SP-D), have been studied in patients with PIF/SSc.

KL-6, a mucin-like glycoprotein, is expressed on type II pneumocytes and respiratory bronchiolar epithelial cells in normal lungs (Kohno et al., 1988). Proliferating and regenerating type II pneumocytes, however, have been found to express the antigen more strongly than normal type II pneumocytes (Kohno et al., 1989; Hamada et al., 1992). KL-6 has been found to be a sensitive indicator of damage to alveolar type II cells. Increased serum levels of KL-6 have been associated with the presence of pulmonary fibrosis in SSc (Yamane et al., 2000; Sato et al., 2000a).

In addition, the levels of KL-6 have also been found to reflect the severity of pulmonary fibrosis, with increased levels correlating inversely with DL_{CO} and FVC. Serial measurements have also suggested that KL-6 might reflect activity of disease (Nakajima et al., 2000; Yanaba et al., 2003). In a longitudinal study of 39 patients with SSc, increasing levels of KL-6 were accompanied by progressive PIF. In contrast, stable levels of KL-6 paralleled non-progressive disease (Yanaba et al., 2003).

Surface protein A and D (SP-D and SP-A) are two of the specific proteins found in pulmonary surfactant. Pulmonary surfactant is a complex material covering the alveolar surface of the lung. Its major function is to reduce surface tension at the air–liquid interface to prevent alveolar collapse during expiration. Like KL-6, elevated levels of both SP-A and SP-D have been found to reflect the presence of PIF/SSc (Takahashi et al., 2000). SP-D levels have also been found to be associated with disease severity (Maeda et al., 2001; Asano et al., 2001).

6.5. Histopathology

Although NSIP is by far the most common histopathologic pattern in PIF/SSc (Fujita et al., 2001; Nicholson et al., 2002; Bouros et al., 2002; Kim et al., 2002), it is not specific for PIF/SSc and can be associated with other aetiologies, including other connective tissue disorders, drug reactions and also idiopathic disease.

NSIP, first described by Katzenstein and Fiorelli in 1994 (Katzenstein and Fiorelli, 1994), is characterised by a temporally homogenous process with varying proportions of interstitial inflammation and fibrosis and is divided into three subgroups: (1) cellular NSIP, consisting predominantly of interstitial inflammation; (2) mixed NSIP, consisting of both interstitial inflammation and fibrosis; and (3) fibrotic NSIP, consisting predominantly of interstitial fibrosis.

In a study of surgical lung biopsies in 80 patients with PIF/SSc, Bouros et al. (2002) confirmed that NSIP was the most prevalent histopathologic pattern in SSc. The histopathologic patterns of UIP and end stage lung (advanced fibrosis) were the next most frequent histopathological patterns. Although not included in the analyses, four patients were found to have the histopathologic features of respiratory bronchiolitis-interstitial lung disease (RB-ILD) (all current smokers); one patient, sarcoidosis (had past history of sarcoidosis) and one patient, organising pneumonia (was taking D-penicillamine).

UIP, the less frequent histopathologic pattern associated with PIF/SSc, in contrast, is characterised by a temporally heterogenous appearance of predominantly interstitial fibrosis with minimal inflammation. The hallmark of UIP is the fibroblastic focus, which consists of actively proliferating myofibroblasts and fibroblasts, which constitute microscopic sites of ongoing alveolar epithelial injury and activation associated with evolving fibrosis (Kuhn et al., 1989; Kuhn and McDonald, 1991; Katzenstein and Myers, 1998). Honeycomb areas are common.

Unlike the idiopathic interstitial pneumonias (IPF and idiopathic NSIP), the prognostic significance of the two histopathologic patterns in SSc remains uncertain (Bouros et al., 2002; Kim et al., 2002; Flaherty et al., 2003a), largely because by far the majority of patients have the NSIP pattern of histopathology.

7. Differential diagnoses

The clinical presentation of PIF in the presence of other features of SSc makes the diagnosis straightforward. However, if interstitial fibrosis precedes all other symptoms and signs, which can occasionally be by years, the underlying systemic disease may be elusive to diagnose. PIF associated with other autoimmune diseases, in particular polymyositis/dermatomyositis (PM/DM) and rheumatoid arthritis (RA), can also present in advance of the systemic process. The identification of specific autoantibodies (anti-Scl-70 for SSc, anti-Jo-1 for PM/DM and rheumatoid factor for RA) greatly assists establishing the true diagnosis. It is suggested that all patients with diffuse fibrosing lung disease should have serological screening with ANA and rheumatoid factor.

Drug associated pneumonitis, although rare, needs to be considered. The pattern is most commonly different from the classical pattern of disease in PIF/SSc and the drugs generally used for SSc uncommonly cause diffuse lung disease. However, there are some reports of lung disease being caused by cyclophosphamide, but generally not with the doses used to treat PIF/SSc. The incidence of cyclophosphamide-induced lung toxicity is difficult to estimate, in part due to the frequent associations with other confounding variables, such as other cytotoxic drugs, opportunistic infections, coexisting lung malignancy and complications from radiation therapy. Cyclophosphamide has been reported to cause ILD that includes the spectrum of DAD, organising pneumonia (OP), and NSIP (Rossi et al., 2000). Reports of cyclophosphamide-induced lung toxicity have been largely associated with treatment of malignancies, in particular lymphomas (Topilow et al., 1973) and Wegener's granulomatosis (Malik et al., 1996); it must be pointed out that there have been no reported cases in patients treated for SSc. The reactions are generally idiosyncratic, with no relationship between development of lung injury and dose or duration of therapy. Reports of lung toxicity have occurred between 2 weeks and 13 years after the commencement of cyclophosphamide (Cooper et al., 1986; Meyers, 1997).

Two distinct patterns of interstitial pneumonitis, early-onset and late-onset, have been described, each with a separate clinical course and outcome. Patients with early-onset interstitial pneumonitis developed acute onset of symptoms of cough and dyspnoea; fever and fatigue were often prominent. Patients were also likely to improve after cessation of cyclophosphamide with good response to corticosteroid treatment. Open lung biopsy specimens have shown an NSIP picture (Spector et al., 1979; Malik et al., 1996). Late-onset interstitial pneumonitis, in contrast, developed in patients who had received prolonged treatment over several months to years, with some cases occurring years after discontinuation of the drug. The patients had an insidious onset of symptoms, of a non-productive cough and dyspnoea. Pleural thickening was often an accompanying feature of diffuse reticulo-nodular infiltrates on CXR (chest X-ray).

There have been rare case reports of lung disease in patients taking azathioprine. In a case series of seven renal transplant patients who had received azathioprine for immunosuppression, open lung biopsies were taken after the development of bilateral pulmonary infiltrates. These showed changes ranging from DAD to UIP culminating in pulmonary fibrosis (Bedrossian et al., 1984).

8. Prognosis

Pulmonary involvement is itself a significant determinant of outcome in SSc (Altman et al., 1991; Steen and Medsger, 2000; Ferri et al., 2002; Scussel-Lonzetti et al., 2002; Simeon et al., 2003); in the last 10 years, it has emerged as the most common disease-related cause of death. In an Italian series containing 1012 patients, a 10-year survival of 70% was observed, and mortality from lung disease, with or without concurrent cardiac disease, was substantially higher (33% of deaths) than mortality from renal disease (12% of deaths) (Ferri et al., 2002).

Progression of PIF/SSc is more likely within the first 5 years of systemic disease (Greenwald et al., 1987; Steen et al., 1994a; Steen, 2003). Hence careful surveillance of disease, especially in the early years, is crucial.

Although pulmonary involvement is associated with a relatively high mortality in patients with SSc, the course of PIF/SSc is variable and can range from indolent to rapidly progressive. It is, therefore, imperative that severity of functional impairment at presentation and subsequent functional longitudinal behaviour are established. Several markers of severity and prognosis in PIF/SSc have emerged:

8.1. Pulmonary function tests

The most widely used index to assess disease severity is pulmonary function testing. The rate of change of lung function has been explored in a number of studies (Greenwald et al., 1987; Steen et al., 1994a; Bouros et al., 2002). Although these changes are often seen within the first 2 years of onset of SSc, careful monitoring in long-standing disease is advocated. A reduction of total gas transfer (DL_{CO}) (Bouros et al., 2002; Scussel-Lonzetti et al., 2002; Morgan et al., 2003) and FVC (Steen et al., 1994a; Steen and Medsger, 2000; Bouros et al., 2002; Morgan et al., 2003) have been observed to predict increased mortality in PIF/SSc. In a study of 80 patients with PIF/SSc, the overall mortality was associated with lower initial DL_{CO} and FVC levels. Increased mortality was associated with lower initial DL_{CO} levels and deterioration in DL_{CO} levels during the next 3 years (Bouros et al., 2002).

8.2. Computed tomography

Although ground glass attenuation on CT can correlate with a biopsy showing predominantly cellular infiltrate and hence reversible disease, it is more likely to be indicative of fine fibrosis in PIF/SSc (Wells et al., 1992, 1993b).

CT features of PIF/SSc have been well correlated with histopathologic subsets (Wells et al., 1993b; MacDonald et al., 2001; Desai et al., 2003); the most common histopathologic subset seen in patients with PIF/SSc is NSIP (Fujita et al., 2001; Bouros et al., 2002; Kim et al., 2002). The major role of CT in predicting prognosis of PIF/SSc appears to be in the assessment of disease severity, which is reflected by the extent of disease on CT (Wells et al., 2003). Increasingly extensive disease on CT has been associated with a shorter time to decline in FVC (Goh et al., 2003b).

8.3. Bronchoalveolar lavage

The pattern of BAL cell profile has been advocated as a predictor of likely progression and as an indicator of the need for treatment (Silver et al., 1990b; Behr et al., 1996; White et al., 2000). A BAL neutrophilia has been linked to more progressive disease, especially in untreated patients. However, patients with a BAL neutrophilia tend to have lower DL_{CO} levels (Wells et al., 1998; White et al., 2000). It has, therefore, been suggested that BAL neutrophilia is linked to the extent of reticular fibrotic abnormalities on CT (Wells et al., 1998). In a comparison between PIF/SSc and IPF, a much more progressive disease, BAL neutrophil levels did not differ between the two diseases after adjustment for the extent of disease on CT and the severity of functional impairment (Wells et al., 1998). Therefore, it would seem likely that a BAL neutrophilia is a reflection of more extensive disease rather than an intrinsic marker of more progressive disease.

A BAL eosinophilia, on the other hand, appears to have prognostic significance independent of disease severity, and has been associated with limited disease in PIF/SSc (Wells et al., 1994b). In addition, Bouros et al. (2002) found that a BAL eosinophilia was linked to a significantly higher mortality in patients with PIF/SSc, despite treatment.

8.4. ^{99m}Tc-DTPA clearance

The rapidity of clearance of ^{99m}Tc-DTPA clearance has been found to be a prognostic indicator in PIF/SSc. Normal ^{99m}Tc-DTPA clearance is strongly predictive of stability of disease over the next 2–3 years, whereas rapid ^{99m}Tc-DTPA clearance (especially persistently rapid clearance) identified an increased likelihood of deterioration (Goh et al., 2003a). The association between increased clearance of ^{99m}Tc-DTPA and a more rapid subsequent deterioration in FVC was independent of morphological severity of disease on CT (Goh et al., 2003a).

8.5. Histopathology

The prognosis of patients with PIF/SSc has been reported to be significantly better than patients with IPF (Wells et al., 1994a, 1997a). This is probably largely due to the fact that the most common histopathological pattern seen in PIF/SSc is NSIP (Bouros et al., 2002; Kim et al., 2002). The significance of the less frequent histopathologic pattern of UIP in PIF/SSc, however, remains uncertain. Bouros et al. (2002) found no difference in survival between patients with NSIP or UIP (5-year survival 91 vs. 82%, respectively). Moreover, survival did not differ significantly between cellular and fibrotic NSIP. However, it must be pointed out that there were only six patients with UIP. In comparison, in a study of 19 patients with PIF/SSc, Kim et al. (2002) suggested that patients with an NSIP pattern had a better prognosis than those with a UIP pattern. Comparing the UIP pattern in IPF and connective tissue disease, Flaherty et al. (2003a) found that connective tissue-associated UIP had fewer fibroblastic foci and a better survival. There were, however, only nine patients with a connective tissue disease, of which only one had SSc, compared to 99 patients with IPF. This does nonetheless probably reflect, in general, a much lower prevalence of UIP associated with connective tissue diseases.

8.6. *Antibody status*

Although autoantibody status has been shown to be predictive of the development of PIF, its role in predicting survival is not as well established. Recent studies, however, have suggested that patients with ACA may have a lower mortality than those with anti-Scl-70 antibodies or ANoA (Ferri et al., 2002; Scussel-Lonzetti et al., 2002).

Although most studies do not find a correlation between disease activity and anti-Scl 70 (de Rooij et al., 1989; Weiner et al., 1991; Hildebrandt et al., 1993; Vazquez-Abad et al., 1995; Henry et al., 2000) and ACA (Tramposch et al., 1984; Weiner et al., 1991; Vazquez-Abad et al., 1995) levels, a study of sequential anti-Scl-70 measurements in 28 patients (Kuwana et al., 2000) found that the antibody had disappeared in six patients over a 10-year period. These patients were found to have a lower frequency of diffuse cutaneous SSc, a less progressive PIF and better survival rates compared with patients in whom anti-Scl-70 persisted.

8.7. *Risk of malignancy*

The association between PM/DM and malignancy is widely reported (Sigurgeirsson et al., 1992; Chow et al., 1995; Davis and Ahmed, 1997; Maoz et al., 1998; Stockton et al., 2001; Hill et al., 2001; Buchbinder et al., 2001; Wakata et al., 2002), with the risk higher in DM than PM; in a population-based, retrospective cohort study from Australia, a standardised incidence ratio of 6.2 was associated with DM and 2.0 with PM (Buchbinder et al., 2001). Although associated with a wide variety of cancers, there have been reports of bronchogenic carcinoma being the most common tumour (Andreev, 1978).

The association between SSc and malignancy is less well recognised. Although several studies have not supported this association (Duncan and Winkelmann, 1979; Black et al., 1982; Chatterjee et al., 2000), the majority of the studies have shown an increased risk for all cancers of about 2-fold (Roumm and Medsger, 1985; Rosenthal et al., 1993, 1995; Abu-Shakra et al., 1993). Breast (Forbes et al., 1989) and lung (Talbott and Barrocas, 1980; Peters-Golden et al., 1985; Yang et al., 2001; Hill et al., 2003) cancers have been most frequently reported, although cancers arising from other sites have also been reported (Mattingly and Mowat, 1979; Bielefeld et al., 1996).

The lung is the site with the greatest reported risk, with relative risks of up to 16.5 (Peters-Golden et al., 1985). In a recent large population-based cohort study (Hill et al., 2003), the relative risk of lung cancer was found to be 5.9. Although both the diffuse and limited forms of SSc were associated with an increased risk of cancer, the diffuse form was linked with a higher relative risk (2.73) compared to the limited form (1.85). This observation is in keeping with another population-based study by Rosenthal et al. (1995). Although the study did not show any association with antibody status, previous studies (Rothfield et al., 1992) have shown an association between the presence of anti-Scl-70 and cancer.

In a review of the literature on the clinical features of patients with SSc who developed lung cancer, Yang et al. (2001) found that there was a significant female predominance, and that there was no relationship between smoking and the development of lung cancer. In contrast with the general population, the most common histopathological subtype was found to be bronchoalveolar and adenocarcinoma, not squamouas cell carcinoma. The cancer was also found to arise more frequently in areas of previously damaged or fibrotic lung. This association with diffuse fibrosis has also been observed in other forms of pulmonary fibrosis, such as IPF (Ma et al., 2001).

9. Treatment

In the absence of any double-blind placebo-controlled trials, there is no conclusive evidence that any drug alters the course of PIF/SSc. Previous small studies have been retrospective and uncontrolled, consisting of heterogenous patient populations; treatment periods were variable with response assessed over a relatively short period, usually 6–12 months.

Treatment options should be individually tailored and the goals made clear at the outset of treatment, both in the minds of the clinician and the patient. In early disease, the need and timing of treatment require careful evaluation of disease prognosis; aiming to obtain significant improvement in this scenario is not unrealistic. In advanced disease, treating to halt disease progression should be viewed as a success. In very advanced disease, supportive therapy, including oxygen, may be the treatment of first choice. In selected cases, referral for transplantation (Rosas et al., 2000) should be considered and the timing of this is crucial. Although there are no clear guidelines, our institution refers for transplantation when the gas transfer (DL_{CO}) falls below 25% of predicted, as long as this is not confounded by significant pulmonary vascular disease or major systemic disease.

9.1. Corticosteroids and cyclophosphamide

The major drugs that are currently used to treat PIF/SSc are corticosteroids and cyclophosphamide. D-penicillamine is of no value in the treatment of PIF/SSc. Although a number of studies suggest that penicillamine might be beneficial (Steen et al., 1985; de Clerck et al., 1987), in a controlled trial of 134 patients on the use of D-penicillamine for skin disease, treatment was not associated with improvement in lung function parameters and some patients developed interstitial fibrosis whilst receiving treatment (Clements et al., 1999).

Historically, corticosteroids have been the mainstay of treatment for PIF/SSc. The evidence for the use of corticosteroids in PIF/SSc, however, is conflicting, with studies both supporting (Kallenberg et al., 1984) and refuting (Rossi et al., 1985) its use. It has been suggested that corticosteroids might be more beneficial if used in combination with cyclophosphamide (Johnson et al., 1989; Silver et al., 1993; White et al., 2000). Recently, however, the use of corticosteroids has been cautioned with reported associations with scleroderma renal crisis (Steen and Medsger, 1998; DeMarco et al., 2002). Doses as low as 7.4 mg/day were an independent risk factor for the development of scleroderma renal crisis, although this occurred only in the presence of high skin scores and large joint contractures (DeMarco et al., 2002).

There have been studies suggesting that oral cyclophosphamide might be efficacious (Silver et al., 1993; Akesson et al., 1994; Steen et al., 1994b; Behr et al., 1996; White et al., 2000), although it has to be pointed out that these studies have limitations, including uncontrolled subjects in small numbers, evaluated in a retrospective fashion. In a study of 103 patients, White et al. (2000) found that patients with a BAL alveolitis (neutrophilia and/or eosinophilia) who received oral cyclophosphamide experienced stabilisation or improvement in FVC and DL_{CO} and a better survival compared to untreated patients. In addition, the outcome of patients who received treatment was as good as in untreated patients without a BAL alveolitis.

Oral cyclophosphamide has been associated with a fairly high percentage of adverse events in the treatment of patients with PIF/SSc; leukopenia, thrombocytopenia, pneumonia and haemorrhagic cystitis have all been reported (Silver et al., 1993; Akesson et al., 1994). The excessive toxicities associated with oral cyclophosphamide have prompted studies of the role of intravenous cyclophosphamide as an alternative. Although the use of intravenous cyclophosphamide in PIF/SSc has shown some promise, the comparative efficacy and toxicity of oral vs. intravenous cyclophosphamide is still to be defined.

Following two promising pilot studies (Varai et al., 1998; Davas et al., 1999), there have been three prospective studies evaluating the efficacy and safety of intravenous cyclophosphamide in PIF/SSc (Pakas et al., 2002; Griffiths et al., 2002; Giacomelli et al., 2002). Both improvements in physiological indices (DL_{CO} and or FVC) (Pakas et al., 2002; Giacomelli et al., 2002) and regression of disease on CT (Pakas et al., 2002; Griffiths et al., 2002) were documented. After receiving a course of pulsed intravenous methylprednisolone and cyclophosphamide over 6 months (six doses, approximately 4 weeks apart), patients were found to have stable lung function indices in the first 12 months. However, the majority deteriorated subsequently on longer follow up (Griffiths et al., 2002).

9.2. Issues

Despite uncontrolled evaluation, there appears to be sufficient evidence to support the use of either oral or intravenous cyclophosphamide in PIF/SSc. However, corticosteroids have been used in conjunction with cyclophosphamide in many studies, thus making it impossible to exclude the possibility that regression of pulmonary disease with cyclophosphamide is, in part, ascribable to corticosteroids. In addition, it is not clear from the literature for how long treatment should be continued and if another immunosuppressive agent should be instituted after pulsed intravenous cyclophosphamide to consolidate any response. Azathioprine with low dose prednisolone is the recommended treatment for IPF (2002) but there is no firm evidence base for this approach at present; azathioprine does, however, have a better side effect profile.

There are two large, ongoing prospective placebo-controlled studies that may offer a more definitive guide to treatment of PIF/SSc in the future. One involves the use of oral cyclophosphamide (multi-centre NIH-sponsored trial in the US) and the other intravenous cyclophosphamide (multi-centre ARC-sponsored trial in the UK).

10. Other forms of ILDs in SSc

Pulmonary fibrosis is by far the most common manifestation of ILD in SSc. Other rarer manifestations include DAD, OP and alveolar haemorrhage.

10.1. Diffuse alveolar damage

Although rare, DAD has been reported to be associated with SSc (Griffin et al., 1990). The histopathologic pattern of DAD can be caused by various insults and may occur as an overlap syndrome with other connective tissue diseases, in particular SLE. Clinically, patients have acute respiratory distress with refractory hypoxaemia and pulmonary oedema, and are rapidly ventilator-dependent. The prognosis is poor. In the exudative phase, the chest radiograph typically shows bilateral airspace opacification with air bronchograms. As the disease progresses, the process becomes less consolidated with the appearance of irregular linear opacities.

High-resolution CT shows ground glass attenuation in the exudative phase, with consolidation, traction bronchiectasis, architectural distortion or cystic lesions in the proliferative/organising phase (Akira, 1999).

10.2. Organising pneumonia

OP is most commonly associated with RA and PM/DM (Wells and du Bois, 1993). There have, however, been rare reports of OP complicating SSc (Bridges et al., 1992; Boehler et al., 1996). In one report, it was noted that the patient was receiving D-penicillamine (Boehler et al., 1996), an association that has been previously described in RA (Anaya et al., 1995).

Patients present with a clinical presentation of pneumonia, multi-focal areas of consolidation both on chest radiography and CT and a restrictive ventilatory defect. Although a good response is generally seen in OP associated with RA and PM/DM, it is difficult to provide any reliable prognostic information about OP in SSc as there have been only a handful of cases reported.

10.3. Alveolar haemorrhage

There have been several case reports of alveolar haemorrhage complicating SSc (Kallenbach et al., 1977; Helfrich et al., 1989; Griffin et al., 1990; Endo et al., 1994; Nishi et al., 1994; Phillips et al., 1998; Chaer et al., 2001).

Recently, SSc has been added to the list of causes of pulmonary renal syndrome (Bar et al., 2001), a combination of diffuse pulmonary haemorrhage and glomerulonephritis. It occurs in a variety of contexts, including Goodpasture's syndrome, various forms of primary systemic vasculitis, cryoglobulinemia, SLE, antiphospholipid syndrome, environmental factors, and drugs (Green et al., 1996).

In a review of pulmonary renal syndrome in SSc, Bar et al. (2001) suggested that previous pulmonary fibrosis and treatment with D-penicillamine might be predisposing factors. It was also noted that pulmonary renal syndrome in SSc occurred on average 6.4 years after the onset of SSc, compared to the shorter interval of 3.2 years between the diagnosis of SSc and scleroderma renal crisis. Renal failure in this context was also noted to be associated with a normal blood pressure. The prognosis in all 11 patients reviewed was poor, all dying within 6 months of diagnosis. It was, however, pointed out that not all patients received corticosteroids and none received cyclophosphamide.

Key points

- The aetiology of SSc is unknown, but it is likely to result from complex interactions between environmental factors in a genetically susceptible host.
- The pathogenesis of SSc is complex but generally involves immune activation, vascular damage and the production of excess ECM.
- Interstitial fibrosis is the most common clinical pulmonary manifestation of SSc; the histopathological pattern is NSIP.
- Pulmonary involvement in SSc is the leading cause of disease-related death.
- The course of PIF/SSc is variable and the assessment of disease severity and likely risk of progression is important in the timing of treatment.
- Current best practise treatment for PIF/SSc consists of low dose corticosteroids with oral or intravenous cyclophosphamide.

References

Abraham, D.J., Vancheeswaran, R., Dashwood, M.R., Rajkumar, V.S., Pantelidis, P., Xu, S.W., du Bois, R.M., Black, C.M. 1997. Increased levels of endothelin-1 and differential endothelin type A and B receptor expression in scleroderma-associated fibrotic lung disease. Am. J. Pathol. 151 (3), 831–841.

Abu-Shakra, M., Guillemin, F., Lee, P. 1993. Cancer in systemic sclerosis. Arthritis Rheum. 36 (4), 460–464.

Agelli, M., Wahl, S.M. 1986. Cytokines and fibrosis. Clin. Exp. Rheumatol. 4 (4), 379–388.

Akesson, A., Scheja, A., Lundin, A., Wollheim, F.A. 1994. Improved pulmonary function in systemic sclerosis after treatment with cyclophosphamide. Arthritis Rheum. 37 (5), 729–735.

Akira, M. 1999. Computed tomography and pathologic findings in fulminant forms of idiopathic interstitial pneumonia. J. Thorac. Imag. 14 (2), 76–84.

Altman, R.D., Medsger, T.A. Jr., Bloch, D.A., Michel, B.A. 1991. Predictors of survival in systemic sclerosis (scleroderma). Arthritis Rheum. 34 (4), 403–413.

American Thoracic Society/European Respiratory Society 2002. American Thoracic Society/European Respiratory Society International Multidisciplinary Consensus Classification of the Idiopathic Interstitial Pneumonias. This Joint Statement of the American Thoracic Society (ATS), and the European Respiratory Society (ERS) was adopted by the ATS Board of Directors, June 2001 and by The ERS Executive Committee, June 2001 Am. J. Respir. Crit. Care Med. 165 (2), 277–304.

Anaya, J.M., Diethelm, L., Ortiz, L.A., Gutierrez, M., Citera, G., Welsh, R.A., Espinoza, L.R. 1995. Pulmonary involvement in rheumatoid arthritis. Semin. Arthritis Rheum. 24 (4), 242–254.

Andreev, V.C. 1978 Skin manifestations in visceral cancer. Curr. Prob. Dermatol. 8, 1–168.

Arnett, F.C., Reveille, J.D., Wilson, R.W., Provost, T.T., Bias, W.B. 1984. Systemic lupus erythematosus: current state of the genetic hypothesis. Semin. Arthritis Rheum. 14 (1), 24–35.

Arnett, F.C., Bias, W.B., McLean, R.H., Engel, M., Duvic, M., Goldstein, R., Freni-Titulaer, L., McKinley, T.W., Hochberg, M.C. 1990. Connective tissue disease in southeast Georgia. A community based study of immunogenetic markers and autoantibodies. J. Rheumatol. 17 (8), 1029–1035.

Arnett, F.C., Howard, R.F., Tan, F., Moulds, J.M., Bias, W.B., Durban, E., Cameron, H.D., Paxton, G., Hodge, T.J., Weathers, P.E., Reveille, J.D. 1996a. Increased prevalence of systemic sclerosis in a Native American tribe in Oklahoma. Association with an Amerindian HLA haplotype. Arthritis Rheum. 39 (8), 1362–1370.

Arnett, F.C., Reveille, J.D., Goldstein, R., Pollard, K.M., Leaird, K., Smith, E.A., Leroy, E.C., Fritzler, M.J. 1996b. Autoantibodies to fibrillarin in systemic sclerosis (scleroderma). An immunogenetic, serologic, and clinical analysis. Arthritis Rheum. 39 (7), 1151–1160.

Arnett, F.C., Cho, M., Chatterjee, S., Aguilar, M.B., Reveille, J.D., Mayes, M.D. 2001. Familial occurrence frequencies and relative risks for systemic sclerosis (scleroderma) in three United States cohorts. Arthritis Rheum. 44 (6), 1359–1362.

Arroliga, A.C., Podell, D.N., Matthay, R.A. 1992. Pulmonary manifestations of scleroderma. J. Thorac. Imag. 7 (2), 30–45.

Artlett, C.M., Smith, J.B., Jimenez, S.A. 1998. Identification of fetal DNA and cells in skin lesions from women with systemic sclerosis. N. Engl. J. Med. 338 (17), 1186–1191.

Artlett, C.M., Cox, L.A., Ramos, R.C., Dennis, T.N., Fortunato, R.A., Hummers, L.K., Jimenez, S.A., Smith, J.B. 2002a. Increased microchimeric CD4 + T lymphocytes in peripheral blood from women with systemic sclerosis. Clin. Immunol. 103 (3 Pt 1), 303–308.

Artlett, C.M., Rasheed, M., Russo-Stieglitz, K.E., Sawaya, H.H., Jimenez, S.A. 2002b. Influence of prior pregnancies on disease course and cause of death in systemic sclerosis. Ann. Rheum. Dis. 61 (4), 346–350.

Asano, Y., Ihn, H., Yamane, K., Kubo, M., Tamaki, K. 2004. Impaired Smad 7-Smurf-mediated negative regulation of TGF-beta signaling in scleroderma fibroblasts. J. Clin. Invest. 113 (2), 253–264.

Asano, Y., Ihn, H., Yamane, K., Yazawa, N., Kubo, M., Fujimoto, M., Tamaki, K. 2001. Clinical significance of surfactant protein D as a serum marker for evaluating pulmonary fibrosis in patients with systemic sclerosis. Arthritis Rheum. 44 (6), 1363–1369.

Atamas, S.P., White, B. 1999. Interleukin 4 in systemic sclerosis: not just an increase. Clin. Diagn. Lab. Immunol. 6 (5), 658–659.

Atamas, S.P., Luzina, I.G., Choi, J., Tsymbalyuk, N., Carbonetti, N.H., Singh, I.S., Trojanowska, M., Jimenez, S.A., White, B. 2003. Pulmonary and activation-regulated chemokine stimulates collagen production in lung fibroblasts. Am. J. Respir. Cell. Mol. Biol. 29 (6), 743–749.

Avila, J.J., Lympany, P.A., Pantelidis, P., Welsh, K.I., Black, C.M., du Bois, R.M. 1999. Fibronectin gene polymorphisms associated with fibrosing alveolitis in systemic sclerosis. Am. J. Respir. Cell Mol. Biol. 20 (1), 106–112.

Bar, J., Ehrenfeld, M., Rozenman, J., Perelman, M., Sidi, Y., Gur, H. 2001. Pulmonary-renal syndrome in systemic sclerosis. Semin. Arthritis Rheum. 30 (6), 403–410.

Bedrossian, C.W., Sussman, J., Conklin, R.H., Kahan, B. 1984. Azathioprine-associated interstitial pneumonitis. Am. J. Clin. Pathol. 82 (2), 148–154.

Beebe, J.L., Lacey, J.V. Jr., Mayes, M.D., et al. 1997. Reproductive history, oral contraceptive use, estrogen replacement therapy and the risk of developing scleroderma. Arthritis Rheum. 40 (Suppl.), S100.

Behr, J., Vogelmeier, C., Beinert, T., Meurer, M., Krombach, F., Konig, G., Fruhmann, G. 1996. Bronchoalveolar lavage for evaluation and management of scleroderma disease of the lung. Am. J. Respir. Crit. Care Med. 154 (2 Pt 1), 400–406.

Bernstein, R.M., Steigerwald, J.C., Tan, E.M. 1982. Association of antinuclear and antinucleolar antibodies in progressive systemic sclerosis. Clin. Exp. Immunol. 48 (1), 43–51.

Bianchi, D.W., Zickwolf, G.K., Weil, G.J., Sylvester, S., DeMaria, M.A. 1996. Male fetal progenitor cells persist in maternal blood for as long as 27 years postpartum. Proc. Natl. Acad. Sci. USA 93 (2), 705–708.

Bielefeld, P., Meyer, P., Caillot, D., Dalac, S., Camus, P., Tavernier, C., Couillaut, G., Chalopin, J.M., Besancenot, J.F. 1996. Systemic scleroderma and cancers: 21 cases and review of the literature. Rev. Med. Int. 17 (10), 810–813.

Black, C.M. 1993. Scleroderma—clinical aspects. J. Intern. Med. 234 (2), 115–118.

Black, K.A., Zilko, P.J., Dawkins, R.L., Armstrong, B.K., Mastaglia, G.L. 1982. Cancer in connective tissue disease. Arthritis Rheum. 25 (9), 1130–1133.

Blaszczyk, M., Jarzabek-Chorzelska, M., Jablonska, S., Chorzelski, T., Kolacinska-Strasz, Z., Beutner, E.H., Kumar, V. 1990. Autoantibodies to nucleolar antigens in systemic scleroderma: clinical correlations. Br. J. Dermatol. 123 (4), 421–430.

Boehler, A., Vogt, P., Speich, R., Weder, W., Russi, E.W. 1996. Bronchiolitis obliterans in a patient with localised scleroderma treated with D-penicillamine. Eur. Respir. J. 9 (6), 1317–1319.

Bolster, M.B., Ludwicka, A., Sutherland, S.E., Strange, C., Silver, R.M. 1997. Cytokine concentrations in bronchoalveolar lavage fluid of patients with systemic sclerosis. Arthritis Rheum. 40 (4), 743–751.

Bouros, D., Wells, A.U., Nicholson, A.G., Colby, T.V., Polychronopoulos, V., Pantelidis, P., Haslam, P.L., Vassilakis, D.A., Black, C.M., du Bois, R.M. 2002. Histopathologic subsets of fibrosing alveolitis in patients with systemic sclerosis and their relationship to outcome. Am. J. Respir. Crit. Care. Med. 165 (12), 1581–1586.

Bramwell, B. 1914. Diffuse scleroderma: its frequency; its occurrence in stonemasons; its treatment by fibrolysin-elevations of temperature due to fibrolysin injections. Edinburgh Med. J. 12, 387.

Bridges, A.J., Hsu, K.C., Dias-Arias, A.A., Chechani, V. 1992. Bronchiolitis obliterans organizing pneumonia and scleroderma. J. Rheumatol. 19 (7), 1136–1140.

Briggs, D.C., Vaughan, R.W., Welsh, K.I., Myers, A., du Bois, R.M., Black, C.M. 1991. Immunogenetic prediction of pulmonary fibrosis in systemic sclerosis. Lancet 338 (8768), 661–662.

Buchbinder, R., Forbes, A., Hall, S., Dennett, X., Giles, G. 2001. Incidence of malignant disease in biopsy-proven inflammatory myopathy. A population-based cohort study. Ann. Intern. Med. 134 (12), 1087–1095.

Bunn, C.C., Denton, C.P., Shi-Wen, X., Knight, C., Black, C.M. 1998. Anti-RNA polymerases and other autoantibody specificities in systemic sclerosis. Br. J. Rheumatol. 37 (1), 15–20.

Cambrey, A.D., Harrison, N.K., Dawes, K.E., Southcott, A.M., Black, C.M., du Bois, R.M., Laurent, G.J., McAnulty, R.J. 1994. Increased levels of endothelin-1 in bronchoalveolar lavage fluid from patients with systemic sclerosis contribute to fibroblast mitogenic activity in vitro. Am. J. Respir. Cell. Mol. Biol. 11 (4), 439–445.

Chaer, R.A., Massad, M.G., Evans, A., Olopade, C., Varga, J. 2001. Systemic sclerosis complicated by diffuse alveolar hemorrhage. Med. Sci. Monit. 7 (5), 1013–1015.

Chandran, G., Smith, M., Ahern, M.J., Roberts-Thomson, P.J. 1995. A study of scleroderma in South Australia: prevalence, subset characteristics and nailfold capillaroscopy. Aust. N. Z. J. Med. 25 (6), 688–694.

Chang, M., Wang, R.J., Yangco, D.T., Sharp, G.C., Komatireddy, G.R., Hoffman, R.W. 1998. Analysis of autoantibodies against RNA polymerases using immunoaffinity-purifed RNA polymerase I, II, and III antigen in an enzyme-linked immunosorbent assay. Clin. Immunol. Immunopathol. 89 (1), 71–78.

Chatterjee, S., Severson, R.K., Weiss, L.K., Kau, T.Y., Mayes, M.D. 2000. Risk of malignancy in Scleroderma [abstract]. Arthritis Rheum. 43 (Suppl), S315.

Chow, W.H., Gridley, G., Mellemkjaer, L., McLaughlin, J.K., Olsen, J.H., Fraumeni, J.F. Jr. 1995. Cancer risk following polymyositis and dermatomyositis: a nationwide cohort study in Denmark. Cancer Causes Control 6 (1), 9–13.

Clements, P.J., Furst, D.E., Wong, W.K., Mayes, M., White, B., Wigley, F., Weisman, M.H., Barr, W., Moreland, L.W., Medsger, T.A. Jr., Steen, V., Martin, R.W., Collier, D., Weinstein, A., Lally, E., Varga, J., Weiner, S., Andrews, B., Abeles, M., Seibold, J.R. 1999. High-dose versus low-dose D-penicillamine in early diffuse systemic sclerosis: analysis of a two-year, double-blind, randomized, controlled clinical trial. Arthritis Rheum. 42 (6), 1194–1203.

Coker, R.K., Laurent, G.J., Jeffery, P.K., du Bois, R.M., Black, C.M., McAnulty, R.J. 2001. Localisation of transforming growth factor beta1 and beta3 mRNA transcripts in normal and fibrotic human lung. Thorax. 56 (7), 549–556.

Collins, C.D., Wells, A.U., Hansell, D.M., Morgan, R.A., MacSweeney, J.E., du Bois, R.M., Rubens, M.B. 1994. Observer variation in pattern type and extent of disease in fibrosing alveolitis on thin section computed tomography and chest radiography. Clin. Radiol. 49 (4), 236–240.

Cooper, J.A. Jr., White, D.A., Matthay, R.A. 1986. Drug-induced pulmonary disease. Part 1. Cytotoxic drugs. Am. Rev. Respir. Dis. 133 (2), 321–340.

Corrin, B., Butcher, D., McAnulty, B.J., du Bois, R.M., Black, C.M., Laurent, G.J., Harrison, N.K. 1994. Immunohistochemical localization of transforming growth factor-beta 1 in the lungs of patients with systemic sclerosis, cryptogenic fibrosing alveolitis and other lung disorders. Histopathology 24 (2), 145–150.

Crilly, A., Hamilton, J., Clark, C.J., Jardine, A., Madhok, R. 2002. Analysis of transforming growth factor beta1 gene polymorphisms in patients with systemic sclerosis. Ann. Rheum. Dis. 61 (8), 678–681.

D'Angelo, W.A., Fries, J.F., Masi, A.T., Shulman, L.E. 1969. Pathologic observations in systemic sclerosis (scleroderma). A study of fifty-eight autopsy cases and fifty-eight matched controls. Am. J. Med. 46 (3), 428–440.

Daniil, Z.D., Gilchrist, F.C., Nicholson, A.G., Hansell, D.M., Harris, J., Colby, T.V., du Bois, R.M. 1999. A histologic pattern of nonspecific interstitial pneumonia is associated with a better prognosis than usual interstitial pneumonia in patients with cryptogenic fibrosing alveolitis. Am. J. Respir. Crit. Care. Med. 160 (3), 899–905.

Davas, E.M., Peppas, C., Maragou, M., Alvanou, E., Hondros, D., Dantis, P.C. 1999. Intravenous cyclophosphamide pulse therapy for the treatment of lung disease associated with scleroderma. Clin. Rheumatol. 18 (6), 455–461.

Davis, M.D., Ahmed, I. 1997. Ovarian malignancy in patients with dermatomyositis and polymyositis: a retrospective analysis of fourteen cases. J. Am. Acad. Dermatol. 37 (5 Pt 1), 730–733.

de Clerck, L.S., Dequeker, J., Francx, L., Demedts, M. 1987. D-penicillamine therapy and interstitial lung disease in scleroderma. A long-term follow-up study. Arthritis Rheum. 30 (6), 643–650.

Deguchi, Y., Kishimoto, S. 1991. Spontaneous activation of transforming growth factor-beta gene transcription in bronchoalveolar mononuclear cells of individuals with systemic autoimmune diseases with lung involvement. Lupus 1 (1), 27–30.

DeMarco, P.J., Weisman, M.H., Seibold, J.R., Furst, D.E., Wong, W.K., Hurwitz, E.L., Mayes, M., White, B., Wigley, F., Barr, W., Moreland, L., Medsger, T.A. Jr., Steen, V., Martin, R.W., Collier, D., Weinstein, A., Lally, E., Varga, J., Weiner, S.R., Andrews, B., Abeles, M., Clements, P.J. 2002. Predictors and outcomes of scleroderma renal crisis: the high-dose versus low-dose D-penicillamine in early diffuse systemic sclerosis trial. Arthritis Rheum. 46 (11), 2983–2989.

Denton, C.P., Xu, S., Black, C.M., Pearson, J.D. 1997. Scleroderma fibroblasts show increased responsiveness to endothelial cell-derived IL-1 and bFGF. J. Invest. Dermatol. 108 (3), 269–274.

de Rooij, D.J., van de Putte, L.B., Habets, W.J., van Venrooij, W.J. 1989. Marker antibodies in scleroderma and polymyositis: clinical associations. Clin. Rheumatol. 8 (2), 231–237.

Desai, S.R., Veeraraghavan, S., Goh, N.S., Hansell, D.M., Nikolakopolou, A., Colby, T.V., Denton, C.P., Black, C., du Bois, R.M., Wells, A.U. 2003. CT features of lung disease in systemic sclerosis: a comparison with the appearances in idiopathic pulmonary fibrosis and non-specific interstitial pneumonitis. Radiology in press.

Desmouliere, A., Geinoz, A., Gabbiani, F., Gabbiani, G. 1993. Transforming growth factor-beta 1 induces alpha-smooth muscle actin expression in granulation tissue myofibroblasts and in quiescent and growing cultured fibroblasts. J. Cell. Biol. 122 (1), 103–111.

Dick, T., Mierau, R., Bartz-Bazzanella, P., Alavi, M., Stoyanova-Scholz, M., Kindler, J., Genth, E. 2002. Coexistence of antitopoisomerase I and anticentromere antibodies in patients with systemic sclerosis. Ann. Rheum. Dis. 61 (2), 121–127.

Dong, C., Zhu, S., Wang, T., Yoon, W., Li, Z., Alvarez, R.J., ten Dijke, P., White, B., Wigley, F.M., Goldschmidt-Clermont, P.J. 2002. Deficient Smad7 expression: a putative molecular defect in scleroderma. Proc. Natl Acad. Sci. USA 99 (6), 3908–3913.

Dubaybo, B.A., Thet, L.A. 1990. Effect of transforming growth factor beta on synthesis of glycosaminoglycans by human lung fibroblasts. Exp. Lung Res. 16 (5), 389–403.

du Bois, E.L., Chandor, S., Friou, G.J., Bischel, M. 1971. Progressive systemic sclerosis (PSS) and localized scleroderma (morphea) with positive LE cell test and unusual systemic manifestations compatible with systemic lupus erythematous (SLE): presentation of 14 cases including one set of identical twins, one with scleroderma and the other with SLE. Review of the literature. Medicine (Baltimore) 50 (3), 199–222.

Duncan, M.R., Berman, B. 1991. Stimulation of collagen and glycosaminoglycan production in cultured human adult dermal fibroblasts by recombinant human interleukin 6. J. Invest. Dermatol. 97 (4), 686–692.

Duncan, S.C., Winkelmann, R.K. 1979. Cancer and scleroderma. Arch. Dermatol. 115 (8), 950–955.

Edworthy, S.M., Martin, L., Barr, S.G., Birdsell, D.C., Brant, R.F., Fritzler, M.J. 1998. A clinical study of the relationship between silicone breast implants and connective tissue disease. J. Rheumatol. 25 (2), 254–260.

Endo, H., Hosono, T., Kondo, H. 1994. Antineutrophil cytoplasmic autoantibodies in 6 patients with renal failure and systemic sclerosis. J. Rheumatol. 21 (5), 864–870.

Englert, H., Small-McMahon, J., Chambers, P., O'Connor, H., Davis, K., Manolios, N., White, R., Dracos, G., Brooks, P. 1999. Familial risk estimation in systemic sclerosis. Aust. N. Z. J. Med. 29 (1), 36–41.

Falkner, D., Wilson, J., Medsger, T.A. Jr., Morel, P.A. 1998. HLA and clinical associations in systemic sclerosis patients with anti-Th/To antibodies. Arthritis Rheum. 41 (1), 74–80.

Falkner, D., Wilson, J., Fertig, N., Clawson, K., Medsger, T.A. Jr., Morel, P.A. 2000. Studies of HLA-DR and DQ alleles in systemic sclerosis patients with autoantibodies to RNA polymerases and U3-RNP (fibrillarin). J. Rheumatol. 27 (5), 1196–1202.

Fallon, P.G., Richardson, E.J., McKenzie, G.J., McKenzie, A.N. 2000. Schistosome infection of transgenic mice defines distinct and contrasting pathogenic roles for IL-4 and IL-13: IL-13 is a profibrotic agent. J. Immunol. 164 (5), 2585–2591.

Fanning, G.C., Welsh, K.I., Bunn, C., Du, B.R., Black, C.M. 1998. HLA associations in three mutually exclusive autoantibody subgroups in UK systemic sclerosis patients. Br. J. Rheumatol. 37 (2), 201–207.

Feghali, C.A., Wright, T.M. 1995. Epidemiologic and clinical study of twins with scleroderma (abstract). Arthritis Rheum. 38, S308.

Ferri, C., Zakrzewska, K., Longombardo, G., Giuggioli, D., Storino, F.A., Pasero, G., Azzi, A. 1999. Parvovirus B19 infection of bone marrow in systemic sclerosis patients. Clin. Exp. Rheumatol. 17 (6), 718–720.

Ferri, C., Valentini, G., Cozzi, F., Sebastiani, M., Michelassi, C., La Montagna, G., Bullo, A., Cazzato, M., Tirri, E., Storino, F., Giuggioli, D., Cuomo, G., Rosada, M., Bombardieri, S., Todesco, S., Tirri, G. 2002. Systemic sclerosis: demographic, clinical, and serologic features and survival in 1,012 Italian patients. Medicine (Baltimore) 81 (2), 139–153.

Fine, A., Goldstein, R.H. 1987. The effect of transforming growth factor-beta on cell proliferation and collagen formation by lung fibroblasts. J. Biol. Chem. 262 (8), 3897–3902.

Flaherty, K.R., Toews, G.B., Travis, W.D., Colby, T.V., Kazerooni, E.A., Gross, B.H., Jain, A., Strawderman, R.L. III, Paine, R., Flint, A., Lynch, J.P. III, Martinez, F.J. 2002. Clinical significance of histological classification of idiopathic interstitial pneumonia. Eur. Respir. J. 19 (2), 275–283.

Flaherty, K.R., Colby, T.V., Travis, W.D., Toews, G.B., Mumford, J., Murray, S., Thannickal, V.J., Kazerooni, E.A., Gross, B.H., Lynch, J.P. III, Martinez, F.J. 2003a. Fibroblastic foci in usual interstitial pneumonia: idiopathic versus collagen vascular disease. Am. J. Respir. Crit. Care. Med. 167 (10), 1410–1415.

Flaherty, K.R., Thwaite, E.L., Kazerooni, E.A., Gross, B.H., Toews, G.B., Colby, T.V., Travis, W.D., Mumford, J.A., Murray, S., Flint, A., Lynch, J.P. III, Martinez, F.J. 2003b. Radiological versus histological diagnosis in UIP and NSIP: survival implications. Thorax 58 (2), 143–148.

Flores, R.H., Stevens, M.B., Arnett, F.C. 1984. Familial occurrence of progressive systemic sclerosis and systemic lupus erythematosus. J. Rheumatol. 11 (3), 321–323.

Forbes, A.M., Woodrow, J.C., Verbov, J.L., Graham, R.M. 1989. Carcinoma of breast and scleroderma: four further cases and a literature review. Br. J. Rheumatol. 28 (1), 65–69.

Fries, K.M., Felch, M.E., Phipps, R.P. 1994. Interleukin-6 is an autocrine growth factor for murine lung fibroblast subsets. Am. J. Respir. Cell. Mol. Biol. 11 (5), 552–560.

Fujita, J., Yoshinouchi, T., Ohtsuki, Y., Tokuda, M., Yang, Y., Yamadori, I., Bandoh, S., Ishida, T., Takahara, J., Ueda, R. 2001. Non-specific interstitial pneumonia as pulmonary involvement of systemic sclerosis. Ann. Rheum. Dis. 60 (3), 281–283.

Furuse, S., Fujii, H., Kaburagi, Y., Fujimoto, M., Hasegawa, M., Takehara, K., Sato, S. 2003. Serum concentrations of the CXC chemokines interleukin 8 and growth-regulated oncogene-alpha are elevated in patients with systemic sclerosis. J. Rheumatol. 30 (7), 1524–1528.

Galindo, M., Santiago, B., Rivero, M., Rullas, J., Alcami, J., Pablos, J.L. 2001. Chemokine expression by systemic sclerosis fibroblasts: abnormal regulation of monocyte chemoattractant protein 1 expression. Arthritis Rheum. 44 (6), 1382–1386.

Giacomelli, R., Valentini, G., Salsano, F., Cipriani, P., Sambo, P., Conforti, M.L., Fulminis, A., De Luca, A., Farina, G., Candela, M., Generini, S., De Francisci, A., Tirri, E., Proietti, M., Bombardieri, S., Gabrielli, A., Tonietti, G., Cerinic, M.M. 2002. Cyclophosphamide pulse regimen in the treatment of alveolitis in systemic sclerosis. J. Rheumatol. 29 (4), 731–736.

Gibbons, G.H., Dzau, V.J. 1990. Endothelial function in vascular remodelling. In: J.B. Warren (Ed.), The Endothelium: An Introduction to Current Research. Wiley-Liss, New York, pp. 81–93.

Gilchrist, F.C., Bunn, C., Foley, P.J., Lympany, P.A., Black, C.M., Welsh, K.I., du Bois, R.M. 2001. Class II HLA associations with autoantibodies in scleroderma: a highly significant role for HLA-DP. Genes Immun. 2 (2), 76–81.

Gladman, D.D., Keystone, E.C., Baron, M., Lee, P., Cane, D., Mervert, H. 1981. Increased frequency of HLA-DR5 in scleroderma. Arthritis Rheum. 24 (6), 854–856.

Goh, N.S., Veeraraghavan, S., Desai, S.R., Hansell, D.M., Anagnostopoulos, C., Denton, C.P., Black, C.M., du Bois, R.M., Wells, A.U. 2003a. The prognostic significance of technetium labeled diethylenetriamine pentacetate (99mTc-DTPA) clearance in patients with the fibrosing alveolitis of systemic sclerosis (FASSc). Am. J. Respir. Crit. Care Med. 167 (7), A475.

Goh, N.S., Veeraraghavan, S., Desai, S.R., Hansell, D.M., Denton, C., Black, C.M., du Bois, R.M., Wells, A.U. 2003b. Fibrosing alveolitis in systemic sclerosis (FASSc): a prognostic evaluation of computed tomography, pulmonary function indices, bronchoalveolar lavage cellularity and clinical data. Am. J. Respir. Crit. Care Med. 167 (7), A475.

Green, R.J., Ruoss, S.J., Kraft, S.A., Duncan, S.R., Berry, G.J., Raffin, T.A. 1996. Pulmonary capillaritis and alveolar hemorrhage. Update on diagnosis and management. Chest 110 (5), 1305–1316.

Greenwald, G.I., Tashkin, D.P., Gong, H., Simmons, M., Duann, S., Furst, D.E., Clements, P. 1987. Longitudinal changes in lung function and respiratory symptoms in progressive systemic sclerosis. Prospective study. Am. J. Med. 83 (1), 83–92.

Griffin, M.T., Robb, J.D., Martin, J.R. 1990. Diffuse alveolar haemorrhage associated with progressive systemic sclerosis. Thorax 45 (11), 903–904.

Griffiths, B., Miles, S., Moss, H., Robertson, R., Veale, D., Emery, P. 2002. Systemic sclerosis and interstitial lung disease: a pilot study using pulse intravenous methylprednisolone and cyclophosphamide to assess the effect on high resolution computed tomography scan and lung function. J. Rheumatol. 29 (11), 2371–2378.

Hagberg, B., Leonhardt, T., Skogh, M. 1961. Familial occurrence of collagen diseases: progressive systemic sclerosis and systemic lupus erythematosus. Acta Med. Scand. 169, 727.

Hahn, B.H. 1998. Antibodies to DNA. N. Engl. J. Med. 338 (19), 1359–1368.

Hall, J.M., Lingenfelter, P., Adams, S.L., Lasser, D., Hansen, J.A., Bean, M.A. 1995. Detection of maternal cells in human umbilical cord blood using fluorescence in situ hybridization. Blood 86 (7), 2829–2832.

Hamada, H., Kohno, N., Akiyama, M., Hiwada, K. 1992. Monitoring of serum KL-6 antigen in a patient with radiation pneumonia. Chest 101 (3), 858–860.

Harrison, N.K., Glanville, A.R., Strickland, B., Haslam, P.L., Corrin, B., Addis, B.J., Lawrence, R., Millar, A.B., Black, C.M., Turner-Warwick, M. 1989. Pulmonary involvement in systemic sclerosis: the detection of early changes by thin section CT scan, bronchoalveolar lavage and 99mTc-DTPA clearance. Respir. Med. 83 (5), 403–414.

Harrison, N.K., McAnulty, R.J., Haslam, P.L., Black, C.M., Laurent, G.J. 1990. Evidence for protein oedema, neutrophil influx, and enhanced collagen production in lungs of patients with systemic sclerosis. Thorax 45 (8), 606–610.

Harrison, N.K., Argent, A.C., McAnulty, R.J., Black, C.M., Corrin, B., Laurent, G.J. 1991a. Collagen synthesis and degradation by systemic sclerosis lung fibroblasts. Responses to transforming growth factor-beta. Chest 99 (Suppl. 3), 71S–72S.

Harrison, N.K., Myers, A.R., Corrin, B., Soosay, G., Dewar, A., Black, C.M., du Bois, R.M., Turner-Warwick, M. 1991b. Structural features of interstitial lung disease in systemic sclerosis. Am. Rev. Respir. Dis. 144 (3 Pt 1), 706–713.

Harrison, N.K., Cambrey, A.D., Myers, A.R., Southcott, A.M., Black, C.M., du Bois, R.M., Laurent, G.J., McAnulty, R.J. 1994. Insulin-like growth factor-I is partially responsible for fibroblast proliferation induced by bronchoalveolar lavage fluid from patients with systemic sclerosis. Clin. Sci. (London) 86 (2), 141–148.

Harvey, G., Black, C., Maddison, P., McHugh, N. 1997. Characterization of antinucleolar antibody reactivity in patients with systemic sclerosis and their relatives. J. Rheumatol. 24 (3), 477–484.

Harvey, G.R., Butts, S., Rands, A.L., Patel, Y., McHugh, N.J. 1999. Clinical and serological associations with anti-RNA polymerase antibodies in systemic sclerosis. Clin. Exp. Immunol. 117 (2), 395–402.

Hasegawa, M., Fujimoto, M., Kikuchi, K., Takehara, K. 1997a. Elevated serum levels of interleukin 4 (IL-4), IL-10, and IL-13 in patients with systemic sclerosis. J. Rheumatol. 24 (2), 328–332.

Hasegawa, M., Fujimoto, M., Kikuchi, K., Takehara, K. 1997b. Elevated serum tumor necrosis factor-alpha levels in patients with systemic sclerosis: association with pulmonary fibrosis. J. Rheumatol. 24 (4), 663–665.

Hasegawa, M., Sato, S., Ihn, H., Takehara, K. 1999a. Enhanced production of interleukin-6 (IL-6), oncostatin M and soluble IL-6 receptor by cultured peripheral blood mononuclear cells from patients with systemic sclerosis. Rheumatology (Oxford) 38 (7), 612–617.

Hasegawa, M., Sato, S., Takehara, K. 1999b. Augmented production of chemokines (monocyte chemotactic protein-1 (MCP-1), macrophage inflammatory protein-1alpha (MIP-1alpha) and MIP-1beta) in patients with systemic sclerosis: MCP-1 and MIP-1alpha may be involved in the development of pulmonary fibrosis. Clin. Exp. Immunol. 117 (1), 159–165.

Hata, R., Akai, J., Kimura, A., Ishikawa, O., Kuwana, M., Shinkai, H. 2000. Association of functional microsatellites in the human type I collagen alpha2 chain (COL1A2) gene with systemic sclerosis. Biochem. Biophys. Res. Commun. 272 (1), 36–40.

Helfrich, D.J., Banner, B., Steen, V.D., Medsger, T.A. Jr. 1989. Normotensive renal failure in systemic sclerosis. Arthritis Rheum. 32 (9), 1128–1134.

Henry, P.A., Atamas, S.P., Yurovsky, V.V., Luzina, I., Wigley, F.M., White, B. 2000. Diversity and plasticity of the anti-DNA topoisomerase I autoantibody response in scleroderma. Arthritis Rheum. 43 (12), 2733–2742.

Hieshima, K., Imai, T., Baba, M., Shoudai, K., Ishizuka, K., Nakagawa, T., Tsuruta, J., Takeya, M., Sakaki, Y., Takatsuki, K., Miura, R., Opdenakker, G., Van Damme, J., Yoshie, O., Nomiyama, H. 1997. A novel human CC chemokine PARC that is most homologous to macrophage-inflammatory protein-1 alpha/LD78 alpha and chemotactic for T lymphocytes, but not for monocytes. J. Immunol. 159 (3), 1140–1149.

Hildebrandt, S., Jackh, G., Weber, S., Peter, H.H. 1993. A long-term longitudinal isotypic study of anti-topoisomerase I autoantibodies. Rheumatol. Int. 12 (6), 231–234.

Hill, C.L., Zhang, Y., Sigurgeirsson, B., Pukkala, E., Mellemkjaer, L., Airio, A., Evans, S.R., Felson, D.T. 2001. Frequency of specific cancer types in dermatomyositis and polymyositis: a population-based study. Lancet 357 (9250), 96–100.

Hill, C.L., Nguyen, A.M., Roder, D., Roberts-Thomson, P. 2003. Risk of cancer in patients with scleroderma: a population based cohort study. Ann. Rheum. Dis. 62 (8), 728–731.

Hochberg, M.C., Perlmutter, D.L. 1996. The association of augmentation mammoplasty with connective tissue disease, including systematic sclerosis (scleroderma): a meta-analysis. Curr. Top. Microbiol. Immunol. 210, 411–417.

Ihn, H., Tamaki, K. 2000. Oncostatin M stimulates the growth of dermal fibroblasts via a mitogen-activated protein kinase-dependent pathway. J. Immunol. 165 (4), 2149–2155.

Ihn, H., Leroy, E.C., Trojanowska, M. 1997. Oncostatin M stimulates transcription of the human alpha2(I) collagen gene via the Sp1/Sp3-binding site. J. Biol. Chem. 272 (39), 24666–24672.

Jacobsen, S., Halberg, P., Ullman, S., van Venrooij, W.J., Hoier-Madsen, M., Wiik, A., Petersen, J. 1998. Clinical features and serum antinuclear antibodies in 230 Danish patients with systemic sclerosis. Br. J. Rheumatol. 37 (1), 39–45.

Janowsky, E.C., Kupper, L.L., Hulka, B.S. 2000. Meta-analyses of the relation between silicone breast implants and the risk of connective-tissue diseases. N. Engl. J. Med. 342 (11), 781–790.

Jelaska, A., Korn, J.H. 2000. Role of apoptosis and transforming growth factor beta1 in fibroblast selection and activation in systemic sclerosis. Arthritis Rheum. 43 (10), 2230–2239.

Jimenez, S.A., Gershwin, M.E. 1996. Animal models of systemic sclerosis. In: P.J. Clements, D.E. Furst (Eds.), Systemic sclerosis, 1st ed., Williams & Wilkins, Baltimore, pp. 251–273.

Johnson, M.A., Kwan, S., Snell, N.J., Nunn, A.J., Darbyshire, J.H., Turner-Warwick, M. 1989. Randomised controlled trial comparing prednisolone alone with cyclophosphamide and low dose prednisolone in combination in cryptogenic fibrosing alveolitis. Thorax 44 (4), 280–288.

Johnson, R.W., Tew, M.B., Arnett, F.C. 2002. The genetics of systemic sclerosis. Curr. Rheumatol. Rep. 4 (2), 99–107.

Kadono, T., Kikuchi, K., Ihn, H., Takehara, K., Tamaki, K. 1998. Increased production of interleukin 6 and interleukin 8 in scleroderma fibroblasts. J. Rheumatol. 25 (2), 296–301.

Kallenbach, J., Prinsloo, I., Zwi, S. 1977. Progressive systemic sclerosis complicated by diffuse pulmonary haemorrhage. Thorax 32 (6), 767–770.

Kallenberg, C.G., Jansen, H.M., Elema, J.D., The, T.H. 1984. Steroid-responsive interstitial pulmonary disease in systemic sclerosis. Monitoring by bronchoalveolar lavage. Chest 86 (3), 489–492.

Kamb, M.L., Murphy, J.J., Jones, J.L., Caston, J.C., Nederlof, K., Horney, L.F., Swygert, L.A., Falk, H., Kilbourne, E.M. 1992. Eosinophilia-myalgia syndrome in L-tryptophan-exposed patients. JAMA 267 (1), 77–82.

Kane, G.C., Varga, J., Conant, E.F., Spirn, P.W., Jimenez, S., Fish, J.E. 1996. Lung involvement in systemic sclerosis (scleroderma): relation to classification based on extent of skin involvement or autoantibody status. Respir. Med. 90 (4), 223–230.

Katzenstein, A.L., Fiorelli, R.F. 1994. Nonspecific interstitial pneumonia/fibrosis. Histologic features and clinical significance. Am. J. Surg. Pathol. 18 (2), 136–147.

Katzenstein, A.L., Myers, J.L. 1998. Idiopathic pulmonary fibrosis: clinical relevance of pathologic classification. Am. J. Respir. Crit Care Med. 157 (4 Pt 1), 1301–1315.

Kikuchi, K., Kadono, T., Furue, M., Tamaki, K. 1997. Tissue inhibitor of metalloproteinase 1 (TIMP-1) may be an autocrine growth factor in scleroderma fibroblasts. J. Invest. Dermatol. 108 (3), 281–284.

Kim, D.S., Yoo, B., Lee, J.S., Kim, E.K., Lim, C.M., Lee, S.D., Koh, Y., Kim, W.S., Kim, W.D., Colby, T.V., Kitiaichi, M. 2002. The major histopathologic pattern of pulmonary fibrosis in scleroderma is nonspecific interstitial pneumonia. Sarcoidosis. Vasc. Diffuse Lung Dis. 19 (2), 121–127.

Kinsella, M.B., Smith, E.A., Miller, K.S., Leroy, E.C., Silver, R.M. 1989. Spontaneous production of fibronectin by alveolar macrophages in patients with scleroderma. Arthritis Rheum. 32 (5), 577–583.

Kirk, T.Z., Mark, M.E., Chua, C.C., Chua, B.H., Mayes, M.D. 1995. Myofibroblasts from scleroderma skin synthesize elevated levels of collagen and tissue inhibitor of metalloproteinase (TIMP-1) with two forms of TIMP-1. J. Biol. Chem. 270 (7), 3423–3428.

Kissin, E.Y., Lemaire, R., Korn, J.H., Lafyatis, R. 2002. Transforming growth factor beta induces fibroblast fibrillin-1 matrix formation. Arthritis Rheum. 46 (11), 3000–3009.

Kohno, N., Akiyama, M., Kyoizumi, S., Hakoda, M., Kobuke, K., Yamakido, M. 1988. Detection of soluble tumor-associated antigens in sera and effusions using novel monoclonal antibodies, KL-3 and KL-6, against lung adenocarcinoma. Jpn. J. Clin. Oncol. 18 (3), 203–216.

Kohno, N., Kyoizumi, S., Awaya, Y., Fukuhara, H., Yamakido, M., Akiyama, M. 1989. New serum indicator of interstitial pneumonitis activity. Sialylated carbohydrate antigen KL-6. Chest 96 (1), 68–73.

Kuhn, C., McDonald, J.A. 1991. The roles of the myofibroblast in idiopathic pulmonary fibrosis. Ultrastructural and immunohistochemical features of sites of active extracellular matrix synthesis. Am. J. Pathol. 138 (5), 1257–1265.

Kuhn, C. III, Boldt, J., King, T.E. Jr., Crouch, E., Vartio, T., McDonald, J.A. 1989. An immunohistochemical study of architectural remodelling and connective tissue synthesis in pulmonary fibrosis. Am. Rev. Respir. Dis. 140 (6), 1693–1703.

Kumagai, Y., Shiokawa, Y., Medsger, T.A. Jr., Rodnan, G.P. 1984. Clinical spectrum of connective tissue disease after cosmetic surgery. Observations on eighteen patients and a review of the Japanese literature. Arthritis Rheum. 27 (1), 1–12.

Kuwana, M., Kaburaki, J., Mimori, T., Tojo, T., Homma, M. 1993a. Autoantibody reactive with three classes of RNA polymerases in sera from patients with systemic sclerosis. J. Clin. Invest. 91 (4), 1399–1404.

Kuwana, M., Kaburaki, J., Okano, Y., Inoko, H., Tsuji, K. 1993b. The HLA-DRand DQ genes control the autoimmune response to DNA topoisomerase I in systemic sclerosis (scleroderma). J. Clin. Invest. 92 (3), 1296–1301.

Kuwana, M., Kaburaki, J., Okano, Y., Tojo, T., Homma, M. 1994. Clinical and prognostic associations based on serum antinuclear antibodies in Japanese patients with systemic sclerosis. Arthritis Rheum. 37 (1), 75–83.

Kuwana, M., Kaburaki, J., Mimori, T., Kawakami, Y., Tojo, T. 2000. Longitudinal analysis of autoantibody response to topoisomerase I in systemic sclerosis. Arthritis Rheum. 43 (5), 1074–1084.

Kuwana, M., Kimura, K., Hirakata, M., Kawakami, Y., Ikeda, Y. 2002. Differences in autoantibody response to Th/To between systemic sclerosis and other autoimmune diseases. Ann. Rheum. Dis. 61 (9), 842–846.

Laing, T.J., Gillespie, B.W., Toth, M.B., Mayes, M.D., Gallavan, R.H. Jr., Burns, C.J., Johanns, J.R., Cooper, B.C., Keroack, B.J., Wasko, M.C., Lacey, J.V. Jr., Schottenfeld, D. 1997. Racial differences in scleroderma among women in Michigan. Arthritis Rheum. 40 (4), 734–742.

Launay, D., Hebbar, M., Hatron, P.Y., Michon-Pasturel, U., Queyrel, V., Hachulla, E., Devulder, B. 2001. Relationship between parity and clinical and biological features in patients with systemic sclerosis. J. Rheumatol. 28 (3), 509–513.

Leask, A., Holmes, A., Abraham, D.J. 2002. Connective tissue growth factor: a new and important player in the pathogenesis of fibrosis. Curr. Rheumatol. Rep. 4 (2), 136–142.

Leroy, E.C., Black, C., Fleischmajer, R., Jablonska, S., Krieg, T., Medsger, T.A. Jr., Rowell, N., Wollheim, F. 1988. Scleroderma (systemic sclerosis): classification, subsets and pathogenesis. J. Rheumatol. 15 (2), 202–205.

Lo, Y.M., Lo, E.S., Watson, N., Noakes, L., Sargent, I.L., Thilaganathan, B., Wainscoat, J.S. 1996. Two-way cell traffic between mother and fetus: biologic and clinical implications. Blood 88 (11), 4390–4395.

Ludwicka, A., Ohba, T., Trojanowska, M., Yamakage, A., Strange, C., Smith, E.A., Leroy, E.C., Sutherland, S., Silver, R.M. 1995. Elevated levels of platelet derived growth factor and transforming growth factor-beta 1 in bronchoalveolar lavage fluid from patients with scleroderma. J. Rheumatol. 22 (10), 1876–1883.

Lunardi, C., Bason, C., Navone, R., Millo, E., Damonte, G., Corrocher, R., Puccetti, A. 2000. Systemic sclerosis immunoglobulin G autoantibodies bind the human cytomegalovirus late protein UL94 and induce apoptosis in human endothelial cells. Nat. Med. 6 (10), 1183–1186.

Luzina, I.G., Atamas, S.P., Wise, R., Wigley, F.M., Xiao, H.Q., White, B. 2002. Gene expression in bronchoalveolar lavage cells from scleroderma patients. Am. J. Respir. Cell Mol. Biol. 26 (5), 549–557.

Ma, Y., Seneviratne, C.K., Koss, M. 2001. Idiopathic pulmonary fibrosis and malignancy. Curr. Opin. Pulm. Med. 7 (5), 278–282.

MacDonald, S.L., Rubens, M.B., Hansell, D.M., Copley, S.J., Desai, S.R., du Bois, R.M., Nicholson, A.G., Colby, T.V., Wells, A.U. 2001. Nonspecific interstitial pneumonia and usual interstitial pneumonia: comparative appearances at and diagnostic accuracy of thin-section CT. Radiology 221 (3), 600–605.

Maddison, P.J., Stephens, C., Briggs, D., Welsh, K.I., Harvey, G., Whyte, J., McHugh, N., Black, C.M. 1993. Connective tissue disease and autoantibodies in the kindreds of 63 patients with systemic sclerosis. The United Kingdom Systemic Sclerosis Study Group. Medicine (Baltimore) 72 (2), 103–112.

Maeda, M., Ichiki, Y., Aoyama, Y., Kitajima, Y. 2001. Surfactant protein D (SP-D) and systemic scleroderma (SSc). J. Dermatol. 28 (9), 467–474.

Malik, S.W., Myers, J.L., DeRemee, R.A., Specks, U. 1996. Lung toxicity associated with cyclophosphamide use. Two distinct patterns. Am. J. Respir. Crit Care Med. 154 (6 Pt 1), 1851–1856.

Maloney, S., Smith, A., Furst, D.E., Myerson, D., Rupert, K., Evans, P.C., Nelson, J.L. 1999. Microchimerism of maternal origin persists into adult life. J. Clin. Invest. 104 (1), 41–47.

Maoz, C.R., Langevitz, P., Livneh, A., Blumstein, Z., Sadeh, M., Bank, I., Gur, H., Ehrenfeld, M. 1998. High incidence of malignancies in patients with dermatomyositis and polymyositis: an 11-year analysis. Semin. Arthritis Rheum. 27 (5), 319–324.

Marguerie, C., Bunn, C.C., Copier, J., Bernstein, R.M., Gilroy, J.M., Black, C.M., So, A.K., Walport, M.J. 1992. The clinical and immunogenetic features of patients with autoantibodies to the nucleolar antigen PM-Scl. Medicine (Baltimore) 71 (6), 327–336.

Masi, A.T., Rodnan, G.P., Medsger, T.A. Jr. 1980. Preliminary criteria for the classification of systemic sclerosis (scleroderma). Arthritis Rheum. 23, 581–590.

Massague, J. 2000. How cells read TGF-beta signals. Nat. Rev. Mol. Cell Biol. 1 (3), 169–178.

Mattingly, P.C., Mowat, A.G. 1979. Rapidly progressive scleroderma associated with carcinoma of the oesophagus. Ann. Rheum. Dis. 38 (2), 177–178.

Mayes, M.D., Lacey, J.V. Jr., Beebe-Dimmer, J., Gillespie, B.W., Cooper, B., Laing, T.J., Schottenfeld, D. 2003. Prevalence, incidence, survival, and disease characteristics of systemic sclerosis in a large US population. Arthritis Rheum. 48 (8), 2246–2255.

McAnulty, R.J., Campa, J.S., Cambrey, A.D., Laurent, G.J. 1991. The effect of transforming growth factor beta on rates of procollagen synthesis and degradation in vitro. Biochim. Biophys. Acta 1091 (2), 231–235.

McHugh, N.J., Whyte, J., Artlett, C., Briggs, D.C., Stephens, C.O., Olsen, N.J., Gusseva, N.G., Maddison, P.J., Black, C.M., Welsh, K. 1994. Anti-centromere antibodies (ACA) in systemic sclerosis patients and their relatives: a serological and HLA study. Clin. Exp. Immunol. 96 (2), 267–274.

Medsger, T.A. 1997. Systemic sclerosis (scleroderma): clinical aspect. In: W.J. Koopman (Ed.), Arthritis and Allied Conditions. A Textbook of Rheumatology, vol. 2, Williams and Wilkins, Philadelphia, pp. 1433–1465.

Meyers, J.L. 1997. Pathology of drug-induced lung disease. In: A.A. Katzenstein, F.B. Askin (Eds.), Katzenstein and Askin's Surgical Pathology of Non-neoplastic Lung Disease, 3rd ed. Saunders, Philadelphia, pp. 81–111.

Minai, O.A., Dweik, R.A., Arroliga, A.C. 1998. Manifestations of scleroderma pulmonary disease. Clin. Chest Med. 19 (4) pp. 713–7ix.

Mogulkoc, N., Brutsche, M.H., Bishop, P.W., Murby, B., Greaves, M.S., Horrocks, A.W., Wilson, M., McCullough, C., Prescott, M., Egan, J.J. 2001. Pulmonary (99m)Tc-DTPA aerosol clearance and survival in usual interstitial pneumonia (UIP). Thorax 56 (12), 916–923.

Moore, B.B., Paine, R. III, Christensen, P.J., Moore, T.A., Sitterding, S., Ngan, R., Wilke, C.A., Kuziel, W.A., Toews, G.B. 2001. Protection from pulmonary fibrosis in the absence of CCR2 signaling. J. Immunol. 167 (8), 4368–4377.

Morel, P.A., Chang, H.J., Wilson, J.W., Conte, C., Falkner, D., Tweardy, D.J., Medsger, T.A. Jr. 1995. HLA and ethnic associations among systemic sclerosis patients with anticentromere antibodies. Hum. Immunol. 42 (1), 35–42.

Morgan, C., Knight, C., Lunt, M., Black, C.M., Silman, A.J. 2003. Predictors of end stage lung disease in a cohort of patients with scleroderma. Ann. Rheum. Dis. 62 (2), 146–150.

Nakajima, H., Harigai, M., Hara, M., Hakoda, M., Tokuda, H., Sakai, F., Kamatani, M., Kashiwazaki, S. 2000. KL-6 as a novel serum marker for interstitial pneumonia associated with collagen diseases. J. Rheumatol. 27 (5), 1164–1170.

Nelson, J.L., Furst, D.E., Maloney, S., Gooley, T., Evans, P.C., Smith, A., Bean, M.A., Ober, C., Bianchi, D.W. 1998. Microchimerism and HLA-compatible relationships of pregnancy in scleroderma. Lancet 351 (9102), 559–562.

Nicholson, A.G., Colby, T.V., du Bois, R.M., Hansell, D.M., Wells, A.U. 2000. The prognostic significance of the histologic pattern of interstitial pneumonia in patients presenting with the clinical entity of cryptogenic fibrosing alveolitis. Am. J. Respir. Crit Care Med. 162 (6), 2213–2217.

Nicholson, A.G., Colby, T.V., Wells, A.U. 2002. Histopathological approach to patterns of interstitial pneumonia in patient with connective tissue disorders. Sarcoidosis. Vasc. Diffuse. Lung Dis. 19 (1), 10–17.

Nietert, P.J., Sutherland, S.E., Silver, R.M., Pandey, J.P., Knapp, R.G., Hoel, D.G., Dosemeci, M. 1998. Is occupational organic solvent exposure a risk factor for scleroderma? Arthritis Rheum. 41 (6), 1111–1118.

Nietert, P.J., Sutherland, S.E., Silver, R.M., Pandey, J.P., Dosemeci, M. 1999. Solvent oriented hobbies and the risk of systemic sclerosis. J. Rheumatol. 26 (11), 2369–2372.

Nishi, K., Myou, S., Ooka, T., Fujimura, M., Matsuda, T. 1994. Diffuse cutaneous systemic sclerosis associated with pan-serositis, disseminated intravascular coagulation, and diffuse alveolar haemorrhage. Respir. Med. 88 (6), 471–473.

Oddis, C.V., Okano, Y., Rudert, W.A., Trucco, M., Duquesnoy, R.J., Medsger, T.A. Jr. 1992. Serum autoantibody to the nucleolar antigen PM-Scl. Clinical and immunogenetic associations. Arthritis Rheum. 35 (10), 1211–1217.

Ohba, T., McDonald, J.K., Silver, R.M., Strange, C., Leroy, E.C., Ludwicka, A. 1994. Scleroderma bronchoalveolar lavage fluid contains thrombin, a mediator of human lung fibroblast proliferation via induction of platelet-derived growth factor alpha-receptor. Am. J. Respir. Cell Mol. Biol. 10 (4), 405–412.

Ohtsuka, T., Miyamoto, Y., Yamakage, A., Yamazaki, S. 2001. Quantitative analysis of microchimerism in systemic sclerosis skin tissue. Arch. Dermatol. Res. 293 (8), 387–391.

Okano, Y., Steen, V.D., Medsger, T.A. Jr. 1993. Autoantibody reactive with RNA polymerase III in systemic sclerosis. Ann. Intern. Med. 119 (10), 1005–1013.

Oriente, A., Fedarko, N.S., Pacocha, S.E., Huang, S.K., Lichtenstein, L.M., Essayan, D.M. 2000. Interleukin-13 modulates collagen homeostasis in human skin and keloid fibroblasts. J. Pharmacol. Exp. Ther. 292 (3), 988–994.

Owens, G.R., Fino, G.J., Herbert, D.L., Steen, V.D., Medsger, T.A. Jr., Pennock, B.E., Cottrell, J.J., Rodnan, G.P., Rogers, R.M. 1983. Pulmonary function in progressive systemic sclerosis. Comparison of CREST syndrome variant with diffuse scleroderma. Chest 84 (5), 546–550.

Pakas, I., Ioannidis, J.P., Malagari, K., Skopouli, F.N., Moutsopoulos, H.M., Vlachoyiannopoulos, P.G. 2002. Cyclophosphamide with low or high dose prednisolone for systemic sclerosis lung disease. J. Rheumatol. 29 (2), 298–304.

Pantelidis, P., Southcott, A.M., Black, C.M., du Bois, R.M. 1997. Up-regulation of IL-8 secretion by alveolar macrophages from patients with fibrosing alveolitis: a subpopulation analysis. Clin. Exp. Immunol. 108 (1), 95–104.

Pantelidis, P., McGrath, D.S., Southcott, A.M., Black, C.M., du Bois, R.M. 2001. Tumour necrosis factor-alpha production in fibrosing alveolitis is macrophage subset specific. Respir. Res. 2 (6), 365–372.

Pardo, A., Smith, K.M., Abrams, J., Coffman, R., Bustos, M., McClanahan, T.K., Grein, J., Murphy, E.E., Zlotnik, A., Selman, M. 2001. CCL18/DC-CK-1/PARC up-regulation in hypersensitivity pneumonitis. J. Leukoc. Biol. 70 (4), 610–616.

Peters-Golden, M., Wise, R.A., Hochberg, M., Stevens, M.B., Wigley, F.M. 1985. Incidence of lung cancer in systemic sclerosis. J. Rheumatol. 12 (6), 1136–1139.

Phan, T.G., Wong, R.C., Adelstein, S. 2002. Autoantibodies to extractable nuclear antigens: making detection and interpretation more meaningful. Clin. Diagn. Lab Immunol. 9 (1), 1–7.

Phillips, D., Phillips, B., Mannino, D. 1998. A case study and national database report of progressive systemic sclerosis and associated conditions. J. Womens Health 7 (9), 1099–1104.

Pisa, F.E., Bovenzi, M., Romeo, L., Tonello, A., Biasi, D., Bambara, L.M., Betta, A., Barbone, F. 2002. Reproductive factors and the risk of scleroderma: an Italian case-control study. Arthritis Rheum. 46 (2), 451–456.

Postlethwaite, A.E., Seyer, J.M. 1990. Stimulation of fibroblast chemotaxis by human recombinant tumor necrosis factor alpha (TNF-alpha) and a synthetic TNF-alpha 31-68 peptide. J. Exp. Med. 172 (6), 1749–1756.

Postlethwaite, A.E., Seyer, J.M. 1991. Fibroblast chemotaxis induction by human recombinant interleukin-4. Identification by synthetic peptide analysis of two chemotactic domains residing in amino acid sequences 70–88 and 89–122. J. Clin. Invest. 87 (6), 2147–2152.

Postlethwaite, A.E., Lachman, L.B., Kang, A.H. 1984. Induction of fibroblast proliferation by interleukin-1 derived from human monocytic leukemia cells. Arthritis Rheum. 27 (9), 995–1001.

Postlethwaite, A.E., Holness, M.A., Katai, H., Raghow, R. 1992. Human fibroblasts synthesize elevated levels of extracellular matrix proteins in response to interleukin 4. J. Clin. Invest. 90 (4), 1479–1485.

Raghu, G., Masta, S., Meyers, D., Narayanan, A.S. 1989. Collagen synthesis by normal and fibrotic human lung fibroblasts and the effect of transforming growth factor-beta. Am. Rev. Respir. Dis. 140 (1), 95–100.

Reddy, R., Tan, E.M., Henning, D., Nohga, K., Busch, H. 1983. Detection of a nucleolar 7–2 ribonucleoprotein and a cytoplasmic 8–2 ribonucleoprotein with autoantibodies from patients with scleroderma. J. Biol. Chem. 258 (3), 1383–1386.

Reimer, G., Rose, K.M., Scheer, U., Tan, E.M. 1987. Autoantibody to RNA polymerase I in scleroderma sera. J. Clin. Invest. 79 (1), 65–72.

Reimer, G., Steen, V.D., Penning, C.A., Medsger, T.A. Jr., Tan, E.M. 1988. Correlates between autoantibodies to nucleolar antigens and clinical features in patients with systemic sclerosis (scleroderma). Arthritis Rheum. 31 (4), 525–532.

Reiser, K.M., Last, J.A. 1986. Early cellular events in pulmonary fibrosis. Exp. Lung Res. 10 (4), 331–355.

Reveille, J.D., Durban, E., MacLeod-St Clair, M.J., Goldstein, R., Moreda, R., Altman, R.D., Arnett, F.C. 1992a. Association of amino acid sequences in the HLA-DQB1 first domain with anti-topoisomerase I autoantibody response in scleroderma (progressive systemic sclerosis). J. Clin. Invest. 90 (3), 973–980.

Reveille, J.D., Owerbach, D., Goldstein, R., Moreda, R., Isern, R.A., Arnett, F.C. 1992b. Association of polar amino acids at position 26 of the HLA-DQB1 first domain with the anticentromere autoantibody response in systemic sclerosis (scleroderma). J. Clin. Invest. 89 (4), 1208–1213.

Reveille, J.D., Fischbach, M., McNearney, T., Friedman, A.W., Aguilar, M.B., Lisse, J., Fritzler, M.J., Ahn, C., Arnett, F.C. 2001. Systemic sclerosis in 3 US ethnic groups: a comparison of clinical, sociodemographic, serologic, and immunogenetic determinants. Semin. Arthritis Rheum. 30 (5), 332–346.

Reveille, J.D., Solomon, D.H., American College of Rhematology Ad Hoc Committee on Immunological Testing Guidelines. 2003. Evidence-based guidelines for the use of immunologic tests: anticentromere, Scl-70, and nucleolar antibodies. Arthritis Rheum. 49 (3), 399–412.

Rom, W.N., Basset, P., Fells, G.A., Nukiwa, T., Trapnell, B.C., Crystal, R.G. 1988. Alveolar macrophages release an insulin-like growth factor I-type molecule. J. Clin. Invest. 82 (5), 1685–1693.

Rosas, V., Conte, J.V., Yang, S.C., Gaine, S.P., Borja, M., Wigley, F.M., White, B., Orens, J.B. 2000. Lung transplantation and systemic sclerosis. Ann. Transplant. 5 (3), 38–43.

Rosenthal, A.K., McLaughlin, J.K., Linet, M.S., Persson, I. 1993. Scleroderma and malignancy: an epidemiological study. Ann. Rheum. Dis. 52 (7), 531–533.

Rosenthal, A.K., McLaughlin, J.K., Gridley, G., Nyren, O. 1995. Incidence of cancer among patients with systemic sclerosis. Cancer 76 (5), 910–914.

Rossi, G.A., Bitterman, P.B., Rennard, S.I., Ferrans, V.J., Crystal, R.G. 1985. Evidence for chronic inflammation as a component of the interstitial lung disease associated with progressive systemic sclerosis. Am. Rev. Respir. Dis. 131 (4), 612–617.

Rossi, S.E., Erasmus, J.J., McAdams, H.P., Sporn, T.A., Goodman, P.C. 2000. Pulmonary drug toxicity: radiologic and pathologic manifestations. Radiographics 20 (5), 1245–1259.

Rothfield, N., Kurtzman, S., Vazques-Abad, D., Charron, C., Daniels, L., Greenberg, B. 1992. Association of anti-topoisomerase I with cancer. Arthritis Rheum. 35 (6), 724.

Roumm, A.D., Medsger, T.A. Jr. 1985. Cancer and systemic sclerosis. An epidemiologic study. Arthritis Rheum. 28 (12), 1336–1340.

Sakkas, L.I., Tourtellotte, C., Berney, S., Myers, A.R., Platsoucas, C.D. 1999. Increased levels of alternatively spliced interleukin 4 (IL-4delta2) transcripts in peripheral blood mononuclear cells from patients with systemic sclerosis. Clin. Diagn. Lab. Immunol. 6 (5), 660–664.

Santiago, B., Galindo, M., Rivero, M., Pablos, J.L. 2001. Decreased susceptibility to Fas-induced apoptosis of systemic sclerosis dermal fibroblasts. Arthritis Rheum. 44 (7), 1667–1676.

Sato, S., Nagaoka, T., Hasegawa, M., Nishijima, C., Takehara, K. 2000a. Elevated serum KL-6 levels in patients with systemic sclerosis: association with the severity of pulmonary fibrosis. Dermatology 200 (3), 196–201.

Sato, S., Nagaoka, T., Hasegawa, M., Tamatani, T., Nakanishi, T., Takigawa, M., Takehara, K. 2000b. Serum levels of connective tissue growth factor are elevated in patients with systemic sclerosis: association with extent of skin sclerosis and severity of pulmonary fibrosis. J. Rheumatol. 27 (1), 149–154.

Schurawitzki, H., Stiglbauer, R., Graninger, W., Herold, C., Polzleitner, D., Burghuber, O.C., Tscholakoff, D. 1990. Interstitial lung disease in progressive systemic sclerosis: high-resolution CT versus radiography. Radiology 176 (3), 755–759.

Scussel-Lonzetti, L., Joyal, F., Raynauld, J.P., Roussin, A., Rich, E., Goulet, J.R., Raymond, Y., Senecal, J.L. 2002. Predicting mortality in systemic sclerosis: analysis of a cohort of 309 French Canadian patients with emphasis on features at diagnosis as predictive factors for survival. Medicine (Baltimore) 81 (2), 154–167.

Shahar, I., Fireman, E., Topilsky, M., Grief, J., Kivity, S., Spirer, Z., Ben Efraim, S. 1996. Effect of IL-6 on alveolar fibroblast proliferation in interstitial lung diseases. Clin. Immunol. Immunopathol. 79 (3), 244–251.

Shimizu, S., Gabazza, E.C., Hayashi, T., Ido, M., Adachi, Y., Suzuki, K. 2000. Thrombin stimulates the expression of PDGF in lung epithelial cells. Am. J. Physiol. Lung. Cell Mol. Physiol. 279 (3), L503–L510.

Shi-Wen, X., Denton, C.P., McWhirter, A., Bou-Gharios, G., Abraham, D.J., du Bois, R.M., Black, C.M. 1997. Scleroderma lung fibroblasts exhibit elevated and dysregulated type I collagen biosynthesis. Arthritis Rheum. 40 (7), 1237–1244.

Sigurgeirsson, B., Lindelof, B., Edhag, O., Allander, E. 1992. Risk of cancer in patients with dermatomyositis or polymyositis. A population-based study. N. Engl. J. Med. 326 (6), 363–367.

Silman, A.J., Jones, S. 1992. What is the contribution of occupational environmental factors to the occurrence of scleroderma in men? Ann. Rheum. Dis. 51 (12), 1322–1324.

Silver, R.M., Heyes, M.P., Maize, J.C., Quearry, B., Vionnet-Fuasset, M., Sternberg, E.M. 1990a. Scleroderma, fasciitis, and eosinophilia associated with the ingestion of tryptophan. N. Engl. J. Med. 322 (13), 874–881.

Silver, R.M., Miller, K.S., Kinsella, M.B., Smith, E.A., Schabel, S.I. 1990b. Evaluation and management of scleroderma lung disease using bronchoalveolar lavage. Am. J. Med. 88 (5), 470–476.

Silver, R.M., Warrick, J.H., Kinsella, M.B., Staudt, L.S., Baumann, M.H., Strange, C. 1993. Cyclophosphamide and low-dose prednisone therapy in patients with systemic sclerosis (scleroderma) with interstitial lung disease. J. Rheumatol. 20 (5), 838–844.

Sime, P.J., Marr, R.A., Gauldie, D., Xing, Z., Hewlett, B.R., Graham, F.L., Gauldie, J. 1998. Transfer of tumor necrosis factor-alpha to rat lung induces severe pulmonary inflammation and patchy interstitial fibrogenesis with induction of transforming growth factor-beta1 and myofibroblasts. Am. J. Pathol. 153 (3), 825–832.

Simeon, C.P., Armadans, L., Fonollosa, V., Solans, R., Selva, A., Villar, M., Lima, J., Vaque, J., Vilardell, M. 2003. Mortality and prognostic factors in Spanish patients with systemic sclerosis. Rheumatology (Oxford) 42 (1), 71–75.

Smith, E.A., Leroy, E.C. 1990. A possible role for transforming growth factor-beta in systemic sclerosis. J. Invest. Dermatol. 95 (6), 125S–127S.

Southcott, A.M., Jones, K.P., Li, D., Majumdar, S., Cambrey, A.D., Pantelidis, P., Black, C.M., Laurent, G.J., Davies, B.H., Jeffery, P.K. 1995. Interleukin-8. Differential expression in lone fibrosing alveolitis and systemic sclerosis. Am. J. Respir. Crit. Care Med. 151 (5), 1604–1612.

Spector, J.I., Zimbler, H. 1982. Cyclophosphamide pneumonitis. N. Engl. J. Med. 307 (4), 251.

Spector, J.I., Zimbler, H., Ross, J.S. 1979. Early-onset cyclophosphamide-induced interstitial pneumonitis. JAMA 242 (26), 2852–2854.

Spencer-Green, G., Alter, D., Welch, H.G. 1997. Test performance in systemic sclerosis: anti-centromere and anti-Scl-70 antibodies. Am. J. Med. 103 (3), 242–248.

Steen, V. 2003. Predictors of end stage lung disease in systemic sclerosis. Ann. Rheum. Dis. 62 (2), 97–99.

Steen, V.D., Medsger, T.A. Jr. 1998. Case-control study of corticosteroids and other drugs that either precipitate or protect from the development of scleroderma renal crisis. Arthritis Rheum. 41 (9), 1613–1619.

Steen, V.D., Medsger, T.A. Jr. 2000. Severe organ involvement in systemic sclerosis with diffuse scleroderma. Arthritis Rheum. 43 (11), 2437–2444.

Steen, V.D., Owens, G.R., Redmond, C., Rodnan, G.P., Medsger, T.A. Jr. 1985. The effect of D-penicillamine on pulmonary findings in systemic sclerosis. Arthritis Rheum. 28 (8), 882–888.

Steen, V.D., Powell, D.L., Medsger, T.A. Jr. 1988. Clinical correlations and prognosis based on serum autoantibodies in patients with systemic sclerosis. Arthritis Rheum. 31 (2), 196–203.

Steen, V.D., Conte, C., Owens, G.R., Medsger, T.A. Jr. 1994a. Severe restrictive lung disease in systemic sclerosis. Arthritis Rheum. 37 (9), 1283–1289.

Steen, V.D., Lanz, J.K. Jr., Conte, C., Owens, G.R., Medsger, T.A. Jr. 1994b. Therapy for severe interstitial lung disease in systemic sclerosis. A retrospective study. Arthritis Rheum. 37 (9), 1290–1296.

Steen, V.D., Oddis, C.V., Conte, C.G., Janoski, J., Casterline, G.Z., Medsger, T.A. Jr. 1997. Incidence of systemic sclerosis in Allegheny County. Pennsylvania. A twenty-year study of hospital-diagnosed cases, 1963–1982. Arthritis Rheum. 40 (3), 441–445.

Stockton, D., Doherty, V.R., Brewster, D.H. 2001. Risk of cancer in patients with dermatomyositis or polymyositis, and follow-up implications: a Scottish population-based cohort study. Br. J. Cancer 85 (1), 41–45.

Suga, M., Iyonaga, K., Ichiyasu, H., Saita, N., Yamasaki, H., Ando, M. 1999. Clinical significance of MCP-1 levels in BALF and serum in patients with interstitial lung diseases. Eur. Respir. J. 14 (2), 376–382.

Susol, E., Rands, A.L., Herrick, A., McHugh, N., Barrett, J.H., Ollier, W.E., Worthington, J. 2000. Association of markers for TGFbeta3, TGFbeta2 and TIMP1 with systemic sclerosis. Rheumatology (Oxford) 39 (12), 1332–1336.

Tabuenca, J.M. 1981. Toxic-allergic syndrome caused by ingestion of rapeseed oil denatured with aniline. Lancet 2, 567–568.

Takahashi, H., Kuroki, Y., Tanaka, H., Saito, T., Kurokawa, K., Chiba, H., Sagawa, A., Nagae, H., Abe, S. 2000. Serum levels of surfactant proteins A and D are useful biomarkers for interstitial lung disease in patients with progressive systemic sclerosis. Am. J. Respir. Crit. Care Med. 162 (1), 258–263.

Talbott, J.H., Barrocas, M. 1980. Carcinoma of the lung in progressive systemic sclerosis: a tabular review of the literature and a detailed report of the roentgenographic changes in two cases. Semin. Arthritis Rheum. 9 (3), 191–217.

Tan, F.K., Stivers, D.N., Arnett, F.C., Chakraborty, R., Howard, R., Reveille, J.D. 1999. HLA haplotypes and microsatellite polymorphisms in and around the major histocompatibility complex region in a Native American population with a high prevalence of scleroderma (systemic sclerosis). Tissue Antigens 53 (1), 74–80.

Tan, F.K., Wang, N., Kuwana, M., Chakraborty, R., Bona, C.A., Milewicz, D.M., Arnett, F.C. 2001. Association of fibrillin 1 single-nucleotide polymorphism haplotypes with systemic sclerosis in Choctaw and Japanese populations. Arthritis Rheum. 44 (4), 893–901.

Topilow, A.A., Rothenberg, S.P., Cottrell, T.S. 1973. Interstitial pneumonia after prolonged treatment with cyclophosphamide. Am. Rev. Respir. Dis. 108 (1), 114–117.

Tormey, V.J., Bunn, C.C., Denton, C.P., Black, C.M. 2001. Anti-fibrillarin antibodies in systemic sclerosis. Rheumatology (Oxford) 40 (10), 1157–1162.

Tramposch, H.D., Smith, C.D., Senecal, J.L., Rothfield, N. 1984. A long-term longitudinal study of anticentromere antibodies. Arthritis Rheum. 27 (2), 121–124.

Vaillant, P., Menard, O., Vignaud, J.M., Martinet, N., Martinet, Y. 1996. The role of cytokines in human lung fibrosis. Monaldi. Arch. Chest Dis. 51 (2), 145–152.

Vancheeswaran, R., Magoulas, T., Efrat, G., Wheeler-Jones, C., Olsen, I., Penny, R., Black, C.M. 1994. Circulating endothelin-1 levels in systemic sclerosis subsets—a marker of fibrosis or vascular dysfunction? J. Rheumatol. 21 (10), 1838–1844.

van Nunen, S.A., Gatenby, P.A., Basten, A. 1982. Post-mammoplasty connective tissue disease. Arthritis Rheum. 25 (6), 694–697.

Varai, G., Earle, L., Jimenez, S.A., Steiner, R.M., Varga, J. 1998. A pilot study of intermittent intravenous cyclophosphamide for the treatment of systemic sclerosis associated lung disease. J. Rheumatol. 25 (7), 1325–1329.

Varga, J., Bashey, R.I. 1995. Regulation of connective tissue synthesis in systemic sclerosis. Int. Rev. Immunol. 12 (2–4), 187–199.

Varga, J., Rosenbloom, J., Jimenez, S.A. 1987. Transforming growth factor beta (TGF beta) causes a persistent increase in steady-state amounts of type I and type III collagen and fibronectin mRNAs in normal human dermal fibroblasts. Biochem. J. 247 (3), 597–604.

Vaughan, M.B., Howard, E.W., Tomasek, J.J. 2000. Transforming growth factor-beta1 promotes the morphological and functional differentiation of the myofibroblast. Exp. Cell. Res. 257 (1), 180–189.

Vazquez-Abad, D., Russell, C.A., Cusick, S.M., Earnshaw, W.C., Rothfield, N.F. 1995. Longitudinal study of anticentromere and antitopoisomerase-I isotypes. Clin. Immunol. Immunopathol. 74 (3), 257–270.

Veltman, G., Lange, C.E., Juhe, S., Stein, G., Bachner, U. 1975. Clinical manifestations and course of vinyl chloride disease. Ann. N. Y. Acad. Sci. 246, 6–17.

Wakata, N., Kurihara, T., Saito, E., Kinoshita, M. 2002. Polymyositis and dermatomyositis associated with malignancy: a 30-year retrospective study. Int. J. Dermatol. 41 (11), 729–734.

Wallaert, B. 1990. Subclinical alveolitis in immunologic systemic disorders. Lung 168, (Suppl.) 974–983.

Wallaert, B., Hatron, P.Y., Grosbois, J.M., Tonnel, A.B., Devulder, B., Voisin, C. 1986. Subclinical pulmonary involvement in collagen-vascular diseases assessed by bronchoalveolar lavage. Relationship between alveolitis and subsequent changes in lung function. Am. Rev. Respir. Dis. 133 (4), 574–580.

Wallaert, B., Bart, F., Aerts, C., Ouaissi, A., Hatron, P.Y., Tonnel, A.B., Voisin, C. 1988. Activated alveolar macrophages in subclinical pulmonary inflammation in collagen vascular diseases. Thorax 43 (1), 24–30.

Weiner, E.S., Hildebrandt, S., Senecal, J.L., Daniels, L., Noell, S., Joyal, F., Roussin, A., Earnshaw, W., Rothfield, N.F. 1991. Prognostic significance of anticentromere antibodies and anti-topoisomerase I antibodies in Raynaud's disease. A prospective study. Arthritis Rheum. 34 (1), 68–77.

Wells, A.U., du Bois, R.M. 1993. Bronchiolitis in association with connective tissue disorders. Clin. Chest Med. 14 (4), 655–666.

Wells, A.U., Hansell, D.M., Corrin, B., Harrison, N.K., Goldstraw, P., Black, C.M., du Bois, R.M. 1992. High resolution computed tomography as a predictor of lung histology in systemic sclerosis. Thorax 47 (9), 738–742.

Wells, A.U., Hansell, D.M., Harrison, N.K., Lawrence, R., Black, C.M., du Bois, R.M. 1993a. Clearance of inhaled 99mTc-DTPA predicts the clinical course of fibrosing alveolitis. Eur. Respir. J. 6 (6), 797–802.

Wells, A.U., Hansell, D.M., Rubens, M.B., Cullinan, P., Black, C.M., du Bois, R.M. 1993b. The predictive value of appearances on thin-section computed tomography in fibrosing alveolitis. Am. Rev. Respir. Dis. 148 (4 Pt 1), 1076–1082.

Wells, A.U., Cullinan, P., Hansell, D.M., Rubens, M.B., Black, C.M., Newman-Taylor, A.J., du Bois, R.M. 1994a. Fibrosing alveolitis associated with systemic sclerosis has a better prognosis than lone cryptogenic fibrosing alveolitis. Am. J. Respir. Crit. Care. Med. 149 (6), 1583–1590.

Wells, A.U., Hansell, D.M., Rubens, M.B., Cullinan, P., Haslam, P.L., Black, C.M., du Bois, R.M. 1994b. Fibrosing alveolitis in systemic sclerosis. Bronchoalveolar lavage findings in relation to computed tomographic appearance. Am. J. Respir. Crit. Care Med. 150 (2), 462–468.

Wells, A.U., Hansell, D.M., Rubens, M.B., Cailes, J.B., Black, C.M., du Bois, R.M. 1997a. Functional impairment in lone cryptogenic fibrosing alveolitis and fibrosing alveolitis associated with systemic sclerosis: a comparison. Am. J. Respir. Crit. Care Med. 155 (5), 1657–1664.

Wells, A.U., Hansell, D.M., Rubens, M.B., King, A.D., Cramer, D., Black, C.M., du Bois, R.M. 1997b. Fibrosing alveolitis in systemic sclerosis: indices of lung function in relation to extent of disease on computed tomography. Arthritis Rheum. 40 (7), 1229–1236.

Wells, A.U., Hansell, D.M., Haslam, P.L., Rubens, M.B., Cailes, J., Black, C.M., du Bois, R.M. 1998. Bronchoalveolar lavage cellularity: lone cryptogenic fibrosing alveolitis compared with the fibrosing alveolitis of systemic sclerosis. Am. J. Respir. Crit. Care Med. 157 (5 Pt 1), 1474–1482.

Wells, A.U., Desai, S.R., Rubens, M.B., Goh, N.S., Cramer, D., Nicholson, A.G., Colby, T.V., du Bois, R.M., Hansell, D.M. 2003. Idiopathic pulmonary fibrosis: a composite physiologic index derived from disease extent observed by computed tomography. Am. J. Respir. Crit. Care Med. 167 (7), 962–969.

White, B., Moore, W.C., Wigley, F.M., Xiao, H.Q., Wise, R.A. 2000. Cyclophosphamide is associated with pulmonary function and survival benefit in patients with scleroderma and alveolitis. Ann. Intern. Med. 132 (12), 947–954.

Whyte, J., Artlett, C., Harvey, G., Stephens, C.O., Welsh, K., Black, C., Maddison, P.J., McHugh, N.J. 1994. HLA-DQB1 associations with anti-topoisomerase-1 antibodies in patients with systemic sclerosis and their first degree relatives. United Kingdom Systemic Sclerosis Study Group. J. Autoimmun. 7 (4), 509–520.

Wiedemann, H.P., Matthay, R.A. 1989. Pulmonary manifestations of the collagen vascular diseases. Clin. Chest Med. 10 (4), 677–722.

Wrana, J.L., Attisano, L. 2000. The Smad pathway. Cytokine Growth Factor Rev. 11 (1–2), 5–13.

Yamakage, A., Kikuchi, K., Smith, E.A., Leroy, E.C., Trojanowska, M. 1992. Selective upregulation of platelet-derived growth factor alpha receptors by transforming growth factor beta in scleroderma fibroblasts. J. Exp. Med. 175 (5), 1227–1234.

Yamamoto, T., Eckes, B., Krieg, T. 2001. High expression and autoinduction of monocyte chemoattractant protein-1 in scleroderma fibroblasts. Eur. J. Immunol. 31 (10), 2936–2941.

Yamane, K., Ihn, H., Kubo, M., Yazawa, N., Kikuchi, K., Soma, Y., Tamaki, K. 2000. Serum levels of KL-6 as a useful marker for evaluating pulmonary fibrosis in patients with systemic sclerosis. J. Rheumatol. 27 (4), 930–934.

Yanaba, K., Hasegawa, M., Hamaguchi, Y., Fujimoto, M., Takehara, K., Sato, S. 2003. Longitudinal analysis of serum KL-6 levels in patients with systemic sclerosis: association with the activity of pulmonary fibrosis. Clin. Exp. Rheumatol. 21 (4), 429–436.

Yang, Y., Fujita, J., Tokuda, M., Bandoh, S., Ishida, T. 2001. Lung cancer associated with several connective tissue diseases: with a review of literature. Rheumatol. Int. 21 (3), 106–111.

Young, V., Ho, M., Vosper, H., Belch, J.J., Palmer, C.N. 2002. Elevated expression of the genes encoding TNF-alpha and thromboxane synthase in leucocytes from patients with systemic sclerosis. Rheumatology (Oxford) 41 (8), 869–875.

Young-Min, S.A., Beeton, C., Laughton, R., Plumpton, T., Bartram, S., Murphy, G., Black, C., Cawston, T.E. 2001. Serum TIMP-1, TIMP-2, and MMP-1 in patients with systemic sclerosis, primary Raynaud's phenomenon, and in normal controls. Ann. Rheum. Dis. 60 (9), 846–851.

Zhang, H.Y., Phan, S.H. 1999. Inhibition of myofibroblast apoptosis by transforming growth factor beta(1). Am. J. Respir. Cell Mol. Biol. 21 (6), 658–665.

Zhang, K., Gharaee-Kermani, M., Jones, M.L., Warren, J.S., Phan, S.H. 1994. Lung monocyte chemoattractant protein-1 gene expression in bleomycin-induced pulmonary fibrosis. J. Immunol. 153 (10), 4733–4741.

Zhang, K., Flanders, K.C., Phan, S.H. 1995. Cellular localization of transforming growth factor-beta expression in bleomycin-induced pulmonary fibrosis. Am. J. Pathol. 147 (2), 352–361.

Handbook of Systemic Autoimmune Diseases, Volume 2
Pulmonary Involvement in Systemic Autoimmune Diseases
A.U. Wells and C.P. Denton, editors

CHAPTER 11

Pulmonary Complications of Polymyositis and Dermatomyositis

Jane Deng[a], Michael P. Keane[b], Joseph P. Lynch III[b,*]

[a]*Division of Pulmonary and Critical Care Medicine, Department of Internal Medicine, University of Michigan Medical Center, Ann Arbor, MI, USA*

[b]*Division of Pulmonary, Critical Care Medicine and Hospitalists, David Geffen School of Medicine at UCLA, Box 951690, Los Angeles, CA 90095-1690, USA*

1. Introduction

Polymyositis (PM) and dermatomyositis (DM) are rare inflammatory myopathies of unknown etiology which may give rise to systemic or pulmonary manifestations (Dalakas, 1991; Schwarz, 1992; Adams-Gandhi et al., 1996; Bohan and Peter, 1975). The estimated prevalence of PM ranges from 0.5 to 8.4 cases per million (Cronin and Plotz, 1990). Polymyositis is 3–4 times more common in women; the age distribution is bimodal, with an early peak at 5–15 years, and a later peak at 50–60 years of age (Adams-Gandhi et al., 1996). Major criteria for the diagnosis of PM include: symmetric proximal muscle weakness; a muscle biopsy showing inflammatory cell infiltrates and necrosis; elevated muscle enzymes (e.g. creatinine (CK) and aldolase); and a characteristic electromyogram (EMG) (Adams-Gandhi et al., 1996; Dalakas, 1991; Bohan and Peter, 1975). Proximal muscle weakness is the most common feature of PM, present in more than 80% of patients at the onset of illness (Dalakas, 1991; Schwarz, 1992; Adams-Gandhi et al., 1996). Patients with PM and a typical rash are considered to have DM (Bohan and Peter, 1975). The rash of DM often exhibits a violaceous discoloration of the upper eyelids (heliotrophic rash) with periorbital edema or an erythematous to violaceous scaly rash (Gottron's papules) involving the knuckles, knees, elbows, or trunk. In DM, the rash antedates clinical myopathy in 56% of patients; myopathy precedes the rash in 16%; the rash and myopathy occur simultaneously in 28% (Adams-Gandhi et al., 1996). Amyotrophic DM (i.e typical cutaneous features of DM but no clinically evident muscle involvement) can also occur (el-Azhary and Pakzad, 2002; Cottin et al., 2003; Caproni et al., 2002; Krain, 1975). Pulmonary complications occur in up to 46% of patients with DM or PM (Dickey and Myers, 1984), and are associated with shortened survival (Lakhanpal et al., 1987; Arsura and Greenberg, 1988; Marie et al., 2002). Other sites of involvement with PM or DM include the gastrointestinal tract (predominantly due to smooth muscle involvement), heart, and joints (Dalakas, 1991; Schwarz, 1992; Adams-Gandhi et al., 1996; Hochberg et al., 1986). Cardiac involvement may give rise to heart block, cardiomyopathy, congestive heart failure, or pericarditis (Hochberg et al., 1986). Malignancy complicates DM in 15–25% of patients, and portends a poor prognosis (Adams-Gandhi et al., 1996; Sigurgeirsson et al., 1992). PM or DM may also occur in patients meeting criteria for other collagen vascular disorders (CVDs) (e.g. rheumatoid arthritis (RA), systemic lupus erythematosus (SLE), or progressive systemic sclerosis (PSS)). In this context, the term Overlap Syndrome is applied. Individuals with Overlap Syndrome and high-titer antibodies to U1 ribonucleoprotein

*Corresponding author.
Tel.: +1-310-825-5988; fax: +1-310-206-8622
E-mail address: jplynch@mednet.ucla.edu (J.P. Lynch).

DOI: 10.1016/S1571-5078(04)02011-2

(the nuclear antigen RNP) have been designated as having mixed connective tissue disease (MCTD) (Sharp et al., 1972; Sullivan et al., 1984), but this designation is not universally accepted.

In this chapter, we limit our discussion to pulmonary complications of DM or PM, with an emphasis on interstitial lung disease (ILD) complicating PM or DM (Takizawa et al., 1987; Lakhanpal et al., 1987; Arsura and Greenberg, 1988; Marie et al., 2002; Lynch et al., 1999). Pulmonary complications and malignancy are the most common causes of death in PM or DM (Benbassat et al., 1985; Lakhanpal et al., 1987; Marie et al., 2001; Sigurgeirsson et al., 1992).

Pulmonary involvement in PM or DM can be classified as follows:

(1) complications of neuromuscular weakness (e.g. aspiration pneumonia, ventilatory insufficiency due to respiratory muscle weakness),
(2) interstitial lung disease,
(3) complications of drug therapy (e.g. drug-induced pneumonitis, opportunistic infections),
(4) primary lung malignancies (Fujita et al., 2001; Hidano et al., 1986, 1992; Manchul et al., 1985; Sigurgeirsson et al., 1992) (these will not be further discussed in this chapter).

2. Respiratory complications of muscular weakness

Muscular weakness can give rise to aspiration pneumonia (as a result of discoordinated swallowing) or respiratory insufficiency (reflecting respiratory muscle dysfunction) (Baumann, 1999). Myopathic inflammation involving the striated muscle of the pharynx and upper esophagus can lead to dysphagia (Baumann, 1999), which has been cited in 12–67% of patients in various series (Benbassat et al., 1985; Dickey and Myers, 1984; Marie et al., 1998; Lakhanpal et al., 1987; Bohan et al., 1977; Hochberg et al., 1986; Baumann, 1999). This, along with respiratory muscle weakness, places patients with DM/PM at considerable risk for aspiration pneumonia (Baumann, 1999). Aspiration pneumonia occurs in 14–20% of patients with PM/DM (Dickey and Myers, 1984; Schwarz, 1998; Medsger et al., 1971; Marie et al., 2001; Benbassat et al., 1985); in this context, dysphagia is invariably present (Dickey and Myers, 1984; Medsger et al., 1971). Dysphagia is independently associated with a greater degree of proximal muscle weakness (Medsger et al., 1971) and is associated with a poor prognosis (Benbassat et al., 1985; Baumann, 1999). Swallowing studies via cineradiography or manometry are the best methods to diagnose esophageal muscle dysfunction (i.e. diminished or absent esophageal peristalsis and laryngeal aspiration) (Turner et al., 1973; Baumann, 1999). Airway protection is critical in PM patients with severe dysphagia; in severe cases, tracheotomy may be necessary while awaiting the impact of medical therapy for the underlying myopathy (Baumann, 1999).

A more unusual manifestation of myopathy is hypercapnic respiratory failure from respiratory muscle weakness (DePalo and McCool, 2002; Gilchrist, 2002; Baumann, 1999). Clinically significant respiratory muscle weakness has been cited in 7–22% of patients with PM/DM (Dickey and Myers, 1984; Marie et al., 1998; Schwarz, 1998). Severe respiratory insufficiency requiring mechanical ventilatory support or leading to death has been described in 2–7% of patients with PM/DM (Blumbergs et al., 1984; Dickey and Myers, 1984; Sano et al., 1994; Astudillo et al., 2001; DeVere and Bradley, 1975). Rarely, bilateral diaphragmatic paralysis has been reported in DM (Schiavi et al., 1984). Respiratory muscle weakness may be the initial presentation of PM, but this is rare (Blumbergs et al., 1984).

Pulmonary function tests (PFTs) in patients with severe neuromuscular weakness reveal a restrictive pattern with reduced lung volumes (e.g. total lung capacity (TLC) and forced vital capacity (FVC) (DePalo and McCool, 2002; Braun et al., 1983). In contrast, residual volume (RV) is increased when expiratory muscle weakness is severe (DePalo and McCool, 2002). Forced expiratory flow rates are reduced proportionate to reductions in FVC; however, the ratio of forced expiratory volume in one second (FEV_1) to FVC is preserved (DePalo and McCool, 2002). Lung volumes are relatively insensitive, as respiratory muscle strength must be reduced nearly by half before changes in VC or TLC are evident (Braun et al., 1983). Reductions in maximal static inspiratory and expiratory pressures (PI max and PE max) are more sensitive than lung volumes for detecting respiratory muscle weakness (DePalo and McCool, 2002; Braun et al., 1983). However, other factors such as sub-maximal effort or air leaks around the mouthpiece may also cause low values. Measurement of PI max during maximal sniff maneuvers enhances accuracy (DePalo and McCool, 2002). Specific tests of diaphragmatic function such as transdiaphragmatic pressures are invasive and uncomfortable. Reductions in maximum voluntary ventilation (MVV) may reflect weakness, poor coordination, or reduced endurance of respiratory muscles, but this is nonspecific (DePalo and McCool, 2002). Diffusing capacity for carbon monoxide (DL_{CO}) may be reduced, but is normal or increased when corrected for alveolar ventilation (V_A). Hypercapnea and hypoxemia are late findings (Braun et al., 1983). Respiratory muscle strength (RMS), calculated by an average of PI max and PE max, is linearly related to $paCO_2$, but only after RMS falls below 50% (Braun et al., 1983). In PM/DM, inspiratory and expiratory muscles are equally affected, whereas *expiratory* muscle weakness is manifest in patients with amyotrophic lateral sclerosis (ALS), myasthenia gravis, and myotonic dystrophies (Braun et al., 1983). Serial measurements of FVC, PI max, and PE max are useful to diagnose respiratory muscle weakness and monitor the course of the disease (DePalo and McCool, 2002; Braun et al., 1983).

On histopathology, the inflammatory and degenerative changes characteristic of PM/DM are present in the intercostal muscles, diaphragm, and accessory muscles (Dickey and Myers, 1984). Atrophy of the diaphragm has been found on autopsy (Lakhanpal et al., 1987). Inflammatory myopathies affecting respiratory muscles usually respond to corticosteroids (CS) and/or immunosuppressive (IS) agents (Bohan and Peter, 1975; Bohan et al., 1977; Dickey and Myers, 1984; Marie et al., 2001). When muscle weakness persists in patients treated with high dose, chronic CS, steroid myopathy should be considered. The presence of type II muscle fiber atrophy when other pathologic features have improved on muscle biopsy or when CK levels have normalized suggests steroid myopathy (Bunch et al., 1980).

3. Interstitial lung disease in PM/DM

3.1. Prevalence

ILD has been cited in 5 to > 30% of patients with PM or DM in retrospective studies (Frazier and Miller, 1974; Bohan et al., 1977; Songcharoen et al., 1980; Salmeron et al., 1981; Dickey and Myers, 1984; Nambu et al., 1994; Hidano et al., 1986, 1992; Takizawa et al., 1987; Grau et al., 1996; Marie et al., 1998, 2002; Douglas et al., 2001; Schnabel et al., 2003; Wells et al., 2003). Prospective studies assessing the prevalence of ILD in PM or DM are lacking. The large variability in reported prevalence likely reflects differences in referral patterns, heterogeneous patient populations, and differences in the sensitivity of diagnostic techniques (Songcharoen et al., 1980; Schwarz, 1998; Schnabel et al., 2003). In three studies comprising 360 patients with PM/DM, aberrations on chest radiographs consistent with ILD were cited in 5–10% (Frazier and Miller, 1974; Dickey and Myers, 1984; Salmeron et al., 1981). However, two small series cited ILD in 47% (7 of 15) and 64% (9 of 14) of patients with PM/DM (Takizawa et al., 1987; Songcharoen et al., 1980). Japanese authors reported prevalence rates of ILD in PM/DM ranging from 40 to 80% (Yoshida et al., 1983; Hirakata and Nagai, 2000; Takizawa et al., 1987). The reason for the discrepancy between the Japanese and Western literature is not clear, but could reflect genetic differences (Fig. 1). The prevalence of ILD may be lower in patients with amyotrophic DM (el-Azhary and Pakzad, 2002; Cottin et al., 2003; Caproni et al., 2002; Krain, 1975). In two recent series comprising 37 (el-Azhary and Pakzad, 2002) and 13 patients (Caproni et al., 2002) with amyotrophic DM, no case of ILD was identified. However, in a recent report, diffuse alveolar damage (DAD) was described in three patients with amyotrophic DM and acute respiratory failure (Lee et al., 2002).

3.2. Epidemiology

As with DM and PM in general, ILD is 3–5 times more common in women than in men (Arsura and Greenberg, 1988; Duncan et al., 1974; Dickey and Myers, 1984; Schwarz et al., 1976; Nambu et al., 1994;

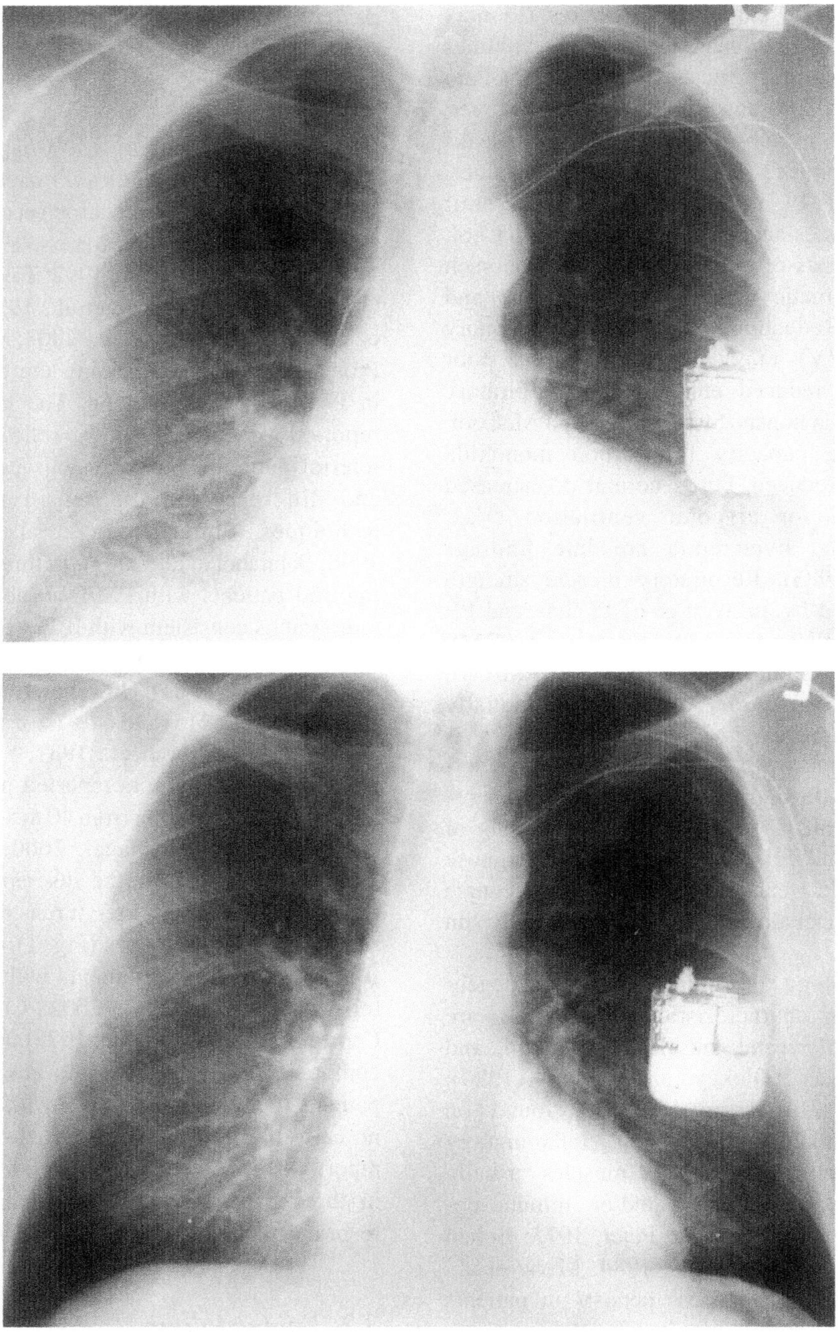

A

B

Figure 1. (a) Polymyositis. PA chest radiograph from a 70-year-old male with polymyositis and a restrictive ventilatory defect reveals bilateral reticular opacities, with a basilar predominance. A left cardiac pacemaker is in place. Transbronchial lung biopsies revealed chronic interstitial inflammation and fibrosis. (b) Polymyositis. PA chest radiograph from the same patient 3 months later following high dose corticosteroid therapy has completely normalized. (Reproduced with permission from Lynch and Chavis, 1992.)

Arakawa et al., 2003; Cottin et al., 2003). The mean age of presentation is 50–55 years, although ILD can present at any age (Duncan et al., 1974; Frazier and Miller, 1974; Schwarz et al., 1976; Dickey and Myers, 1984; Douglas et al., 2001; Arakawa et al., 2003; Cottin et al., 2003). ILD is more common with PM than DM (Schwarz, 1992; Schwarz et al., 1976; Dickey and Myers, 1984; Arsura and Greenberg, 1988). As will be discussed in detail later, circulating autoantibodies to transfer RNA (tRNA) synthetases (particularly anti-Jo-1) are present in 70–85% of patients with PM and ILD, and are typically associated with a constellation of features including myositis, ILD, arthritis, and various cutaneous and vascular components (Marguerie et al., 1990; Yoshida et al., 1983; Schmidt et al., 2000) (Table 1).

3.3. Clinical manifestations

Although the spectrum of PM/DM-associated ILD is broad, the onset is usually insidious, progressing over weeks to months (Schwarz et al., 1976; Dickey and Myers, 1984; Grau et al., 1996; Schwarz, 1998; Marie et al., 2002). Dyspnea and nonproductive cough are the primary symptoms (Schwarz et al., 1976; Dickey and Myers, 1984; Grau et al., 1996; Schwarz, 1998; Marie et al., 2002). Physical examination typically reveals crackles; clubbing is uncommon (Arsura and Greenberg, 1988; Dickey and Myers, 1984; Grathwohl et al., 1995; Grau et al., 1996; Schwarz et al., 1976). Raynaud's phenomenon is present in 50–60% of PM patients with anti-Jo-1 syndrome

Table 1
PM-associated ILD: typical clinical features

Restrictive ventilatory defect, low DL_{CO}
Abnormalities on HRCT (e.g. thickened interlobular septa; reticulation; GGO; consolidation)
Nonspecific interstitial pneumonia (NSIP) most common histological pattern
Raynaud's phenomenon (50–60%)
Arthralgias (>70%)
Auto-antibodies to transfer RNA (tRNA) synthetase (e.g. anti-Jo-1, anti-PL7, antiPL12)
BAL lymphocytosis and/or neutrophilia
Course of ILD does not correlate with severity of muscle or systemic disease

(Schmidt et al., 2000) or ILD (Hidano et al., 1992; Schnabel et al., 2003) and is associated with a worse survival (Arsura and Greenberg, 1988; Schwarz, 1992). Importantly, the severity and extent of pulmonary parenchymal involvement does *not* correlate with the course of the muscle disease, muscle enzymes, or systemic features (Lakhanpal et al., 1987; Tazelaar et al., 1990). However, arthritis and arthralgias are far more common in PM patients with ILD (48–100% prevalence) (Schwarz, 1998; Marie et al., 2002; Dickey and Myers, 1984; Lakhanpal et al., 1987; Hidano et al., 1992; Grau et al., 1996; Douglas et al., 2001; Yoshida et al., 1983; Schnabel et al., 2003) compared to patients *without* ILD (5–39% prevalence) (Lakhanpal et al., 1987; Schnabel et al., 2003; Grau et al., 1996). The arthritis mostly involves the hands, wrists, or knees in a symmetrical fashion (Grau et al., 1996; Yoshida et al., 1983; Schumacher et al., 1979; Delbrel et al., 2001).

ILD can occur at any point in the course of the disease (Schwarz et al., 1976; Dickey and Myers, 1984; Marie et al., 2002; Yang et al., 2002). In a series of 156 consecutive patients with DM/PM, 35 (23%) patients developed ILD (Marie et al., 2002). ILD onset preceded PM/DM in 7 (20%); it developed concurrently with PM/DM in 15 (42%), and after PM/DM onset in 14 (38%). However, in another series of DM patients with ILD, pulmonary disease preceded the onset of muscular symptoms in 75% of patients (Grau et al., 1996). The diagnosis may be missed in patients presenting with predominant respiratory symptoms. Furthermore, treatment with CS or IS agents for presumed idiopathic ILD may mask the myopathy, delaying the diagnosis for weeks or even years (Douglas et al., 2001). ILD developing concurrently or within 6 months of the onset of DM has been associated with a rapidly progressive course in some patients; in contrast, ILD occurring before or at least 1 year after the onset of DM has a better prognosis (Hidano et al., 1986, 1992).

Rarely, patients present more acutely, with fevers, dyspnea, and cough evolving over a few days or weeks (Marie et al., 2002; Lee et al., 2002). In this context, fulminant progression to acute respiratory failure may occur. This syndrome resembles idiopathic acute interstitial pneumonia (AIP) and is associated with a histopathological pattern of DAD on lung biopsy or necropsy (Arsura and Greenberg, 1988;

Frazier and Miller, 1974; Tazelaar et al., 1990; Duncan et al., 1974; Schwarz et al., 1976; Dickey and Myers, 1984). High dose 'pulse' intravenous (IV) methylprednisolone in this context may be lifesaving (Lee et al., 2002; Marie et al., 2002).

3.4. Diagnostic investigations

3.4.1. Radiographic studies

Chest radiographs in PM-associated ILD typically demonstrate diffuse reticular (interstitial) infiltrates with a basilar predominance (Schwarz et al., 1976; Dickey and Myers, 1984). Alveolar opacities may also be observed (Schwarz et al., 1976; Grau et al., 1996). Pleural effusions or intrathoracic lymphadenopathy are *not* found. High-resolution computed tomographic (HRCT) scans are far more sensitive than chest radiographs in detecting ILD (Schurawitzki et al., 1990; Wells et al., 2003; Mino et al., 1997) and have prognostic and diagnostic value (discussed later) (Akira et al., 1999; Ellis and Hansell, 2002; Arakawa et al., 2003; Schnabel et al., 2003; Marie et al., 2002).

Salient CT features of PM-associated ILD include: thickened interlobular septa (>90%); linear (reticular) opacities (43–92%); irregular interfaces (80%); ground-glass opacities (GGO) (33–100%); parenchymal nodules (27–73%); patchy consolidation (22–100%); honeycomb change (0–19%); and traction bronchiectasis or bronchiolectasis (0–17%) (Ikezoe et al., 1996; Mino et al., 1997; Douglas et al., 2001; Saito et al., 2002; Arakawa et al., 2003; Akira et al., 1999; Kim et al., 2002b; Cottin et al., 2003; Marie et al., 2002) (see Table 2). Similar to idiopathic and CVD-associated pulmonary fibrosis, PM/DM-associated ILD exhibits a predilection for basilar and peripheral regions (Mino et al., 1997; Douglas et al., 2001; Arakawa et al., 2003; Schnabel et al., 2003; Saito et al., 2002). The prevalence of specific CT features is difficult to assess since terminology and CT features evaluated were not uniform and patient populations were heterogeneous in the various publications (Fig. 2).

Certain CT features correlate with histological patterns. Airspace consolidation is a prominent feature of bronchiolitis obliterans organizing pneumonia (BOOP), nonspecific interstitial pneumonia (NSIP), or DAD (Cottin et al., 2003; Arakawa et al., 2003; Marie et al., 2002). However, consolidation is more uniform and extensive with DAD (Cottin et al., 2003; Ikezoe et al., 1996). A combination of patchy GGO, intra-lobular reticular opacities, and traction bronchiectasis without HC suggests NSIP (Cottin et al., 2003; Arakawa et al., 2003). Subpleural lines, parenchymal bands, traction bronchiectasis, HC, and minimal or no GGO suggest usual interstitial pneumonia (UIP) (Ikezoe et al., 1996; Mino et al., 1997; Akira et al., 1999; Kim et al., 2002b). Specific features on CT have prognostic value. Consolidation or GGO often reverse with CS or IS therapy whereas HC never improves and may progress (Schnabel et al., 2003; Mino et al., 1997; Akira et al., 1999; Arakawa et al., 2003). In one study, serial CT scans improved with treatment in 16 of 17 (94%) patients with PM-associated ILD (Mino et al., 1997).

Table 2
Polymyositis-associated ILD: CT features

HRCT feature	Reference and number of patients			
	Ikezoe et al. (1996), $N = 25$	Mino et al. (1997), $N = 19$	Saito et al. (2002), $N = 42$	Marie et al. (2002), $N = 36$
Thickened interlobular septa	92%	100%	100%	NA
Ground glass opacities	92%	100%	33%	50%
Linear opacities	92%	NA	43%	75%
Irregular interfaces	88%	79%	NA	83%
Consolidation	52%	100%	45%	NA
Parenchymal micronodules	28%	NA	73%	30%
Honeycomb change	16%	0	19%	6%

A

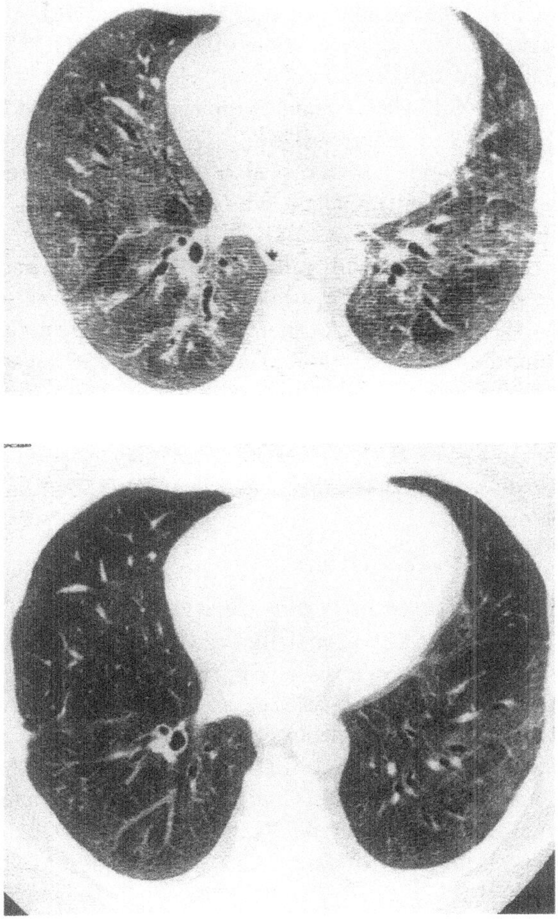

B

Figure 2. (a) Dermatomyositis. HRCT demonstrates diffuse ground-glass attenuation in a patient with DM, dyspnea, and a restrictive ventilatory defect. (b) HRCT from the same patient 3 weeks after institution of high dose corticosteroid therapy showing marked improvement. (Reproduced with permission from Lynch et al., 1999.)

Patchy consolidation, parenchymal bands, and peribronchovascular thickening resolved, but were often replaced by prominent interlobular septa, subpleural lines, or GGO. In another study, serial CT scans were performed in 14 patients with PM/DM and NSIP; after institution of CS or IS therapy, CT scans improved in 13 (93%) (Arakawa et al., 2003). Using semi-quantitative analyses, improvement was noted in the following parameters: GGO (12 of 14); reticular opacities (11 of 14); consolidation (5 of 6); and traction bronchiectasis (4 of 12). However, *complete* resolution of *all* radiographic abnormalities was never seen. When consolidation improved, it evolved into GGO mixed with variable degrees of reticulation. No patient developed HC at a mean follow-up of 27.6 months. A decrease in total area of increased opacities, GGO, or reticular opacities correlated with improvement in FVC. Although long-term data are sparse, we believe CT scans are invaluable to identify patterns that are amenable to therapy and monitor evolution of the disease.

3.4.2. Pulmonary function tests

PFTs in PM/DM-associated ILD reveal a restrictive pattern, with decreased lung volumes and DL_{CO} (Salmeron et al., 1981; Dickey and Myers, 1984; Lakhanpal et al., 1987; Schwarz, 1998; Grau et al., 1996; Cottin et al., 2003; Marie et al., 2002). In a recent study, severe reduction in DL_{CO} ($\leq$45% of predicted values) was associated with a heightened mortality (Marie et al., 2002). Airflow obstruction is not a feature of PM-ILD (Dickey and Myers, 1984; Grau et al., 1996). Arterial blood gases may demonstrate hypoxemia at rest, which worsens upon exertion (Duncan et al., 1974; Schwarz et al., 1976; Songcharoen et al., 1980; Dickey and Myers, 1984; Salmeron et al., 1981; Schwarz, 1992; Cottin et al., 2003). With CS and/or IS therapy, PFTs may improve (Arakawa et al., 2003). In one recent study, physiological improvement coincided with regression (on CT scan) of total lung opacities, reticular opacities, or GGO (Arakawa et al., 2003). In 13 patients, the total area of increased opacity (on CT) improved; the decrease in CT extent correlated inversely with changes in FVC ($r = -0.65$, $p = 0.03$). The decrease in GGO correlated inversely with changes in FVC ($r = 0.76$, $p = 0.012$) and DL_{CO} ($r = -0.67$, $p = 0.04$).

3.4.3. Histological features

Early reports of PM-associated ILD described varying degrees of interstitial lymphoplasmacytic and mononuclear inflammation and fibrosis (Salmeron et al., 1981; Takizawa et al., 1987; Lakhanpal et al., 1987; Tazelaar et al., 1990; Schwarz, 1992; Duncan et al., 1974). The distribution of lesions was often heterogeneous, with normal lung parenchyma interspersed with areas of pathology (Salmeron et al., 1981; Lakhanpal et al., 1987; Takizawa et al., 1987). Additional features cited included: hyperplasia of type II pneumocytes (Salmeron et al., 1981; Lakhanpal et al., 1987; Takizawa et al., 1987; Tazelaar et al., 1990); foamy macrophages (Salmeron et al., 1981; Takizawa et al., 1987; Lakhanpal et al., 1987); and germinal centers (Tazelaar et al., 1990).

More recent studies categorized PM-associated ILD according to histopathological patterns endorsed by recent International Consensus Statements of idiopathic interstitial pneumonias (IIPs) (American Thoracic Society, 2000, 2002) (Katzenstein and Myers, 1998). Although PM or DM may give rise to diverse histological patterns, NSIP is most common (comprising 45–82% of cases); BOOP, UIP, DAD, and lymphocytic interstitial pneumonia (LIP) may also be observed (Douglas et al., 2001; Marie et al., 2002; Cottin et al., 2003; Takizawa et al., 1987; Tazelaar et al., 1990) (see Table 3). Importantly, NSIP can occur in other CVDs (Cottin et al., 1998; Katzenstein and Fiorelli, 1994; Kim et al., 2002a; Bouros et al., 2002). In two recent series of patients with PSS who had SLBx, NSIP was observed in 62 of 80 (77%) (Bouros et al., 2002) and 13 of 19 patients (68%) (Kim et al., 2002a); only 7 and 26% of cases, respectively, exhibited UIP pattern. Histological features of NSIP complicating CVD are similar to idiopathic disease (Martinez et al., 2003). Defining features include: temporal homogeneity; diffuse involvement of alveolar walls with varying degrees of inflammation or fibrosis; preservation of the alveolar architecture; and minimal or no fibroblastic foci (Douglas et al., 2001; Martinez et al., 2003).

Since prospective studies assessing the prevalence of histological subtypes in PM-associated ILD are lacking, over-representation of NSIP or BOOP in published data could reflect a selection bias, since patients with HRCT features typical of UIP would be less likely to undergo SLBx.

Histological patterns also correlate with the clinical presentation and prognosis. Acute onset of lung disease suggests BOOP or DAD whereas an insidious onset usually reflects NSIP or UIP (Schwarz, 1998). Furthermore, the histologic patterns of BOOP or NSIP are far more responsive to treatment than the UIP pattern (Tazelaar et al., 1990; Schwarz, 1992; Clawson and Oddis, 1995; Grau et al., 1996; Douglas et al., 2001; Marie et al., 2002). The prognosis of DAD is variable, but may respond to IV pulse methylprednisolone (Lee et al., 2002; Marie et al., 2002).

3.4.4. Bronchoalveolar lavage

The use of bronchoalveolar lavage (BAL) in assessing severity and prognosis is controversial (Arsura and Greenberg, 1988; Marie et al., 2002). Both BAL lymphocytosis and neutrophilia have been described in DM/PM-associated ILD (Wallaert et al., 1986; Enomoto et al., 2003; Grau et al., 1996; Yamadori et al., 2001; Cottin et al., 2003; Marie et al., 2002). In one recent study of 14 patients with PM or DM and ILD, BAL revealed lymphocytosis (>25% lymphocytes) in seven (50%); neutrophilia (>10% neutrophils) in three (21%); mixed pattern in two (14%); and eosinophilia in one; BAL was normal in one patient (Cottin et al., 2003). Several groups noted

Table 3
Polymyositis-associated ILD: histological patterns

Reference (number of surgical lung biopsies)	Histological pattern number (percent)				
	NSIP	UIP	BOOP	DAD	LIP
Tazelaar et al. (1990) ($n = 15$)	1 (7%)	5 (33%)	6 (40%)	3 (20%)	0
Douglas et al. (2001) ($n = 22$)	18 (82%)	1 (4.5%)	1 (4.5%)	2 (9%)	0
Arakawa et al. (2003) ($n = 22$)	18 (82%)	2 (9%)	1 (4.5%)	1 (4.5%)	0
Cottin et al. (2003) ($n = 18$)	11 (65%)	2 (11%)	2 (11%)	0	1 (5%)
Marie et al. (2002) ($n = 11$)	4 (36%)	5 (45%)	2 (18%)	0	0

NSIP, nonspecific interstitial pneumonia; UIP, usual interstitial pneumonia; BOOP, bronchiolitis obliterans organizing pneumonia; DAD, diffuse alveolar damage; LIP, lymphocytic interstitial pneumonia.

elevated CD8 + cells and low CD4/CD8 ratios in PM-associated ILD (Sauty et al., 1997; Kourakata et al., 1999; Komocsi et al., 2001; Enomoto et al., 2003; Yamadori et al., 2001). BAL neutrophilia appears to predict a worse prognosis. In one recent study, BAL was performed in 20 patients with PM/DM-associated ILD; lymphocytosis was noted in seven (35%); neutrophilia in 13 (65%). Importantly, all nine patients whose ILD deteriorated manifested BAL neutrophilia; in contrast, among patients whose disease *improved or stabilized*, seven had lymphocytic alveolitis; four, neutrophilic alveolitis (Marie et al., 2002). In another study of 20 patients with PM-associated ILD, 10 worsened and 10 stabilized or improved (Schnabel et al., 2003). Median BAL neutrophil counts were higher (10.5%) in the cohort exhibiting disease progression (worsening) compared to the nonprogressive group (mean of 2.5%) ($p = 0.002$) (Schnabel et al., 2003). BAL neutrophilia was present in 8 of 10 patients whose disease worsened but in only 2 of 10 in the nonprogressive group. These data support previous studies in fibrosing alveolitis complicating other CVDs that BAL neutrophilia identifies a subset of patients who are more likely to deteriorate (Silver et al., 1990; Wallaert et al., 1986; White et al., 2000; Komocsi et al., 2001).

3.4.5. Laboratory tests

The likelihood of developing ILD does not correlate with the severity of muscular or cutaneous disease (Frazier and Miller, 1974; Dickey and Myers, 1984; Schwarz, 1992). Although one study noted that patients with high levels of CK, aldolase, and muscle necrosis had an increased risk for developing ILD (Songcharoen et al., 1980), several studies found no such relationship (Frazier and Miller, 1974; Schwarz et al., 1976; Hidano et al., 1992; Dickey and Myers, 1984; Grau et al., 1996; Marie et al., 1998; Yang et al., 2002). In fact, in one study, the incidence of ILD was higher (65%) in patients with normal CK levels at the onset of myositis compared to patients with elevated CK (20% incidence) (Nawata et al., 1999). Similarly, in another study, 77% of DM patients with normal CK levels developed ILD (Takizawa et al., 1987).

The presence of low CK in PM/DM has been associated with a worse outcome in ILD. In one study of PM/DM-associated ILD, 17 of 19 (89%) with high CK levels responded to CS compared to only 3 of 17 (18%) with normal CK levels (Nawata et al., 1999). One-year survival rates were 89 and 31%, respectively. Lee and colleagues reported five patients with fulminant DM–PM associated ILD (all died within 5 months of onset of symptoms); CK levels were normal in all five (Lee et al., 2002). Several reports affirm that DM patients with low CK levels have more rapidly progressive ILD (Fudman and Schnitzer, 1986; Takizawa et al., 1987, 1996; Yamanishi et al., 1999; Hirakata and Nagai, 2000; Sontheimer and Miyagawa, 2003; Kuroda et al., 2003; High et al., 2003). In addition, ILD associated with amyopathic DM (i.e. dermatomyositis sine myositis (Euwer and Sontheimer, 1994)) appears to have a worse prognosis (Sontheimer and Miyagawa, 2003).

3.4.6. Autoantibodies to t-RNA synthetases

Antibodies to a group of cellular enzymes, transfer RNA (tRNA) synthetases (anti-Jo1, anti-PL7, anti-PL12) (Marguerie et al., 1990), KJ (Targoff et al., 1989; Sauty et al., 1997; Targoff, 1994), or Mi-2 (Adams-Gandhi et al., 1996) are present in only 30% of PM/DM patients, but correlate *strongly* with the presence of ILD (Targoff, 1994; Schmidt et al., 2000). ILD is present in 75–100% of PM/DM patients with antibodies to these various tRNA synthetases but in only 3–37% of PM/DM patients *without* these antibodies (Marguerie et al., 1990; Targoff et al., 1989; Hirakata et al., 1992; Yoshida et al., 1983; Hochberg et al., 1984; Grau et al., 1996; Marie et al., 1998; Schnabel et al., 2003; Schmidt et al., 2000; Arnett et al., 1981). These auto-antibodies are rarely present in other CVDs (Marguerie et al., 1990; Targoff et al., 1989; Schnabel et al., 2003; Schmidt et al., 2000). In one study of 213 patients with scleroderma, anti-tRNA synthetase antibodies were never found (Vazquez-Abad and Rothfield, 1996). The most common of these auto-antibodies is directed against the Jo-1 antigen, a cytoplasmic histidyl-t-RNA synthetase (Marguerie et al., 1990; Bernstein et al., 1984; Hirakata and Nagai, 2000; Delbrel et al., 2001; Arnett et al., 1981; Yoshida et al., 1983; Hochberg et al., 1984; Schmidt et al., 2000). The presence of this circulating antibody is usually associated with a *clinical syndrome* characterized by ILD, polyarthritis, myositis, and additional cutaneous or vascular features (Schmidt et al., 2000; Targoff, 1994). Auto-antibodies directed at other cytoplasmic aminoacyl- or glycyl-tRNA synthetases (e.g. PL-7, PL-12, EJ, OJ), are associated with clinical features similar to the anti-Jo-1 syndrome (Targoff, 1990, 1994; Cottin et al., 2003; Marguerie et al., 1990), but in the aggregate are 5–6 times less common than anti-Jo-1 (Schmidt et al., 2000; Targoff, 1994; Hirakata et al., 1992).

Studies from Europe, the United States, and Japan affirmed a strong relationship between anti-Jo1 antibodies and ILD among patients with PM or DM (Bernstein et al., 1984; Yoshida et al., 1983; Hochberg et al., 1984; Grau et al., 1996; Marie et al., 1998; Schnabel et al., 2003). In one sentinel Japanese study, ILD was present on chest radiographs in all nine PM/DM patients with anti-Jo-1 antibodies but in only 5 of 23 patients (22%) lacking these antibodies (Yoshida et al., 1983). Similarly, a study in the United States cited ILD in 5 of 10 patients (50%) with anti-Jo-1 antibody but in only 5 of 34 (13%) anti-Jo-1 negative patients (Hochberg et al., 1984). In Europe, anti-Jo-1 antibodies were detected in 75% of PM/DM patients with ILD but in only 3 (Grau et al., 1996) and 12% (Schnabel et al., 2003) of PM/DM patients lacking these antibodies. Cases of rapidly progressive and treatment-refractory ILD may occur among anti-Jo-1 positive patients (Clawson and Oddis, 1995), but two retrospective studies of PM/DM patients *with ILD* noted similar long-term survival rates (Douglas et al., 2001) and clinical course (Marie et al., 2002) among anti-Jo-1 positive and anti-Jo-1 negative patients with ILD. Although ILD is the most common pulmonary feature observed in PM patients with anti-Jo-1 antibodies, anecdotal cases of organizing pneumonia (OP) (Chan et al., 1995), acute respiratory distress syndrome (ARDS) (Clawson and Oddis, 1995), and capillaritis with diffuse alveolar hemorrhage (Schwarz et al., 1995) have been described; these manifestations are rare.

The salient clinical and laboratory features of anti-Jo-1 syndrome were detailed in a comprehensive review of 231 patients with anti-Jo1 antibodies gleaned from 46 publications (Schmidt et al., 2000) (Table 4). Concomitant laboratory features included: elevated erythrocyte sedimentation rate (ESR) (77%); elevated C-reactive protein (CRP) (73%); antinuclear antibody (ANA) (36%); and rheumatoid factor (RF) (27%). Importantly, the following auto-antibodies were rarely evident (0–5%): anti-centromere, anti-U1-RNP; anti-La; anti-double-stranding (ds) DNA, antinuclear cytoplasmic antibody (ANCA) (Table 5). Anti-SCL-70 was never found (Schmidt et al., 2000). Similarly, in two series comprising 58 patients with anti-tRNA syntetases (including 44 with anti-Jo-1 antibodies), anti-SCL-70 was never found; anti-La, anti-U1-RNP, anti-centromere, anti-DNA, and anti-Sm antibodies were detected in 4–11% (Love et al., 1991; Hausmanowa-Petrusewicz et al., 1997).

Although not specific for DM/PM, other serum markers may be biomarkers of ILD. KL-6 is a mucinous glycoprotein present in the circulation and on alveolar type II pneumocytes (Ohnishi et al., 2002). Elevated levels of serum KL-6 have been noted in CVD-associated ILD, hypersensitivity pneumonia, and idiopathic interstitial pneumonias

Table 4
Clinical features of anti-Jo-1 syndrome (adapted from Schmidt et al., 2000)

Clinical features (231 patients)	Percent
Myositis	91
Interstitial lung disease	75
Arthritis	74
Raynaud's phenomenon	50
Sicca syndrome	34
Sclerodactyly	26
Dermatomyositis	22
Mechanic's hands	21
Telangiectasia	18

Table 5
Laboratory features of anti-Jo-1 syndrome (adapted from Schmidt et al., 2000)

Clinical features (231 patients)	Number of patients/percent
Elevated ESR	57 of 74 (77%)
Elevated C-reactive protein (CRP)	46 of 63 (73%)
Antinuclear antibody (ANA)	41 of 114 (36%)
Anti-Ro	7 of 89 (8%)
Anti-U1-RNP	4 of 88 (5%)
Anti-La	1 of 31 (3%)
Anti-double stranded DNA	2 of 71 (2%)
Anti-SCL-70	0 of 26 (0%)
ANCA	0 of 26 (0%)

compared to patients without ILD (Kobayashi and Kitamura, 1995; Nakajima et al., 2000; Ohnishi et al., 2002). Furthermore, serum levels may correlate with disease activity (Kobayashi and Kitamura, 1995; Nakajima et al., 2000; Ohnishi et al., 2002) These findings also extend to patients with ILD complicating PM/DM (Bandoh et al., 2000; Kubo et al., 2000). High serum levels of surfactant protein-D are also associated with various ILDs (Honda et al., 1995; Takahashi et al., 2000a,b; Ohnishi et al., 2002) but sensitivity and diagnostic accuracy is less than KL-6 (Ohnishi et al., 2002). Like KL-6, SP-D appears to be a marker for PM/DM-associated ILD (Ihn et al., 2002).

3.4.7. Differential diagnosis

Pulmonary infiltrates in the setting of *treated* patients with PM or DM can reflect opportunistic infections or even drug-induced pulmonary toxicity. Both methotrexate (MTX) and cyclophosphamide (CP) can cause lung injury. Methotrexate-induced pneumonitis occurs in 0.5–14% of patients receiving low doses of the medication (Zisman et al., 2001). Methotrexate most commonly causes hypersensitivity pneumonia with dry cough, fever, dyspnea, and peripheral eosinophilia (Lynch and McCune, 1997; Zisman et al., 2001). The toxic effects of MTX on the lung can occur at any time during the course of therapy, at any dose, and with any route of administration. Treatment includes stopping MTX and, in severe cases, initiating CS therapy.

Cyclophosphamide-induced lung toxicity is characterized by either acute pneumonitis or chronic, progressive pulmonary fibrosis (Lynch and McCune, 1997; Malik et al., 1996). The acute form usually occurs within the first 6 months of treatment, while the chronic fibrosing pneumonitis occurs with long-term use (Malik et al., 1996). The diagnosis may go unrecognized for years after cessation of the drug. Acute pneumonitis usually improves with CS therapy, but the chronic pattern generally is progressive and often fatal (Malik et al., 1996). Fortunately, CP-induced pneumonitis is rare in the absence of other possible risk factors, such as radiation therapy and concurrent use of cytotoxic agents (e.g. bleomycin).

3.4.8. Treatment

Optimal treatment for PM-associated ILD has not been elucidated, as randomized, controlled therapeutic trials have not been done. As has been discussed, the clinical course and prognosis of PM-associated ILD is heterogeneous, and treatment needs to be individualized. Nonetheless, ILD is a serious and potentially fatal complication of PM/DM. In two separate retrospective surveys of dermatologic institutions in Japan, fatality rates among patients with DM-associated ILD were 45 and 42% (Hidano et al., 1986, 1992). Similarly, retrospective studies in the USA and France cited 5-year mortality rates exceeding 40% (Arsura and Greenberg, 1988; Douglas et al., 2001; Marie et al., 2002). The presence of ILD complicating PM/DM was associated with heightened mortality in some (Lakhanpal et al., 1987; Arsura and Greenberg, 1988; Cottin et al., 2003), but not all (Marie et al., 2002; Grau et al., 1996), studies. Survival depends upon the underlying lung histology in PM/DM-associated ILD; the prognosis of UIP pattern is worse than NSIP (Arakawa et al., 2003; Clawson and Oddis, 1995; Grau et al., 1996; Douglas et al., 2001; Marie et al., 2002) or BOOP (Tazelaar et al., 1990) patterns.

The decision to treat PM-associated ILD depends upon numerous factors including the acuity and severity of the disease, extent of pulmonary dysfunction, type and extent of aberrations on HRCT, and presence or absence of contraindications to CS or IS therapy. For patients requiring treatment, most authors consider CS as the preferred initial therapy (DeVere and Bradley, 1975; Caproni et al., 2002; Frazier and Miller, 1974; Duncan et al., 1974; Schwarz et al., 1976; Salmeron et al., 1981; Saito et al., 2002; Tazelaar et al., 1990; Nawata et al., 1999). Optimal dose and duration have not been studied in randomized trials, but initial therapy with oral prednisone 0.75–1.0 mg/kg per day (or equivalent), with gradual taper is reasonable. For more severe or fulminant disease, high-dose IV methylprednisolone (1.0 gm daily for 3 days) may be administered (Hirakata and Nagai, 2000; Oddis, 2000; Sauty et al., 1997; Nawata et al., 1999). Patients failing CS or experiencing adverse effects from CS should be treated with IS or cytotoxic agents (Douglas et al., 2001; Yamadori et al., 2001; Cottin et al., 2003;

Marie et al., 2002). Although data are limited to small series and case reports, responses have been noted with: cyclophosphamide (CP) (IV or oral) (al-Janadi et al., 1989; Marie et al., 1998, 2002; Schnabel et al., 1998; Knoell et al., 1999; Yoshida et al., 1999; Tanaka et al., 2000; Sugisaki et al., 2002; Mok et al., 2003; Maccioni and Colebatch, 1990; Shinohara et al., 1997); azathioprine (AZA) (Rowen and Reichel, 1983; Sauty et al., 1997; Marie et al., 1998, 2002; Mok et al., 2003; Grau et al., 1996), methotrexate (MTX) (Chang and Lee, 2003; Itoh et al., 1999; Songcharoen et al., 1980), cyclosporin A (CsA) (Gruhn and Diaz-Buxo, 1987; Sauty et al., 1997; Stedeford and Wordsworth, 1991; Mehregan and Su, 1993; Maeda et al., 1997; Nawata et al., 1999; Sugisaki et al., 2002; Miyake et al., 2002; Kuroda et al., 2003), and tacrolimus (Oddis et al., 1999), even in patients failing CS.

Early reports suggested a relatively poor prognosis and response to therapy among patients with PM-associated ILD (Lynch and Hunninghake, 1992; Arsura and Greenberg, 1988; Hidano et al., 1986, 1992), but recent studies suggest the prognosis is favorable provided treatment is initiated early (Cottin et al., 2003; Arakawa et al., 2003; Mino et al., 1997; Nawata et al., 1999). In two studies evaluating serial CT scans in PM-associated ILD, short-term improvement was noted with medical therapy in 16 of 17 (94%) (Mino et al., 1997) and 13 of 14 (93%) patients, respectively (Arakawa et al., 2003). In another study, favorable responses were achieved with CS in 20 of 36 (56%) patients with PM-associated ILD; however, responses were much lower (3 of 17 (18%) among patients with normal CK levels) (Nawata et al., 1999). Investigators from the Mayo Clinic retrospectively reviewed 70 patients with PM/DM and ILD (Douglas et al., 2001). Initial treatment included CS in 67 patients (96%); additional agents were added when response to CS was suboptimal. The most commonly employed IS agents included: AZA ($n = 25$); MTX ($n = 14$); hydroxychloroquine ($n = 10$); CP ($n = 7$); CsA ($n = 3$). Efficacy of individual treatment regimens was not analyzed. Among 58 patients diagnosed after 1989, 3- and 5-year survival rates were 74 and 60%, respectively (Douglas et al., 2001). French investigators described clinical outcomes in 17 patients with PM-associated ILD treated with various regimens (CS ($n = 16$); IS ($n = 12$); IV polyclonal gamma-globulins ($n = 5$); plasma exchange ($n = 1$) (Cottin et al., 2003). The pulmonary disease improved in 11 (complete in two), but five relapses occurred in three patients with taper or discontinuation of therapy. At long-term follow-up, 12 patients were alive; five died of respiratory failure (at a mean of 3.5 years following SLBx); one patient underwent transplantation. One-, two- and five-year survival rates were 100, 93, and 50%, respectively. Importantly, the outcome of the muscle disease was not always concordant with the pulmonary process. Marie et al. retrospectively evaluated 36 patients with PM/DM and ILD (Marie et al., 2002). All patients received CS; half of the patients also received CP ($n = 10$) or AZA ($n = 8$). During a median follow-up of 53 months, ILD resolved completely in 27 (75%) (partial in 20; complete in 7) and worsened in 9 (25%) (Marie et al., 2002). Survival rates at 3- and 5-years were 90 and 86.5%, respectively (Marie et al., 2002). In another recent study, 14 patients with NSIP complicating PM were treated with CS *combined with* IS (Arakawa et al., 2003). One patient died of respiratory failure; the remaining 13 patients improved (by CT or PFT parameters). In one study, 12 patients with PM/DM and NSIP were treated with pulse methylprednisolone (followed by a CS taper) *plus* pulse CP (once weekly × 3 weeks) (Yamadori et al., 2001). All 12 'improved' but no additional data were provided. Favorable responses have been noted with the calcineurin inhibitors, cyclosporin A (CsA) or tacrolimus. In one study, five of five patients with CS-recalcitrant ILD responded to CsA (Nawata et al., 1999). In another study, three patients with CS-recalcitrant NSIP complicating PM responded to a combination of CsA *plus* AZA (Sauty et al., 1997).

4. What is the role of lung biopsy in patients with PM-associated ILD?

Management and treatment of ILD in the setting of PM/DM is complex and should be individualized. For patients with mild disease or an indolent course, we recommend baseline studies to include PFTs and HRCT. Invasive studies (e.g. flexible fiberoptic bronchoscopy (FFB) with BAL and transbronchial lung biopsies (TBBs) or surgical lung biopsy) are reserved for selected patients. We perform FFB with BAL and TBBs in PM/DM patients with new-onset pulmonary infiltrates, particularly when the disease is focal or consolidation is present. When bronchoscopic findings are not definitive, SLBx should be considered. Histological confirmation is mandatory when an infectious process is suspected (e.g. when fever, sweats or chills are present), particularly when patients have received CS or IS therapy. Bronchoscopy with appropriate cultures and biopsies may establish a diagnosis of BOOP or infection in some patients, but cannot unequivocally diagnose other IIPs such as NSIP or UIP. Surgical lung biopsy often provides a definitive diagnosis, but its role to diagnose PM-associated ILD is controversial. Histological findings on SLBx are prognostically useful (i.e. discriminating BOOP, NSIP, UIP, etc.), but may have minimal impact on treatment. Further, SLBx is associated with potential morbidity and (rarely) mortality (Tazelaar et al., 1990). For these reasons, indications for SLBx should be circumscribed. We see little role for SLBx in previously untreated patients with classic DM/PM, positive anti-Jo-1 antibody, reticular (interstitial) infiltrates, and an indolent course. In this context, empirical treatment with CS is reasonable after obtaining appropriate baseline studies (e.g. PFTs, serologies, or HRCT scan) (Duncan et al., 1974; Schwarz, 1992). Conversely, the development of focal pulmonary infiltrates in PM or DM patients on high dose CS or IS therapy could reflect opportunistic infection. In this setting, an invasive approach, employing FFB or video-assisted thoracoscopic surgical lung biopsy (VATS), is advised.

When infection has been definitely excluded, treatment with high dose CS is warranted, particularly for patients with a subacute course or severe disease. However, not all PM patients with ILD should be treated, particularly when surrogate markers of inflammation are lacking. Findings on HRCT scan may be invaluable to identify best or worst candidates for treatment. Extensive GGO on CT suggests the presence of an active inflammatory alveolitis, and warrants prompt treatment with CS and/or IS agents (provided infection has been excluded). By contrast, the presence of a *pure* reticular pattern or HC and no GGO suggests a low likelihood of responsiveness to therapy. In this context, aggressive treatment is usually ill advised. In this context, particularly among patients with mild to moderate symptoms and an indolent course, treatment may be withheld pending an observation period (weeks to months). Serial PFTs and CT scans should be performed to monitor the course of the disease. When the disease progresses (worsens), aggressive treatment with CS and/or IS agents should be considered.

As we have discussed, optimal therapy of DM-associated ILD has not been investigated in controlled, randomized trials. Unless specific contraindications to CS exist, we initiate treatment with CS and assess response clinically and by PFTs. Patients failing or experiencing adverse effects from CS are treated with IS agents. In this setting, oral AZA or MTX are first-line agents for in less severe cases. We reserve CP (IV or oral) for patients failing AZA or MTX or with life-threatening disease. Calcineurin inhibitors (e.g. cyclosporin A or tacrolimus) are reserved for patients failing CS and/or additional IS agents.

Key points

- ILD can complicate PM or DM at any point in the disease, and is associated with significant potential morbidity and mortality.
- Predominant physiological aberrations of PM-associated ILD include a restrictive ventilatory defect, impaired gas transfer and impaired oxygenation.
- Respiratory failure due to neuromuscular weakness can also give rise to a restrictive ventilatory defect and hypoxemia and needs to be excluded.
- The clinical presentation and course of PM-associated ILD is variable, and in part depends upon underlying the histological pattern (assessed by surgical lung biopsy).
- NSIP is the most common histological pattern observed in patients with ILD complicating PM or DM, but other patterns can be seen.
- Surgical lung biopsy may be important to exclude opportunistic infections and establish a precise histological diagnosis, but is not always essential provided other features are characteristic.

- The course and evolution of ILD is not necessarily concordant with the extent and activity of muscular or systemic components.
- High resolution thin-section computed tomographic scans are useful to identify the nature and extent of disease and assess a predominant pattern.
- Auto-antibodies to transfer RNA synthetases (particularly anti-Jo-1) are a marker for ILD in patients with PM or DM, and are associated with a characteristic syndrome displaying myositis, ILD, polyarthritis, and diverse cutaneous and vascular features.
- Optimal treatment of PM-associated ILD has not been well defined, as randomized, controlled therapeutic trials have not been performed. However, corticosteroids, alone or combined with immunosuppressive agents, are usually efficacious if initiated early.

References

Adams-Gandhi, L.B., Boyd, A.S., King, L.E. Jr. 1996. Diagnosis and management of dermatomyositis. Compr. Ther. 22, 156–164.

Akira, M., Hara, H., Sakatani, M. 1999. Interstitial lung disease in association with polymyositis–dermatomyositis: long-term follow-up CT evaluation in seven patients. Radiology 210, 333–338.

al-Janadi, M., Smith, C.D., Karsh, J. 1989. Cyclophosphamide treatment of interstitial pulmonary fibrosis in polymyositis/dermatomyositis. J. Rheumatol. 16, 1592–1596.

American Thoracic Society (ATS), 2000. American Thoracic Society. Idiopathic pulmonary fibrosis: diagnosis and treatment. International consensus statement. Am. J. Respir. Crit. Care Med. 161, 646–664.

American Thoracic Society (ATS), 2002. American Thoracic Society/European Respiratory Society International Multidisciplinary Consensus Classification of the Idiopathic Interstitial Pneumonias. This joint statement of the American Thoracic Society (ATS), and the European Respiratory Society (ERS) was adopted by the ATS board of directors, June 2001 and by the ERS Executive Committee, June 2001. Am. J. Respir. Crit. Care Med. 165, 277–304.

Arakawa, H., Yamada, H., Kurihara, Y., Nakajima, Y., Takeda, A., Fukushima, Y., Fujioka, M. 2003. Nonspecific interstitial pneumonia associated with polymyositis and dermatomyositis: serial high-resolution CT findings and functional correlation. Chest 123, 1096–1103.

Arnett, F.C., Hirsch, T.J., Bias, W.B., Nishikai, M., Reichlin, M. 1981. The Jo-1 antibody system in myositis: relationships to clinical features and HLA. J. Rheumatol. 8, 925–930.

Arsura, E.L., Greenberg, A.S. 1988. Adverse impact of interstitial pulmonary fibrosis on prognosis in polymyositis and dermatomyositis. Semin. Arthritis Rheum. 18, 29–37.

Astudillo, L.M., Carreiro, M., Sailler, L., Dingremont, C.F., Arlet, P.M. 2001. Hypercapnic coma due to diaphragmatic involvement in a patient with dermatomyositis. Clin. Exp. Rheumatol. 19, 456–458.

Bandoh, S., Fujita, J., Ohtsuki, Y., Ueda, Y., Hojo, S., Tokuda, M., Dobashi, H., Kurata, N., Yoshinouchi, T., Kohno, N., Takahara, J. 2000. Sequential changes of KL-6 in sera of patients with interstitial pneumonia associated with polymyositis/dermatomyositis. Ann. Rheum. Dis. 59, 257–262.

Baumann, M.H. 1999. The lung in polymyositis and dermatomyositis. Semin. Respir. Crit. Care Med. 20, 131–138.

Benbassat, J., Gefel, D., Larholt, K., Sukenik, S., Morgenstern, V., Zlotnick, A. 1985. Prognostic factors in polymyositis/dermatomyositis. A computer-assisted analysis of ninety-two cases. Arthritis Rheum. 28, 249–255.

Bernstein, R.M., Morgan, S.H., Chapman, J., Bunn, C.C., Mathews, M.B., Turner-Warwick, M., Hughes, G.R. 1984. Anti-Jo-1 antibody: a marker for myositis with interstitial lung disease. Br. Med. J. (Clin. Res. Ed.) 289, 151–152.

Blumbergs, P.C., Byrne, E., Kakulas, B.A. 1984. Polymyositis presenting with respiratory failure. J. Neurol. Sci. 65, 221–229.

Bohan, A., Peter, J.B. 1975. Polymyositis and dermatomyositis (first of two parts). N. Engl. J. Med. 292, 344–347.

Bohan, A., Peter, J.B., Bowman, R.L., Pearson, C.M. 1977. Computer-assisted analysis of 153 patients with polymyositis and dermatomyositis. Medicine (Baltimore) 56, 255–286.

Bouros, D., Wells, A.U., Nicholson, A.G., Colby, T.V., Polychronopoulos, V., Pantelidis, P., Haslam, P.L., Vassilakis, D.A., Black, C.M., du Bois, R.M. 2002. Histopathologic subsets of fibrosing alveolitis in patients with systemic sclerosis and their relationship to outcome. Am. J. Respir. Crit. Care Med. 165, 1581–1586.

Braun, N.M., Arora, N.S., Rochester, D.F. 1983. Respiratory muscle and pulmonary function in polymyositis and other proximal myopathies. Thorax 38, 616–623.

Bunch, T.W., Worthington, J.W., Combs, J.J., Ilstrup, D.M., Engel, A.G. 1980. Azathioprine with prednisone for polymyositis. A controlled, clinical trial. Ann. Intern. Med. 92, 365–369.

Caproni, M., Cardinali, C., Parodi, A., Giomi, B., Papini, M., Vaccaro, M., Marzano, A., De Simone, C., Fazio, M., Rebora, A., Fabbri, P. 2002. Amyopathic dermatomyositis: a review by the Italian Group of Immunodermatology. Arch. Dermatol. 138, 23–27.

Chan, W.M., Ip, M., Lau, C.S., Wang, E., Peh, W.C. 1995. Anti-Jo-1 syndrome presenting as cryptogenic organizing pneumonia. Respir. Med. 89, 639–641.

Chang, H.K., Lee, D.H. 2003. Successful combination therapy of cyclosporine and methotrexate for refractory polymyositis with anti-jo-1 antibody: a case report. J. Korean Med. Sci. 18, 131–134.

Clawson, K., Oddis, C.V. 1995. Adult respiratory distress syndrome in polymyositis patients with the anti-Jo-1 antibody. Arthritis Rheum. 38, 1519–1523.

Cottin, V., Donsbeck, A.V., Revel, D., Loire, R., Cordier, J.F. 1998. Nonspecific interstitial pneumonia. Individualization of a clinicopathologic entity in a series of 12 patients. Am. J. Respir. Crit. Care Med. 158, 1286–1293.

Cottin, V., Thivolet-Bejul, F., Reynaud-Gaubert, M., Cadranel, J., Delaval, P., Ternamian, P.-J., Cordier, J.-F. 2003. Interstitial lung disease in amyopathic dermatomyositis, dermatomyositis, and polymyositis. Eur. Respir. J. 22, 245–250.

Cronin, M.E., Plotz, P.H. 1990. Idiopathic inflammatory myopathies. Rheum. Dis. Clin. North Am. 16, 655–665.

Dalakas, M.C. 1991. Polymyositis, dermatomyositis and inclusion-body myositis. N. Engl. J. Med. 325, 1487–1498.

Delbrel, X., Schaeverbeke, T., Lifermann, F., Dehais, J. 2001. Arthropathy associated with anti-Jo-1 antibody. Joint Bone Spine 68, 166–169.

DePalo, V., McCool, F. 2002. Respiratory muscle evaluation of the patient with neuromuscular disease. Semin. Respir. Crit. Care Med. 23, 201–209.

DeVere, R., Bradley, W.G. 1975. Polymyositis: its presentation, morbidity and mortality. Brain 98, 637–666.

Dickey, B.F., Myers, A.R. 1984. Pulmonary disease in polymyositis/dermatomyositis. Semin. Arthritis Rheum. 14, 60–76.

Douglas, W.W., Tazelaar, H.D., Hartman, T.E., Hartman, R.P., Decker, P.A., Schroeder, D.R., Ryu, J.H. 2001. Polymyositis–dermatomyositis-associated interstitial lung disease. Am. J. Respir. Crit. Care Med. 164, 1182–1185.

Duncan, P.E., Griffin, J.P., Garcia, A., Kaplan, S.B. 1974. Fibrosing alveolitis in polymyositis. A review of histologically confirmed cases. Am. J. Med. 57, 621–626.

el-Azhary, R.A., Pakzad, S.Y. 2002. Amyopathic dermatomyositis: retrospective review of 37 cases. J. Am. Acad. Dermatol. 46, 560–565.

Ellis, S.M., Hansell, D.M. 2002. Idiopathic interstitial pneumonias: imaging–pathology correlation. Eur. Radiol. 12, 610–626.

Enomoto, K., Takada, T., Suzuki, E., Ishida, T., Moriyama, H., Ooi, H., Hasegawa, T., Tsukada, H., Nakano, M., Gejyo, F. 2003. Bronchoalveolar lavage fluid cells in mixed connective tissue disease. Respirology 8, 149–156.

Euwer, R.L., Sontheimer, R.D. 1994. Dermatologic aspects of myositis. Curr. Opin. Rheumatol. 6, 583–589.

Frazier, A.R., Miller, R.D. 1974. Interstitial pneumonitis in association with polymyositis and dermatomyositis. Chest 65, 403–407.

Fudman, E.J., Schnitzer, T.J. 1986. Dermatomyositis without creatine kinase elevation. A poor prognostic sign. Am. J. Med. 80, 329–332.

Fujita, J., Tokuda, M., Bandoh, S., Yang, Y., Fukunaga, Y., Hojo, S., Ueda, Y., Dobashi, N., Dohmoto, K., Ishida, T., Takahara, J. 2001. Primary lung cancer associated with polymyositis/dermatomyositis, with a review of the literature. Rheumatol. Int. 20, 81–84.

Gilchrist, J. 2002. Overview of neuromuscular disorders affected respiratory function. Semin. Respir. Crit. Care Med. 23, 191–200.

Grathwohl, K.W., Thompson, J.W., Riordan, K.K., Roth, B.J., Dillard, T.A. 1995. Digital clubbing associated with polymyositis and interstitial lung disease. Chest 108, 1751–1752.

Grau, J.M., Miro, O., Pedrol, E., Casademont, J., Masanes, F., Herrero, C., Haussman, G., Urbano-Marquez, A. 1996. Interstitial lung disease related to dermatomyositis. Comparative study with patients without lung involvement. J. Rheumatol. 23, 1921–1926.

Gruhn, W.B., Diaz-Buxo, J.A. 1987. Cyclosporine treatment of steroid resistant interstitial pneumonitis associated with dermatomyositis/polymyositis. J. Rheumatol. 14, 1045–1047.

Hausmanowa-Petrusewicz, I., Kowalska-Oledzka, E., Miller, F.W., Jarzabek-Chorzelska, M., Targoff, I.N., Blaszczyk-Kostanecka, M., Jablonska, S. 1997. Clinical, serologic, and immunogenetic features in Polish patients with idiopathic inflammatory myopathies. Arthritis Rheum. 40, 1257–1266.

Hidano, A., Kaneko, K., Arai, Y., Kikuchi, R. 1986. Survey of the prognosis for dermatomyositis, with special reference to its association with malignancy and pulmonary fibrosis. J. Dermatol. 13, 233–241.

Hidano, A., Torikai, S., Uemura, T., Shimizu, S. 1992. Malignancy and interstitial pneumonitis as fatal complications in dermatomyositis. J. Dermatol. 19, 153–160.

High, W.A., Cohen, J.B., Murphy, B.A., Costner, M.I. 2003. Fatal interstitial pulmonary fibrosis in anti-Jo-1-negative amyopathic dermatomyositis. J. Am. Acad. Dermatol. 49, 295–298.

Hirakata, M., Nagai, S. 2000. Interstitial lung disease in polymyositis and dermatomyositis. Curr. Opin. Rheumatol. 12, 501–508.

Hirakata, M., Mimori, T., Akizuki, M., Craft, J., Hardin, J.A., Homma, M. 1992. Autoantibodies to small nuclear and cytoplasmic ribonucleoproteins in Japanese patients with inflammatory muscle disease. Arthritis Rheum. 35, 449–456.

Hochberg, M.C., Feldman, D., Stevens, M.B., Arnett, F.C., Reichlin, M. 1984. Antibody to Jo-1 in polymyositis/dermatomyositis: association with interstitial pulmonary disease. J. Rheumatol. 11, 663–665.

Hochberg, M.C., Feldman, D., Stevens, M.B. 1986. Adult onset polymyositis/dermatomyositis: an analysis of clinical and laboratory features and survival in 76 patients with a review of the literature. Semin. Arthritis Rheum. 15, 168–178.

Honda, Y., Kuroki, Y., Matsuura, E., Nagae, H., Takahashi, H., Akino, T., Abe, S. 1995. Pulmonary surfactant protein D in sera and bronchoalveolar lavage fluids. Am. J. Respir. Crit. Care Med. 152, 1860–1866.

Ihn, H., Asano, Y., Kubo, M., Yamane, K., Jinnin, M., Yazawa, N., Fujimoto, M., Tamaki, K. 2002. Clinical significance of serum surfactant protein D (SP-D) in patients with polymyositis/dermatomyositis: correlation with interstitial lung disease. Rheumatology (Oxford) 41, 1268–1272.

Ikezoe, J., Johkoh, T., Kohno, N., Takeuchi, N., Ichikado, K., Nakamura, H. 1996. High-resolution CT findings of lung disease in patients with polymyositis and dermatomyositis. J. Thorac. Imaging 11, 250–259.

Itoh, T., Mitsuoka, S., Uji, M., Matsushita, H. 1999. Successful combination chemotherapy with low-dose methotrexate and steroids for dermatomyositis complicated by interstitial pneumonitis. Nihon Kokyuki Gakkai Zasshi 37, 636–640.

Katzenstein, A.L., Fiorelli, R.F. 1994. Nonspecific interstitial pneumonia/fibrosis. Histologic features and clinical significance. Am. J. Surg. Pathol. 18, 136–147.

Katzenstein, A.L., Myers, J.L. 1998. Idiopathic pulmonary fibrosis: clinical relevance of pathologic classification. Am. J. Respir. Crit. Care Med. 157, 1301–1315.

Kim, D.S., Yoo, B., Lee, J.S., Kim, E.K., Lim, C.M., Lee, S.D., Koh, Y., Kim, W.S., Kim, W.D., Colby, T.V., Kitiaichi, M. 2002a. The major histopathologic pattern of pulmonary fibrosis in scleroderma is nonspecific interstitial pneumonia. Sarcoidosis Vasc. Diffuse Lung Dis. 19, 121–127.

Kim, E.A., Lee, K.S., Johkoh, T., Kim, T.S., Suh, G.Y., Kwon, O.J., Han, J. 2002b. Interstitial lung diseases associated with collagen vascular diseases: radiologic and histopathologic findings. Radiographics 22, S151–S165.

Knoell, K.A., Hook, M., Grice, D.P., Hendrix, J.D. Jr. 1999. Dermatomyositis associated with bronchiolitis obliterans organizing pneumonia (BOOP). J. Am. Acad. Dermatol. 40, 328–330.

Kobayashi, J., Kitamura, S. 1995. KL-6: a serum marker for interstitial pneumonia. Chest 108, 311–315.

Komocsi, A., Kumanovics, G., Zibotics, H., Czirjak, L. 2001. Alveolitis may persist during treatment that sufficiently controls muscle inflammation in myositis. Rheumatol. Int. 20, 113–118.

Kourakata, H., Takada, T., Suzuki, E., Enomoto, K., Saito, I., Taguchi, Y., Tsukada, H., Nakano, M., Arakawa, M. 1999. Flowcytometric analysis of bronchoalveolar lavage fluid cells in polymyositis/dermatomyositis with interstitial pneumonia. Respirology 4, 223–228.

Krain, L. 1975. Dermatomyositis in six patients without initial muscle involvement. Arch. Dermatol. 111, 241–245.

Kubo, M., Ihn, H., Yamane, K., Kikuchi, K., Yazawa, N., Soma, Y., Tamaki, K. 2000. Serum KL-6 in adult patients with polymyositis and dermatomyositis. Rheumatology (Oxford) 39, 632–636.

Kuroda, T., Morikawa, H., Satou, T., Tanabe, Y., Murakami, S., Ito, S., Nakan, M., Gejyo, F. 2003. A case of dermatomyositis complicated with pneumomediastinum successfully treated with cyclosporin A. Clin. Rheumatol. 22, 45–48.

Lakhanpal, S., Lie, J.T., Conn, D.L., Martin, W.J. 2nd 1987. Pulmonary disease in polymyositis/dermatomyositis: a clinicopathological analysis of 65 autopsy cases. Ann. Rheum. Dis. 46, 23–29.

Lee, C.S., Chen, T.L., Tzen, C.Y., Lin, F.J., Peng, M.J., Wu, C.L., Chen, P.J. 2002. Idiopathic inflammatory myopathy with diffuse alveolar damage. Clin. Rheumatol. 21, 391–396.

Love, L.A., Leff, R.L., Fraser, D.D., Targoff, I.N., Dalakas, M., Plotz, P.H., Miller, F.W. 1991. A new approach to the classification of idiopathic inflammatory myopathy: myositis-specific autoantibodies define useful homogeneous patient groups. Medicine (Baltimore) 70, 360–374.

Lynch, J.P. 3rd, Chavis, A. 1992. Chronic interstitial pulmonary disorders. In: L. Victor (Ed.), Clinical Pulmonary Medicine. Little Brown, Boston, MA, pp. 193–264.

Lynch, J.P. 3rd, Hunninghake, G.W. 1992. Pulmonary complications of collagen vascular disease. Annu. Rev. Med. 43, 17–35.

Lynch, J.P. 3rd, McCune, W.J. 1997. Immunosuppressive and cytotoxic pharmacotherapy for pulmonary disorders. Am. J. Respir. Crit. Care Med. 155, 395–420.

Lynch, J.P. 3rd, Orens, J., Kazerooni, E. 1999. Collagen vascular disease. In: M. Sperber (Ed.), Diffuse Lung Disorders: A Comprehensive Clinical–Radiological Overview. Springer, London.

Maccioni, F.J., Colebatch, H.J. 1990. Management of fibrosing alveolitis with polymyositis dermatomyositis. Aust. NZ J. Med. 20, 806–810.

Maeda, K., Kimura, R., Komuta, K., Igarashi, T. 1997. Cyclosporine treatment for polymyositis/dermatomyositis: is it possible to rescue the deteriorating cases with interstitial pneumonitis? Scand. J. Rheumatol. 26, 24–29.

Malik, S.W., Myers, J.L., DeRemee, R.A., Specks, U. 1996. Lung toxicity associated with cyclophosphamide use. Two distinct patterns. Am. J. Respir. Crit. Care Med. 154, 1851–1856.

Manchul, L.A., Jin, A., Pritchard, K.I., Tenenbaum, J., Boyd, N.F., Lee, P., Germanson, T., Gordon, D.A. 1985. The frequency of malignant neoplasms in patients with polymyositis–dermatomyositis. A controlled study. Arch. Intern. Med. 145, 1835–1839.

Marguerie, C., Bunn, C.C., Beynon, H.L., Bernstein, R.M., Hughes, J.M., So, A.K., Walport, M.J. 1990. Polymyositis, pulmonary fibrosis and autoantibodies to aminoacyl-tRNA synthetase enzymes. Q. J. Med. 77, 1019–1038.

Marie, I., Hatron, P.Y., Hachulla, E., Wallaert, B., Michon-Pasturel, U., Devulder, B. 1998. Pulmonary involvement in polymyositis and in dermatomyositis. J. Rheumatol. 25, 1336–1343.

Marie, I., Hachulla, E., Hatron, P.Y., Hellot, M.F., Levesque, H., Devulder, B., Courtois, H. 2001. Polymyositis and dermatomyositis: short term and longterm outcome, and predictive factors of prognosis. J. Rheumatol. 28, 2230–2237.

Marie, I., Hachulla, E., Cherin, P., Dominique, S., Hatron, P.Y., Hellot, M.F., Devulder, B., Herson, S., Levesque, H., Courtois, H. 2002. Interstitial lung disease in polymyositis and dermatomyositis. Arthritis Rheum. 47, 614–622.

Martinez, F., Flaherty, K., Travis, W., Lynch, J.P. 3rd 2003. Nonspecific interstitial pneumonia. In: J.P. Lynch, III (Ed.), Idiopathic Pulmonary Fibrosis. Marcel Dekker, New York, pp. 101–136.

Medsger, T.A. Jr., Robinson, H., Masi, A.T. 1971. Factors affecting survivorship in polymyositis. A life-table study of 124 patients. Arthritis Rheum. 14, 249–258.

Mehregan, D.R., Su, W.P. 1993. Cyclosporine treatment for dermatomyositis/polymyositis. Cutis 51, 59–61.

Mino, M., Noma, S., Taguchi, Y., Tomii, K., Kohri, Y., Oida, K. 1997. Pulmonary involvement in polymyositis and dermatomyositis: sequential evaluation with CT. AJR Am. J. Roentgenol. 169, 83–87.

Miyake, S., Ohtani, Y., Sawada, M., Inase, N., Miyazaki, Y., Takano, S., Miyasaka, N., Yoshizawa, Y. 2002. Usefulness of cyclosporine A on rapidly progressive interstitial pneumonia in dermatomyositis. Sarcoidosis Vasc. Diffuse Lung Dis. 19, 128–133.

Mok, C.C., To, C.H., Szeto, M.L. 2003. Successful treatment of dermatomyositis-related rapidly progressive interstitial pneumonitis with sequential oral cyclophosphamide and azathioprine. Scand. J. Rheumatol. 32, 181–183.

Nakajima, H., Harigai, M., Hara, M., Hakoda, M., Tokuda, H., Sakai, F., Kamatani, N., Kashiwazaki, S. 2000. KL-6 as a novel serum marker for interstitial pneumonia associated with collagen diseases. J. Rheumatol. 27, 1164–1170.

Nambu, Y., Mouri, M., Toga, H., Ohya, N., Iwata, T., Kobashi, Y. 1994. Gender and underlying diseases affect the frequency of the concurrence of adult polymyositis/dermatomyositis and interstitial pneumonia. Chest 106, 1931–1932.

Nawata, Y., Kurasawa, K., Takabayashi, K., Miike, S., Watanabe, N., Hiraguri, M., Kita, Y., Kawai, M., Saito, Y., Iwamoto, I. 1999. Corticosteroid resistant interstitial pneumonitis in dermatomyositis/polymyositis: prediction and treatment with cyclosporine. J. Rheumatol. 26, 1527–1533.

Oddis, C.V. 2000. Current approach to the treatment of polymyositis and dermatomyositis. Curr. Opin. Rheumatol. 12, 492–497.

Oddis, C.V., Sciurba, F.C., Elmagd, K.A., Starzl, T.E. 1999. Tacrolimus in refractory polymyositis with interstitial lung disease. Lancet 353, 1762–1763.

Ohnishi, H., Yokoyama, A., Kondo, K., Hamada, H., Abe, M., Nishimura, K., Hiwada, K., Kohno, N. 2002. Comparative study of KL-6, surfactant protein-A, surfactant protein-D, and monocyte chemoattractant protein-1 as serum markers for interstitial lung diseases. Am. J. Respir. Crit. Care Med. 165, 378–381.

Rowen, A.J., Reichel, J. 1983. Dermatomyositis with lung involvement, successfully treated with azathioprine. Respiration 44, 143–146.

Saito, Y., Terada, M., Takada, T., Ishida, T., Moriyama, H., Ooi, H., Hasegawa, T., Tsukada, H., Suzuki, E., Gejyo, F., Kihara, Y. 2002. Pulmonary involvement in mixed connective tissue disease: comparison with other collagen vascular diseases using high resolution CT. J. Comput. Assist. Tomogr. 26, 349–357.

Salmeron, G., Greenberg, S.D., Lidsky, M.D. 1981. Polymyositis and diffuse interstitial lung disease. A review of the pulmonary histopathologic findings. Arch. Intern. Med. 141, 1005–1010.

Sano, M., Suzuki, M., Sato, M., Sakamoto, T., Uchigata, M. 1994. Fatal respiratory failure due to polymyositis. Intern. Med. 33, 185–187.

Sauty, A., Rochat, T., Schoch, O.D., Hamacher, J., Kurt, A.M., Dayer, J.M., Nicod, L.P. 1997. Pulmonary fibrosis with predominant CD8 lymphocytic alveolitis and anti-Jo-1 antibodies. Eur. Respir. J. 10, 2907–2912.

Schiavi, E.A., Roncoroni, A.J., Puy, R.J. 1984. Isolated bilateral diaphragmatic paresis with interstitial lung disease. An unusual presentation of dermatomyositis. Am. Rev. Respir. Dis. 129, 337–339.

Schmidt, W.A., Wetzel, W., Friedlander, R., Lange, R., Sorensen, H.F., Lichey, H.J., Genth, E., Mierau, R., Gromnica-Ihle, E. 2000. Clinical and serological aspects of patients with anti-Jo-1 antibodies—an evolving spectrum of disease manifestations. Clin. Rheumatol. 19, 371–377.

Schnabel, A., Reuter, M., Gross, W.L. 1998. Intravenous pulse cyclophosphamide in the treatment of interstitial lung disease due to collagen vascular diseases. Arthritis Rheum. 41, 1215–1220.

Schnabel, A., Reuter, M., Biederer, J., Richter, C., Gross, W.L. 2003. Interstitial lung disease in polymyositis and dermatomyositis: clinical course and response to treatment. Semin. Arthritis Rheum. 32, 273–284.

Schumacher, H.R., Schimmer, B., Gordon, G.V., Bookspan, M.A., Brogadir, S., Dorwart, B.B. 1979. Articular manifestations of polymyositis and dermatomyositis. Am. J. Med. 67, 287–292.

Schurawitzki, H., Stiglbauer, R., Graninger, W., Herold, C., Polzleitner, D., Burghuber, O.C., Tscholakoff, D. 1990. Interstitial lung disease in progressive systemic sclerosis: high-resolution CT versus radiography. Radiology 175, 755–759.

Schwarz, M.I. 1992. Pulmonary and cardiac manifestations of polymyositis–dermatomyositis. J. Thorac. Imaging 7, 46–54.

Schwarz, M.I. 1998. The lung in polymyositis. Clin. Chest Med 19, 701–712, viii.

Schwarz, M.I., Matthay, R.A., Sahn, S.A., Stanford, R.E., Marmorstein, B.L., Scheinhorn, D.J. 1976. Interstitial lung disease in polymyositis and dermatomyositis: analysis of six cases and review of the literature. Medicine (Baltimore) 55, 89–104.

Schwarz, M.I., Sutarik, J.M., Nick, J.A., Leff, J.A., Emlen, J.W., Tuder, R.M. 1995. Pulmonary capillaritis and diffuse alveolar hemorrhage. A primary manifestation of polymyositis. Am. J. Respir. Crit. Care Med. 151, 2037–2040.

Sharp, G.C., Irvin, W.S., Tan, E.M., Gould, R.G., Holman, H.R. 1972. Mixed connective tissue disease—an apparently distinct rheumatic disease syndrome associated with a specific antibody to an extractable nuclear antigen (ENA). Am. J. Med. 52, 148–159.

Shinohara, T., Hidaka, T., Matsuki, Y., Ishizuka, T., Takamizawa, M., Kawakami, M., Kikuma, H., Suzuki, K., Nakamura, H. 1997. Rapidly progressive interstitial lung disease associated with dermatomyositis responding to intravenous cyclophosphamide pulse therapy. Intern. Med. 36, 519–523.

Sigurgeirsson, B., Lindelof, B., Edhag, O., Allander, E. 1992. Risk of cancer in patients with dermatomyositis or polymyositis. A population-based study. N. Engl. J. Med. 326, 363–367.

Silver, R.M., Miller, K.S., Kinsella, M.B., Smith, E.A., Schabel, S.I. 1990. Evaluation and management of scleroderma lung disease using bronchoalveolar lavage. Am. J. Med. 88, 470–476.

Songcharoen, S., Raju, S.F., Pennebaker, J.B. 1980. Interstitial lung disease in polymyositis and dermatomyositis. J. Rheumatol. 7, 353–360.

Sontheimer, R.D., Miyagawa, S. 2003. Potentially fatal interstitial lung disease can occur in clinically amyopathic dermatomyositis. J. Am. Acad. Dermatol. 48, 797–798.

Stedeford, J., Wordsworth, B.P. 1991. Cyclosporin A treatment of dermatomyositis. Arthritis Rheum. 34, 933.

Sugisaki, K., Takeda, I., Iwadate, H., Kanno, T., Nishimaki, T., Kasukawa, R. 2002. Prevention of progression of interstitial lung lesions by early combination therapy with corticosteroids and cyclosporine/cyclophosphamide in two patients with amyopathic dermatomyositis. Fukushima J. Med. Sci. 48, 103–110.

Sullivan, W.D., Hurst, D.J., Harmon, C.E., Esther, J.H., Agia, G.A., Maltby, J.D., Lillard, S.B., Held, C.N., Wolfe, J.F., Sunderrajan, E.V., Maricq, H.R., Sharp, G.R. 1984. A prospective evaluation emphasizing pulmonary involvement in patients with mixed connective tissue disease. Medicine (Baltimore) 63, 92–107.

Takahashi, H., Fujishima, T., Koba, H., Murakami, S., Kurokawa, K., Shibuya, Y., Shiratori, M., Kuroki, Y., Abe, S. 2000a. Serum surfactant proteins A and D as prognostic factors in idiopathic pulmonary fibrosis and their relationship to disease extent. Am. J. Respir. Crit. Care Med. 162, 1109–1114.

Takahashi, H., Kuroki, Y., Tanaka, H., Saito, T., Kurokawa, K., Chiba, H., Sagawa, A., Nagae, H., Abe, S. 2000b. Serum levels of surfactant proteins A and D are useful biomarkers for interstitial lung disease in patients with progressive systemic sclerosis. Am. J. Respir. Crit. Care Med. 162, 258–263.

Takizawa, H., Shiga, J., Moroi, Y., Miyachi, S., Nishiwaki, M., Miyamoto, T. 1987. Interstitial lung disease in dermatomyositis: clinicopathological study. J. Rheumatol. 14, 102–107.

Takizawa, H., Suzuki, N., Yanagawa, T., Okazaki, H., Satoh, M., Akiyama, N., Kohyama, T., Kawasaki, S., Ito, K., Oka, T. 1996. Outcome in patients with interstitial lung disease and polymyositis–dermatomyositis—a subgroup with poor prognosis. Nihon Kyobu Shikkan Gakkai Zasshi 34, 1093–1097.

Tanaka, F., Origuchi, T., Migita, K., Tominaga, M., Kawakami, A., Kawabe, Y., Eguchi, K. 2000. Successful combined therapy of cyclophosphamide and cyclosporine for acute exacerbated interstitial pneumonia associated with dermatomyositis. Intern. Med. 39, 428–430.

Targoff, I.N. 1990. Autoantibodies to aminoacyl-transfer RNA synthetases for isoleucine and glycine. Two additional synthetases are antigenic in myositis. J. Immunol. 144, 1737–1743.

Targoff, I.N. 1994. Immune manifestations of inflammatory muscle disease. Rheum. Dis. Clin. North Am. 20, 857–880.

Targoff, I.N., Arnett, F.C., Berman, L., O'Brien, C., Reichlin, M. 1989. Anti-KJ: a new antibody associated with the syndrome of polymyositis and interstitial lung disease. J. Clin. Invest. 84, 162–172.

Tazelaar, H.D., Viggiano, R.W., Pickersgill, J., Colby, T.V. 1990. Interstitial lung disease in polymyositis and dermatomyositis. Clinical features and prognosis as correlated with histologic findings. Am. Rev. Respir. Dis. 141, 727–733.

Turner, R., Lipshutz, W., Miller, W., Rittenberg, G., Schumacher, H.R., Cohen, S. 1973. Esophageal dysfunction in collagen disease. Am. J. Med. Sci. 265, 191–199.

Vazquez-Abad, D., Rothfield, N.F. 1996. Sensitivity and specificity of anti-Jo-1 antibodies in autoimmune diseases with myositis. Arthritis Rheum. 39, 292–296.

Wallaert, B., Hatron, P.Y., Grosbois, J.M., Tonnel, A.B., Devulder, B., Voisin, C. 1986. Subclinical pulmonary involvement in collagen-vascular diseases assessed by bronchoalveolar lavage. Relationship between alveolitis and subsequent changes in lung function. Am. Rev. Respir. Dis. 133, 574–580.

Wells, A.U., du Bois, R.M., Nicholson, A. 2003. Pulmonary fibrosis in connective tissue disease. In: J.P. Lynch, III (Ed.), Idiopathic Pulmonary Fibrosis. Marcel Dekker, New York, pp. 273–302.

White, B., Moore, W.C., Wigley, F.M., Xiao, H.Q., Wise, R.A. 2000. Cyclophosphamide is associated with pulmonary function and survival benefit in patients with scleroderma and alveolitis. Ann. Intern. Med. 132, 947–954.

Yamadori, I., Fujita, J., Kajitani, H., Bandoh, S., Tokuda, M., Ohtsuki, Y., Yoshinouchi, T., Okahara, M., Yamaji, Y., Tanimoto, Y., Sato, Y., Ishida, T. 2001. Lymphocyte subsets in lung tissues of interstitial pneumonia associated with untreated polymyositis/dermatomyositis. Rheumatol. Int. 21, 89–93.

Yamanishi, Y., Maeda, H., Konishi, F., Hiyama, K., Yamana, S., Ishioka, S., Yamakido, M. 1999. Dermatomyositis associated with rapidly progressive fatal interstitial pneumonitis and pneumomediastinum. Scand. J. Rheumatol. 28, 58–61.

Yang, Y., Fujita, J., Tokuda, M., Bandoh, S., Ishida, T. 2002. Chronological evaluation of the onset of histologically confirmed interstitial pneumonia associated with polymyositis/dermatomyositis. Intern. Med. 41, 1135–1141.

Yoshida, S., Akizuki, M., Mimori, T., Yamagata, H., Inada, S., Homma, M. 1983. The precipitating antibody to an acidic nuclear protein antigen, the Jo-1, in connective tissue diseases. A marker for a subset of polymyositis with interstitial pulmonary fibrosis. Arthritis Rheum. 26, 604–611.

Yoshida, T., Koga, H., Saitoh, F., Sakamoto, M., Harada, M., Yoshida, H., Sakisaka, S., Sata, M. 1999. Pulse intravenous cyclophosphamide treatment for steroid-resistant interstitial pneumonitis associated with polymyositis. Intern. Med. 38, 733–738.

Zisman, D.A., McCune, W.J., Tino, G., Lynch, J.P. 3rd 2001. Drug-induced pneumonitis: the role of methotrexate. Sarcoidosis Vasc. Diffuse Lung Dis. 18, 243–252.

Handbook of Systemic Autoimmune Diseases, Volume 2
Pulmonary Involvement in Systemic Autoimmune Diseases
A.U. Wells and C.P. Denton, editors

CHAPTER 12

Pulmonary Involvement in Miscellaneous Connective Tissue Diseases

Athol U. Wells*, Gary Davies
Royal Brompton Hospital, Chelsea, London, UK.

1. Introduction

This chapter covers the lung manifestations of a number of miscellaneous connective tissue disorders: mixed connective tissue disease (MCTD), relapsing polychondritis (with the exception of the associated vasculitis, which is discussed elsewhere in this volume), ankylosing spondylitis (AS) and the Marfan syndrome (MS). These conditions have in common the fact that pulmonary involvement is well recognised, may be life threatening, but is infrequently encountered in routine clinical practice, either because the systemic disorder is rare (especially relapsing polychondritis), or because lung involvement occurs infrequently.

2. Mixed connective tissue disease

Disorders with overlapping features of more than one rheumatological disease have long caused classification difficulties. The terminology used to describe the mixture of features of systemic lupus erythematosus (SLE), systemic sclerosis (SSc) and polymyositis/dermatomyositis (PM/DM) has included overlap syndrome, undifferentiated connective tissue disease and mixed collagenosis (Ginsburg et al., 1983; Prakash, 1992, 1998). The concept that this spectrum of disease can be unified into a single disorder has fuelled considerable debate. It has been argued that overlap syndromes should be viewed as intermediate disorders, with many patients ultimately meeting criteria for a single predominant rheumatological disorder (SLE, SSc or PM/DM) (van den Hoogen et al., 1994), with differentiation into an individual disorder in part genetically determined (Gendi et al., 1995; Kallenberg, 1993). However, it is now broadly accepted that serological data justify the use of the term 'mixed connective tissue disease' (MCTD), first proposed in 1972 (Sharp et al., 1972). The presence of high titres of circulating autoantibodies to a nuclear ribonucleoprotein antigen (anti-(U1)-Sn-RNP) is a prerequisite for the diagnosis of MCTD (Maddison, 1991). In the initial classification of Sharp (Sharp and Anderson, 1980), diagnostic criteria for MCTD were as follows.

Major criteria:

(1) severe myositis
(2) lung involvement (DLco $< 70\%$ or proliferative vascular lesions on biopsy)
(3) Raynaud's phenomenon or esophageal dysmotility
(4) swollen hands or sclerodactyly
(5) anti-RNA $> 1/10,000$, with positive anti-RNP and negative anti-Sm antibodies.

Minor criteria: alopecia, leukopenia, anaemia, pleuritis, pericarditis, arthritis, trigeminal neuralgia,

*Corresponding author.
Tel.: +44-207-351-8327; fax: +44-207-351-8336
E-mail address: a.wells@rbh.nthames.nhs.uk (A.U. Wells).

DOI: 10.1016/S1571-5078(04)02012-4

malar rash, thrombocytopenia, mild myositis, history of swollen hands.

In this classification system, MCTD is considered to be definite if four major criteria are met, anti U1 RNP titres exceed 1/4000 and anti-Sm antibodies are absent. MCTD is considered to be probable if anti U1 RNP titres exceed 1/4000 and *either* three major criteria are met and anti-Sm antibodies are absent *or* two major criteria and one minor criterion are met. However, the ephemeral nature of the clinical features of MCTD is amply illustrated by the existence of three alternative classification systems (Amigues et al., 1996), all requiring the presence of anti U1 RNP antibodies, but a variable selection of clinical features.

The most pragmatic classification, that of Kahn (Amigues et al., 1996), consists of:

(1) serological criteria: presence of high titre anti-RNP, corresponding to speckled ANA at titres $>1/2000$
(2) clinical criteria: (a) Raynaud's phenomenon; (b) synovitis; (c) myositis; (d) swollen fingers.

The diagnosis of MCTD requires positive serological criteria, Raynaud's phenomenon and satisfaction of two of the remaining three clinical criteria.

The distinctive features of the Kahn criteria are that precision in the designation of clinical features is not required, and histological evaluation is unnecessary. This has obvious advantages in a disorder which tends to evolve clinically as disease progresses, and in which individual clinical criteria may be ephemeral. The drawback of the multiplicity of classification systems, applying especially to the Kahn criteria, is that published series necessarily contain highly variable patient sub-groups and it is, therefore, difficult to compare populations and standardise clinical evaluation. The prevalence of MCTD, more than three decades after the syndrome was proposed, has not been precisely defined but probably approximates 1 in 10,000 (Venables, 1998). The disease develops most frequently in females in the fourth decade and no racial predilection has been documented. In addition to the clinical features proposed by Sharp, generalised lymphadenopathy is present in up to 50% and renal involvement in 10–20% (Sullivan et al., 1984). Cardiac manifestations include pericarditis and, less commonly, myocarditis and left ventricular impairment, occasionally resulting in left ventricular failure (Alpert et al., 1983).

Pulmonary involvement in MCTD encompasses the full range of lung disease seen in SSc, PM / DM and SLE, described in detail elsewhere in this volume. Amongst a large number of manifestations of lung involvement, the three most frequent are pleural effusion, interstitial fibrosis and pulmonary hypertension, in keeping with the most prevalent pulmonary complications of SSc, PM/DM and SLE (Table 1). The prevalence of pulmonary disease in MCTD is critically dependent upon the level and duration of evaluation. In a retrospective series of 81 MCTD patients, only 25% were considered to have pleuropulmonary disease, most commonly basal interstitial fibrosis (Prakash et al., 1985). However, in a prospective study of 34 patients, abnormal infiltrates on chest radiography compatible with interstitial lung disease were present in 85% (Sullivan et al., 1984). The marked differences between these two reports may reflect variations in patient subsets in a notoriously heterogeneous disorder, but also differences in the duration of follow-up.

Pleural disease in MCTD occurs most frequently in MCTD patients with predominantly SLE-like clinical features; the pleura are very seldom involved in SSc or PM / DM. Pleuritic pain is reported in up to 40% of patients (Sullivan et al., 1984), but despite this high prevalence, pleural abnormalities are very seldom the initial manifestation of disease (unlike SLE) (Beier et al., 1992). In the few reported cases in which

Table 1
In MCTD, it is clinically useful to characterise the nature of lung involvement as typical of SSc, PM/DM or SLE

	SLE	PM / DM	SSc
Interstitial fibrosis	+	++	+++
Organising pneumonia	±	++	±
Lymphocytic interstitial pneumonia	±	±	±
Obliterative bronchiolitis	±	±	
Bronchiectasis	±		
Pleural involvement	+++		
Respiratory muscle weakness	++	++	±
Pulmonary hypertension	++	+	+++
Diffuse alveolar haemorrhage	+	±	±

The prevalence of pulmonary complications in these three disorders is shown semi-quantitatively: +++: common; ++: fairly frequent; +: occasional; ±: rare.

pleural involvement is the primary presenting feature of MCTD, exudative effusions have tended to be associated with pericarditis (Beier et al., 1992; Richard et al., 1996), although this is not invariably the case (Hoogsteden et al., 1985). Pleural effusions may be unilateral or bilateral, are usually small and generally resolve spontaneously (Prakash, 1998).

Interstitial fibrosis is probably the most prevalent pulmonary complication in MCTD (Prakash, 1992) and is predominantly basal in distribution on lung auscultation (Sullivan et al., 1984) and on chest radiography (Prakash et al., 1985). Histological abnormalities consist of alveolar septal infiltration by lymphocytes, plasma cells and type III collagen, with appearances similar to those in SSc (Wiener-Kronish et al., 1981); this description is compatible with an underlying histological pattern of non-specific interstitial pneumonia, the most frequent fibrotic interstitial pattern in SSc (Bouros et al., 2002) and PM / DM (Douglas et al., 2001). Perhaps surprisingly, organising pneumonia appears to be relatively infrequent in MCTD, despite a high prevalence in PM / DM. In a recent high resolution CT evaluation of 41 patients with MCTD and overt lung involvement, appearances were typical of non-specific interstitial pneumonia, with prominent ground-glass attenuation and fine fibrotic abnormalities but little honeycombing (Kozuka et al., 2001). In this series, air-space consolidation (compatible with organising pneumonia) was present in a quarter of cases but was very limited in extent. Thus, interstitial disease in MCTD appears to be largely fibrotic and irreversible, most closely resembling interstitial lung involvement in SSc, although there are no definitive evaluations of the rapidity of disease progression on MCTD.

Pulmonary function studies suggest a high prevalence of sub-clinical interstitial lung abnormalities in MCTD. Gas transfer (DLco) levels are reduced in two-thirds of patients with no respiratory symptoms, and a restrictive ventilatory defect is present in a large minority (Sharp and Anderson, 1980). Bronchoalveolar lavage abnormalities have also been reported in asymptomatic MCTD patients (believed to denote subclinical alveolitis), although the nature of the abnormality has been variably neutrophilic (Wallaert et al., 1990) and lymphocytic (Enomoto et al., 2003). The clinical significance of mild lung function impairment, limited CT abnormalities and increased bronchoalveolar lavage cellularity in asymptomatic MCTD patients is often difficult to judge; there is no evidence, as yet, that subclinical alveolitis is a precursor of progressive interstitial fibrosis.

Pulmonary vascular disease is well recognised in MCTD, with fatal pulmonary hypertension reported in a number of cases, typically in women aged less than 40 (King, 1998). Underlying mechanisms may include vasoconstriction due to pulmonary artery hyper-reactivity (Ueda et al., 1984), severe pulmonary vasculitis (Alpert et al., 1983; Wiener-Kronish et al., 1981; Demedts, 1990), and pulmonary thromboembolism, especially in MCTD with SLE-like features, with or without circulating prothrombotic antibodies (Hainaut et al., 1986). Overall, it appears that pulmonary vascular histological abnormalities in MCTD most often resemble those of SSc, with marked intimal and medial thickening in small to medium-sized arteries and endarteritis obliterans (Wiener-Kronish et al., 1981; Ueda et al , 1984; Hosoda et al., 1987); vasculitis and thromboembolism, both features of pulmonary vascular disease in SLE, are less prevalent. Although clinically overt pulmonary vascular disease is less frequent than interstitial fibrosis, it is an important cause of morbidity and mortality in MCTD.

Other pulmonary disorders in MCTD vary with the nature of systemic disease. In patients with a predominant picture of PM/DM, respiratory muscle weakness is occasionally a manifestation of inflammatory myositis and may even result in respiratory failure (Martyn et al., 1988), although respiratory muscle function is normal in most patients (Derderian et al., 1985). In patients with an SLE-like disease, severe diffuse alveolar haemorrhage has occurred (Germain and Davidman, 1984; Sanchez-Guerrero et al., 1989). When the systemic profile is predominantly that of SSc or PM / DM, esophageal dysmotility, hypotonicity and dilatation are common (Prakash et al., 1985). Evidence of small airways involvement, as judged by studies of dynamic compliance, was frequent in one report (Izumiyama et al., 1993), but tests of small airways function are notoriously difficult to interpret in early interstitial lung disease and in any case, clinical significant obliterative bronchiolitis has yet to be reported in MCTD. Finally, opportunistic infection may complicate immunosuppressive therapy, exactly as in other connective tissue diseases; lung infection has presented as cavitary lung nodules in a number of cases (Webb and Gamsu, 1981).

There are no controlled data on which to base therapy for lung involvement in MCTD but the same reservation largely applies to other connective tissue diseases. It is generally accepted that lung involvement should be characterised as most closely resembling lung disease in SSc, PM / DM or SLE; this exercise provides a guide to likely prognosis and allows the accumulated therapeutic experience in these disorders to be applied to MCTD. Thus, pleural effusions can usefully be treated as in SLE, organising pneumonia as in PM / DM, and interstitial fibrosis or pulmonary hypertension as in SSc. The nature of the predominant lung process is often obvious when pulmonary function tests, echocardiography and high resolution CT are evaluated in conjunction, and it is now seldom necessary to resort to a surgical lung biopsy in most MCTD patients. The regimens used for the various lung disorders of MCTD are described in detail elsewhere in this volume, in sections dealing with SLE, SSc and PM/DM. Broadly, most disorders are treated with corticosteroids and/or immunosuppressive agents, in keeping with an autoimmune pathogenesis. Interstitial fibrosis is irreversible but, as in other connective tissue diseases, treatment may be warranted in the hope of preventing or slowing disease progression. Regimens used for interstitial fibrosis in SSc (Latsi and Wells, 2003) appear appropriate and usually consist of low dose steroids in combination with an immunosuppressive agent such as cyclophosphamide or azathioprine.

In general, pleural effusions and organising pneumonia often respond well to corticosteroid therapy, although an immunosuppressive agent may need to be added when organising pneumonia is refractory.

The exceptions to immunosuppressive treatment are pulmonary hypertension and opportunistic infection. Pulmonary hypertension will occasionally partially respond to vasodilating agents such as captopril (Alpert et al., 1992) and nifedipene (Alpert et al., 1991) and the more recently discovered Bosentan (Kenyon and Nappi, 2003) and Epoprostenol (Strange et al., 2000). Pulmonary hypertension is seldom completely reversible, except in occasional cases with a vasculitic pathogenesis.

Long-term outcome has not been quantified with any precision. However, it is clear that the natural history and treated course of the various lung disorders are highly heterogeneous. In some cases, involvement is limited, indolent or responds well to treatment; a good outcome with immunosuppressive treatment was seen in the majority of cases in a prospective evaluation of 34 cases (Sullivan et al., 1984). However, a minority of patients progresses inexorably in spite of intervention, and this applies especially to those with pulmonary hypertension (Wiener-Kronish et al., 1981) or an SSc-like systemic profile (Sullivan et al., 1984).

3. Relapsing polychondritis

Relapsing polychondritis is a rare multi-system disease in which recurrent progressive inflammation of cartilaginous structures results in widespread degenerative change. Sites involved include the elastic cartilage of the nose and ears, the hyaline cartilage of peripheral joints, and fibrocartilage at axial sites (such as the ribs). Pulmonary involvement consists of degradation of cartilage in the tracheobronchial tree. The disease is generally multifocal; inflammation may also develop in other structures rich in proteoglycans, including the blood vessels, eyes, inner ear, heart and kidneys. The spectrum of systemic and pulmonary disease in relapsing polychondritis is reviewed in a number of articles (Tanoue, 1992; Lee-Chiong, 1998; Letko et al., 2002).

Relapsing polychondritis was first reported as 'polychondropathia' by Jaksch-Wartenhorst (1923) and the widespread nature of the disease was documented by Alther (1936). Synonyms have included chondromalacia, diffuse perichondritis, chronic atrophic polychondritis, diffuse chondrolysis and dyschondroplasia; the term "relapsing polychondritis" was coined in an influential article by Pearson et al. (1960). It was, by then, apparent that the disease was exceedingly rare; the accumulated experience of relapsing polychondritis now amounts to over 700 published cases. Cartilaginous involvement occurs most frequently in the ears (85–95%), nose (50–60%), upper respiratory tract (30–50%), and ribs; the other most frequent complications consist of ocular inflammation, non-erosive arthropathy, and vestibulo-cochlear dysfunction (Zeuner et al., 1997; Isaak et al., 1986).

The compilation of sites of involvement in relapsing polychondritis is complicated by the high prevalence of other autoimmune disorders; thus, it is uncertain, in many cases, whether apparent sites of disease activity merely represent the manifestations of associated diseases. Vasculitis of small and large arteries is extremely common (Burlew et al., 1992) and is discussed in detail elsewhere in this volume, in the chapter by Bennett and D'Cruz. Other autoimmune diseases, fulfilling formal diagnostic criteria, are present in approximately 30% of cases and these include rheumatoid arthritis, SLE, Sjogren's syndrome, AS, polyarteritis nodosa, Wegener's granulomatosis, Bechet's disease and Reiter's syndrome (Tanoue, 1992; Eng and Sabanathan, 1991; Hunninghake and Fauci, 1979; Higenbottam and Dixon, 1979; Small et al., 1980). Thus, although the cause of relapsing polychondritis is unknown, an autoimmune pathogenesis appears likely, with possible triggers including trauma, infection, allergy and altered enzyme proteolysis (Burlew et al., 1992). The frequent presence of both autoantibodies and cellular immune reactions to type II collagen in relapsing polychondritis (Dolan et al., 1966; Ebringer et al., 1981; Foidart et al., 1978) lends further support to an autoimmune aetiology. The fact that titres against native type II collagen are higher than titres against constituent alpha-1 chains suggests that antibody formation to type II collagen is likely to be pivotal, rather than a non-specific result of inflammation (Foidart et al., 1978).

An incidence of 3.5 cases per million has been estimated (Luthra, 1988). It is believed by some that the disease has a predilection for Caucasians (Trentham and Le, 1998), although this view has been challenged (Luthra, 1988). The peak prevalence occurs in the fifth and sixth decades, with reported range from 5 to 84 years of age. There is a slight male predominance. No strong genetic predisposition has been identified, although an association with HLA-DR4 (with no predominant sub-type) has been reported (Lang et al., 1993). Survival rates of 70% at 4 years, 74% at 5 years and 55% at 10 years have been reported (McAdam et al., 1976; Michet et al., 1986). A recent improvement in survival to 94% at 8 years (Trentham and Le, 1998) may be attributable to improvements in medical and surgical treatment.

The difficulties in characterising relapsing polychondritis are cogently summarised by Letko et al. (2002), and these apply equally to pulmonary and systemic disease. In common with other rare diseases, the diagnosis tends to be made when involvement is obvious, resulting in a bias towards severe disease. Cases tend to be reported shortly after diagnosis and, thus, the prevalence of involvement of specific sites is understated; in most patients, involvement becomes more extensive as disease progresses. The paucity of follow-up information has led to uncertainties about the natural history and treated course. To these constraints can be added the difficulty in making a secure diagnosis in many cases, especially when relapsing polychondritis is associated with other autoimmune disorders. The single most useful diagnostic test is a cartilage biopsy, but appearances are sometimes indeterminate and, therefore, the diagnosis is generally clinical. The most widely applied diagnostic criteria are those first proposed by McAdam et al. (1976) and Zeuner et al. (1997). The presence of three or more of the following clinical features is required:

(1) bilateral auricular chondritis
(2) non-erosive, sero-negative inflammatory polyarthritis
(3) nasal chondritis
(4) ocular inflammation
(5) respiratory tract involvement (either upper or lower respiratory tract)
(6) cochlear with or without vestibular abnormality.

Biopsy of affected cartilage is not amongst the McAdam criteria and is often unnecessary, although pivotal to diagnosis in some cases; auricular biopsy is the most frequent procedure, but it is sometimes necessary to biopsy the tracheal rings. Similarly, specific laboratory tests are not a formal part of diagnosis, although the presence of anti-cartilage antibodies may be helpful; it is likely that this serological feature will be incorporated when the diagnostic criteria are eventually revised. Other abnormalities in laboratory tests include anaemia, elevation of inflammatory markers, and autoantibodies found in associated autoimmune diseases (e.g. positive serology for rheumatoid factor or antinuclear antibodies, hypergammaglobulinaemia).

Involvement of the respiratory tract accounted for over half of deaths ascribable to relapsing polychondritis in the series of McAdam et al. (1976). As the condition became increasingly recognised and the diagnosis was made in less severe disease, mortality from lung involvement became less frequent; although no definitive estimates exist, respiratory complications (tracheal involvement or pneumonia) are the primary cause of death in perhaps 10–15% of patients (Michet et al., 1986). Laryngotracheal involvement is now widely recognised as a malignant prognostic determinant, especially in patients aged below 50. Involvement of the glottis, trachea and larger bronchi is the primary presenting feature in up to 25% of cases (Michet et al., 1986), occurring more frequently in females (Adliff et al., 1997). Respiratory tract involvement may be generalised or limited to focal areas; the most frequent focal site is the larynx and upper trachea, but isolated single large bronchial or small airways abnormalities have been reported (Eng and Sabanathan, 1991). Pulmonary parenchymal disease is rare with the exception of vasculitis, which is often present but is not always clinically overt.

The histological appearances in involved areas in the respiratory tract are typical of those seen in involved cartilage in other sites (Kaye and Sones, 1964). Early in disease, inflammation predominates; the latter course is characterised by replacement of cartilage by granulation tissue and, eventually, by marked tissue thickening, cyst formation, calcification and, occasionally, bone formation. The clinical profile mirrors the histological evolution of disease (Arkin and Masi, 1975). At presentation, tracheal or laryngeal tenderness, wheezing and hoarseness are typical (McAdam et al., 1976). Subsequently, severe airway compromise may supervene, due to stricture formation, leading to fixed airflow obstruction, dyspnoea and, ultimately, to respiratory failure and death. Lower respiratory tract infection is a common late complication and is largely ascribable to retention of secretions, due equally to airway narrowing and ineffective cough (resulting from dynamic upper airway collapse) (Mohsenifar et al., 1982). Therefore, symptoms suggestive of respiratory tract involvement should prompt immediate radiological assessment of the airways (radiography and CT) and pulmonary function evaluation (McAdam et al., 1976; Mohsenifar et al., 1982).

Chest and lateral neck radiographic evaluation may reveal ectopic calcification in tracheal or laryngeal cartilage and occasionally reveals narrowing of the trachea or large bronchi (although this is seldom overt on plain radiography) (Kilman, 1978). The chest radiograph may also show evidence of pneumonia or atelectasis, resulting from airway narrowing or collapse (Michet et al., 1986). However, in many cases, chest and lateral neck radiography is insensitive, even in patients with prominent symptoms. Laryngography, as a means of delineating the upper airways, is contraindicated because of the risk of acute airway compromise (Tanoue, 1992). Thus, the most useful radiological procedures is CT, which commonly discloses smooth thickening of airway walls as well as increased airway wall attenuation, with or without calcification (Behar et al., 2002). Abnormalities may extend to the lobar and segmental airways and this is readily appreciated on high resolution CT. Focal or diffuse narrowing of airways (including the trachea) is seen less frequently on inspiratory CT; tracheal and bronchial abnormalities are more readily visualised by expiratory CT which may unmask airway collapse or lobar air-trapping (Behar et al., 2002). Dynamic CT scanning (cineradiography) may also help to localise large airway disease by demonstrating airway collapse during expiration (Tanoue, 1992).

Pulmonary function tests are an essential part of evaluation, both in initial diagnosis and as an aid to monitoring disease progression. Tracheal involvement is characterised by a reduction in expiratory and inspiratory flow rates, with a plateau pattern in early to mid inspiration and expiration (Gibson and Davis, 1974; Mohsenifar et al., 1982). This typical finding is present in a minority of patients but expiratory airflow obstruction is frequent; reductions in expiratory flow rates in association with preservation of static recoil pressures are highly suggestive of intrinsic structural airway abnormalities (as opposed to parenchymal disease) (Krell et al., 1986). In general, non-fixed extra-thoracic airway abnormalities tend to have their greatest effect upon inspiratory flow rates, whereas dynamic intra-thoracic disease causes expiratory airflow obstruction. Thus, pulmonary function tests help to identify the predominate site of disease and to

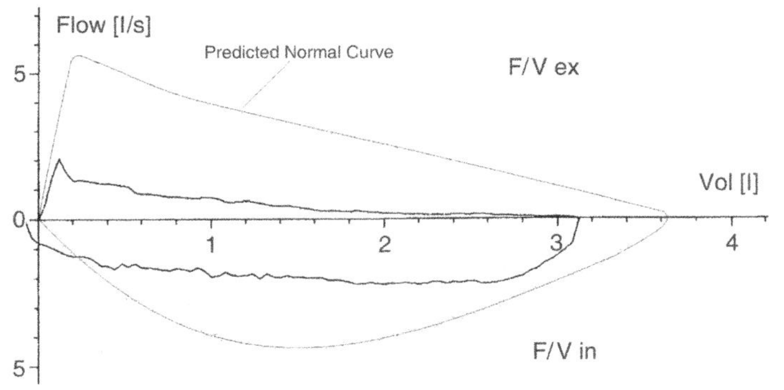

Figure 1. Flow volume loop of a patient with relapsing polychondritis. The patient's predicted normal curve is also drawn for comparison. This shows reduction in expiratory and inspiratory flow rates.

distinguish between fixed and dynamic abnormalities (Fig. 1).

Bronchoscopy may demonstrate severe endobronchial inflammation or obvious airway stenosis or collapse (Eng and Sabanathan, 1991), but seldom adds usefully to pulmonary function testing in the evaluation of disease severity. Generally, spirometric findings correlate well with intrathoracic bronchoscopic observations (Krell et al., 1986) and have obvious advantages in routine monitoring. Furthermore, bronchoscopic appearances are often misleading in the evaluation of the upper respiratory tract; the larynx may appear normal despite major reductions in inspiratory flow rates. Nonetheless, bronchoscopic evaluation is probably worthwhile at presentation to confirm that expiratory airflow obstruction is due to airway-centred disease, and also because Wegener's granulomatosis, which can mimic the clinical features of respiratory tract involvement in relapsing polychondritis, is occasionally diagnosed by biopsy of an endobronchial mass. In severe disease, bronchoscopic evaluation should be undertaken with great caution as it has been reported to precipitate acute airway obstruction (Eng and Sabanathan, 1991).

The decision to treat and the selection of therapeutic agent is entirely dependent upon disease severity. Because of the paucity of cases and wide variety of presentations, there are no universally accepted regimens and no controlled treatment data. The episodic nature of disease, with unpredictable relapses and spontaneous remissions, justifies the institution of treatment on a symptomatic basis. Mild inflammation of the joints or respiratory tract may be controlled by non-steroidal anti-inflammatory agents, colchicine or dapsone, and in systemic disease, dapsone has been efficacious in several reports (Matoba et al., 1984; Barranco et al., 1976; Ridgway et al., 1979). Systemic corticosteroid therapy is used in acute exacerbations and it is sometimes possible to withdraw treatment without relapse. In acute airway involvement, high dose intravenous corticosteroid therapy (pulsed methyl-prednisolone) is warranted. In life-threatening disease, steroid-resistant disease and with repeated relapses, corticosteroid therapy in combination with an immunosuppressive agent, such

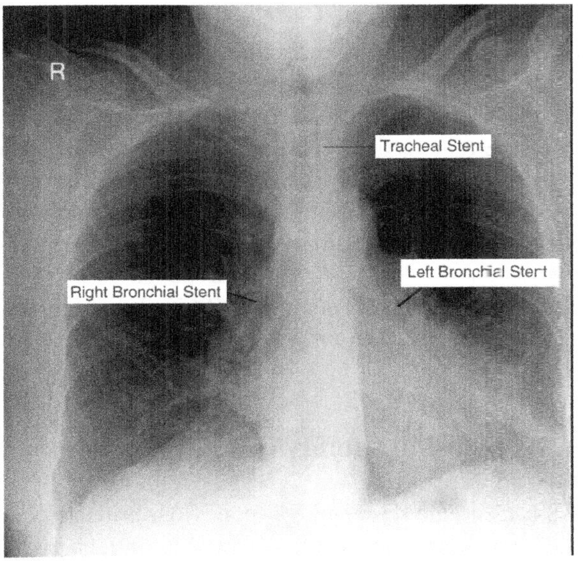

Figure 2. The chest X-ray shows the same patient as in Fig. 1, following surgery and the insertion of a tracheal stent and right and left bronchial stents.

as cyclophosphamide, is usual (Mohsenifar et al., 1982; Mahindrakar et al., 1970; Dolan et al., 1966). However, although inflammation generally regresses with corticosteroid treatment in the short-term and the likelihood of relapse is reduced by prolonged immunosuppression, disease progression and vital organ involvement are not prevented. In the most definitive review of published experience, encompassing 159 reported cases, 75% of patients required prolonged treatment and although this was symptomatically effective in the intermediate term, there was little evidence that the long-term course of disease was materially influenced (McAdam et al., 1976).

Surgical intervention, in order to provide and maintain airway patency, is occasionally life-saving in severe focal respiratory tract involvement. Tracheostomy may be required for severe glottic or subglottic obstruction (Eng and Sabanathan, 1991). Stenting (Figs. 2–4) is occasionally indicated for airway collapse or refractory airway stenosis; self-expanding stents can be inserted through a rigid bronchoscope under general anaesthesia (Shah et al., 1995). Tracheal strictures have been successfully resected, with end-to-end anastomoses (Eng and Sabanathan, 1991; Spraggs et al., 1997). Major airway obstruction has occasionally been dealt with by resection of an inflammatory mass (Eng and Sabanathan, 1991). However, surgical intervention is impracticable in many cases, due to the diffuse nature of respiratory tract involvement, as it often triggers flares in inflammation and sometimes results in devastating infection. Intraluminal stenting may be complicated by haemorrhage due to erosion through the trachea, sudden asphyxia due to stent displacement, mucosal ulceration or scarring, or retention of secretions due to ineffective cough (Eng and Sabanathan, 1991; Montgomery, 1965). Thus, surgery should be undertaken only as a last resort.

4. Ankylosing spondylitis

AS is a chronic seronegative spondyloarthritis associated with the major histocompatibility antigen HLA B27 (Schlosstein et al., 1973). The prevalence of AS is much higher in Caucasian males (approximately 0.15% (Calin and Fries, 1975)) than in black males and the male to female ratio is 10:1 (Tanoue, 1992). The cardinal site of disease is the vertebral column. In early disease, sacroiliac inflammation is usual, with or without more widespread vertebral involvement. As the disease progresses, inflammation progresses to fibrosis and ossification, resulting in calcification of the spinal ligaments, syndesmophyte formation and joint ankylosis. The peripheral joints are affected in approximately a third of patients (Hunninghake and Fauci, 1979).

The cause of AS remains uncertain but associated disorders include ulcerative colitis, psoriasis and SSc and, therefore, an autoimmune pathogenesis appears likely. A microbial trigger, cross-reacting with histocompatability antigens, has been proposed, based upon the identification of Klebsiella related antigens. AS is a multi-system disorder with involvement of a number of extra-articular sites. Non-granulomatous anterior uveitis occurs in up to 25% of patients and is often an early feature of disease (Hunninghake and Fauci, 1979). Asymptomatic inflammation of the thoracic aorta is present in 20–30%, with echocardiographic evidence of dilatation of the aortic root (LaBresh et al., 1985); in 10% of AS patients, clinically important aortic incompetence or dilatation of the ascending aorta develops (Graham and Smythe, 1958). Other less frequent systemic features include renal disease, urethritis, chronic prostatism and spinal cord stenosis. Pulmonary disease may take the form of extra-pulmonic restriction or parenchymal disease.

Extra-pulmonic restriction results from immobilisation of the chest wall, due to fusion of the costovertebral joints or sternoclavicular joint involvement, which is frequently present (Fournie et al., 1997). These abnormalities are often asymptomatic and functional impairment is generally mild, consisting of reductions in vital capacity, total lung capacity and maximal inspiratory and expiratory pressures (Hunninghake and Fauci, 1979). The residual volume is increased, denoting fixation of the chest wall at a high resting volume. The surprisingly mild reduction in pulmonary function indices may reflect the fact that the diaphragm is able to compensate for chest wall immobilisation when the resting volume is elevated (Hunninghake and Fauci, 1979). Gas transfer levels are almost always preserved in the absence of parenchymal disease (Franssen et al., 1986). Exercise tolerance is usually unimpaired provided that an active lifestyle is maintained, despite a restrictive ventilatory pattern and limitation of chest wall movement (Seckin et al., 2000). Chest wall fixation tends to increase in prevalence and severity in disease of longer duration and is not influenced by anti-inflammatory treatment (Franssen et al., 1986). Thus, intervention is confined to the maintenance of general fitness with exercise programmes, and spinal extension exercises.

Parenchymal disease in AS is rare and, when present, is often mild. Typically, fibrobullous abnormalities are confined to the lung apices, with or without cavitation (Rosenow et al., 1977; Appelrouth and Gottlieb, 1975; Hillerdal, 1983). The prevalence of apical fibro-bullous disease in AS has been overstated in some small series, probably as a result of selection biases. In the largest chest radiographic series of 2080 patients followed at the Mayo Clinic, pleuropulmonary abnormalities were evident in only 28 patients (1.3%), including 26 cases of apical fibrosis (Rosenow et al., 1977). In that series, serial radiographic evaluation established that disease generally begins unilaterally and progresses to bilateral apical bullous and cystic disease, associated with fibrosis and, in advanced disease, cavitation with hilar distortion. Apical pleural thickening is common and may be striking in advanced disease, but is confined to lung regions in which there is adjacent interstitial fibrosis (Rosenow et al., 1977). Disease is seldom extensive, except in severe spinal disease (Chakera et al., 1975) and in patients with a long history of AS. Apical fibrobullous disease in AS is almost exclusively seen in males (Boulware et al., 1985) and develops an average of 15 years after the onset of systemic disease (Rumancik et al., 1984), although it occasionally precedes systemic manifestations. Despite having a low prevalence of apical fibrosis, AS is an important cause of predominantly apical interstitial fibrosis at large, being present in over 20% of patients with progressive apical fibrocystic disease (Kentala et al., 1978; Repo et al., 1981).

As in other connective tissue disorders, the prevalence of parenchymal disease is critically dependent upon the investigative modality used. In a prospective study, lung abnormalities were seen on high resolution CT in 18 of 26 AS patients (69%) and in all but four cases, chest radiographic appearances were normal. Findings on CT included interstitial lung disease ($n = 6$), bronchial wall thickening with or without bronchiectasis ($n = 6$) and paraseptal emphysema ($n = 3$); interstitial lung disease was confined to the apices in only two cases (Fenlon et al., 1997). In two subsequent series containing AS patients with normal chest radiographs, CT abnormalities were evident in 15 of 21 patients (71%) (Turetschek et al., 2000) and in 18 of 28 patients (64%) (Kiris et al., 2003), including mosaic attenuation (denoting uneven regional ventilation), bronchial wall thickening and parenchymal abnormalities, ranging from septal thickening to areas of interstitial fibrosis. As observed in chest radiographic studies, parenchymal abnormalities, on high resolution CT, increase in prevalence in long-standing disease, being present in 11 of 12 patients with a disease duration of over 11 years in a recent report (Senocak et al., 2003). Similarly, bronchoalveolar lavage studies have shown that a sub-clinical lymphocytic alveolitis is frequent in AS (Jeandel et al., 1994). The clinical importance of these findings is difficult to interpret. However, there is no evidence that 'subclinical alveolitis' progresses to clinically important pulmonary fibrosis in connective tissue disease and the significance of limited abnormalities on high resolution CT, in the absence of symptoms or radiographic abnormalities, is equally uncertain. Thus, it is difficult to justify routine CT or bronchoalveolar lavage as screening procedures in AS; rather, both modalities should be reserved for the

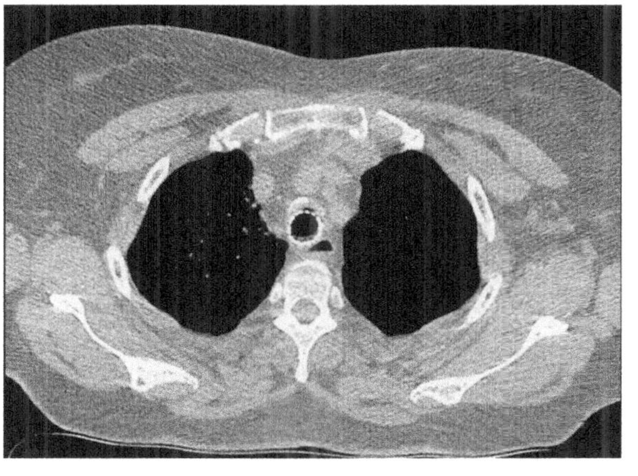

Figure 3. This shows the corresponding CT scan to the chest X-ray and illustrates the tracheal stent in situ. Mucus can also be seen posteriorly within the stent.

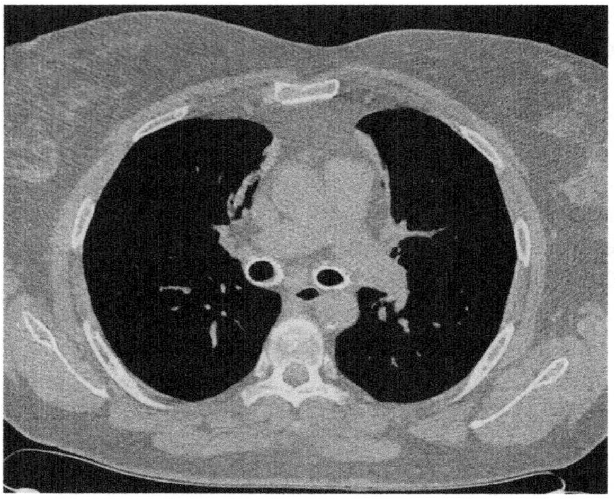

Figure 4. This again shows the corresponding CT scan to the chest X-ray and illustrates the right and left bronchial stents.

evaluation of AS patients with respiratory symptoms or evidence of lung disease on chest radiography.

The pathogenesis of apical fibro-bullous disease is likely to represent evolution from inflammation to fibrosis, as in other extra-articular manifestations such as uveitis and aortitis. Histological evaluation reveals fragmented elastic tissue with degeneration of connective tissue and intra-alveolar fibrosis, without vasculitis or granulomatous disease (Jessamine, 1968; Cohen et al., 1971). However, the particular vulnerability of the lung apices is unexplained. Diminished upper lobe ventilation was believed to be an important contributing factor, based on the observation of a regional reduction in apical ventilation, as judged by xenon-133 scanning, in AS (Stewart et al., 1976). However, this finding was not reproduced in a larger group of AS patients (Parkin et al., 1982). There is no evidence that infection plays a role in pathogenesis, although it becomes a major source of morbidity and mortality in advanced pulmonary disease; in a large cohort of 88 AS patients, lung infection was found to be very infrequent (Zorab, 1962). The most plausible explanation is that the thoracic spinal immobilisation results in increased apical mechanical stress, leading to bullous degeneration, secondary fibrosis and an increased prevalence of pneumothoraces (Rosenow et al., 1977).

Many AS patients with lung involvement are asymptomatic (Hunninghake and Fauci, 1979). Cough, sputum production and dyspnoea are manifestations of advanced disease and often reflect secondary bacterial or fungal infection. Haemoptysis, which may be massive, is a feature of intracavitary mycetoma formation. Thus, life-threatening complications of lung involvement in AS most commonly result from secondary infection in cavities, which have developed within distorted fibrotic apical tissue (Rosenow et al., 1977; Hunninghake and Fauci, 1979; Jewkes et al., 1983). Chronic, clinically overt, infection by fungi or mycobacteria occurs in up to 30% of AS patients with apical cavitation (Rumancik et al., 1984), with *Aspergillus fumigatus* isolated in up to 60% (although not always associated with morbidity) (Davies, 1972). Other organisms found less frequently include atypical mycobacteria species (*Mycobacterium kansasii*, *Mycobacterium avium complex*, *Mycobacterium fortuitum*, *Mycobacterium scrofulaceum*) and fungi (*Candida albicans*, *Aspergillus niger*, *Aspergillus terreus*) (Rosenow et al., 1977; Hunninghake and Fauci, 1979; Hillerdal, 1983; Gacad and Hamosh, 1973; Kennedy et al., 1972; Levy et al., 1988). It is not clear that tuberculosis is increased in prevalence in AS, despite initial reports (Dunham and Kautz, 1941; Campbell and Macdonald, 1965); empirical anti-tuberculous therapy is often instituted in AS, without confirmation by culture, because the radiological manifestations of lung involvement closely resemble those of tuberculosis (Hillerdal, 1983; Jessamine, 1968; editorial, 1971), and this led to an erroneous perception that tuberculosis might be responsible for the apical fibrocystic pulmonary disease of AS (Tanoue, 1992).

Respiratory mortality in AS is largely ascribable to secondary infection. In AS at large, parenchymal disease is the primary cause of death in less than 4% of fatal outcomes, whereas cardiovascular involvement is responsible for 35% of fatalities (Lehtinen, 1980). Mortality due to lung disease in AS has been reported in two contexts.

In AS patients treated with radiation for spinal disease, death from respiratory infection or other respiratory disease is 2.5 times higher than expected (Brown and Doll, 1965), whereas in patients not receiving radiotherapy, respiratory mortality is only 1.5 times higher than expected (Radford et al., 1977).

It has been argued that radiotherapy may predispose to subsequent pulmonary infection or bronchogenic carcinoma (Brown and Doll, 1965), but this hypothesis is contentious. It is equally possible that therapeutic radiotherapy and advanced lung involvement are both associated with prolonged severe AS and are linked for that reason, and not because of a causative relationship.

In the largest published series, severe pulmonary infection occurred only in patients with lung cavitation (Rosenow et al., 1977). Thus, for practical therapeutic purposes, the risk of a fatal respiratory outcome in AS can be viewed as largely restricted to this clinical context.

Therapeutic intervention in parenchymal disease is confined to infective complications. No treatment exists to retard the development of apical fibrosis; resistance to corticosteroid therapy is the rule (Hunninghake and Fauci, 1979; Boulware et al., 1985). Thus, in most patients, careful observation without treatment is appropriate, with specific antimicrobial therapy based upon organisms isolated in the context of symptomatic cavitatary disease. Due to the paucity of cases, it is inconceivable that intervention will ever be based on controlled data. It is usual to resort to the empirical administration of anti-bacterial or antifungal agents, given systemically or by intracavitary instillation. However, although medical treatment may be efficacious in invasive aspergillosis, it is seldom successful when cavities harbour *Aspergillus fumigatus* (Hunninghake and Fauci, 1979). For this reason, treatment of asymptomatic aspergilloma is generally unnecessary and futile. The greatest therapeutic dilemma is the patient with major haemoptysis, which is sometimes but not always controllable by medical treatment, bronchial artery embolisation or direct intracavitary instillation (Jewkes et al., 1983; Stiksa et al., 1976; Elliott et al., 1989; Hargis et al., 1980). There may be no option but to proceed to surgical resection of the cavity (usually by means of lobectomy) but this should be regarded as a treatment of last resort. There is an exceedingly high prevalence of up to 50% of post-operative bronchopleural fistula or empyema, and a high risk of a fatal outcome (Hunninghake and Fauci, 1979; Jewkes et al., 1983; Boushea and Sundstrom, 1989).

5. Marfan syndrome

MS is the inherited disorder of connective tissue constitute in which the respiratory system is most frequently involved. MS is an autosomal dominant disorder of variable penetrance, with 15% of cases resulting from spontaneous mutation. The prevalence of classic MS is approximately 5/100,000 (Pyeritz and McKusick, 1979), but with the inclusion of milder variants, the real prevalence is probably much higher. There is no predilection for race or gender. MS is characterised by abnormalities of fibrous connective tissue with abundant type I collagen, in association, in some cases, with mutations on chromosome 15 (Kainulainen et al., 1990). The most frequent sites of involvement are the skeleton (joint laxity long limbs, arachnodactyly, pectus excavatum, and kyphoscoliosis), eyes (subluxation of the lens, retinal detachment) and cardiovascular system (aortic or mitral regurgitation, aneurysm of the ascending aorta). The diagnosis is made when two of the four diagnostic criteria of Pyeritz and McKusick (1979) are present:

(1) positive family history
(2) skeletal abnormalities
(3) cardiovascular abnormalities
(4) ocular abnormalities.

Cardiovascular abnormalities are present in over 60% and are largely responsible for the reduced life expectancy of MS. No effective treatment exists to reverse disease or slow disease progression.

Pulmonary involvement in MS can be subdivided into extra-pulmonary (thoracic cage) abnormalities and parenchymal disease. As the lung has a high collagen content, it is somewhat surprising that pulmonary involvement in MS is relatively infrequent and seldom severe; pulmonary abnormalities are apparent in approximately 10–15% of MS patients (Dwyer and Troncale, 1965; Wood et al., 1984). In MS patients without major chest wall deformity or overt parenchymal disease, lung volumes are normal (Streeten et al., 1987; Fuleihan et al., 1963).

Thoracic cage involvement in MS, present in over 50% of patients (Pyeritz and McKusick, 1979), takes the form of pectus excavatum or scoliosis. Lung volumes, gas transfer and arterial gases are usually normal in isolated pectus excavatum (Weg et al., 1967). By contrast, severe scoliosis is generally associated with lung restriction; the functional effects of scoliosis in MS do not appear to differ from those of scoliosis in the general population (Pyeritz, 1985). However, nocturnal desaturation may amplify hypoxia in MS patients with scoliosis; increased upper airway collapsibility during sleep is common in MS and is probably responsible for an association between MS and obstructive sleep apnoea (Cistulli and Sullivan, 1995). This mechanism may also account for the development of fatal cor pulmonale in MS (Wanderman et al., 1975).

The most frequent *parenchymal abnormality* in MS, pneumothorax, has a prevalence of 5–10% (Wood et al., 1984; Hall et al., 1984), which is over a 100-fold higher than in the non-MS population. Pneumothoraces in MS are often recurrent and bilateral. The presenting features (pleuritic chest pain, dyspnoea, and, in tension pneumothoraces, haemodynamic compromise) are typical of pneumothorax in the general population but in MS, the differential diagnosis of dissection of the ascending aorta should not be forgotten. Pneumothoraces are likely to result from the rupture of sub-pleural bullae. In many MS patients with pneumothoraces, there is chest radiographic evidence of underlying emphysema (Wood et al., 1984; Hall et al., 1984). The long thin body habitus and consequent increases in mechanical stress in the lung apices of MS may be an additional predisposing factor, as observed in pneumothoraces in the general population.

Emphysema in MS, occurring in a small minority, is believed to result from the underlying connective tissue defect in some cases; in two series, alveolar elastic tissue was characterised by distorted and fragmented elastic fibres (Reye and Bale, 1973; Sayers et al., 1975). However, these abnormalities are not invariably present in MS patients with emphysema and it has been suggested that increased small airway collapsibility resulting from subtle abnormalities in the supporting tissue might lead to hyperinflation and emphysema (Bolande and Tucker, 1964). Generalised emphysema in non-smoking MS patients has been reported in adults and children and is sometimes fatal in early childhood (Dominguez et al., 1987). Localised bulla formation in the lung apices, which may be striking, has been reported in adults and children (Wood et al., 1984; Hall et al., 1984; Turner and Stanley, 1976).

Other pulmonary parenchymal abnormalities in MS are rare. Otherwise unexplained bilateral upper lobe pulmonary fibrosis has been described (Wood et al., 1984), and there are occasional reports of bronchiectasis, although it is not clear whether this results from the underlying connective tissue disease or is unrelated. Rare congenital pulmonary malformations associated with MS include absence of the right middle lobe and abnormal lobulation of the left lung (Dwyer and Troncale, 1965).

No medical treatment exists that reverses the pulmonary abnormalities of MS. Scuba-diving is contraindicated in patients with pulmonary parenchymal disease because of the risk of bullous rupture. Pneumothoraces should be treated as in the general population with pleurodesis and pleurectomy warranted if episodes are recurrent. Surgical intervention is seldom necessary for isolated pectus excavatum but may be required in severe scoliosis, on symptomatic grounds or in the setting of increasing lung restriction.

6. Summary

Mixed connective tissue disease

- Lung involvement should be characterised as most closely resembling the lung disease of SLE, SSc or PM/DM, as this approach gives the best guide as to prognosis and treatment.
- Interstitial lung disease is the most frequent complication and has a highly variable prognosis.
- Pulmonary vascular disease is less frequent but not uncommon, and is often lethal.

Relapsing polychondritis

- There is a frequent association with other autoimmune diseases, which should be detected and characterised.
- Respiratory tract disease is common and often severe. Symptoms and signs of stricture formation/airway laxity should be investigated urgently with CT and pulmonary function tests.

- All patients should be routinely staged and monitored for respiratory tract involvement using pulmonary function tests.

Ankylosing Spondylitis

- Extra-pulmonic restriction is frequently mild and though a restrictive ventilatory pattern may be present, exercise tolerance is rarely affected if patient stays active.
- Interstitial lung disease is rare and largely consists of fibro-bullous apical abnormalities.
- Secondary infection is the major determinant of a fatal respiratory outcome. Treatment of parenchymal disease should be aimed at infective complications only, as no treatment is effective at slowing rate of fibrosis.

Marfan syndrome

- Pectus excavatum and scoliosis are common. The former is generally benign. The latter may cause a restrictive pattern and can lead to fatal cor pulmonale.
- Pneumothorax is the only frequent parenchymal lung disorder.

References

Adliff, M., Ngato, D., Keshavjee, S., Brenaman, S., Granton, J.T. 1997. Treatment of diffuse tracheomalacia secondary to relapsing polychondritis with continuous positive airway pressure. Chest 112, 1701–1704.

Alpert, M.A., Goldberg, S.H., Singsen, B.H., Durham, J.B., Sharp, G.C., Ahmad, M., Madigan, N.P., Hurst, D.P., Sullivan, W.D. 1983. Cardiovascular manifestations of mixed connective tissue disease in adults. Circulation 68, 1182–1193.

Alpert, M.A., Pressly, T.A., Mukerji, V., Lambert, C.R., Mukerji, B., Panayiotou, H., Sharp, G.C. 1991. Acute and long-term effects of nifedipine on pulmonary and systemic hemodynamics in patients with pulmonary hypertension associated with diffuse systemic sclerosis, the CREST syndrome and mixed connective tissue disease. Am. J. Cardiol. 68, 1687–1691.

Alpert, M.A., Pressly, T.A., Mukerji, V., Lambert, C.R., Mukerji, B. 1992. Short- and long-term hemodynamic effects of captopril in patients with pulmonary hypertension and selected connective tissue disease. Chest 102, 1407–1412.

Alther, F. 1936. Uber einen fall von systematisierter chondromalacie. Virchows Archiv Pathological Anatomy and Histopathology 297, 445–479.

Amigues, J.M., Cantagrel, A., Abbal, M., Mazieres, B. 1996. Comparative study of 4 diagnosis criteria sets for mixed connective tissue disease in patients with anti-RNP antibodies. Autoimmunity Group of the Hospitals of Toulouse. J. Rheumatol. 23, 2055–2062.

Anonymous, 1971. The lungs in ankylosing spondylitis. Br. Med. J. 3, 492–493.

Appelrouth, D., Gottlieb, N.L. 1975. Pulmonary manifestations of ankylosing spondylitis. J. Rheumatol. 2, 446–453.

Arkin, C.R., Masi, A.T. 1975. Relapsing polychondritis: review of current status and case report. Semin. Arthritis Rheum. 5, 41–62.

Barranco, V.P., Minor, D.B., Soloman, H. 1976. Treatment of relapsing polychondritis with dapsone. Arch. Dermatol. 112, 1286–1288.

Behar, J.V., Choi, Y.W., Hartman, T.A., Allen, N.B., McAdams, H.P. 2002. Relapsing polychondritis affecting the lower respiratory tract. Am. J. Roentgenol. 178, 173–177

Beier, J.M., Nielsen, H.L., Nielsen, D. 1992. Pleuritis-pericarditis—an unusual initial manifestation of mixed connective tissue disease. Eur. Heart J. 13, 859–861.

Bolande, R.P., Tucker, A.S. 1964. Pulmonary emphysema and other cardiorespiratory lesions as part of the Marfan abiotrophy. Pediatrics 33, 356–366.

Boulware, D.W., Weissman, D.N., Doll, N.J. 1985. Pulmonary manifestations of the rheumatic diseases. Clin. Rev. Allergy 3, 249–267.

Bouros, D., Wells, A.U., Nicholson, A.G., Colby, T.V., Polychronopoulos, V., Pantelidis, P., Haslam, P.L., Vassilakis, D.A., Black, C.M., du Bois, R.M. 2002. Histopathologic subsets of fibrosing alveolitis in patients with systemic sclerosis and their relationship to outcome. Am. J. Respir. Crit. Care Med. 165, 1581–1586.

Boushea, D.K., Sundstrom, W.R. 1989. The pleuropulmonary manifestations of ankylosing spondylitis. Semin. Arthritis Rheum. 18, 277–281.

Brown, W.M., Doll, R. 1965. Mortality from cancer and other causes after radiotherapy for ankylosing spondylitis. Br. Med. J. 5474, 1327–1332.

Burlew, B.P., Lippton, H., Klinestiver, D., Haponik, E.J. 1992. Relapsing polychondritis: new pulmonary manifestations. J. La State Med. Soc. 144, 58–62.

Calin, A., Fries, J.F. 1975. Striking prevalence of ankylosing spondylitis in 'healthy' w27 positive males and females. N. Engl. J. Med. 293, 835–839.

Campbell, A.H., Macdonald, C.B. 1965. Upper lobe fibrosis associated with ankylosing spondylitis. Br. J. Dis. Chest 59, 90–101.

Chakera, T.M., Howarth, F.H., Kendall, M.J., Lawrence, D.S., Whitfield, A.G. 1975. The chest radiograph in ankylosing spondylitis. Clin. Radiol. 26, 455–459.

Cistulli, P.A., Sullivan, C.E. 1995. Sleep apnea in Marfan's syndrome. Increased upper airway collapsibility during sleep. Chest 108, 631–635.

Cohen, A.A., Natelson, E.A., Fechner, R.E. 1971. Fibrosing interstitial pneumonitis in ankylosing spondylitis. Chest 59, 369–371.

Davies, D. 1972. Ankylosing spondylitis and lung fibrosis. Q. J. Med. 41, 395–417.

Demedts, M. 1990. Pulmonary hypertension in connective tissue disease. Clin. Rheumatol. 9, 20–21.

Derderian, S.S., Tellis, C.J., Abbrecht, P.H., Welton, R.C., Rajagopal, K.R. 1985. Pulmonary involvement in mixed connective tissue disease. Chest 88, 45–48.

Dolan, D.L., Lemmon, G.B. Jr., Teitelbaum, S.L. 1966. Relapsing polychondritis. Analytical literature review and studies on pathogenesis. Am. J. Med. 41, 285–299.

Dominguez, R., Weisgrau, R.A., Santamaria, M. 1987. Pulmonary hyperinflation and emphysema in infants with the Marfan syndrome. Pediatr. Radiol. 17, 365–369.

Douglas, W.W., Tazelaar, H.D., Hartman, T.E., Hartman, R.P., Decker, P.A., Schroeder, D.R., Ryu, J.H. 2001. Polymyositis–dermatomyositis-associated interstitial lung disease. Am. J. Respir. Crit. Care Med. 164, 1182–1185.

Dunham, C., Kautz, F. 1941. Spondylarthritis ankylopoietica: a review and report of 20 cases. Am. J. Med. Sci 201, 232–250.

Dwyer, E.M. Jr., Troncale, F. 1965. Spontaneous pneumothorax and pulmonary disease in the Marfan syndrome. Report of two cases and review of the literature. Ann. Intern. Med. 62, 1285–1292.

Ebringer, R., Rook, G., Swana, G.T., Bottazzo, G.F., Doniach, D. 1981. Autoantibodies to cartilage and type II collagen in relapsing polychondritis and other rheumatic diseases. Ann. Rheum. Dis. 40, 473–479.

Elliott, J.A., Milne, L.J., Cumming, D. 1989. Chronic necrotising pulmonary aspergillosis treated with itraconazole. Thorax 44, 820–821.

Eng, J., Sabanathan, S. 1991. Airway complications in relapsing polychondritis. Ann. Thorac. Surg. 51, 686–692.

Enomoto, K., Takada, T., Suzuki, E., Ishida, T., Moriyama, H., Ooi, H., Hasegawa, T., Tsukada, H., Nakano, M., Gejyo, F. 2003. Bronchoalveolar lavage fluid cells in mixed connective tissue disease. Respirology 8, 149–156.

Fenlon, H.M., Casserly, I., Sant, S.M., Breatnach, E. 1997. Plain radiographs and thoracic high-resolution CT in patients with ankylosing spondylitis. Am. J. Roentgenol. 168, 1067–1072.

Foidart, J.M., Abe, S., Martin, G.R., Zizic, T.M., Barnett, E.V., Lawley, T.J., Katz, S.I. 1978. Antibodies to type II collagen in relapsing polychondritis. N. Engl. J. Med. 299, 1203–1207.

Fournie, B., Boutes, A., Dromer, C., Sixou, L., Le Guennec, P., Granel, J., Railhac, J.J. 1997. Prospective study of anterior chest wall involvement in ankylosing spondylitis and psoriatic arthritis. Rev. Rhum. Engl. Ed. 64, 22–25.

Franssen, M.J., van Herwaarden, C.L., van de Putte, L.B., Gribnau, F.W. 1986. Lung function in patients with ankylosing spondylitis. A study of the influence of disease activity and treatment with nonsteroidal antiinflammatory drugs. J. Rheumatol. 13, 936–940.

Fuleihan, F.J., Suh, S.K., Shepard, R.H. 1963. Some aspects of pulmonary function in the Marfan syndrome. Bull. Johns Hopkins Hosp. 113, 320–329.

Gacad, G., Hamosh, P. 1973. The lung in ankylosing spondylitis. Am. Rev. Respir. Dis. 107, 286–289.

Gendi, N.S., Welsh, K.I., van Venrooij, W.J., Vancheeswaran, R., Gilroy, J., Black, C.M. 1995. HLA type as a predictor of mixed connective tissue disease differentiation. Ten-year clinical and immunogenetic followup of 46 patients. Arthritis Rheum. 38, 259–266.

Germain, M.J., Davidman, M. 1984. Pulmonary hemorrhage and acute renal failure in a patient with mixed connective tissue disease. Am. J. Kidney Dis. 3, 420–424.

Gibson, G.J., Davis, P. 1974. Respiratory complications of relapsing polychondritis. Thorax 29, 726–731.

Ginsburg, W.W., Conn, D.L., Bunch, T.W., McDuffie, F.C. 1983. Comparison of clinical and serologic markers in systemic lupus erythematosus and overlap syndrome: a review of 247 patients. J. Rheumatol. 10, 235–241.

Graham, D.C., Smythe, H.A. 1958. The carditis and aortitis of ankylosing spondylitis. Bull. Rheum. Dis. 9, 171–174.

Hainaut, P., Lavenne, E., Magy, J.M., Lebacq, E.G. 1986. Circulating lupus type anticoagulant and pulmonary hypertension associated with mixed connective tissue disease. Clin. Rheumatol. 5, 96–101.

Hall, J.R., Pyeritz, R.E., Dudgeon, D.L., Haller, J.A. Jr. 1984. Pneumothorax in the Marfan syndrome: prevalence and therapy. Ann. Thorac. Surg. 37, 500–504.

Hargis, J.L., Bone, R.C., Stewart, J., Rector, N., Hiller, F.C. 1980. Intracavitary amphotereicin B in the treatment of symptomatic pulmonary aspergillomas. Am. J. Med. 68, 389–394.

Higenbottam, T., Dixon, J. 1979. Chondritis associated with fatal intramural bronchial fibrosis. Thorax 34, 563–564.

Hillerdal, G. 1983. Ankylosing spondylitis lung disease—an underdiagnosed entity? Eur. J. Respir. Dis. 64, 437–441.

Hoogsteden, H.C., van Dongen, J.J., van der Kwast, T.H., Hooijkaas, H., Hilvering, C. 1985. Bilateral exudative pleuritis, an unusual pulmonary onset of mixed connective tissue disease. Respiration 48, 164–167.

Hosoda, Y., Suzuki, Y., Takano, M., Tojo, T., Homma, M. 1987. Mixed connective tissue disease with pulmonary hypertension:a clinical and pathological study. J. Rheumatol. 14, 826–830.

Hunninghake, G.W., Fauci, A.S. 1979. Pulmonary involvement in the collagen vascular diseases. Am. Rev. Respir. Dis. 119, 471–503.

Isaak, B.L., Liesegang, T.J., Michet, C.J. Jr. 1986. Ocular and systemic findings in relapsing polychondritis. Ophthalmology 93, 681–689.

Izumiyama, T., Hida, W., Ichinose, M., Inoue, H., Takishima, T., Okazaki, T., Shirato, K. 1993. Small airway involvement in mixed connective tissue disease. Tohoku J. Exp. Med. 170, 273–283.

Jaksch-Wartenhorst, R. 1923. Polychondropathia. Wien. Arch. Int. Med. 6, 93–100.

Jeandel, P., Bonnet, D., Chouc, P.Y., Molinier, S., Raphenon, G., Martet, G., Merouze, F., de Muizon, H. 1994. Demonstration of subclinical pulmonary alveolitis in spondylarthropathies. Rev. Rhum. Ed. Fr. 61, 301–309.

Jessamine, A.G. 1968. Upper lung lobe fibrosis in ankylosing spondylitis. Can. Med. Assoc. J. 98, 25–29.

Jewkes, J., Kay, P.H., Paneth, M., Citron, K.M. 1983. Pulmonary aspergilloma: analysis of prognosis in relation to haemoptysis and survey of treatment. Thorax 38, 572–578.

Kainulainen, K., Pulkkinen, L., Savolainen, A., Kaitila, I., Peltonen, L. 1990. Location on chromosome 15 of the gene defect causing Marfan syndrome. N. Engl. J. Med. 323, 935–939.

Kallenberg, C.G. 1993. Overlapping syndromes, undifferentiated connective tissue disease, and other fibrosing conditions. Curr. Opin. Rheumatol. 5, 809–815.

Kaye, R.L., Sones, D.A. 1964. Relapsing polychondritis. Clinical and pathologic features in fourteen cases. Ann. Intern. Med. 60, 653–664.

Kennedy, W.P., Milne, L.J., Blyth, W., Crompton, G.K. 1972. Two unusual organisms, *Aspergillus terreus* and *Metschnikowia pulcherrima*, associated with the lung disease of ankylosing spondylitis. Thorax 27, 604–610.

Kentala, E., Repo, U.K., Lehtipuu, A.L., Vuornos, T. 1978. HLA-antigens and pulmonary upper lobe fibrocystic changes with and without ankylosing spondylitis. A report of seven cases. Scand. J. Respir. Dis. 59, 8–12.

Kenyon, K.W., Nappi, J.M. 2003. Bosentan for the treatment of pulmonary arterial hypertension. Ann. Pharmacother. 37, 1055–1062.

Kilman, W.J. 1978. Narrowing of the airway in relapsing polychondritis. Radiology 126, 373–376.

King, T. 1998. In: M.I. Schwarz, T. King (Eds.), Interstitial Lung Disease. BC Decker Inc., Hamilton, London, pp. 451–505.

Kiris, A., Ozgocmen, S., Kocakoc, E., Ardicoglu, O., Ogur, E. 2003. Lung findings on high resolution CT in early ankylosing spondylitis. Eur. J. Radiol. 47, 71–76.

Kozuka, T., Johkoh, T., Honda, O., Mihara, N., Koyama, M., Tomiyama, N., Hamada, S., Nakamura, H., Ichikado, K. 2001. Pulmonary involvement in mixed connective tissue disease: high-resolution CT findings in 41 patients. J. Thorac. Imag. 16, 94–98.

Krell, W.S., Staats, B.A., Hyatt, R.E. 1986. Pulmonary function in relapsing polychondritis. Am. Rev. Respir. Dis. 133, 1120–1123.

LaBresh, K.A., Lally, E.V., Sharma, S.C., Ho, G. Jr. 1985. Two-dimensional echocardiographic detection of preclinical aortic root abnormalities in rheumatoid variant diseases. Am. J. Med. 78, 908–912.

Lang, B., Rothenfusser, A., Lanchbury, J.S., Rauh, G., Breedveld, F.C., Urlacher, A., Albert, E.D., Peter, H.H., Melchers, I. 1993. Susceptibility to relapsing polychondritis is associated with HLA-DR4. Arthritis Rheum. 36, 660–664.

Latsi, P.I., Wells, A.U. 2003. Evaluation and management of alveolitis and interstitial lung disease in scleroderma. Curr. Opin. Rheumatol. 15, 748–755.

Lee-Chiong, T.L. Jr. 1998. Pulmonary manifestations of ankylosing spondylitis and relapsing polychondritis. Clin. Chest Med. 19, ix, 747–757.

Lehtinen, K. 1980. Cause of death in 79 patients with ankylosing spondylitis. Scand. J. Rheumatol. 9, 145–147.

Letko, E., Zafirakis, P., Baltatzis, S., Voudouri, A., Livir-Rallatos, C., Foster, C.S. 2002. Relapsing polychondritis: a clinical review. Semin. Arthritis Rheum. 31, 384–395.

Levy, H., Hurwitz, M.D., Strimling, M., Zwi, S. 1988. Ankylosing spondylitis lung disease and Mycobacterium scrofulaceum. Br. J. Dis. Chest 82, 84–87.

Luthra, H. 1988. In: J. Klippel, P. Dieppe (Eds.), Rheumatology, vol. 27. Mosby, St Louis, pp. 1–4.

Maddison, P.J. 1991. Overlap syndromes and mixed connective tissue disease. Curr. Opin. Rheumatol. 3, 995–1000.

Mahindrakar, N.H., Libman, L.J. 1970. Relapsing polychondritis. J. Laryngol. Otol. 84, 337–342.

Martyn, J.B., Wong, M.J., Huang, S.H. 1988. Pulmonary and neuromuscular complications of mixed connective tissue disease: a report and review of the literature. J. Rheumatol. 15, 703–705.

Matoba, A., Plager, S., Barber, J., McCulley, J.P. 1984. Keratitis in relapsing polychondritis. Ann. Ophthalmol. 16, 367–370.

McAdam, L.P., O'Hanlan, M.A., Bluestone, R., Pearson, C.M. 1976. Relapsing polychondritis: prospective study of 23 patients and a review of the literature. Medicine (Baltimore) 55, 193–215.

Michet, C.J. Jr., McKenna, C.H., Luthra, H.S., O'Fallon, W.M. 1986. Relapsing polychondritis. Survival and predictive role of early disease manifestations. Ann. Intern. Med. 104, 74–78.

Mohsenifar, Z., Tashkin, D.P., Carson, S.A., Bellamy, P.E. 1982. Pulmonary function in patients with relapsing polychondritis. Chest 81, 711–717.

Montgomery, W.W. 1965. T-tube tracheal stent. Arch. Otolaryngol. 82, 320–321.

Parkin, A., Robinson, P.J., Hickling, P. 1982. Regional lung ventilation in ankylosing spondylitis. Br. J. Radiol. 55, 833–836.

Pearson, C.M., Kline, H.M., Newcomer, V.D. 1960. Relapsing polychondritis. N. Engl. J. Med. 263, 51–58.

Prakash, U.B. 1992. Lungs in mixed connective tissue disease. J. Thorac. Imag. 7, 55–61.

Prakash, U.B. 1998. Respiratory complications in mixed connective tissue disease. Clin. Chest Med. 19, ix, 733–746.

Prakash, U.B., Luthra, H.S., Divertie, M.B. 1985. Intrathoracic manifestations in mixed connective tissue disease. Mayo Clin. Proc. 60, 813–821.

Pyeritz, R.E. 1985. Connective tissue in the lung: lessons from the Marfan syndrome. Ann. Intern. Med. 103, 289–290.

Pyeritz, R.E., McKusick, V.A. 1979. The Marfan syndrome: diagnosis and management. N. Engl. J. Med. 300, 772–777.

Radford, E.P., Doll, R., Smith, P.G. 1977. Mortality among patients with ankylosing spondylitis not given X-ray therapy. N. Engl. J. Med. 297, 572–576.

Repo, U.K., Kentala, E., Koistinen, J., Lehtipuu, A.L., Miettinen, A., Pyrhonen, S., Tiilikainen, A., Vuornos, T. 1981. Pulmonary apical fibrocystic disease. A serologic study. Eur. J. Respir. Dis. 62, 46–55.

Reye, R.D., Bale, P.M. 1973. Elastic tissue in pulmonary emphysema in Marfan syndrome. Arch. Pathol. 96, 427–431.

Richard, P., Sabouret, P., Vayre, F., Desrame, J., Ollivier, J.P. 1996. Pleuropericarditis complicated of tamponade disclosing mixed connective tissue disease. Remission with non-steroidal anti-inflammatory agents. Apropos of a case. Ann. Cardiol. Angeiol. (Paris) 45, 513–515.

Ridgway, H.B., Hansotia, P.L., Schorr, W.F. 1979. Relapsing polychondritis: unusual neurological findings and therapeutic efficacy of dapsone. Arch. Dermatol. 115, 43–45.

Rosenow, E., Strimlan, C.V., Muhm, J.R., Ferguson, R.H. 1977. Pleuropulmonary manifestations of ankylosing spondylitis. Mayo Clin. Proc. 52, 641–649.

Rumancik, W.M., Firooznia, H., Davis, M.S. Jr., Leitman, B.S., Golimbu, C., Rafii, M., McCauley, D.I. 1984. Fibrobullous disease of the upper lobes: an extraskeletal manifestation of ankylosing spondylitis. J. Comput. Tomogr. 8, 225–229.

Sanchez-Guerrero, J., Cesarman, G., Alarcon-Segovia, D. 1989. Massive pulmonary hemorrhage in mixed connective tissue diseases. J. Rheumatol. 16, 1132–1134.

Sayers, C.P., Goltz, R.W., Mottiaz, J. 1975. Pulmonary elastic tissue in generalized elastolysis (cutis laxa) and Marfan's syndrome: a light and electron microscopic study. J. Invest. Dermatol. 65, 451–457.

Schlosstein, L., Terasaki, P.I., Bluestone, R., Pearson, C.M. 1973. High association of an HL-A antigen, W27, with ankylosing spondylitis. N. Engl. J. Med. 288, 704–706.

Seckin, U., Bolukbasi, N., Gursel, G., Eroz, S., Sepici, V., Ekim, N. 2000. Relationship between pulmonary function and exercise tolerance in patients with ankylosing spondylitis. Clin. Exp. Rheumatol. 18, 503–506.

Senocak, O., Manisali, M., Ozaksoy, D., Sevinc, C., Akalin, E. 2003. Lung parenchyma changes in ankylosing spondylitis: demonstration with high resolution CT and correlation with disease duration. Eur. J. Radiol. 45, 117–122.

Shah, R., Sabanathan, S., Mearns, A.J., Featherstone, H. 1995. Self-expanding tracheobronchial stents in the management of major airway problems. J. Cardiovasc. Surg. (Torino) 36, 343–348.

Sharp, G.C., Anderson, P.C. 1980. Current concepts in the classification of connective tissue diseases. Overlap syndromes and mixed connective tissue disease (MCTD). J. Am. Acad. Dermatol. 2, 269–279.

Sharp, G.C., Irvin, W.S., Tan, E.M., Gould, R.G., Holman, H.R. 1972. Mixed connective tissue disease—an apparently distinct rheumatic disease syndrome associated with a specific antibody to an extractable nuclear antigen (ENA). Am. J. Med. 52, 148–159.

Small, P., Black, M., Davidman, M., de Champlain, M.L., Kapusta, M.A., Kreisman, H. 1980. Wegener's granulomatosis and relapsing polychondritis: a case report. J. Rheumatol. 7, 915–918.

Spraggs, P.D., Tostevin, P.M., Howard, D.J. 1997. Management of laryngotracheobronchial sequelae and complications of relapsing polychondritis. Laryngoscope 107, 936–941.

Stewart, R.M., Ridyard, J.B., Pearson, J.D. 1976. Regional lung function in ankylosing spondylitis. Thorax 31, 433–437.

Stiksa, G., Eklundh, G., Riebe, I., Simonsson, B.G. 1976. Bilateral pulmonary aspergilloma in ankylosing spondylitis treated with transthoracic intracavitary instillations of antifungal agents. Scand. J. Respir. Dis. 57, 163–170.

Strange, C., Bolster, M., Mazur, J., Taylor, M., Gossage, J.R., Silver, R. 2000. Hemodynamic effects of epoprostenol in patients with systemic sclerosis and pulmonary hypertension. Chest 118, 1077–1082.

Streeten, E.A., Murphy, E.A., Pyeritz, R.E. 1987. Pulmonary function in the Marfan syndrome. Chest 91, 408–412.

Sullivan, W.D., Hurst, D.J., Harmon, C.E., Esther, J.H., Agia, G.A., Maltby, J.D., Lillard, S.B., Held, C.N., Wolfe, J.F., Sunderrajan, E.V., et al. 1984. A prospective evaluation emphasizing pulmonary involvement in patients with mixed connective tissue disease. Medicine (Baltimore) 63, 92–107.

Tanoue, L.T. 1992. Pulmonary involvement in collagen vascular disease: a review of the pulmonary manifestations of the Marfan syndrome, ankylosing spondylitis, Sjogren's syndrome, and relapsing polychondritis. J. Thorac. Imag. 7, 62–77.

Trentham, D.E., Le, C.H. 1998. Relapsing polychondritis. Ann. Intern. Med. 129, 114–122.

Turetschek, K., Ebner, W., Fleischmann, D., Wunderbaldinger, P., Erlacher, L., Zontsich, T., Bankier, A.A. 2000. Early pulmonary involvement in ankylosing spondylitis: assessment with thin-section CT. Clin. Radiol. 55, 632–636.

Turner, J.A., Stanley, N.N. 1976. Fragile lung in the Marfan syndrome. Thorax 31, 771–775.

Ueda, N., Mimura, K., Maeda, H., Sugiyama, T., Kado, T., Kobayashi, K., Fukuzaki, H. 1984. Mixed connective tissue disease with fatal pulmonary hypertension and a review of literature. Virchows Arch. A Pathol. Anat. Histopathol. 404, 335–340.

van den Hoogen, F.H., Spronk, P.E., Boerbooms, A.M., Bootsma, H., de Rooij, D.J., Kallenberg, C.G., van de Putte, L.B. 1994. Long-term follow-up of 46 patients with anti-(U1)snRNP antibodies. Br. J. Rheumatol. 33, 1117–1120.

Venables, P. 1998. In: J.H. Klippel, P. Dieppe (Eds.), Rheumatology. Mosby, London, pp. 33.1–33.8.

Wallaert, B., Dugas, M., Dansin, E., Perez, T., Marquette, C.H., Ramon, P., Tonnel, A.B., Voisin, C. 1990. Subclinical alveolitis in immunological systemic disorders. Transition between health and disease? Eur. Respir. J. 3, 1206–1216.

Wanderman, K.L., Goldstein, M.S., Faber, J. 1975. Letter: cor pulmonale secondary to severe kyphoscoliosis in Marfan's syndrome. Chest 67, 250–251.

Webb, W.R., Gamsu, G. 1981. Cavitary pulmonary nodules with systemic lupus erythematosus: differential diagnosis. Am. J. Roentgenol. 136, 27–31.

Weg, J.G., Krumholz, R.A., Harkleroad, L.E. 1967. Pulmonary dysfunction in pectus excavatum. Am. Rev. Respir. Dis. 96, 936–945.

Wiener-Kronish, J.P., Solinger, A.M., Warnock, M.L., Churg, A., Ordonez, N., Golden, J.A. 1981. Severe pulmonary involvement in mixed connective tissue disease. Am. Rev. Respir. Dis. 124, 499–503.

Wood, J.R., Bellamy, D., Child, A.H., Citron, K.M. 1984. Pulmonary disease in patients with Marfan syndrome. Thorax 39, 780–784.

Zeuner, M., Straub, R.H., Rauh, G., Albert, E.D., Scholmerich, J., Lang, B. 1997. Relapsing polychondritis: clinical and immunogenetic analysis of 62 patients. J. Rheumatol. 24, 96–101.

Zorab, P. 1962. The lungs in ankylosing spondylitis. Q. J. Med. 31, 267–280.

PART VI

Drug-Induced Respiratory Disease

Handbook of Systemic Autoimmune Diseases, Volume 2
Pulmonary Involvement in Systemic Autoimmune Diseases
A.U. Wells and C.P. Denton, editors

CHAPTER 13

Drug-Induced Respiratory Disease in Connective Tissue Diseases

Philippe Camus

Department of Pulmonary and Intensive Care, University Medical Center Le Bocage and Medical School, Université de Bourgogne, F-21034 Dijon, France

1. Introduction

Approximately 350 drugs can cause respiratory injury (http://www.pneumotox.com, 1997), and the list of drugs and patterns of involvement continues to increase inexorably (http://www.pneumotox.com, 1997). Drug-induced lung diseases (DILDs) vary in severity from mild to life threatening. Generally, DILDs subside upon drug discontinuance, and leave permanent sequelae in a minority of patients. Less frequently, DILDs persist unabated, or progress despite drug withdrawal, requiring specific management.

The classic drugs used to treat connective tissue disease (CTD) and related autoimmune conditions, i.e. aspirin, other nonsteroidal antiinflammatory drugs (NSAIDs), azathioprine, chlorambucil, colchicine, cyclophosphamide, gold, methotrexate, minocycline, D-penicillamine and sulfasalazine, have long been known to produce lung injury (White and Ward, 1985; Cannon, 1990; Zitnik and Cooper, 1990; Cannon, 1997; Roux and Zitnik, 1997; Tomioka and King, 1997; http://www.pneumotox.com, 1997; Libby and White, 1998). Novel agents now available to treat CTD also can cause distinct toxic or hypersensitivity pulmonary or systemic reactions (Libby and White, 1998; http://www.pneumotox.com, 1997; Loorand- Stiver and Murty, 2002). Novel treatment strategies proposed in the treatment of CTD have changed the profile of adverse pulmonary reactions to drugs: methotrexate pneumonitis and adverse effects of anti-TNF agents or interferons have become more common, while the adverse reactions to penicillamine and gold have become increasingly infrequent.

Diagnosing DILD in CTD is an increasingly complex exercise. Patients may be exposed to more than one drug causing adverse pulmonary reactions, and drugs can cause more than one pattern of injury (http://www.pneumotox.com, 1997). Response to drug withdrawal is not always convincing (Persoz et al., 2001), and corticosteroids may complicate the evaluation of drug dechallenge. The background disease can involve the lung in a manner (Dawson et al., 2002; Freemer and King, 2003) and with an incidence rate (Thomeer et al., 2001a,b) similar to that of DILD. Conversely, the pattern of injury produced by drugs can mimic the pulmonary involvement of naturally occurring CTD, and drugs can produce systemic conditions (Choi et al., 2000a). Lastly, several of the drugs used to treat CTD (e.g. azathioprine, corticosteroids, cyclophosphamide, etanercept, infliximab, leflunomide and methotrexate) are immunosuppressive agents, and exposure to these agents increases the risk of developing opportunistic pulmonary infections (Lionakis and Kontoyiannis, 2003; Metzler et al., 2004; White, 2004). The combined effect of background disease (Ward and Donald, 1999), type of drug (especially corticosteroids, cyclophosphamide and methotrexate) (White, 2004), dosage or timing of drugs (high-dose induction vs. low-dose maintenance therapy) (Koselj-Kajtna et al., 2002), as well as

E-mail address: philippe.camus@chu-dijon.fr (P. Camus).

DOI: 10.1016/S1571-5078(04)02013-6

country of residence (for instance as regards background rates of tuberculosis, or the risk of airborne diseases such as histoplasmosis), may impose distinct risks of opportunistic infections in CTD. Drug-induced opportunistic infections remain a strong competing diagnosis, as DILDs are notoriously difficult to reliably differentiate from an infection (Lewis et al., 1978; Logan et al., 1995; Cleverley et al., 2002). Iatrogenic infections have been reviewed elsewhere (Min and Monaco, 1991; Libby and White, 1998; Hill et al., 1999; Starzl, 1999a,b; Rolston, 2001; Lionakis and Kontoyiannis, 2003; White, 2004), and are not covered here in great detail.

This chapter discusses respiratory and systemic disease induced by drugs used in CTD, including drugs used to treat the complications of CTD, and other drugs commonly used in the age range of such patients (e.g. amiodarone, oral anticoagulants, anticonvulsants, angiotensin converting enzyme inhibitors (ACEI) and diuretic drugs) (http://www.pneumotox.com, 1997).

2. Diagnostic criteria

Criteria for the diagnosis of drug-induced respiratory disease include (Irey, 1976b; Camus, 2003; Flieder and Travis, 2004) the following:

(1) *Correct identification of the drug*. This requires a meticulous drug history, including dose and duration of treatment, and exposure to over-the-counter medications (Ashar et al., 2003), illicit drugs, dietary compounds (Drazen, 2003), home-made products (Gaine et al., 2000), herbs (Ernst, 1998; Kessler, 2000; Matsushima et al., 2002; Samenuk et al., 2002; Adachi et al., 2003) and odd substances (Yel et al., 2004), the innocuity of which is seriously challenged (Egermayer, 2000; Matsushima et al., 2002; Samenuk et al., 2002; Adachi et al., 2003; Ashar et al., 2003; Kanda et al., 2003; Lontos et al., 2003; Yoshida, 2003).

(2) *Temporal eligibility*. Time from the beginning of treatment to onset of the reaction (also called the latency period) varies from a few seconds or minutes in drug-induced anaphylaxis or asthma attacks, to months or years in treatment with anticonvulsants, cyclophosphamide, gold, methotrexate and other drugs. The shorter the latency period, the easier the recognition of the drug etiology.

(3) *Singularity of drug*. Patients with CTD are often exposed to several potentially pneumotoxic drugs (e.g. combined treatments with multiple disease-modifying drugs in patients with rheumatoid arthritis (RA)), and this creates confusion about which drug is responsible for the pulmonary reaction. However, weighing the respective responsibility of each drug is critical to enable selective drug withdrawal, which minimizes the risk of relapse of the background disease. A rough estimate of the incidence of adverse effects from a particular drug is given by the number of reports in the literature (http://www.pneumotox.com, 1997).

(4) *Characteristic clinical imaging and physiologic pattern of the reaction to the specific drug*. Many drug reactions are associated with a distinctive imaging pattern (Padley et al., 1992; Taylor, 1990; Kuhlman, 1991; Ellis et al., 2000; Rossi et al., 2000; Collins, 2001; Cleverley et al., 2002; Erasmus et al., 2002a,b; Camus and Gibson, 2003; Camus, 2003; Lindell and Hartman, 2004), and this enables easier recognition of the drug condition. High-resolution CT (HRCT) is more sensitive than plain chest radiograph in the detection of mild or early drug-induced involvement (Padley et al., 1992; Siniakowicz et al., 2001), and can be used to chose the area of biopsy.

(5) *Characteristic histopathological pattern of reaction to the specific drug*. A lung biopsy is necessary in a small subset of patients suspect of having DILD, and a risk-benefit evaluation is not available (Malhorta et al., 2003). If appropriately sampled and processed, the lung biopsy will exclude the presence of underlying disease or infection, and determine whether the pulmonary reaction is appropriate for a particular drug (Walker-Smith, 1990; Pietra, 1991; Colby et al., 1991; Flieder and Travis, 2004).

(6) *Exclusion of other causes for the lung disease*. This is a difficult exercise, especially in patients with infiltrative lung disease (ILD), because drugs and the background disease can produce similar imaging-pathologic patterns of parenchymal involvement (Prakash, 1984; Murin et al., 1998; Primack and Muller, 1998; Schwarz, 1998; Sullivan and

Hoffman, 1998; Tanoue, 1998; Mayberry et al., 2000; Franquet, 2001; Freemer and King, 2003). Adequate sampling of blood and lung fluids should be performed to exclude an infection (Shelhamer et al., 1996).

(7) *Remission of signs and symptoms with removal of the drug*. Ideally, all signs and symptoms should clear after drug withdrawal. Where possible, corticosteroids should not be given, to better evaluate the effects of drug dechallenge. However, patients with fulminant ILD may not improve after removal of the drug (Lévy et al., 1997), and also drug-induced fibrotic conditions (e.g. pulmonary or pleural fibrosis, pulmonary hypertension, *bronchiolitis obliterans* (BO)) do not generally respond convincingly to drug discontinuance.

(8) *Quantification of drug levels in blood or lung tissue*. This may be necessary to confirm adverse reactions resulting from drug overdose (Irey, 1976a; Heffner and Sahn, 1981; Merigian and Blaho, 1995).

(9) *In vitro tests*. In vitro tests of monocyte migration, or proliferation and transformation of lymphocytes harvested in peripheral blood or, less often, bronchoalveolar lavage (BAL) have been used (Ripps and Fellner, 1966; Vischer, 1966; Sarkany, 1967; Denman and Denman, 1968; Walzer et al., 1972; Pearsall et al., 1974; Houwerzijl et al., 1977; Pirmohamed et al., 1991; Hertl et al., 1995; Mauri- Hellweg et al., 1995; Bentur et al., 1997; Schreiber et al., 1999; Adkinson et al., 2002; Pichler, 2003). Cytotoxicity and proliferative assays in the presence of the drug, or the drug and a metabolic activating system, have yielded positive results in patients with adverse skin reactions (Hertl et al., 1995). However, the lack of standardization of these tests, coupled to difficulties inherent to the rarity and diversity of adverse reactions to drugs, has not yet yielded consistent results. Also these tests may lack sensitivity (Drory and Korczyn, 1993).

(10) *Recurrence with rechallenge*. Recurrence with rechallenge is central to the diagnosis of DILD, but seldom is performed intentionally, as pulmonary reactions of increased severity and death may ensue (Kremer et al., 1997). This raises evident safety and ethical issues, and many will recommend against deliberate re-exposure, inasmuch as authentic DILD may not relapse after rechallenge (Fehr et al., 2003). Rechallenge with increasing amounts of a vital drug with the purpose of desensitization can be contemplated (Shepherd, 2003).

3. Patterns of respiratory involvement caused by drugs used to treat CTD

3.1. Infiltrative lung diseases

Drug-induced ILD (DI-ILD) is a group of conditions characterized by dyspnea, pulmonary infiltrates on chest film and HRCT (Akira et al., 2002; Erasmus et al., 2002a,b; Lindell and Hartman, 2004), a physiology of low lung volumes, hypoxemia, derangements of BAL cell populations, and inflammation and fibrosis in variable proportions on lung histology. Patients with DI-ILD present with the signs and symptoms of cough, dyspnea and, often, fever. The diagnosis is suggested on imaging (Ansell, 1969; Kormano, 1974; Morrison and Goldman, 1979; Bargon, 1984; Taylor, 1990; Kuhlman, 1991; Ellis et al., 2000; Rossi et al., 2000; Cleverley et al., 2002; Erasmus et al., 2002a,b; Lindell and Hartman, 2004), and is supported by BAL, drug dechallenge and, in some patients, a lung biopsy (Flieder and Travis, 2004). Disease severity ranges from simple pulmonary infiltrates and an asymptomatic state to diffuse consolidation with acute respiratory failure, or an ARDS picture (Akira et al., 2002). Obliteration of the airspaces by the pathologic process of cellular interstitial-, eosinophilic- and organizing pneumonia, and the associated features of diffuse alveolar damage (DAD) or alveolar hemorrhage, characterize those cases with severe involvement.

It is at times difficult to separate DI-ILD from ILD resulting from the background CTD, and imaging does not always aid in this distinction (Logan et al., 1995). There is, however, a tendency for pulmonary manifestations of the background disease to slowly progress with time, except those in *lupus erythematosus*, whereas the pulmonary manifestations of DI-ILD have a more protracted course, and are generally reversible.

3.1.1. Nonspecific, or cellular, interstitial pneumonia

Drug-induced nonspecific interstitial pneumonia, also called cellular interstitial pneumonia, alveolitis or hypersensitivity pneumonitis, is a common pattern of drug-induced pulmonary involvement. Drugs causing the syndrome in patients with CTD include azathioprine, chlorambucil, chrysotherapy, cyclophosphamide, interferon alpha and beta, possibly leflunomide, methotrexate, penicillamine and propylthiouracil (http://www.pneumotox.com, 1997); Loorand-Stiver and Murty, 2002 #18638]. Many drugs used outside the context of CTD (e.g. nitrofurantoin) also produce the condition (http://www.pneumotox.com, 1997; Camus, 2003).

Time to onset is from a few days to years into treatment and is unpredictable, except perhaps for gold-induced lung disease, which generally occurs within the first 6 months of treatment (Tomioka and King, 1997). Onset of the disease is progressive over a few weeks, or abrupt, especially in patients with methotrexate lung. Signs and symptoms include increasing dyspnea, a dry cough, high fevers and sometimes a skin rash. Changes in liver chemistry are thought to reflect concomitant liver toxicity (Gomez et al., 1992; Yalçin et al., 1997). The spectrum of severity ranges from mild symptoms and ill-defined pulmonary opacities to extensive consolidation and respiratory failure, especially with the use of gold or methotrexate (Tomioka and King, 1997; Imokawa et al., 2000). Radiographic studies indicate bilateral, approximately symmetrical, interstitial or alveolar opacities. A miliary pattern has been reported in a few patients with the use of chrysotherapy, methotrexate and sirolimus. The infiltrates may localize in the lung bases or mid-lung zones, or be diffuse, and the radiographic density can be discrete haze, ground-glass, or dense bilateral consolidation with air bronchograms and volume loss. Pleural effusions and mediastinal lymphadenopathy are occasional findings. The CT examination can show thickening of interlobular or intralobular septa, a crazy-paving-, ground-glass-, or mosaic pattern, and in cases with extensive disease, patchy or diffuse dense alveolar shadowing. Restrictive ventilatory impairment and hypoxemia correlate with the extent of radiographic involvement (Akira et al., 2002). The diffusing capacity may be lower in DI-ILD than in ILD of other causes (Thomeer et al., 2001a). In azathioprine pneumonitis, a restrictive physiology and hypoxemia can coexist with limited radiographic changes (Rubin et al., 1972).

Fiberoptic bronchoscopy and BAL are indicated. Appropriate stains, cultures and molecular techniques should be negative in BAL and other fluids to exclude an opportunistic infection (Shelhamer et al., 1996). The BAL usually shows a lymphocyte predominance. The contribution of lymphocyte typing is unclear, because increases in CD4+ or in CD8+ subsets have been observed (Akoun et al., 1986; White et al., 1989; Salaffi et al., 1997; Fuhrman et al., 2001). A very low ratio of CD4+ to CD8+ lymphocytes is suggestive, but not specific for the drug etiology. Other BAL findings include a neutrophilia, or a combined pattern of lymphocytosis with neutrophilia or eosinophilia (Pfitzenmeyer et al., 1992; Leduc et al., 1993; Costabel et al., 2004).

A lung biopsy may be required in selected cases. The main histologic features include mild to extensive interstitial inflammation (Myers, 1993). Pulmonary granulomas have been described with etanercept, interferons and methotrexate (Imokawa et al., 2000) (in addition to intracavitary BCG used to treat bladder carcinoma (Mooren et al., 2000; Schattner et al., 2002)). Interstitial fibrosis may also be seen, but is not the dominant histopathological feature (Imokawa et al., 2000; Tomioka and King, 1997). The distinctive pattern of desquamative interstitial pneumonia suggests exposure to nitrofurantoin (Bone et al., 1976). Alveolar edema or hemorrhage may be found as a manifestation of severe pneumonitis from gold (Noseworthy et al., 1983), methotrexate (Lisbona et al., 1973), or nitrofurantoin (Bucknall et al., 1987).

Overall, the prognosis of cellular drug-induced pneumonitis is good. High-dose corticosteroids are recommended in patients with acute respiratory failure although in some, the disease can subside after simple drug withdrawal (Berkani et al., 2003). Fatalities have been reported in patients with severe gold or methotrexate lung (Tomioka and King, 1997; Imokawa et al., 2000), in patients who were not given corticosteroids in time (Smith et al., 1993), and in a sizable fraction of those who were rechallenged with the drug (Kremer et al., 1997). Irreversible lung fibrosis following recognition and treatment of this problem is unusual (van der Veen et al., 1995). Patients should be properly instructed to avoid inadvertent reexposure to the drug, or to structurally or pharmacologically related compounds. Rechallenge with the drug will often lead to relapse, and is not generally recommended because of risks inherent with the procedure (Kremer et al., 1997).

3.1.2. Pulmonary infiltrates and eosinophilia

Pulmonary infiltrates and eosinophilia (PIE), also known as eosinophilic pneumonia, can be caused by multiple chemically-unrelated drugs (http://www.pneumotox.com, 1997). The disease was first reported in the 1940s in patients exposed to sulfonamides (Ellis and McKinlay, 1941), and there was a concern that sulfone drugs might cause systemic vasculitis and *polyarteritis nodosa* (Rich, 1942). Many sulfone antibiotic and non-antibiotic drugs (e.g. chlorothiazide, chlorpropamide, dapsone, furosemide, sulfasalazine), as well as sulfa drugs (sulfadiazine, sulfamethoxazole), are still in use today, and can cause systemic and pulmonary adverse reactions (van der Klauw et al., 1996; Oshitani et al., 1998; Russian and Levine, 2001; Strom et al., 2003; Dominguez-Ortega et al., 2003). Most members of certain drug *classes* (e.g. antibiotics, antidepressants, ACEI and NSAIDs) cause PIE. Drugs causing PIE in patients with CTD and allied conditions include antidepressants (amitriptylline, clomipramine, maprotilin, sertraline, trazodone and venlafaxine), aspirin and other NSAIDs, carbamazepine, chloroquine, interferon, mesalazine, minocycline, inhaled or parenteral pentamidine, phenytoin, radiographic contrast material, and sulfa drugs (http://www.pneumotox.com, 1997). Recently, cyclooxygenase-2 (COX-2) inhibitors and infliximab also were implicated (http://www.pneumotox.com, 1997; Mehandru et al., 2002; Riegert-Johnson et al., 2002). Methotrexate lung is often associated with mild eosinophilia in the blood and BAL (Imokawa et al., 2000), but is not an eosinophilic pneumonia. Some patients with PIE exhibit clinical features which overlap with the systemic angiitis and eosinophilia of Churg–Strauss syndrome (CSS) (Sitbon et al., 1994; Oermann et al., 2000), and distinguishing the two conditions may be problematic. A few drugs, mainly leukotriene receptor antagonists (LTRA), can produce both conditions (Weller et al., 2001; Lilly et al., 2002) (see below). The possibility of a parasitic infection should be considered in any patient with PIE, because this requires specific management.

Typically, the syndrome of PIE develops *during* oral or parenteral treatments with the causative drug (http://www.pneumotox.com, 1997); rarely does the condition develop *after* termination of treatment (Cauchie et al., 1989; Riegert-Johnson et al., 2002). Drugs administered topically (Kohlhäufl et al., 2003), or via inhalation (Dupon et al., 1993), can also cause PIE. Risk factors include prior atopy or asthma, a history of allergic reactions to other or related drugs, and repeated courses of treatment with the drug, which can sensitize patients (Sitbon et al., 1994; Berkes, 2003). Onset is difficult to predict; for instance NSAIDs-induced PIE develops after 1 week to 3 years (average 17 weeks) into treatment (Pfitzenmeyer et al., 1994).

Typical signs and symptoms of PIE include dyspnea, a dry cough, fever, chest discomfort and a skin rash (Sitbon et al., 1994). The intensity of respiratory symptoms and hypoxemia correlate with the extent of pulmonary infiltrates, and in some patients, acute eosinophilic pneumonia develops with or without pleural effusion and respiratory failure (Fujimori et al., 1999; Riegert-Johnson et al., 2002). Symptoms are more prominent if an eosinophilic bronchitis is present, and this is suspected if wheezing is heard at auscultation (Mahatma et al., 1989). Systemic symptoms can be present in patients with elevated levels of blood eosinophils (Diffee et al., 1986). An eosinophilic pleural effusion (Bravo et al., 1977; Ueda et al., 2002) and involvement of distant organs have been described in a few patients (Grcevska et al., 1993; Zaacks et al., 1999; Hayashi et al., 2001).

On imaging, the pulmonary infiltrates of PIE are typically alveolar and symmetrical. The pattern of 'photographic negative of pulmonary edema' is distinctive (Gaensler and Carrington, 1977), but is not found in all cases. The opacities of PIE may be diffuse (Tohyama et al., 2002), or migratory (Fiegenberg et al., 1967), or may appear as faint shadowing or discrete ground-glass. Kerley 'B' lines suggesting the presence of interstitial fluid have been consistently described in PIE due to NSAIDs or other drugs (Pfitzenmeyer et al., 1994; Fleisch et al., 2000). On CT, the opacities of PIE range in density from a discrete haze to patchy subpleural or diffuse shadowing or consolidation (Pfitzenmeyer et al., 1994). Enlargement of peripheral or mediastinal lymph nodes is an occasional finding in PIE associated with exposure to minocycline (Bando et al., 1994) or certain NSAIDs (Oishi et al., 2001).

PIE is diagnosed by the presence of increased percentages or numbers of eosinophils in blood (which can be as high as 80% (Goodwin and Glenny, 1992)), BAL, or lung tissue, although a lung biopsy is rarely required for diagnosis (Sitbon et al., 1994). Peripheral eosinophilia is transiently suppressed if corticosteroids are given (Benzaquen-Forner et al., 1998). BAL commonly shows an increase in both eosinophils and lymphocytes (Fujimura et al., 1998; Pfitzenmeyer et al., 1994). On histology, an interstitial infiltrate of eosinophils admixed with mononuclear cells is seen (Myers, 1993), and a Giemsa stain may help identify eosinophils. Inconspicuous foci of organizing pneumonia may be present (Myers, 1993). Eosinophils may cluster around arterioles without, however, invading their walls (Myers, 1993). An active vasculitis raises the suspicion of CSS (Katzenstein, 2000).

While eosinophilic pneumonia is a common complication of treatments with drugs, it is a rather unusual presenting feature of CTD or autoimmune conditions, except CSS (Freemer and King, 2003). Therefore, relating PIE to drug exposure is generally straightforward, especially if patients are exposed to one single eligible drug, and if drug withdrawal is followed by improvement. Drug withdrawal may not translate into improvement in patients with acute eosinophilic pneumonia (Lévy et al., 1997). If drug therapy withdrawal is without effect, or if acute respiratory failure is present, corticosteroids are indicated and generally quickly reverse all manifestations of PIE (Fleisch et al., 2000). Death in PIE is the exception (Hara et al., 1998).

Rechallenge with the drug leads to recurrence of the clinical manifestations of drug-induced PIE, blood or BAL eosinophilia, and pulmonary infiltrates (Chetty et al., 1993; Jedynak et al., 1997). However, the diagnostic contribution of rechallenge is questionable. Patients with inflammatory bowel disease who develop PIE as a result of exposure to sulfasalazine or mesalazine can deliberately be rechallenged with incremental doses of the drug (Camus et al., 1993). This has resulted in desensitization, reinstatement of the drug and maintained control of the basic disease (Sullivan, 1987; Camus et al., 1993; Greenberger, 2000; Parry et al., 2002). Patients who relapse after graded rechallenge can be rechallenged again, using smaller doses of the drug, achieving successful desensitization (Miller and Green, 1962).

3.1.3. Organizing pneumonia—BOOP

Drug-induced organizing pneumonia or bronchiolitis obliterans organizing pneumonia (OP/BOOP) is a distinctive pattern of lung response to drugs. However, the syndrome can also occur as a presenting feature, or later in the course of CTD, inflammatory bowel disease and autoimmune or hematologic conditions (Ryu et al., 2003). Drug-induced OP was initially reported as a life-threatening event in patients treated with the early antihypertensive drugs hexamethonium (Doniach et al., 1954) and mecamylamine (Rosketh and Storstein, 1960). Later, nodular OP simulating pulmonary metastases on imaging was described during treatments with bleomycin (Santrach et al., 1989). Eventually, amiodarone (Camus et al., 1989; Rossi et al., 2000), β-blocking agents (Camus et al., 1989; Faller et al., 1997), carbamazepine (Milesi-Lecat et al., 1997; Banka and Ward, 2002), gold (Morley et al., 1984; Costabel et al., 1992; Cohen et al., 1994), interferons (Ferriby and Stojkovic, 2001; Kumar et al., 2001), methotrexate (Elsasser et al., 1989; Hollingsworth, 1994), nitrofurantoin (Cameron et al., 2000; Fawcett and Ibrahim, 2001), penicillamine (Lohr et al., 1997), 3-hydroxy-3-methyl glutaryl-coenzyme A (HMG-CoA) reductase inhibitors (statins) (Nizami et al., 1995), and sulindac (Hollingsworth, 1994) were recognised to produce an OP pattern. Several other drugs used outside the context of CTD and allied conditions can also cause OP (http://www.pneumotox.com, 1997; Ryu et al., 2003). The association of OP with ACEI or other NSAIDs is circumstantial at this time (Nizami et al., 1995).

Clinically, drug-induced OP manifests with dyspnea, low-grade fever and, sometimes, lancinating or acute pleuritic chest pain if the foci of OP abut the pleural surface. Rarely increasing dyspnea culminates in acute respiratory failure (Cohen et al., 1994; Nizami et al., 1995; Kumar et al., 2001). On imaging, the disease is suspected when migratory opacities are seen on chest films taken sequentially over a few weeks (Camus et al., 1989; Faller et al., 1997). There may be intervening periods of significant duration with a normal chest radiograph, despite continued exposure to the causative drug. The opacities of OP are in the form of a mass or masses, which may contain air bronchograms (Moreau et al., 1998; Cameron et al., 2000). The masses may have a recognizable segmental or lobar distribution (Camus et al., 1989), or appear as patchy shadows along the bronchovascular bundles, a pattern suggestive of exposure to nitro drugs (Pfitzenmeyer et al., 1992; Fawcett and Ibrahim, 2001) and, possibly, penicillamine. Other patterns include biapical masses (Camus et al., 1993), diffuse ill-defined infiltrates (Ogata et al., 1994), multiple nodules (Milesi-Lecat et al., 1997), and a pattern of dense diffuse and severe ILD, with volume loss and acute respiratory failure (Cohen et al., 1994; Nizami et al., 1995).

No distinctive BAL pattern has been described in association with drug-induced OP (Majori et al., 2000; Costabel et al., 2004). Often, however, the percentage of lymphocytes and sometimes of neutrophils or eosinophils is increased in BAL (Costabel et al., 2004). If a lung biopsy is deemed necessary to reliably establish the diagnosis, the surgical approach is preferred to transbronchial lung biopsy and is guided by the results of CT (Flieder and Travis, 2004). Histology reveals interstitial inflammation and alveolar collapse, superimposed on the dominant background of alveolar and ductal fibrosis (Myers and Colby, 1993; Camus et al., 1993; Ryu et al., 2003; Epler, 2004). In a fraction of patients, significant tissue eosinophilia is present, making the differentiation of *organizing* from *eosinophilic* pneumonia difficult, and overlapping features of the two conditions may be present in the same lung specimen (Faller et al., 1997).

Acute fibrinous OP is a recently recognized pattern of lung involvement (Beasley et al., 2002), which shares some features with classic OP, including exposure to drugs (Beasley et al., 2002). On histology in the former, there is the dominant pattern of intra-alveolar fibrin and OP, associated with varying amounts of type 2 pneumocyte hyperplasia, interstitial edema and acute or chronic inflammation. The clinical impact of acute fibrinous OP is more severe than that of classic OP (Beasley et al., 2002).

Distinguishing OP due to drugs from that due to the background disease can be problematic, as the condition has been described in association with multiple CTD as well as inflammatory diseases such as *polymyalgia rheumatica*, inflammatory bowel disease and other conditions (Camus et al., 1993; Cordier, 2000; Epler, 2001; Freemer and King, 2003). If patients have moderate symptoms, drug discontinuance is justified, and follow-up will indicate whether symptoms of OP abate, supporting the drug etiology.

Not all patients with migratory pulmonary opacities and a background of compatible exposure to drugs actually have OP, as the same imaging pattern can be seen in patients with drug-induced PIE, and BAL may not separate the two conditions well. In patients with migrating opacities and mild symptoms, the risks of lung biopsy may not be justified. The patient is observed after drug withdrawal, which serves as a diagnostic test. Should drug discontinuance not be followed by improvement within a few weeks, then a lung biopsy or a trial of steroids is considered (Portel et al., 1998). Multiple relapses of drug-induced OP can occur, requiring repeated courses of corticosteroids when the drug condition is not recognized, and the drug is continued. Organizing pneumonia associated with amiodarone may relapse after several weeks or months despite drug withdrawal, especially during steroid tapering or after steroid weaning. This is due to the persistence of amiodarone in lung tissue, and prolonged use or reinstatement of corticosteroid therapy is indicated (Camus et al., 2004).

Management of CTD patients with severe OP while being treated with drugs is more complex, as the response to drug discontinuance is limited, or the lung disease can progress despite drug withdrawal (Sullivan, 1987). Discontinuation of treatment and institution of corticosteroids are recommended, even though this complicates the evaluation of drug, as opposed to background disease, as the cause of OP. Elevated dosages of i.v. corticosteroids and sometimes cyclophosphamide have been used in patients with severe OP and in some, this treatment has failed (Cohen et al., 1994).

3.1.4. Amiodarone pulmonary toxicity

Patients with CTD may require amiodarone for the treatment of dysrhythmias associated with their background disease (Doherty and Siegel, 1985; Moder et al., 1999), or for incidental reasons. Amiodarone pulmonary toxicity (APT) is a distinctive DI-ILD (Martin and Rosenow, 1988a,b; Zitnik, 1996; Camus et al., 2004). Amiodarone pulmonary toxicity, a major and common adverse effect of the drug, is mainly a disease in adults, and is difficult to predict even if pulmonary function is measured serially (Ohar et al., 1989). Amiodarone pulmonary toxicity may occur at any time between a few weeks and several years of treatment. Time to onset may be shorter in patients who have been exposed to elevated dosages, or who have been exposed to a loading dose of amiodarone. Amiodarone pulmonary toxicity may develop rapidly following cardiac or pulmonary surgery (van Mieghem et al., 1994; Liverani et al., 2001; Handschin et al., 2003). An elevated erythrocyte sedimentation rate can precede the clinical onset of APT (Marchlinski et al., 1982). Onset is insidious, with dyspnea, crackles, constitutional symptoms, sometimes a pleuritic chest pain, friction rub and moderate fever. Classic amiodarone pneumonitis manifests with bilateral, generally asymmetrical infiltrates, which may assume a recognizable lobar distribution. Involvement of the right upper lobe is suggestive. On CT, involvement is often patchy and asymmetrical, with areas of haze, ground-glass, intralobular linear or alveolar opacities, or dense consolidation with high attenuation numbers (Kuhlman et al., 1987; Ren et al., 1990; Olshansky, 1997; Vernhet et al., 2001; Erasmus et al., 2002b). Pleural thickening is a common finding en face the areas of parenchymal involvement. Amiodarone pulmonary toxicity also can manifest as irreversible pulmonary fibrosis, multiple nodules, wandering opacities, a lone mass or masses with a center of decreased attenuation, or a lone exudative pleural effusion.

A restrictive lung dysfunction and arterial hypoxemia are generally present, and are more severe in patients with extensive disease. The presence of tobacco-related emphysema may alter the radiographic expression of APT, and complicate the interpretation of pulmonary function tests (Cockcroft and Fisher, 1999). Acute APT manifests with diffuse alveolar shadowing or mottling, with respiratory failure or sometimes an ARDS picture. Foamy macrophages reflecting abnormal phospholipid turnover are present in BAL or lung tissue (Myers et al., 1987; Olshansky, 1997; Malhorta et al., 2003). An increase of lymphocytes, neutrophils or both cell types can be found in BAL. Elevated lymphocytes characterize those cases with early onset and marked symptoms of the disease. Lung biopsy is rarely needed to confirm the diagnosis of APT (Malhorta et al., 2003), and shows distinctive amiodarone-induced dyslipidotic changes, on a background of inflammation and fibrosis (Myers et al., 1987). There is general agreement that corticosteroids positively influence the outcome of APT. Corticosteroids should be given for months, otherwise APT may recur, owing to the sequestration of amiodarone in lung tissue, and a relapse of APT may prove more difficult to control than the first bout of the disease. Overall, the mortality is $<10\%$, but it is substantially higher in patients requiring admission to hospital (20–33%) (Camus et al., 2004).

3.1.5. Diffuse alveolar damage

DAD is a common reaction to chemotherapeutic agents (Limper, 2004); it is an unusual complication of treatments with noncytotoxic agents (Lock et al., 2004). In CTD, DAD is particularly associated with aspirin (Gonzolez et al., 1998), azathioprine (Bedrossian et al., 1984), carbamazepine (Wilschut et al., 1997), cyclophosphamide (Anonymous, 1972), nitrofurantoin (Cameron et al., 2000), narcotics (Savici and Katzenstein, 2001), penicillamine (Camus et al., 1982), and simvastatin (Hill et al., 1995). DAD manifests with dyspnea, pulmonary infiltrates and hypoxemia or respiratory failure (Camus, 2003). Widespread symmetrical infiltrates are present on imaging, and the density ranges from diffuse haze or ground-glass to white lungs. Some patients develop acute lung injury, or an ARDS picture (Bedrossian et al., 1984; Wilschut et al., 1997; Woolley et al., 1997; Gonzolez et al., 1998; Grabe et al., 1999).

DAD is defined histopathologically by the findings of hyaline membranes, alveolar and interstitial edema and dysplasia of type 2 pneumocytes (Colby et al., 1991; Colby, 2000). The abnormal type 2 cells may be retrieved by BAL (Beskow et al., 2000).

Determining the histopathologic background in cases with severe involvement is problematic (Chevrolet et al., 1991), as severe ILD, pulmonary edema, and hemorrhage can be undistinguishable from DAD, and patients may be too ill to undergo a confirmatory lung biopsy. Corticosteroids may bring some benefit. However, the prognosis of this condition, when it relates to chemotherapeutic agents, is poor (Bedrossian et al., 1984).

3.1.6. Pulmonary fibrosis

Drug-induced pulmonary fibrosis can develop in patients with CTD during or after treatments with (http://www.pneumotox.com, 1997) amiodarone (Kharabsheh et al., 2002), cyclophosphamide (Stentoft, 1987; Hamada et al., 2003), gold (Tomioka and King, 1997), methotrexate (Imokawa et al , 2000) and, possibly, sulfasalazine (Camus et al., 1993). Given the high incidence of pulmonary fibrosis in several CTDs, including RA and scleroderma (Minai et al., 1998), and the fact that pulmonary fibrosis can also occur sporadically (Gross and Hunninghake, 2001), it is generally difficult to assess drug causality, unless there is a close temporal association between drug exposure and the onset of pulmonary fibrosis. Thus, chest radiographs taken prior to the onset of treatment should be reviewed. The disease manifests with basilar or diffuse streaky opacities and loss of volume. Honeycombing and apical opacities are unusual findings. Drug withdrawal is rarely followed by measurable benefit. The response to steroids is largely unpredictable, and often limited in magnitude or duration.

A few patients with CTD develop the accelerated variant of pulmonary fibrosis known as acute interstitial pneumonia, or the Hamman and Rich syndrome (Jacobs, 1975; Bedrossian et al., 1979). The syndrome has been reported in patients exposed to gold, methotrexate, penicillamine, or other disease-modifying drugs (Coblyn and Weinblatt, 1981; Camus et al., 1982). However, accelerated pulmonary fibrosis can also develop without reasons related to drugs (Pratt et al., 1979). The prognosis of accelerated lung fibrosis remains poor, despite drug withdrawal and institution of high-dose corticosteroids.

3.1.7. Lipoid pneumonia

Alveolar filling by mineral oil can occur in patients chronically exposed to paraffin to combat constipation (Volk et al., 1951). Inexplicably, the oil is often given at night (Rachappa et al., 1984). This may favor lipid spreading down the airways during sleep. Patients with swallowing difficulties and the elderly are at risk (Volk et al., 1951). Lipoid pneumonia may manifest as basilar or widespread shadowing of low attenuation (Gondouin et al., 1996). The pulmonary vasculature may be visible within the areas of parenchymal involvement on contrast non-enhanced CT (Gondouin et al., 1996). Ideally, the diagnosis is suggested at history taking, and is confirmed by the finding of oil and lipid droplets in fluid and/or cells retrieved in sputum (Volk et al., 1951), or BAL (Gondouin et al., 1996). Mineral lipids in BAL cells can be stained using oil red-0 or Sudan black (Gondouin et al., 1996), or lipids can be evidenced on BAL fluid chromatography (Dongay et al., 1986). A lung biopsy is rarely needed. Patients may not improve after drug withdrawal (Gondouin et al., 1996). Corticosteroids generally offer limited benefit.

3.2. Pulmonary edema

Pulmonary edema has been reported during treatments with many chemically unrelated drugs (Reed and Glauser, 1991; http://www.pneumotox.com, 1997), and following an overdose of several drugs (Marshall and Moore, 1973; Hill et al., 1975; Kitson and Wauchob, 1988; Varnell et al., 1989; Humbert et al., 1991; Wilschut et al., 1997; Li and Gefter, 1992; Sporer and Dorn, 2001; Kelly et al., 2003) or illicit substances (Sporer and Dorn, 2001; Piastra et al., 2002; Hutter, 2003). Overall, pulmonary edema is unusual as a complication of treatments with drugs (Reed and Glauser, 1991; Albertson et al., 1995). In the setting of CTD, pulmonary edema can be caused by aspirin, other NSAIDs (Schooley et al., 1977; Heffner and Sahn, 1981; Chetty et al., 1993; Figueras et al., 1994; Beji et al., 1995; Gonzolez et al., 1998; Resta et al., 1999), blood transfusions (Wallis, 2003), colchicine (Hill et al., 1975), minor analgesics (Beji et al., 1995; Resta et al., 1999), hydrochlorothiazide (Biron et al., 1991; Almoosa, 1999), methotrexate (Lisbona et al., 1973; Lascari et al., 1977), nitrofurantoin (Murray and Kronenberg, 1965; Frankenfeld, 1967; Sovijärvi et al., 1977; Formgren et al., 1980; Nyvad and Jensen, 1987), noramidopyrine (Resta et al., 1999), opiates (Flacke et al., 1977; Partridge and Ward, 1986; Stadnyk and Grossman, 1986; Bruera and Miller, 1989; Lao, 1997), quinine (Krantz et al., 2002), and radiographic contrast material (Vandenplas et al., 1990; Lieberman and Seigle, 1999; Bristedt and Tylén, 1998). The attack rate differs between drugs, and the most common offenders include aspirin, blood and blood products, hydrochlorothiazide, and opiates (Cannon, 1990; Reed and Glauser, 1991; http://www.pneumotox.com, 1997; Wallis, 2003). Pulmonary edema can occur as a complication of severe hypersensitivity pneumonitis, e.g. from gold or methotrexate (Lascari et al., 1977). Nifedipine, prostacyclin and nitric oxide used to treat pulmonary hypertension in CTD can also produce acute pulmonary edema and pleural effusion (Palmer et al., 1998; Farber et al., 1999; Humbert et al., 1999; Gugnani et al., 2000). A few cases of drug-induced myocarditis complicated by left ventricular dysfunction and pulmonary edema have been reported (Fenoglio et al., 1981; Morrow et al., 1989; Kwon et al., 2003). Other causes or contexts associated with pulmonary edema include drug-induced anaphylaxis (James and Austen, 1964; Delage and Irey, 1972; Carlson et al., 1981; Daumal et al., 1984; Shkutin et al., 1989; Vandenplas et al., 1990; Knowles et al., 1996; Vucicevic and Suskoovic, 1997; Kumar et al., 2002b), administration of adrenaline/epinephrine (Ersoz and Finestone, 1971; Pumphrey, 2000), and treatments with glitazones in type 2 diabetes (Hirsch et al., 1999; Inoue and Sano, 2000; Kelly et al., 2000; Wang et al., 2002; Buse, 2003; Kermani and Garg, 2003). The latter medicines produce weight gain, fluid retention and pulmonary edema, suggesting a generalized increase in capillary permeability (Idris et al., 2003).

Most cases of drug-induced pulmonary edema are non-cardiac, and result from a drug-mediated increase in capillary permeability, followed by leakage of intravascular fluids into the interstitial and alveolar space (Sovijärvi et al., 1977; Reed and Glauser, 1991). Accordingly, heart size on imaging, pulmonary capillary wedge pressure, and cardiac echocardiography are essentially normal. The opacities of pulmonary edema can develop within a minute of the first exposure to the drug (Vandenplas et al., 1990; Biron et al., 1991; Bristedt and Tylén, 1998), or later, during chronic treatment (Heffner and Sahn, 1981; Gonzolez et al., 1998). Pulmonary edema manifests with dyspnea, and sometimes develops into acute respiratory failure, or an ARDS picture (Gonzolez et al., 1998). Fever, neurologic symptoms, obtundation and shock are possible associated features (Hoegholm et al., 1990). On imaging, there are bilateral symmetrical hazy or ground-glass opacities, and a crazy paving pattern is visible on HRCT (Bristedt and Tylén, 1998). The manifestations of drug-induced pulmonary edema recur after rechallenge (Gonzolez et al., 1998), and it is not unusual for the diagnosis to be raised by the patient or family after several relapses have occurred. Disease severity tends to increase with sequential rechallenge (Jara Chinarro et al., 2003).

Management includes drug discontinuation and, if needed, positive pressure breathing. The beneficial role of corticosteroids is unclear. Diuresis may be detrimental in dehydrated patients (Wallis, 2003). The pulmonary opacities of pulmonary edema usually clear rapidly. Rechallenge with the drug leads to recurrence, and may require repeated hospital admission until the drug etiology is eventually recognized.

Transient pulmonary infiltrates closely associated with a single drug exposure have been referred to as 'allergic pneumonitis' or pulmonary edema (Johnson et al., 1990; Basoglu et al., 1997; Maillard et al., 1999; Krantz et al., 2002). However, transient pulmonary infiltrates are not synonymous with pulmonary edema, as ILD, vasculitis and alveolar damage have been documented (Geller et al., 1976; Formgren et al., 1980).

3.3. Alveolar hemorrhage

Diffuse alveolar hemorrhage (DAH) is an unusual complication of drugs, which consists of diffuse and probably synchronous bleeding from pulmonary capillaries. This may or may not be associated with histologically demonstrable capillaritis (Schwarz and Fontenot, 2004). Since BAL is an excellent and minimally invasive diagnostic tool, lung biopsy has been performed in a minority of patients with this condition (Dhillon et al., 1999; Schwarz and Fontenot, 2004). Establishing the responsibility of drugs in CTD patients who develop DAH is difficult, since DAH also can develop in the untreated course of many systemic conditions, including *lupus erythematosus*, RA, mixed CTD, systemic sclerosis, polymyositis, the antiphospholipid syndrome, Henoch–Schönlein purpura, Behçet disease, Goospasture syndrome, Wegener's granulomatosis (WG), IgA nephropathy, idiopathic glomerulonephritis, *myasthenia gravis*, cryoglobulinemia, and primary ANCA-positive or -negative micropolyangitis (Horiki et al., 1998; Fontenot and Schwarz, 2003). DAH is not a feature of drug-induced *lupus*, as opposed to naturally occurring systemic *lupus erythematosus* (Santos-Ocampo et al., 2000). Drug-induced DAH occurs in isolation, or in association with involvement of the kidney or other internal organs (Choi et al., 2000a).

Drugs causing DAH in patients with CTD include oral anticoagulants, the inhibitor of platelet glycoprotein IIb/III abciximab (Kalra et al., 2001), allopurinol (Choi et al., 1998), aspirin (Gopalakrishnan et al., 1997), azathioprine (Stetter et al., 1994), clopicogrel (Kilraru et al., 2001), methotrexate (Kokelj et al., 1999), and phenytoin (Polman et al., 1998). Drugs causing thrombocytopenia also can produce bleeding in the lung (LeBlanc, 1980; Polman et al., 1998). Occasionally, DAH occurs as a complication of severe gold-, methotrexate or nitrofurantoin pneumonitis (Noseworthy et al., 1983; Meyer and Meyer, 1994; Kokelj et al., 1999). Hydralazine, penicillamine, propylthiouracil and, less often, azathioprine, leflunomide, and phenytoin can produce a pneumorenal syndrome, which mimics Goodpasture's or WG (Stetter et al., 1994; Ohtsuka et al., 1997; Phillips et al., 1998; Polman et al., 1998; Dhillon et al., 1999; Katayama et al., 2002; Derk and Jimenez, 2003; Bruyn et al., 2003) (see drug-induced angiitis below). Patients with DAH resulting from treatments with these agents may present with a perinuclear p-ANCA staining pattern and a anti-myeloperoxidase, -lactoferrin, or -elastase specificity (Choi et al., 1998, 1999, 2000a), contrasted with the cytoplasmic ANCA (c-ANCA) staining pattern and anti-proteinase 3 specificity of naturally occurring Wegener's (van der Geld et al., 2001). Antiglomerular basement membrane (anti-GBM) antibodies are rarely found in drug-induced DAH (Choi et al., 2000a; Bruyn et al., 2003), as opposed to naturally occurring Goodpasture's disease (Kluth and Rees, 1999; Salama et al., 2001).

DAH can be subclinical or rapidly progressive, and requires expeditious management to avoid irreversible intra-alveolar clotting (Mark and Ramirez, 1985; Horiki et al., 1998; Schwarz and Fontenot, 2004). The spectrum of severity ranges from discrete subclinical opacities on imaging to an ARDS picture with or without renal failure. Full-blown disease may cause general symptoms, arthralgias, dyspnea, alveolar infiltrates which may assume a batwing distribution, and anemia (Schwarz and Fontenot, 2004). Hemoptysis is not a constant feature, even in patients with significant alveolar bleeding. An increase in the diffusing capacity for carbon monoxide suggesting free hemoglobin in alveolar spaces has been found in a few patients with DAH (Schwarz and Fontenot, 2004). This indicates massive bleeding, but is not a reliable or consistent finding. Macroscopically, BAL is hemorrhagic and demonstrates increased staining in sequential aliquots (Schwarz and Fontenot, 2004). Microscopically, BAL shows increased numbers of red cells. Hemosiderin-laden macrophages, if present, indicate a background of sub-acute or chronic bleeding. A search for ANAs, ANCAs, and anti-GBM autoantibodies is essential in all cases, to classify drug-induced DAH (autoimmune vs. non-autoimmune) and separate drug-induced DAH from DAH related to CTD and systemic illnesses (Choi et al., 1999; Schwarz and Fontenot, 2004).

Drug causality is suggested when DAH occurs during treatments with drugs which intentionally produce coagulation defects, even though coagulation studies are within an acceptable therapeutic range (Rostand et al., 1977). Otherwise, causality assessment is more difficult, because DAH can occur in so many systemic conditions (Fontenot and Schwarz, 2003). Patients who present with DAH and positive antinuclear (ANA), especially the anti-double strand DNA subtype, ANCAs with a cytoplasmic staining and PR3 specificity, or anti-GBM antibodies, are more likely to have naturally-occurring *lupus erythematosus*, Wegener's or Goodpasture's disease, respectively, rather than a drug condition. A temporal association of drug exposure, p-ANCA titers, and DAH is consistent with the drug etiology. A change in ANCA specificity in a patient with WG during follow-up may indicate drug-induced disease, rather than relapse of the background condition (Choi et al., 1999).

Drug therapy withdrawal is generally advised and may suffice in patients with anticoagulant-induced bleeding. Patients with other forms of DAH and extensive or persistent bleeding, or evidence of renal failure, are considered for treatment with corticosteroids or immunosuppressive agents, in a manner similar to autoimmune disease (Schwarz and Fontenot, 2004). However, no current guidelines exist. The role of factor VIIa is not established (Hicks et al., 2002). One patient was rechallenged with azathioprine, and this was promptly followed by relapse of anti-GBM-negative DAH (Stetter et al., 1994).

3.4. Airway involvement

3.4.1. Upper airway

Upper airway obstruction (UAO) is a rapidly evolving and potentially life-threatening complication of drugs. UAO results from edema of the mouth floor, tongue, laryngeal area, or tracheal walls (Berkes, 2003). This entity can occur in isolation, or in the context of drug-induced bronchospasm or anaphylaxis (Delage and Irey, 1972; Israili and Hall, 1992; Assadi et al., 1999). Rarely, UAO following exposure to drugs unravels C1-esterase deficiency (Wong and Gadsden, 2003). Crucially, ACEI (Zanoletti et al., 2003), less often angiotensin II antagonists (Chiu et al., 2001a), azathioprine (Jungling and Shangraw, 2000), betalactams (Romano et al., 2003), NSAIDs and COX-2 inhibitors (Figueras et al., 1994; Mommens et al., 2003), methotrexate (Alkins et al., 1996), metoclopramide (MacLaren and Shields, 1998) and sulfasalazine (Collins, 1968) can cause UAO with or without bronchospasm and anaphylaxis. UAO can develop very shortly after the first exposure to the drug (Seidman et al., 1990; Israili and Hall, 1992), or unexpectedly later, after a falsely reassuring period of treatment (Chin and Buchan, 1990; Schuster et al., 1999; Mchaourab et al., 1999). UAO can occasion severe airway compromise (Chiu et al., 2001a,b), and this requires timely laryngotracheal intubation or emergency tracheostomy to restore airway patency (Chiu et al., 2001a; Chiyo et al., 2003), otherwise fatal asphyxia can occur (Giannocarro et al., 1989; Ulmer and Garvey, 1992). Prior episodes of tongue swelling or hoarseness suggestive of the diagnosis may be overlooked (Israili and Hall, 1992). Usually, the condition resolves within 48 h of treatment with corticosteroids and antihistamines (Berkes, 2003). Drug withdrawal is mandatory: drug continuation exposes patients to recurrence after variable periods of further treatment (Gregory and Davis, 1996).

Anticoagulants can produce lingual or mediastinal hematoma, and this also can result in life-threatening UAO (Rosenbaum et al., 1979; Gupta et al., 2003).

Anticoagulants and aspirin increase the risk of bleeding associated with bronchial biopsies (van Sonnenberg and Wittich, 1998). Hemoptysis in patients exposed to these drugs may unmask underlying bronchial lesions (O'Reilly et al., 1994).

3.4.2. Lower airways

3.4.2.1. Bronchospasm—asthma. Bronchospasm is a common adverse reaction to drugs, and is prevalent in patients with CTD. In a series of 187 bronchospastic episodes reported to the Swiss Monitoring Center for Adverse Effects of Medicines, 24% were caused by NSAIDs and analgesics (Leuppi et al., 2001). Asthma aggravated by therapeutic drugs used to treat rheumatic conditions is usually seen against a background of pre-existing asthma. Less commonly, drug-induced asthma occurs de novo, producing sudden or catastrophic bronchospasm. Rarely it persists after exposure to the drug has ceased. The symptoms of asthma can occur in isolation, or in association with such symptoms as flushing, alterations in heart rate, back pain, fever, pruritus, nausea, a skin rash, shock, or anaphylaxis.

3.4.2.1.1. Aspirin and NSAIDs. Aspirin sensitivity, known as 'aspirin-induced or exacerbated asthma', is the most widely known form of drug-induced bronchospasm (Samter and Beers, 1968; Berkes, 2003). Aspirin and many other first-generation NSAIDs are inhibitors of prostaglandin H1 and H2 synthase (cyclooxygenase-1 or COX1). COX-1 inhibition diverts the metabolic pathway of arachidonic acid towards bronchoconstrictor leukotrienes (Stevenson and Zuraw, 2003). This shared effect of COX-inhibition is also the mechanism for shared adverse effects (Berkes, 2003). Therefore, to some extent, aspirin-induced asthma is a misnomer, because patients cross-react adversely to all COX-1-inhibiting NSAIDs, not just aspirin, even though these drugs are structurally dissimilar. Only a few patients specifically react to a single NSAID, via allergic IgE-dependent mechanisms (Berkes, 2003). The risk of bronchospasm following exposure to aspirin and NSAIDs is probably enhanced in patients using the drug on an intermittent basis, and in those with a prior history of drug allergy or intolerance (Berkes, 2003). Heteroaryl acetic acids are more likely to induce adverse reactions than arylpropionic acids (Berkes, 2003). The weak inhibitors of COX-1 acetaminophen and salsalate require higher concentrations to trigger bronchospasm (Berkes, 2003). The preferential COX-2 inhibitors nimesulide and meloxicam cross-react poorly with aspirin (Berkes, 2003). The newer and selective COX-2 inhibitors (celecoxib, rofecoxib) (FitzGerald and Patrono, 2001) cross-react with aspirin in 1.5–2% of ASA/NSAID-sensitive individuals (Perrone et al., 2003). The lower incidence rate of adverse response to COX-2 inhibitors is corroborated by the absence of release of leukotrienes after in vitro exposure of peripheral blood leukocytes from aspirin-intolerant asthmatics to celecoxib, as opposed to aspirin (Kowalski et al., 2003). The above pathophysiology has received substantial clinical, experimental and genetic support. However, the failure of leukotriene inhibitors to inhibit the adverse reactions to COX-1 suggests that other mechanisms may play a role (Menéndez et al., 1998). Also, the sudden explosive nature of aspirin/NSAID-induced bronchospasm is difficult to reconcile with mere inhibition of prostaglandin synthesis by these agents.

Aspirin-exacerbated asthma is characterized clinically by recalcitrant sinusitis/polyposis, asthma and precipitation of asthma after ingestion of aspirin and most COX-1 inhibitor NSAIDs (Figueras et al., 1994; Namazy and Simon, 2002). A cross-reaction between ASA and NSAIDs often occurs with first exposure to the drug, unlike IgE-mediated allergic drug reactions or anaphylaxis, which involve an IgE-mediated response to a specific drug due to prior sensitization (Berkes, 2003). A fraction of patients with ASA-intolerance may remain asymptomatic until challenged with the drug (Szczeklik et al., 2000). The gravity of drug-induced bronchoconstriction resides in its unpredictability, the explosive nature of the asthmatic attack, the possible association with anaphylaxis, and the consequent respiratory failure, which may lead to irreversible brain damage or death (Samter and Beers, 1968). Although most accidents occur after oral intake or parenteral injections, dermal applications and rectal or ophthalmic administration of NSAIDs also can trigger an asthma attack (Kashiwabara and Nakamura, 2001; Berkes, 2003).

The prevalence of aspirin and NSAID sensitivity is higher than that of other drug-induced respiratory disease. It is also easier to ascertain, because temporal relationships are more straightforward and the diagnosis can be confirmed by drug challenge (Szczeklik and Stevenson, 2003). The prevalence of aspirin-exacerbated asthma varies appreciably, depending on diagnostic criteria (Hailemeskel et al., 1997; Stevenson, 1998). Estimates based on history alone suggest sensitivity in 1–3% of all asthmatic subjects, but if challenge tests are performed, the prevalence lies between 5 and 10% (Vally et al., 2002; Kasper et al., 2003). Prevalence is higher (about 20%) among subjects prone to chronic rhino-sinusitis, rhinorrhea or nasal polyps (Larsen, 1996), and in those with a history of acute asthma attacks (about 25%) (Marquette et al., 1992; Plaza et al., 2002). Typically, aspirin-sensitive asthma develops in the third or fourth decade of life, although sensitivity also occurs in childhood (Fischer et al., 1983). Aspirin-sensitive asthma is more common in women than men (in a ratio of about 2 to 1), and approximately 60% of the patients have nasal polyps (Szczeklik et al., 2000). Rhinitis and rhinorrhea usually precede the development of asthma, with aspirin sensitivity becoming apparent subsequently (Szczeklik et al., 2000). Patients with aspirin sensitivity often have difficult-to-control asthma, with about 50% requiring regular treatment with oral corticosteroids (Szczeklik and Sanak, 2000). At its most dramatic, the response to a single tablet of aspirin or other NSAID is anaphylactoid (Figueras et al., 1994; Sturtevant, 1999), with a rapid onset of malaise, urticaria, angioedema and, variably, upper airway compromise, abdominal cramping, diarrhea, shock, life-threatening bronchoconstriction, locked lung, and severe nasal symptoms leading to a choking sensation, rapid loss of consciousness, and death within minutes of exposure to the drug (Ibanez et al., 1991; Pumphrey, 2000). There is an increase in circulating levels of histamine and tryptase during the adverse event, and also during controlled challenge with the drug (Szczeklik et al., 1996; Stevenson and

Zuraw, 2003), but this is not specific for intolerance, as opposed to anaphylaxis (Berkes, 2003). Less sensitive individuals show more gradual development of ocular and nasal symptoms and bronchospasm (Bini and Weinshel, 1999).

Treatment of acute bronchospasm induced by intake of an NSAID requires antihistamines H2 blockers, corticosteroids, and sometimes epinephrine or ventilatory support (Marquette et al., 1992; Berkes, 2003; Mommens et al., 2003). In many subjects, the history is sufficiently clear for further investigation to be unnecessary. When the association is less definite, or when treatment with an NSAID or aspirin is desirable, carefully controlled challenge tests are justified. Challenge is best performed in the intensive care unit, the patient should have a venous access placed, and all therapy drugs and resuscitation equipment should be available. Bronchial challenge can be performed by using inhaled lysine-aspirin, which is safe and more rapid than oral challenge, although a little less sensitive (Nizankowska et al., 2000). A simpler alternative is nasal challenge with lysine-aspirin, but this is rather less reliable for confident exclusion of sensitivity (Milewski et al., 1998). Since aspirin-exacerbated airways disease very seldom resolves (Rosado et al., 2003), patients with a clear history of intolerance to aspirin should be formally advised to avoid all aspirin-containing products and other COX-1 inhibitors, and be given a comprehensive list of prohibited drugs to keep at all times. Paracetamol (acetaminophen) is safe in normal therapeutic doses in most patients with NSAID sensitivity, as only large doses produce reactions in a minority (Settipane et al., 1995). Patients may take a COX-2 inhibitor, with a substantially lower risk of adverse effects (Szczeklik et al., 2001; Marks et al., 2001; Woessner et al., 2002; Berkes, 2003; Perrone et al., 2003; Mommens et al., 2003; Layton et al., 2003). Nevertheless, the prescription of COX-2 inhibitors should be done with caution, since these drugs can produce severe systemic reactions, including anaphylaxis in a minority (Gagnon et al., 2003; Layton et al., 2003; Mommens et al., 2003).

Desensitization to aspirin can be practiced in CTD patients who are intolerant to aspirin or NSAIDs, and need these drugs for the treatment of their basic rheumatic condition (Berges-Gimeno et al., 2003; Stevenson, 2003; Szczeklik and Stevenson, 2003). The observation that a single NSAID challenge results in a refractory period which can last for up to 5 days (van Arsdel, 1984) led to desensitizing schedules using gradually increasing doses, followed by regular treatment. If desensitization to aspirin is achieved, intake of aspirin or NSAID is not followed by detectable bronchospasm or elevations of tryptase and/or histamine, and there is cross-tolerance to other NSAIDs as well (Pleskow et al., 1982). In addition, desensitization improves nasal and sinus signs and symptoms (Sweet et al., 1990), allows reductions in corticosteroid dosage, and improves both the control of asthma and the quality of life (Sweet et al., 1990). If there is a need to continue NSAID or aspirin for the treatment of the background inflammatory disease, daily treatment is required to maintain the refractory state as otherwise sensitivity returns in a few days (Pleskow et al., 1982).

The likely pathogenetic mechanisms of NSAID-induced asthma would suggest that drugs which inhibit leukotrienes or antagonize their effects might be useful. Some protection has been shown in single exposure challenges and in a double-blind study of the 5-lipoxygenase inhibitor, zileuton (Dahlén et al., 1998). A recent study has shown subjective and objective improvement in symptom scores and airway function in aspirin-intolerant asthmatics after 6 months of montelukast (Paganin et al., 2003), but not all studies confirmed the efficacy of this class of compounds (Volkman and Pontikes, 2002). Severe aspirin sensitivity may not be countered by leukotriene antagonists (Enrique et al., 1999; Broadfoot et al., 2002; Volkman and Pontikes, 2002). Subjects with NSAID sensitivity may not derive greater benefit from these agents than those with non-ASA-sensitive asthma.

3.4.2.1.2. β-blockers. β-blockers are commonly prescribed to patients with a history of myocardial infarction or systemic hypertension, and these account for most cases of drug-induced bronchospasm (Hoigné et al., 1997). Fatal bronchospastic reactions still occur following exposure to these agents, especially the older and less selective β-blockers (Fallowfield and Marlow, 1996). Although meta-analyses suggest that short-term treatments with cardioselective β1-blockers are safe in patients with moderate asthma or chronic obstructive pulmonary disease (COPD) (Salpeter et al., 2002, 2003; Anonymous, 2002; Chen et al., 2001), many challenge this view, pointing out that the likelihood, magnitude and time course of bronchospasm during treatments with β-blockers is unpredictable (Williams and Millard, 1980; Im Hof, 1995; Chafin et al., 1999; Shulan et al., 2003). Patients who do not exhibit significant bronchospasm when challenged with β-blockers in the clinic may present with severe bronchospasm later during treatment with the β-blocker, due to the unstable nature of their asthma, or after an encounter with an asthma trigger (Chafin et al., 1999). Chronic treatments with β-blockers may increase the risk of anaphylactoid reactions to radiographic contrast material (Lang et al., 1991), or following anesthesia (Wagner et al., 1994). β-blockers also may blunt the therapeutic response to β2-agonists, should these drugs be required for the treatment of an asthma attack or anaphylaxis (Reid et al., 1993).

Ophthalmic preparations of β-blockers produce similar adverse bronchial reactions (Diggory and Franks, 1994; Novack et al., 2002).

3.4.2.1.3. Miscellaneous drugs. ACEIs (Lunde et al., 1994), antibiotics (Gibbs et al., 2003), cyclophosphamide (Salles et al., 1991), interferons (Bini and Weinshel, 1999), methotrexate (Jones et al., 1991), narcotics (Assem, 1976), penicillamine (Camus, 1982), inhaled (Katzman et al., 1992) and, less commonly, intravenous pentamidine (Gearhart and Bhutani, 1992), ribavirin (Zucker and Meadow, 1995), and radiographic contrast material can also sometimes cause severe bronchospasm (Morcos, 2003). There is no clear pathophysiologic link with ASA/NSAID-exacerbated asthma.

Occasionally patients with aspirin sensitivity react adversely to intravenous hydrocortisone sodium succinate (Partridge and Gibson, 1978; Dajani et al., 1981; Hölz et al., 2002). This effect appears to be related to the succinate ester, and may be avoided by using hydrocortisone sodium phosphate or a different corticosteroid. Rare patients demonstrate allergy to inhaled corticosteroids (Kilpiö and Hannuksela, 2003), which can be substantiated by skin testing (Kilpiö and Hannuksela, 2003).

3.4.2.2. Bronchiolitis obliterans. BO has been particularly associated with penicillamine treatment of RA in women in the 1970s and 1980s (Geddes et al., 1977). The nature of the association remains speculative, and a reporting bias cannot be excluded (Geddes et al., 1977). Chrysotherapy and tiopronine were also associated with BO (Schwartzman et al., 1995), but the incidence seems less. Clinically, patients with BO develop rapidly progressive and irreversible obstruction to airflow, with FEV1.0 down to less than 1.0 l and decreased FEV1.0/FVC. The chest radiograph may remain normal. A discrete mosaic pattern may be visualized on HRCT examination (Higenbottam, 1997). Although lung biopsy is not necessary for diagnosis, which is strongly suggested by history and the results of pulmonary function tests, the histology shows diffuse narrowing of small airways by endoluminal plugs of granulation tissue or by fibrotic constriction of the airway walls (Yokoi et al., 1997). The airflow obstruction rarely improves after drug therapy withdrawal and the addition of bronchodilators, steroids or immunosuppressive agents (van de Laar et al., 1985). Although most cases of drug-induced BO are irreversible, early diagnosis and withdrawal of the drug has been followed by stabilization or improvement (Le Loet et al., 1983). Lung transplantation is an option in patients with severe drug-induced or dietary BO (Hsu et al., 2000).

Only a handful of patients developed BO while receiving penicillamine for the treatment of CTD other than RA (Camus, 1982; Boehler et al., 1996). BO also can develop in patients with RA during treatments with gold or tiopronine (Demaziere et al., 1993). On the other hand, BO has been reported in patients with RA who had never been exposed to drugs (Epler et al., 1979). For these reasons, the responsibility of penicillamine, as opposed to the background RA, remains elusive (Epler et al., 1979). The issue is likely to remain unresolved, as penicillamine is less in use nowadays than it once was.

Several Taiwanese patients developed severe and irreversible BO after exposure to extracts of the Malaysian herb *Sauropus androgynus* (Higenbottam, 1997; Chang et al., 1998; Wang et al., 2000).

3.4.2.3. Sustained coughing. The majority of cases of drug-induced cough correspond to an adverse reaction to ACEI (Lee et al., 2000). Three to 20% of patients taking an ACEI develop the cough (Özkan et al., 2001). The cough is more common in women with no history of asthma or atopy, and may be associated with certain ACE genotypes (Takahashi et al., 2001). The cough develops after variable periods of treatment with the ACEI, and sometimes follows an episode of upper respiratory tract infection. The cough is typically nonproductive and annoying, and interferes with daily activities and sleep (Poole and Postma, 1991). Patients may suffer stress rib fractures (Lee et al., 2000), urinary incontinence, or cough syncope (Ishizuka et al., 2000). Features characteristic of asthma, such as wheeze or reversible airway obstruction, are usually absent. Before considering ACEI-induced cough, other causes of cough must be ruled out, as ACEI can unravel tussigenic diseases such as lung cancer. Cough may also be a presenting feature of the background CTD, particularly Sjögren's syndrome (Birring et al., 2003).

Although bronchodilators, cromolyn, and thromboxane inhibitors have been suggested as therapeutic interventions in ACEI-induced cough, no drug reliably controls this form of coughing. Withdrawal of ACEI is followed by the gradual disappearance of the cough within a few weeks. The cough will continue or relapse if patients are switched to another ACEI or rechallenged. The incidence rate of cough with the angiotensin II antagonists valsartan, candesartan or losartan is not dissimilar to that with a placebo (Benz et al., 1997; Conigliaro and Gleason, 2000). However, these drugs can induce coughing in a minority of patients (Mackay et al., 1999; Conigliaro and Gleason, 1999).

Patients on methotrexate can develop cough due to methotrexate-induced airway irritation (Schnabel et al., 1996). As opposed to patients with methotrexate pneumonitis, those with methotrexate-induced cough typically have no evidence of ILD on imaging or lung biopsy, and results of pulmonary function tests are normal (Schnabel et al., 1996). Although BAL cellularity is typically lymphocytic, the percentage of lymphocytes is less than in those with overt methotrexate pneumonitis (Schnabel et al., 1996). The cough is controlled by antitussives and drug withdrawal (Schnabel et al., 1996). Importantly, in some patients with RA, the cough abated despite continuation of methotrexate (Schnabel et al., 1996).

There are anecdotal reports of cough during treatments with interferon (Pileire et al., 1999), and paroxetine (Hamel et al., 2000), with abatement after withdrawal, and recurrence after rechallenge.

Explosive coughing has been reported as a complication of general anesthesia with fentanyl, isoflurane, propofol, or sulfentanyl (Tweed and Dakin, 2001). Inhaled antiasthma medications may minimize this form of coughing (Agarwal et al., 2003).

3.5. Pleural involvement

In general, pleural effusion or pleuritis is more often related to the background CTD (e.g. RA or systemic *lupus erythematosus*) (Sahn, 1988; Freemer and King, 2003) than to drugs. The drug etiology is supported by the slow diminution of pleural effusion after drug discontinuance, and meticulous exclusion of other causes.

3.5.1. Eosinophilic pleural effusions

Dantrolene, mesalazine, nitrofurantoin, propylthiouracil, sulfasalazine, L-tryptophan (the drug was recalled in the 1990s) and valproate can produce lone eosinophilic pleural or pleuropericardial effusion (Sahn, 1988; Morelock and Sahn, 1999; http://www.pneumotox.com, 1997; Camus, 2004; Huggins and Sahn, 2004). Eosinophilia can be present in blood, BAL and pleural tissue, concomitant with eosinophilia in the pleural fluid (Morelock and Sahn, 1999; Huggins and Sahn, 2004). Rechallenge causes a recurrence of symptoms (Huggins and Sahn, 2004). Overall, the prognosis of drug-induced lone eosinophilic effusions is good after withdrawal of the causative drug (Camus, 2004).

Eosinophilic pleural effusions can develop in conjunction with extensive eosinophilic pneumonia due to ACEI (Benzaquen-Forner et al., 1998), diflunisal (Rich and Thomas, 1997), minocycline (Toyoshima et al., 1996), nevirapine (Bourezane et al., 1998), L-tryptophan (Shore, 1990), and dietary supplements (Yamawaki et al., 1996; Nakanishi et al., 2001). Signs and symptoms of eosinophilic pneumonia and pleural effusion improve in parallel after drug withdrawal, and quickly return after rechallenge (Brander and Selroos, 1969; Braun et al., 1993; Melloni et al., 1994; Bayliff et al., 1997).

3.5.2. Pleural thickening

Pleural or pleuropericardial thickening is a common complication of long-term treatments with ergoline drugs (e.g. bromocriptine or ergotamine) used to treat migraine and Parkinson's disease (http://www.pneumotox.com, 1997; Pfitzenmeyer et al., 1996; Bleumink et al., 2002). In some patients, this has resulted in pulmonary encasement by bilateral pleural fibrosis, with consequent restrictive lung function defect. The disease is common, with 2–4% of the treated population affected. Diagnosis is often raised late in the history (Pfitzenmeyer et al., 1996). Pleural effusion and thickening are slowly improved upon drug withdrawal. Residual pleural thickening and restrictive physiology often persist indefinitely (Camus, 2004).

Pleural thickening also is a manifestation of the drug-induced *lupus* (Camus, 2004).

3.5.3. Other effusions

Approximately 3% of patients with acute nitrofurantoin lung present with transient bilateral pleural effusions of small volume, which are manifested by acute chest pain and blunting of cardiophrenic angles (Holmberg and Boman, 1981). Chest pain and the effusion quickly return upon re-exposure to the drug (Bayliff et al., 1997).

Pleural effusions develop as an associated feature in about 10% of patients with methotrexate lung (Massin et al., 1990), and in about 3% of those with gold lung (Baethge and Wolf, 1988; Tomioka and King, 1997). The effusions are often evident a few days after the height of the pneumonitis.

Pleural effusion is an unusual finding in the course of drug-induced pulmonary edema: amongst all reported cases of hydrochlorothiazide-and aspirin-induced pulmonary edema, pleural effusion was present in only one patient (Reed and Glauser, 1991; Camus, 2004).

Pleural effusion has been reported in CTD patients with pulmonary hypertension or venoocclusive disease receiving calcium-channel blocking agents or prostacyclin (Chaouat et al., 1996; Gugnani et al., 2000).

Hemothorax can complicate treatments with oral anticoagulants, ticlopidine, and aspirin (Simon et al., 1969; Rostand et al., 1977, 1995; Cafri et al., 1997; Quinn and Dillard, 1999). Early recognition is warranted, as the pleural space can accommodate substantial amounts of blood, and this complication can be life-threatening or fatal (Simon et al., 1969).

4. Systemic reactions and CTD induced by drugs

Drugs have long been known to produce systemic autoimmune conditions such as the *lupus* syndrome (Sahn, 1988; Brogan and Olsen, 2003). Specifically, drugs used to treat CTD or their complications (e.g. anticonvulsants for seizures in *lupus* patients) can produce systemic inflammatory or autoimmune disease including anaphylaxis, drug fever, vasculitis, myositis, and the 'drug hypersensitivity syndrome' (Choi et al., 2000a; Pumphrey, 2000; Adkinson et al., 2002; Sicherer, 2003). These reactions are likely immune-mediated, and can involve varying target organs, including the lung and serosal surfaces (Abbondazo et al., 1995; De Vriese et al., 1995; Christ et al., 1996; Choi et al., 2000a; Verma et al., 2000; Sheikhzadeh et al., 2002). Except for anaphylaxis, the drug etiology in drug-induced systemic syndromes may be recognized late, at a time when progressive or irreversible tissue damage has occurred, and drug therapy withdrawal may not be as effective as it is earlier in the course of the disease. Early clinical recognition and testing for autoantibodies (ANAs, ANCAs, and anti-GBM) are essential to classify these peculiar adverse reactions to drugs properly. Improvement follows drug withdrawal.

4.1. Anaphylaxis

Anaphylaxis is an explosive reaction, which generally results from IgE-mediated release of preformed mediators in response to insect stings, antigens, foods (e.g. nuts) and drugs (James and Austen, 1964; Bochner and Lichtenstein, 1991; van der Klauw et al., 1996; Pumphrey, 2000). Drugs may cause up to 20–40% of anaphylactic episodes (Kemp et al., 1995). Exposure to analgesics, anesthetic agents, antibiotics (amoxicillin, ciprofloxacin, penicillin, sulfamides, sulfamethoxazole, trimethoprime, vancomycin), aspirin, colloid plasma expanders, cortisone, NSAIDs (e.g. diclofenac), COX-2 inhibitors, curares, fluorescein, immunoglobulins, latex, methotrexate, opiates, heterologous proteins and radiographic contrast media can cause anaphylaxis (Johnson et al., 1990; Bochner and Lichtenstein, 1991; Deamer et al., 1992; Alkins et al., 1996; van der Klauw et al., 1996; http://www.pneumotox.com, 1997; Bijl et al., 1998; Pumphrey, 2000; Berkes, 2003). Most accidents, however, occur after administration of analgesics, NSAIDs, and penicillin (van der Klauw et al., 1993). Disease incidence is greater in females (Youlten, 1989), in atopics (Kemp et al., 1995), and in patients with systemic mastocytosis (Pumphrey, 2000). Clinical manifestations include the sudden onset of urticaria, itching of the nose or palate, abdominal pain, vomiting, diarrhea, nasal, ocular or asthmatic symptoms, and shock. Full-blown reaction is characterized by hypotension, laryngeal and/or tracheal angioedema with consequent UAO, bronchospasm, frothy sputum, hemoptysis, internal organ edema, shock and seizures, followed by cardiac arrest and death within 15 min of exposure to the causative drug (Lamson, 1929; Delage and Irey, 1972; Gregory and Davis, 1996; Pumphrey, 2000). Autopsy studies indicate marked edema of the epiglottis, larynx and trachea, pulmonary hyperinflation, edema and hemorrhage (Lamson, 1929; Delage and Irey, 1972). These changes account for the airway compromise and respiratory difficulties (James and Austen, 1964; Delage and Irey, 1972).

A recent series indicates that about 20 deaths from anaphylaxis occur each year in the UK, of which half are iatrogenic (Pumphrey, 2000). The time to respiratory or cardiac arrest averaged 5 min. Even though 28% of the patients were resuscitated, most died 3–30 h later from hypoxic brain damage (Pumphrey, 2000). Anaphylaxis was mistaken for panic attack in some patients, and the diagnosis was unnecessarily delayed. Complications of treatment included fluid overload, adrenaline-induced vomiting followed by inhalation of the gastric content, adrenaline-induced myocardial infarction, and pulmonary edema (Pumphrey, 2000).

Management of anaphylaxis requires preparedness and prompt recognition. Management of the full-blown disease includes parenteral adrenaline, to be repeated every 15 min, high-dose corticosteroids, and correction of hypovolemia and cardiac arrhythmias. Ensuring early and adequate access to the airway is critical, as when laryngeal edema has developed beyond a certain extent attempts at laryngotracheal intubation may be unsuccessful (Berkes, 2003).

4.2. Drug hypersensitivity—the ‘anticonvulsant syndrome’

Drug hypersensitivity is a potentially life-threatening syndrome with many possible clinical patterns and significant morbidity. DHS is characterised by fever, a cutaneous rash, eosinophilia and internal organ involvement. Prompt recognition and early identification and withdrawal of all suspect medicines are vital. Avoidance of re-exposure to the responsible agent is essential, otherwise relapse will occur. Cross-reactivity to structurally related drugs is common, and first-degree relatives may be predisposed to developing this syndrome as well. The paucity of reports in the recent past does not help maintain clinical awareness. Drug hypersensitivity is also called ‘drug rash with eosinophilia and systemic symptoms’, the ‘sulfone syndrome’, ‘glandular fever’ or ‘anticonvulsant’ or ‘carbamazepine hypersensitivity syndrome’, depending on the causative drug. DHS is an idiosyncratic reaction defined by the clinical triad of fever, rash and organ involvement such as hepatitis, myocarditis, nephritis, or pneumonitis. The disease typically develops within the first 8 weeks into treatment with anticonvulsants, with an attack rate of 1 out of 5000–10,000 patients on the drug (Rademaker and Maling, 2003).

The variable presentations of DHS lead to considerable diagnostic confusion and delay in diagnosis, because dermatological, hematologic (anemia, thrombopenia, leukemic reactions), lymphatic, or internal organ involvement can mimic systemic diseases or an infection (Olmer et al., 1952; De Vriese et al., 1995; Anonymous, 1996). Therefore, a high index of suspicion is required in patients receiving drugs, which cause the syndrome (Pichler, 2003; Shepherd, 2003; Rademaker and Maling, 2003). These include allopurinol, aromatic anticonvulsants (particularly carbamazepine and phenytoin), and sulfonamides. Less common inducers include abacavir, atenolol, azathioprine, captopril, diltiazem, gold salts, minocycline, nevirapine, oxicam NSAIDs, sulfasalazine, and trimethoprim (http://www.pneumotox.com, 1997; Pichler, 2003; Rademaker and Maling, 2003). Recently, bupropion and leflunomide were shown to cause the syndrome (Bagshaw et al., 2003; Mohty et al., 2003).

Onset is gradual, with fever and skin reactions as the first indicators. Fever is a common early feature of DHS, followed by a widespread and long-lasting papulopustular, erythematous skin eruption (Rademaker and Maling, 2003), which may progress to exfoliative dermatitis (Roujeau and Stern, 1994). The severity or extent of the skin-related changes does not correlate well with the severity or extent of internal organ involvement, which may remain asymptomatic, or be life-threatening. Eosinophilia and atypical lymphocytosis occur in up to 30% of cases (Rademaker and Maling, 2003; Dosch et al., 1982). DHS can also be manifested by cytopenia (Cacatian and Rando, 1981; Gerson et al., 1983; Brain et al., 1984), hemolytic anemia (Sinnige et al., 1990), transient antibody deficiency (Dosch et al., 1982), or hypogammaglobulinemia (Lillie et al., 1983), or can mimic acute leukemia (Ray-Chaudhuri et al., 1989; Anonymous, 1996) or a viral infection (Brain et al., 1984). Organ involvement in DHS is manifold. Shear et al. reported 53 patients with DHS to different anticonvulsants (Shear and Spielberg, 1988). The clinical profile of DHS was similar, regardless of which anticonvulsant drug was taken. Fever was present in 94% of patients, a skin rash in 87%, hepatitis in 51%, and in 62% there was involvement of more than one organ. The thoracic manifestations of DHS include lymphoid interstitial pneumonia (Chamberlain et al., 1986), ILD (de Swert et al., 1984), eosinophilic pneumonia (Stephan et al., 1978), and pleural effusion (Bourezane et al., 1998; Corp and Ghishan, 1998; Thompson et al., 1998). Radioactive gallium is taken up in lung in about a third of patients taking phenytoin, but the contribution of this test in routine practice is unclear (Lentle et al., 1983). Other organ involvements in DHS include hepatosplenomegaly (Boissier et al., 1983), eosinophilic myocarditis (Salzman et al., 1997), colitis (Eland et al., 1999), granulomatous angiitis (Gaffey et al., 1986), a systemic *lupus erythematosus*-like picture with organizing pneumonia (Milesi-Lecat et al., 1997), and multiple organ dysfunction (Marik, 1999).

Four cases of carbamazepine-hypersensitivity syndrome were examined by De Vriese et al. (1995). Signs and symptoms developed 1 week to 3 months into treatment (average 4 weeks), and included fever, lymphadenopathy, a characteristic edema of the hands and face, hepatitis with a laboratory profile resembling viral hepatitis, acute tubulo-interstitial nephritis, hypersensitivity vasculitis in the kidney, and increased blood eosinophils (up to 36% of 55,000 cells in one case). Variegated autoantibodies (ANA, rheumatoid factor, antithyroid and anti-smooth muscle) were present.

Patients taking anticonvulsants may present with diffuse lymph node enlargement as a prominent manifestation of DHS (Saltzstein and Ackerman, 1959), and sometimes this is more visible in the mediastinum (Heitzman, 1967). Histopathology shows hyperplasia, or Reed–Sternberg cells and necrosis-mimicking Hodgkin's disease (De Vriese et al., 1995). Earlier reports or small series indicate reactive hyperplasia, immunoblastic lymphadenopathy, malignant lymphoma or Hodgkin's disease during treatments with anticonvulsants (Saltzstein and Ackerman, 1959; Hyman and Sommers, 1966; Schreiber and McGregor, 1968; Anthony, 1970; Sorell and Forbes, 1975). One recent series collated 25 patients (14 women) with lymphadenopathy during treatments with Dilantin (phenytoin) (Abbondazo et al., 1995). Patients' age ranged from 24 to 81 years, and lymphadenopathy developed 1 week to 30 years into treatment (Abbondazo et al., 1995). Fifteen of 25 cases showed a benign histology (reactive hyperplasia), seven were non-Hodgkin's lymphoma, and three were Hodgkin's disease (Abbondazo et al., 1995). Progression from paracortical hyperplasia to malignant lymphoma was evidenced in two out of five cases for which sequential biopsies were available (Abbondazo et al., 2000). Pseudolymphoma or lymphoma can diminish after drug therapy withdrawal but in some patients there is relapse to uncontrollable lymphoma (Gams et al., 1968). The development of lymphoma in the skin or internal organs during exposure to anticonvulsants is unusual (Rubinstein et al., 1985; Bocquet et al., 1996).

Underlying mechanisms causing DHS include enhanced metabolic activation of the drug (Pirmohamed et al., 1991), defective detoxification of reactive arene oxide metabolites (Spielberg et al., 1981), and slow acetylation. All these may lead to increased or persistent levels of toxic metabolites. Since these factors are likely controlled under genetic influences (Evans and McLeod, 2003), this may explain why the disease develops in only a few patients. In vitro tests have evidenced increased cell death in the presence of activated drug metabolites (Spielberg et al., 1981), blast transformation of drug-challenged cells (Virolainen, 1971; de Swert et al., 1984; Horneff et al., 1992), and cross-reaction between different drugs (Shear and Spielberg, 1988). These and other data (Mauri-Hellweg et al., 1995) suggest that there is an expansion of drug-specific T-cells, which may inflict damage to skin and internal organs (Mauri-Hellweg et al., 1995; Pichler, 2003). In the absence of skin lesions, a positive patch test may support the diagnosis (De Vriese et al., 1995). Circulating antibodies to the drug have been detected in a few cases (Kleckner et al., 1975), suggesting that the drug serves as a hapten (Pichler, 2003). A role for co-infection with the human herpes virus 6 acting as a danger signal is suspected (Pirmohamed et al., 2002; Descamps et al., 2003).

Treatment consists of immediate withdrawal of all suspect drugs, followed by supportive care of symptoms and corticosteroid drugs. Drug withdrawal is generally followed by significant improvement in a few days (Lewis and Rosenbloom, 1982). However, in a few patients, the disease accelerates a few weeks after withdrawal (De Vriese et al., 1995). The mortality rate is 8–10% (Bocquet et al., 1996; Rademaker and Maling, 2003). Relapse may occur as corticosteroid doses are tapered, and treatment may need to be continued for several months. Patients who develop DHS must avoid re-exposure to the causative medication and to related aromatic compounds (phenytoin, carbamazepine, phenobarbitone). Rechallenge produces relapse with increased severity (De Vriese et al., 1995). Cross-reaction can occur with oxicam NSAIDs. Because genetic factors are suspected in DHS, relatives should be instructed as regards the symptoms of DHS, and their enhanced risk of developing similar adverse reactions, should they take similar medications.

4.3. Drug-induced lupus erythematosus and antiphospholipid antibodies

Drug-induced *lupus* was first described in 1945 in a patient treated with sulfadiazine (Hoffman, 1945). Subsequently, many cases of drug-induced *lupus* were reported in the 1950s, when hydralazine became generally available for the treatment of systemic hypertension (Dustan et al., 1954). Hydralazine produces fever, arthralgias, and serositis, along with high titers of circulating ANA. It is estimated that after 4 years of treatment, 80–100% of patients develop ANA and 30–50% eventually develop symptoms of *lupus* (Goldberg et al., 1980).

At the time, the clustering of cases of drug-induced *lupus* produced a measurable increase in the prevalence of *lupus* above the background prevalence of idiopathic disease (Siegel et al., 1967). Later, isoniazid and procainamide were also recognized to cause the drug-induced *lupus*, and the latter drug is still considered the most potent *lupus*-inducing drug. Drug-induced *lupus* has now been reported with about 60 chemically and pharmacologically unrelated drugs (Adkinson et al., 2002) including amiodarone, ACEI, anticonvulsants (carbamazepine, ethosuximide, phenytoin, primidone, trimethadone, and valproate, but not benzodiazepines or phenobarbital), anti-TNF agents, β-blockers (mainly acebutolol), chlorpromazine, oral contraceptives, recombinant cytokines or antibodies, dihydralazine, interferon, mesalazine, methyldopa, minocycline, nitrofurantoin, propylthiouracil, statins, sulfasalazine and ticlopidine (Hess, 1981; Cush and Goldings, 1985; Skaer, 1992; Stevens, 1992; Price and Venables, 1995; http://www.pneumotox.com, 1997; Hannhahs Hahn, 1998; Yee and Pochapin, 2001; Jarrett et al., 2003). Although hydralazine and procainamide are now less in use, drug-induced *lupus* continues to occur in clinical practice (Gordon and Porter, 2001). Some of the cases with the drug *lupus* possibly would now be reclassified as having drug-induced vasculitis on the basis of ANCA testing, which was not available at the time (see below).

Overall, the prevalence of drug-induced *lupus* is 0.8 per 100,000 population, and it is estimated that drugs cause approximately 30% of all cases of *lupus*. Minocycline increases the risk of developing *lupus*

8.5-fold, compared to the background rate (Gordon and Porter, 2001). Generally, drugs induce a form of *lupus* which is *clinically* (milder course, absence of flares, rare kidney or neurological involvement, frequent reversal upon discontinuance of drug therapy, equal distribution in men and women, as opposed to the 90% female predominance in idiopathic *lupus*) and *biologically* (anti-double-strand-DNA antibodies distinctly unusual, normal complement levels) dissimilar to idiopathic *lupus* (Cohen and Prowse, 1989).

Risk factors for the development of drug-induced *lupus* are drug- and patient-related and include

- type of drug (e.g. arylamine and hydrazine drugs are potent *lupus*-inducing agents)
- the degree of exposure (i.e. dose and duration) to the drug
- acetylator phenotype

Patients with the slow hydralazine acetylator phenotype produce more oxidative and unconjugated metabolites, have a higher liability to disease, and develop *lupus*-related symptoms earlier than do those with rapid acetylators. In contrast, patients with the rapid acetylator phenotype rapidly metabolize hydralazine into conjugated metabolites, which are less potent inducers of *lupus* (Hofstra, 1994).

- genetic and ethnic background.

Relatives of patients with DI-*lupus* are more prone to the development of idiopathic autoimmune conditions, and the drug *lupus* develops more often in whites than it does in dark-skinned people.

As the disease develops insidiously after months or years into treatment, the diagnosis is often established late. The drug *lupus* manifests with chest pain, a dry hacking cough, dyspnea, arthralgias, skin changes, fever and malaise. In some patients the chest pain is excruciating or the cough is exhausting. Approximately half the patients with drug-induced *lupus* present with pneumonitis, rarely an ARDS picture (Sridhar and Abdulla, 1998), pleuritis, pleural thickening or effusion (Özkan et al., 2001), and up to a third present with pericardial effusion (Siddiqui and Khan, 2002), or tamponade (Verma et al., 2000). As in idiopathic *lupus*, the pleural fluid is an exudate (Good et al., 1983). Cells counts range from 230 to 55,000 cells/μl (Good et al., 1983; Smith and Nacht, 1992), the percentage of neutrophils from 10 to 100% (Good et al., 1983; Morelock and Sahn, 1999), and pleural levels of LDH from 200 to 550 IU/l. Elevated titers of ANA in the pleural fluid are a useful marker of *lupus* (Kaplan et al., 1978; Hiraoka et al., 1998), but may not separate drug-induced *lupus* from the idiopathic disease well. In one report, 11 of 13 patients with *lupus* pleuritis (two drug-induced) had pleural fluid ANA $\geq$1:160, and in 9, the pleural fluid-to-serum ANA ratio was greater than unity (Good et al., 1983). Antinuclear antibodies are specifically present in the pleural tissue of patients with drug *lupus* pleuritis, as opposed to pleural effusions of other causes (Chandrasekhar et al., 1978). Antinuclear antibodies are also found in the pericardial fluid of patients with pericardial effusion (Goldberg et al., 1980). Rare patients presented with peripheral eosinophilia as an associated feature (Paladini et al., 1982; Khosla et al., 1998).

Circulating antinuclear and antihistone antibodies are nearly always present in patients with drug-induced *lupus*, if appropriate techniques are employed. There is no relationship between ANA levels and the likelihood of developing *lupus*, or the type or severity of symptoms. Some patients with drug-induced *lupus* lack ANA, with only antihistone antibodies present (Carter et al., 2001). Antihistone antibodies are not specific for the drug etiology, and have different specificities, depending on the causative drug (H2A, H2B, or H2A-H2B-complex in procainamide-induced *lupus*, and H3 and H4 in hydralazine-induced *lupus*, respectively (Portanova et al., 1987)). Anti-double-strand-DNA antibodies have been described in a few patients with acebutolol-, hydralazine-, infliximab-, penicillamine-, and procainamide-induced *lupus*. Hypocomplementemia and anti-myeloperoxidase antibodies also are unusual findings in patients with typical drug-induced *lupus* (Pape et al., 2002). However, testing for ANCAs, especially anti-MPO, antilactoferrin or antielastase antibodies, is required, as the clinical features of drug-induced *lupus* and vasculitis occasionally overlap (Martinez-Vea et al., 1987; Choi et al., 2000a). The *lupus* anticoagulant and antiphospholipid antibodies are present in a few patients (Pape et al., 2002), and may associate with thromboembolic phenomena or the hypercoagulable state (Asherson et al., 1989; Yee and Pochapin, 2001). The diagnosis of drug-induced *lupus* may be difficult when elevated ANA titers are an expected feature of a background disease. Examples include the association of pleural effusion and elevated ANA titers in patients with ulcerative colitis, RA, or tuberculosis treated with mesalazine, penicillamine, or isoniazide, respectively. In such cases, changes in pleural involvement and ANA during treatment and/or upon drug withdrawal will help determine whether the condition is drug related.

Treatment consists mainly of discontinuation of the drug, with corticosteroid therapy reserved for severe reactions. Upon stoppage of drug therapy, all symptoms diminish within a few days or weeks (Gordon and Porter, 2001). This is followed by a more gradual decrease in circulating ANA towards lower or normal levels. In a fraction of patients, ANA and/or symptoms persist for longer periods (Gordon and Porter, 2001). Rechallenge leads to recurrence of symptoms within shorter periods (Gordon and Porter, 2001). Patients with subclinical ANA levels during treatments with drugs known to induce *lupus* need simple follow-up. The drug needs not be discontinued, unless an alternate treatment is available, or symptoms suggestive of autoimmune disease develop (Rubin et al., 1986).

4.4. Drug-induced vasculitis

Drugs of nearly all pharmacologic classes can cause hypersensitivity vascular reactions that may include cutaneous leukocytoclastic vasculitis (Mullick et al., 1979). Systemic vasculitis with internal organ involvement, in contrast, is considerably less common (Calabrese and Duna, 1996; Doyle and Cuellar, 2003). Early reports described systemic angiitis during treatments with sulfonamides and sulfamides (Rich, 1942; Tompson and Zeek, 1945; Lichtenstein and Fox, 1946). The list of drugs at the origin of systemic angiitis with pulmonary involvement has grown, and now includes allopurinol (Jarzobski et al., 1970), antithyroid drugs (Wing and Fantus, 1987; Merkel, 1998), anti-tumor necrosis factor-alpha therapy (Calabrese and Duna, 1996; Jarrett et al., 2003), celecoxib (Schneider et al., 2002), hematopoietic growth factors (Merkel, 1998), hydralazine (Merkel, 1998), minocycline (Elkayam et al., 1996; Schrodt and Callen, 1999), penicillamine (Merkel, 1998) and phenytoin (Yermakov et al., 1983; Michael and Rudin, 1981; Doyle and Cuellar, 2003). The quality of the evidence for proving causality with these agents is wide-ranging, from circumstantial in case reports, to supportive in larger series of patients (Choi et al., 2000a; Doyle and Cuellar, 2003). Not all patients who develop vasculitis from these agents present with pulmonary involvement, however.

The advent of ANCA testing in the 1990s has challenged previous clinical classifications (Drory and Korczyn, 1993), and may allow for reclassification of drug-induced angiitides (Merkel, 1998; Doyle and Cuellar, 2003). For most cases published before 1990, especially of penicillamine-associated pseudo-Goopasture syndrome, the exact etiopathogenesis of the vasculitis (i.e. ANCA-positive or not) is likely to remain out of reach. Currently, drug-induced p-ANCA-positive vasculitis and CSS emerge as the most prominent patterns of drug-induced pulmonary angiitis, whereas the possibility that drugs produce authentic Wegener's remains circumstantial (Choi et al., 2000a). As for any vasculitic process, early diagnosis is encouraged, otherwise loss of tissue and compromised function may occur. Treatment of drug-induced vasculitis consists of drug withdrawal, corticosteroids, immunosuppressive drugs and, sometimes, plasmapheresis.

4.4.1. Drug-induced ANCA-positive vasculitis

The antithyroid thionamides (propylthiouracil, carbimazole, methimazole and thiamazole (Gunton et al., 1999; Morita et al., 2000; Choi et al., 1999)), allopurinol (Choi et al., 1998), hydralazine (Nässberger et al., 1991; Merkel, 1998; Choi et al., 1999), minocycline (Merkel, 1998), penicillamine (Merkel, 1998) and sulfasalazine (Salerno et al., 1996; Choi et al., 2000a) produce systemic angiitis with possible pulmonary involvement. Out of 250 new patients with systemic vasculitis and pANCA antibodies, Choi et al. (2000a) examined the 30 with the highest antibody titers. There was long-term (>9 months) exposure to hydralazine in 10 (33%) and propylthiouracil in three (10%), and in five (17%) there was exposure to penicillamine, allopurinol, or sulfasalazine (Choi et al., 2000a). Half the patients with hydralazine-associated antibody-positive vasculitis had pulmonary involvement, with hemoptysis in four (Choi et al., 2000a). The two patients who developed ANCA during treatment with penicillamine also presented with pulmonary hemorrhage, which was fatal in both patients (Choi et al., 2000a). There was a strong association between the presence of antielastase and/or antilactoferrin antibodies and exposure to the above candidate drugs (Choi et al., 2000a). Anti-TNF-alpha therapy also produces p-ANCA-positive vasculitis, with cross-reaction between infliximab and etanercept suggesting a class effect (Jarrett et al., 2003). Extrapulmonary signs and symptoms of drug-induced vasculitis include constitutional symptoms, arthralgias, purpuric skin lesions or leukocytoclastic vasculitis, glomerulonephritis, renal failure, upper respiratory tract or ear, nose and throat involvement in addition to pleural effusion, chest pain, pulmonary infiltrates, alveolar hemorrhage, and lung nodules or cavitation (Cassorla et al., 1983; Stankus and Johnson, 1992; D'Cruz et al., 1995; Ohtsuka et al., 1997; Gunton et al., 1999; Chastain et al., 1999; Erten et al., 2002; Dinmezel et al., 2003) (for review of organs affected in drug-induced angiitis, see Chastain et al., 1999). Thus, drug-induced vasculitis can clinically imitate naturally occurring systemic vasculitis (Merkel, 1998).

The histopathologic background in patients with skin or kidney involvement shows active vasculitis, and this is similar to idiopathic vasculitis (Choi et al., 2000a). Capillaritis has been evidenced on the lung biopsy in one patient with DAH during treatment with propylthiouracil (Dhillon et al., 1999). Bland hemorrhage has been demonstrated in other cases (Choi et al., 2000a). Histopathology was unavailable in many cases (Schwarz and Fontenot, 2004).

The p-ANCA staining pattern coupled to myeloperoxidase (MPO), antilactoferrin or antielastase specificity (Ohtsuka et al., 1997) will separate most cases of drug-induced vasculitis from classic Wegener's, a condition associated with c-ANCAs positivity and PR3 specificity (Choi et al., 1999). In patients with ANCA-positive vasculitis, antinuclear (ANA) antibodies may be present, raising the possibility of drug-induced *lupus*. However, the high titers of anti-MPO antibodies and the highly distinctive clinical profile of ANCA-positive vasculitis with, notably, alveolar hemorrhage and necrotizing or crescentic glomerulonephritis usually enable the distinction with the drug-induced *lupus*.

p-ANCAs are thought to have pathogenic relevance, at least above a certain threshold (Noh et al., 2001), as they are temporally associated with flares of vasculitis (Choi et al., 1999). However, clinical disease can predate the rise in p-ANCAs (Morita et al., 2000). Prompt resolution of the vasculitis generally occurs after drug discontinuance. If dechallenge is followed by normalization of clinical manifestations of the disease and a fall in antibody titers, this is taken as strong supportive evidence for the drug etiology (Chastain et al., 1999; Choi et al., 1999). About 4% of patients taking propylthiouracil long-term develop ANCA, but vasculitis develops in only a few (Noh et al., 2001). No ANCA seroconversion was detected in patients with RA or systemic sclerosis treated with minocycline, penicillamine or sulfasalazine (Choi et al., 2000b). Low levels of ANCA generally are associated with absence of clinical disease, whereas higher levels of ANCA require close follow-up (Noh et al., 2001). In patients with naturally occurring ANCA-positive vasculitis or CTD (Merkel et al., 1997), treatment with drugs known to raise ANCA titers and/or to produce antibody-positive vasculitis (e.g. hydralazine, propylthiouracil) requires close monitoring. The development of c-ANCAs as opposed to p-ANCAs during treatments with therapy drugs is a rare occurrence (D'Cruz et al., 1995; Morita et al., 2000). The possibility that drugs induce Wegener's disease cannot be dismissed at this time (Dolman et al., 1993).

4.4.2. Drug-induced Churg–Strauss syndrome

The use of LTRA in the treatment of asthma has been associated with the development of CSS. Early reports described the occurrence of CSS in patients receiving zafirlukast (Knoell et al., 1998), and these were followed by reports of CSS in association with montelukast, pranlukast, and zileuton (Tuggey and

Hosker, 2000; Mukhopadhyay and Stanley, 2001). Patients presented with eosinophilia, pulmonary infiltrates, rarely DAH (Solans et al., 2002), cardiomyopathy, muscle pain, mononeuritis and, less often, digestive or dermatological involvement (Pedvis et al., 1999; Sabio et al., 2001). Symptoms occurred a few weeks or months into treatment with the LTRA (Weller et al., 2001). In 67–88% of the patients (Stirling and Chung, 1999; Weller et al., 2001), corticosteroids were being tapered at the time of onset of the CSS, whereas corticosteroid dosage was not altered in the remainder of patients. The temporal association of corticosteroid tapering and onset or relapse of symptoms of CSS has been described in the past in asthmatics who were unexposed to LTRA (Churg et al., 1995). Consequently, it was hypothesized that it is the tapering of corticosteroid that triggered the onset of CSS (Wechsler et al., 1998). However, several facts need be explained before this hypothesis can be accepted. Firstly, some studies have shown a 10-fold increase in the incidence of CSS in association with novel asthma-modifying drugs (Martin et al., 1999). Secondly, CSS has been observed in patients in whom corticosteroid dosage had not been altered before or after the introduction of the LTRA (Tang and Yosipovitch, 2003). Thirdly, CSS developed in patients who were not exposed to oral corticosteroids (Tuggey and Hosker, 2000; Green and Vayonis, 1999), or who had never been exposed to corticosteroids (Sabio et al., 2001). Fourthly, all manifestations of CSS reversed promptly after withdrawal of montelukast in one patient (Mukhopadhyay and Stanley, 2001). Furthermore, other steroid sparing agents are rarely associated with the development of CSS, despite their use for over 30 years (Stirling and Chung, 1999; Stoloff and Stempel, 2000). Lastly, one patient with a previous diagnosis of CSS relapsed after the introduction of montelukast to control the symptoms of asthma (Solans et al., 2002). Conversely, a few patients with CSS during treatments with LTRA reportedly could resume treatment with the drug without suffering relapse of CSS (Wechsler and Drazen, 2000). CSS has also been reported in asthma after systemic steroids tapering concomitant with the introduction of inhaled corticosteroids (Wechsler et al., 1999; Cooper et al., 2002). As for any novel adverse effect, a reporting bias cannot be excluded. Current estimates of the incidence of CSS in asthma are reassuring (Wechsler and Drazen, 2000; Lilly et al., 2002; Keogh and Specks, 2003).

The diagnosis of naturally occurring CSS is often established from clinical findings or biopsy of extrapulmonary sites, and lung biopsy is performed infrequently. Lung biospy is generally unavailable in patients with drug-induced CSS. According to Katzenstein, the classic pathologic findings in the lung include a combination of eosinophilic pneumonia, granulomatous inflammation and vasculitis. However, these three features are not all present in every case (Katzenstein, 2000).

There is some evidence linking treatments with macrolide antibiotics (Hübner et al., 1997), aspirin (Schmitz Schumann et al., 1998), vaccination against hepatitis B (Beretta et al., 2001) and immunotherapy (M'Raihi and Zegaya, 1990) with the development of CSS.

4.5. Sarcoidosis

Most cases of granulomatous lung disease result from treatments with interferon (IFN) alpha or beta. Interferon-induced sarcoidosis was first described in 1987 in a patient with renal cancer treated with IFN-beta (Abdi et al., 1987). This was followed by cases of sarcoidosis during treatments with IFN-alpha (Otte et al., 1997). IFN-induced sarcoidosis can also occur with pegylated IFNs (Rocca et al., 2002; Kumar et al., 2002a), and when ribavirin is combined with IFN in chronic hepatitis C infection (Hoffmann et al., 1998). Sarcoidosis has not been described in patients receiving ribavirin or IFN-gamma in isolation (Hoffmann et al., 1998). A literature review on IFN-alpha- and beta-induced sarcoidosis is available (Tahan et al., 2003). Interferon-induced sarcoidosis typically develops after a few months of treatment, and rarely after drug withdrawal (Hoffmann et al., 1998). Patients can be asymptomatic, or complain of fatigue, breathlessness and cough. These manifestations can be obscured by the flu-like symptoms and fatigue that usually accompany the first weeks of treatment with IFNs (Hoffmann et al., 1998). In some patients, IFN produced relapse of previously diagnosed sarcoidosis, which had been quiescent for many years (Wandl et al., 1992). Interferon-induced sarcoidosis reproduces the naturally occurring form of the disease, with involvement of mediastinal lymph nodes, lung parenchyma (Hoffmann et al., 1998; Ravenel et al., 2001), skin (including *erythema nodosum* and Löfgren syndrome) (Yavorkovsky et al., 1998; Hoffmann et al., 1998; Eberlein-König et al., 1999; Leveque et al., 2001), liver (Propst et al., 1995; Veerabagu et al., 1997), central nervous system, kidney and possibly calcium homeostasis, producing organ-targeted symptoms or dysfunction. Lymphocytes are increased in BAL (Moriya et al., 1994). However, BAL lymphocytes also are increased in untreated chronic viral hepatitis C, and the lymphocyte count decreases during uncomplicated treatments of this condition with IFN (Yamaguchi et al., 1997). The diagnosis of IFN-induced sarcoidosis is established by the demonstration of noncaseating granulomas in lung, bronchial mucosa, mediastinal lymph nodes or other organs. Interferon-induced sarcoidosis is improved with reduction in drug dosage, drug withdrawal, or institution of corticosteroids (Anderson et al., 2003). Thoracic and other manifestations of IFN-induced sarcoidosis tend to disappear in a few months (Hoffmann et al., 1998). In some patients, the granulomatous process may progress with time despite drug withdrawal, and corticosteroids are required as an adjunctive therapy for several months. No patient with IFN-induced sarcoidosis has progressed to the late fibrotic stage seen in naturally occurring pulmonary sarcoidosis.

Granulomas are an occasional finding in lung tissue or in lymph nodes of patients exposed to etanercept (Peno-Green et al., 2002), methotrexate (Verdich and Christensen, 1979), phenylbutazone (Goldstein, 1963), phenytoin (Rubinstein et al., 1986) and sirolimus (Avitzur et al., 2003).

4.6. Myopathies

Many drugs can produce myopathies (Le Quintrec and Le Quintrec, 1991; Zuckner, 1994; Cacoub et al., 1999; Dourmishev and Dourmishev, 1999; Dalakas and Hohlfeld, 2003). However, drugs rarely cause myositis with concomitant pulmonary involvement.

Hill et al. (1995) described a 76-year-old woman exposed to the HMG-CoA reductase inhibitor simvastatin. The patient developed limb weakness, a skin rash and pulmonary infiltrates. Laboratory investigation revealed increased levels of creatine kinase and antinuclear antibodies. Antisynthetase antibodies were not tested. Creatine kinase levels diminished after drug dechallenge, and the patient was given corticosteroids. Despite this, the lung disease progressed to DAD, and the patient died after 12 weeks. According to these investigators, the picture was consistent with dermatomyositis (Hill et al., 1995).

A 68-year-old man developed a clinical picture suggestive of the antisynthetase syndrome, with mechanic's fingers and fibrosing alveolitis after 2 months of treatment with valsartan (Thickett and Millar, 1997). There was, however, no serologic documentation of antisynthetase antibodies.

Whether the combination of polymyalgias and pulmonary infiltrates in patients exposed to statins (Liebhaber et al., 1999) is an early manifestation of polymyositis is unclear.

4.7. The eosinophilia-myalgia syndrome

In the 1980s L-tryptophan was a popular dietary supplement. The contamination of L-tryptophan with 1,1′-ethylenebis-L-tryptophan during the bacteria-driven synthesis of L-tryptophan in one plant produced a disabling condition known as eosinophilia-myalgia syndrome (EMS), which emerged as a novel disease in the late 1980s (Kilbourne, 1992; Sidransky, 1994). Over 1500 patients were affected, of whom 31 had died by 1992 (Hedberg et al., 1992). The incidence culminated in the late months of 1989 (Kilbourne, 1992), and diminished abruptly once L-tryptophan-containing products were recalled (Kilbourne et al., 1996). Affected patients presented with the insidious or more rapid onset of constitutional symptoms, myalgias, low muscle force, skin changes, fasciitis, neurologic involvement, cardiomyopathy, and eosinophilia. Respiratory involvement included pulmonary infiltrates, eosinophilic pneumonia, pulmonary angiitis, persistent pulmonary hypertension, and pleural effusion (Tazelaar et al., 1990, 1993). Long-term studies showed that eosinophilia, dermatological involvement, neuromuscular changes, and pulmonary hypertension could persist beyond 1 year (Hedberg et al., 1992; Hertzman et al., 1995; Pincus, 1996). One potential explanation for EMS lies in the possibility of 1,1′-ethylenebis-L-tryptophan being incorporated as an essential amino acid into peptides (Buss et al., 1996), and functionally activating eosinophils (Yamaoka et al., 1994).

5. Specific drugs causing respiratory involvement

5.1. Anti-TNF therapy

TNF-alpha is a proinflammatory cytokine which plays an important role in the pathogenesis of several CTDs including RA, WG, Behçet's disease, and inflammatory bowel disease. A chimeric monoclonal anti-TNF antibody (infliximab) and a recombinant TNF receptor fusion protein (etanercept) are available to inhibit TNF-alpha activity in these conditions.

Adverse effects *common to both agents* include opportunistic infections, mainly tuberculosis, acute and delayed hypersensitivity infusion reactions (Riegert-Johnson et al., 2002), rare instances of drug-induced *lupus* (Shakoor et al., 2002; Favalli et al., 2002; Carlson and Rothfield, 2003; Lepore et al., 2003), systemic vasculitis with ANA or p-ANCA positivity (Jarrett et al., 2003) and, possibly, malignant lymphoma (Aithal and Mansfield, 2001; Day, 2002).

Treatments with *etanercept* have rarely been associated with sterile caseating (Vavricka et al., 2003) and noncaseating (Peno-Green et al., 2002) pulmonary granulomas. In one patient, rheumatoid nodules developed after the introduction of etanercept (Hübscher et al., 2003).

Seven days after the second infusion of *infliximab*, a patient developed arthralgias, myalgias, fever, and respiratory failure requiring ventilatory support. Acute eosinophilic pneumonia was diagnosed on lung biopsy, and high concentrations of human antichimeric antibodies were present in lung tissue. The patient improved after drug withdrawal and intravenous corticosteroids (Riegert-Johnson et al., 2002). Infliximab was temporally associated with the development of acute methotrexate pneumonitis after the third infusion in three patients (Kramer et al., 2002), and with rapidly evolving pulmonary fibrosis in one patient. A drug-drug interaction is suggested (Kramer et al., 2003). In one patient with RA, treatment with infliximab was associated with deterioration of obstructive sleep apnea (Zamarron et al., 2004).

Time will tell whether anti-TNF agents cause specific lung disease, interact with other disease modifying anti-rheumatic drugs in terms of adverse pulmonary effects, or promote some pulmonary manifestations of RA.

The novel anti-TNF agents infliximab and, to a lesser degree, etanercept increase the risk of pulmonary and extrapulmonary tuberculosis (Gardam et al., 2003; Gardam and Iverson, 2003). Keane et al. (2001) reviewed 70 cases of tuberculosis after treatment with infliximab. Time to onset averaged 12 weeks, and in 48 patients, tuberculosis developed after three or fewer infusions. Forty patients had extrapulmonary tuberculosis and 17 had disseminated disease. Sixty-four patients were from countries with a low incidence of tuberculosis. Gomez-Reino et al. conducted a multicenter prospective study in Spain on 1578 treatment with anti-TNF agents (infliximab in 86%, etanercept in 14% of 1540 patients, respectively) (Gomez-Reino et al., 2003). They identified 17 cases of tuberculosis in patients treated with infliximab. The incidence of tuberculosis associated with infliximab in RA was 1893 and 1113 per 100,000 in the years 2000 and 2001, respectively, a significantly increased risk. The percentages of extra-pulmonary tuberculosis and mortality were greater than in non-infliximab-related tuberculosis. The excess rate of tuberculosis decreased in 2002, after guidelines for prevention and treatment of latent tuberculosis were implemented before treatment of RA with anti-TNF agents.

It is important to evaluate the risk of drug-induced tuberculosis in any patient with RA before starting treatment with these agents (Hamilton, 2003; Gardam et al., 2003; Gardam and Iverson, 2003). Consideration of background incidence in the general population of the country concerned, BCG vaccination earlier in the patient's life, prior history of tuberculosis, radiographic evidence of 'healed' tuberculosis, ethnicity and country of origin, and tuberculin skin testing is required. However, patients with RA are often anergic, due to background disease and ongoing treatments with methotrexate and corticosteroids. Thus, a 5-mm cut-off of tuberculin skin test positivity has been suggested. With this, one can evaluate whether chemoprophylaxis with isoniazid or isoniazid plus rifampin is required. It is safer to start infliximab 1 month into chemoprophylaxis for tuberculosis, so that INH tolerability and hepatotoxicity is evaluated, since overlapping medication toxicities can occur. Tuberculosis in patients being treated with anti-TNF agents is diagnosed and treated as it is in other contexts (Hamilton, 2003).

Pulmonary infections with *Aspergillus* (Warris et al., 2001), *Histoplasma* (Nakelchik and Mangino, 2002), and viruses (Smith and Letendre, 2002) have been described as a complication of therapy with anti-TNF agents in isolated reports.

5.2. Aspirin

In addition to producing bronchospasm in predisposed subjects (see under 'asthma'), chronic and 'excessive' intake of salicylate can produce pulmonary edema (Heffner and Sahn, 1981). The complication occurs preferentially in chronically exposed elderly patients, and not all cases are recognized (Anderson et al., 1976). Pulmonary edema is present in 10–15% of patients with an aspirin overdose (Heffner and Sahn, 1981). Clues to the diagnosis include exposure to the drug, dyspnea, bilateral pulmonary infiltrates, confusion, lactic acidosis, and sometimes shock or multiple organ failure (Leatherman and Schmitz, 1991; Matuschak, 1991). When present, proteinuria is thought to reflect an increase in capillary permeability (Matuschak, 1991; Gonzolez et al., 1998), a hypothesis, which has received experimental support (Glauser et al., 1978). Clinical examination reveals crackles and wheeze, and in cases with severe disease, cough productive of frothy sputum, cyanosis, arterial hypoxemia, hypotension or shock can be present (Gonzolez et al., 1998). A few patients developed pseudo-sepsis with shock and multiple organ dysfunction, including an ARDS picture, acute renal failure, diffuse intravascular coagulation, and encephalopathy (Pei and Thompson, 1987; Leatherman and Schmitz, 1991). On the chest radiograph, vague or bilateral fluffy infiltrates, Kerley B lines and, rarely, pleural effusion are present (Heffner and Sahn, 1981). Septal thickening and ground-glass or alveolar shadows are seen on HRCT (Bernal and Patarca, 1999). A BAL neutrophilia has been reported (Suarez and Krieger, 1986). The histopathologic appearance, available in a few patients, is that of interstitial or alveolar edema, with alveolar filling with proteinaceous fluid or DAD (Heffner and Sahn, 1981; Gonzolez et al., 1998). The diagnosis of salicylate pulmonary edema is supported by measurements of salicylate blood levels above 40–45 mg/dl, if obtained close to the time of admission. The disease may recur on rechallenge or continued exposure to ASA (Heffner and Sahn, 1981). The very quick return of pulmonary opacities along with a rise in temperature and neurologic symptoms upon rechallenge is characteristic, and led some authors to propose the term allergic pneumonitis or pulmonary edema.

Circumstantial evidence relates chronic exposure to aspirin with hemoptysis, DAH, or hemothorax (Gonzalo Hernandez et al., 1987; Gopalakrishnan et al., 1997; Kahn, 1998; van Sonnenberg and Wittich, 1998).

5.3. Azathioprine

Azathioprine is the nitroimidazole derivative of 6-mercaptopurine. The drug is used to treat several CTD, inflammatory bowel disease and, as a steroid-sparing agent, in CTD and pulmonary fibrosis. Treatments with azathioprine have been associated with a reversible restrictive pattern of lung dysfunction (Rubin et al., 1972), and with ILD with a lymphocytic BAL (Perreaux et al., 2000). Azathioprine can also produce DAD, which may evolve to irreversible pulmonary fibrosis (Bedrossian et al., 1984). A patient with Crohn's disease developed necrotizing vasculitis, which reversed after drug withdrawal (Attila et al., 2002). In one patient with Goodpasture's syndrome, treatment with azathioprine produced anti-GBM-negative flares of DAH (Stetter et al., 1994).

5.4. Corticosteroids

Corticosteroid drugs impact on the respiratory system in a number of ways.

Long-term corticosteroid therapy can lead to mediastinal lipomatosis, a radiographic curiosity in most patients, and a cause for cough (Sorhage et al., 1996) or mediastinal hemorrhage in a few (Taillé et al., 2001).

Corticosteroid drugs may induce respiratory muscle weakness. This may result in diminished force and pressure generated by the respiratory muscles, with consequent restrictive lung dysfunction (Decramer et al., 1996; Similowski and Strauss, 2004).

Cortisone allergy is rare (Kilpiö and Hannuksela, 2003).

Corticosteroids exert a broad range of immunosuppressive activities (Lionakis and Kontoyiannis, 2003). The risk of opportunistic infections is particularly increased for daily or cumulated doses of prednisolone above 10 and 700 mg, respectively (White, 2004). High-dose corticosteroids such as, for instance, intravenous boluses substantially increase the risk of opportunistic bacterial and fungal infections (Lionakis and Kontoyiannis, 2003). In patients on steroids, biological abnormalities (Agusti et al., 2003) and tissue response resulting from infection with microorganisms may be attenuated or altered (Lionakis and Kontoyiannis, 2003). Corticosteroids also may prevent the expected rise in body temperature in response to infectious agents (Lionakis and Kontoyiannis, 2003). Accordingly, the recognition of opportunistic infections is delayed (Lionakis and Kontoyiannis, 2003), with a consequent increase in mortality (Agusti et al., 2003). Microorganisms specifically associated with corticosteroid drug treatments now include *Mycobacterium tuberculosis*, *Staphylococcus*, *Aspergillus*, *Mucorales*, *Candida*, *Cryptococcus*, and *Pneumocystis carinii* (Agusti et al., 2003; Lionakis and Kontoyiannis, 2003; White, 2004) causing life-threatening staphylococcal infection or invasive aspergillosis. Agusti et al. (2003) reviewed 33 patients with pulmonary infiltrates while receiving corticosteroids. *Aspergillus* and *Staphylococcus* were the most common pathogens, at 30 and 20%, respectively. Overall, mortality was 45%, and was greater if there was bilateral involvement, delayed diagnosis, or requirement for mechanical ventilation (Agusti et al., 2003). Yale and Limper analyzed 116 non-AIDS patients with a first episode of *Pneumocystis carinii* pneumonia (Yale and Limper, 1996). Twenty-two percent of these patients had an inflammatory condition, and in 90% of the patients there was a history of treatment with corticosteroids. The median daily corticosteroid dose was equivalent to 30 mg of prednisone, 25% of patients had received as little as 16 mg of prednisone daily, and the median duration of corticosteroid therapy was 12 weeks before the development of *Pneumocystis carinii* pneumonia. About half the patients developed respiratory failure, and a third of the patients died from this complication. In addition to treatment-related factors, the background disease plays a role, as *Pneumocystis carinii* pneumonia occurs more frequently in systemic *lupus erythematosus*, WG, polymyositis, or *periarteritis nodosa* than in RA (Ward and Donald, 1999).

There are several case reports of fungal infection of the lung and airways following the regular use of inhaled and topical corticosteroids (Fairfax et al., 1999; Baratz and Hattenhauer, 1999; Leav et al., 2000; Peter et al., 2002; Zhou et al., 2003).

5.5. Cyclophosphamide

Like busulfan and nitrosoureas, cyclophosphamide is an alkylating agent used in the treatment of various solid tumors, leukemias, lymphomas, CTDs, and Wegener's or Churg–Strauss vasculitis. Although most cases of cyclophosphamide pneumonitis occur in malignant conditions, patients with WG (Anonymous, 1978; Stentoft, 1987), glomerulonephritis (Mark et al., 1978), *periarteritis nodosa* (Medrano San Ildefonso et al., 1986; Diaz-Gonzalez et al., 1992), and micropolyangiitis (Gromnica-Ihle, 2000) also develop the condition. Cyclophosphamide pneumonitis may differ little from the background disease for which the drug is given (Malik et al., 1996). When administered intravenously, cyclophosphamide can induce early pulmonary toxicity, in association with a BAL lymphocytosis (Cuguillière et al., 1999). Although sometimes severe (Woolley et al., 1997), early cyclophosphamide pneumonitis is largely reversible upon removal of the drug (Malik et al., 1996), except in a few patients who develop the ARDS picture (Woolley et al., 1997). Late toxicity mostly follows chronic oral exposure (Burke et al., 1982), and can occur with up to 13 years of treatment (Abdel Karim et al., 1983).

Chronic pneumonitis takes the form of progressive pulmonary fibrosis with, sometimes, digital clubbing (Topilow et al., 1973). It is mostly irreversible, even with drug withdrawal and the institution of corticosteroid therapy (Malik et al., 1996). In some patients, the peculiar features of late cyclophosphamide pulmonary toxicity are a pattern of fibrosis which also involves the upper and lateral aspects of the pleura, in addition to more typical changes of pulmonary fibrosis (Malik et al., 1996). In children, changes include the progressive narrowing of the anteroposterior diameter of the thorax, which contributes to a restrictive ventilatory defect during lung growth and development (Tucker et al., 1977; Alvarado et al., 1978). In patients in whom the diagnosis of cyclophosphamide pneumonitis is entertained, it is important to rule out an infection (Scheinman and Stamler, 1969; Kattwinkel et al., 1991; Kulke and Vance, 1997). *Pneumocystis carinii* pneumonia is difficult to differentiate from acute cyclophosphamide pneumonitis, and the two diseases can even coexist (Anonymous, 1984).

5.6. Gold

The gold salts aurothiomalate, aurothioglucose, and auranofin are among the first drugs recognized as causing eosinophilic pneumonia and hypersensitivity pneumonitis (Vaccarezza and Pavlovsky, 1945; Garrell, 1960). Hydrocortisone was efficacious in early cases (Garrell, 1960). Gold lung has received increasing attention following the paper by Winterbauer et al. (1976), who noted that rechallenge was quickly followed by recurrence of symptoms, and that too early a withdrawal of corticosteroids led to relapse (Winterbauer et al., 1976). Cocke and Bamji (1981) confirmed these findings in a review of 16 case reports. Gold lung has been the subject of a recent review summarizing 140 published cases, which were compared with 208 cases of rheumatoid lung (Tomioka and King, 1997).

Gold lung is unusual; for instance there was no case of gold lung in a series of 1019 patients exposed to the drug (Lockie and Smith, 1985). Gold lung is likely to become even less frequent as novel and more efficacious therapies such as methotrexate and anti-TNF drugs are available for the treatment of RA. Most patients with gold lung have RA, with only a few receiving the drug for asthma, unspecified arthritis, or *pemphigus* (Tomioka and King, 1997). Gold lung occurs largely in women, and tends to develop within the first 6 months of treatment, with a total dose of less than 1300 mg (range 30–3000 mg (average 677 mg) of drug) (Tomioka and King, 1997). Patients with certain HLA haplotypes may be at increased risk (Partanen et al., 1987). Symptoms include the rapid onset of dyspnea (in >90% of the patients), cough (in two-thirds), fever (in 50%), and a skin rash (in about 40%) (Tomioka and King, 1997). A restrictive ventilatory defect with decreased diffusing capacity and hypoxemia are common. Chest imaging shows bibasilar shadowing in about a third, and this is sometimes accompanied by severe volume loss (Weaver and Law, 1978; Hellebrand et al., 1979; Podell et al., 1980). Other imaging patterns include apical (Terho et al., 1979), butterfly-or batwing-shaped subpleural (Baethge and Wolf, 1988) or diffuse opacities, which can obscure both lung fields (Garrell, 1960). A few reports described a miliary pattern (Autran et al., 1978; Hellebrand et al., 1979). In the few reported CT studies, patchy opacities center along bronchovascular bundles (Vernhet et al., 1995; Nomura et al., 1997), a pattern reminiscent of nitrofurantoin lung, but clearly different from untreated rheumatoid lung (Tomioka and King, 1997; Freemer and King, 2003). Moderate peripheral eosinophilia is noted in about 40% of cases, but does not necessarily indicate parenchymal eosinophilic pneumonia. BAL findings show an increased lymphocyte count in about two-thirds of cases, with an inverted CD4+/CD8+ ratio in 80% (Tomioka and King, 1997), and a normal BAL in 15% (Tomioka and King, 1997). Several reports described positive stimulation when blood lymphocytes are challenged with gold in vitro (McCormick et al., 1980; Tomioka and King, 1997).

Pathology material was available in 85 of the 140 cases reviewed by Tomioka and King (1997), although this is not generally required for diagnosis. Patterns seen on histopathology include septal inflammation, which would probably now be classified as cellular or nonspecific interstitial pneumonia, and eosinophilic or organizing pneumonia, superimposed on a background of interstitial fibrosis (Tomioka and King, 1997).

The pulmonary manifestations of intolerance to gold can progress despite cessation of exposure, and this is occasionally fatal with 12% of patients dying from respiratory failure (Levinson et al., 1981; Usuba et al., 1989). Corticosteroids induce complete remission in two-thirds of cases (Tomioka and King, 1997), but treatment may be required for up to 18 months for a complete response (Slingerland et al., 1987).

Two main issues confounded the diagnosis and recognition of gold lung in RA. Concomitant NSAIDs can also cause severe eosinophilic pneumonia (Fujimori et al., 1999), and it may be necessary to stop NSAIDs in patients not improving after cessation of gold (McFadden et al., 1989). Rapidly progressive rheumatoid lung may produce acute respiratory failure and simulate gold lung (Noseworthy et al., 1983; Chatzigiannis et al., 1984), but is characterized by BAL neutrophilia and resistance to the administration of corticosteroid drugs (Freemer and King, 2003), unlike gold lung (Tomioka and King, 1997). However, in accelerated disease, it can be difficult to distinguish between rheumatoid and gold lung.

5.7. Interferons

Interferons may become a therapeutic option in patients with CTD (Tatsis et al., 1998), in addition to their established use for the treatment of chronic hepatitis C virus infection, multiple sclerosis, and malignant or nonmalignant hematologic conditions. Interferon-gamma has been used experimentally to treat lung cancer, malignant pleural effusions, multidrug resistant tuberculosis, and as a salvage therapy of corticosteroid-resistant pulmonary toxicity syndrome following BCNU-based chemotherapy in bone marrow transplantees (Antoniou et al., 2003; Suratt et al., 2003). Recently, IFN-gamma has been tried in patients with idiopathic pulmonary fibrosis (IPF) (Raghu et al., 2004).

While the most distinctive adverse pulmonary effect of *IFNs alpha and beta* is a sarcoidosis reaction (Kumar et al., 2002a) (see above), IFNs also can produce cellular, eosinophilic (Hoffman et al., 2003) or, less often, fibrotic ILD (Kamisako et al., 1993). Respiratory failure was present in several patients with IFN-induced pneumonitis (Chin et al., 1994; Wolf et al., 1997; Kumar et al., 2002a). On imaging, diffuse, sometimes streaky shadows are present bilaterally, and have a predilection for the lung bases (Ishizaki et al., 1996). At the height of the pulmonary reaction, CD8 + lymphocytes are increased in BAL (Moriya et al., 1994; Ishizaki et al., 1996). Interferon-induced ILD responds favorably to corticosteroids (Moriya et al., 1994). One patient with IFN-induced ILD died within a few weeks with multiple organ dysfunction syndrome (Abi-Nassif et al., 2003). Other patterns of IFN-induced ILD include BOOP (Ferriby and Stojkovic, 2001; Patel et al., 2001), which manifests with diffuse infiltrates (Ogata et al., 1994; Kumar et al., 2001) or a solitary mass (Ferriby and Stojkovic, 2001), and a desquamative interstitial pneumonia pattern (Kamisako et al., 1993). Less common adverse effects of IFNs alpha and beta include deterioration of asthma (Krasnowska et al., 1992), which relapses after rechallenge with the drug (Bini and Weinshel, 1999), cough (Pileire et al., 1999), pleural effusion (Takeda et al., 2000), and pulmonary hypertension (Fruehauf et al., 2001). Drug withdrawal may reverse these conditions.

Treatments with *IFN-gamma* have been associated with serious adverse pulmonary reactions (Shaw et al., 1995). More recently, precipitous deterioration of the respiratory status has been reported in four patients with IPF during treatment with IFN-gamma-1b (Honoré et al., 2003). The four patients had advanced IPF with baseline TLC of 46%, diffusing capacity of less than 30% of predicted, and a PaO_2 of 57 mm Hg. The patients developed hypoxemic respiratory failure corresponding to DAD after 2–35 injections of IFN-gamma. They did not respond to corticosteroids, and the disease was fatal in three patients, with one patient successfully transplanted (Honoré et al., 2003). No patient in three recent series of IFN-gamma in IPF developed this complication (Prasse et al., 2003; Raghu et al., 2004; Nathan et al., 2004).

5.8. Methotrexate

Methotrexate pneumonitis complicates the treatment of various neoplastic and nonneoplastic conditions with an incidence rate between 0.3 and 11.6%

(Imokawa et al., 2000), 0.5 and 14% (Zisman et al., 2001), 0.3 and 18% (Salaffi et al., 1997), or 1.5% per year (Cottin et al., 1996). The high incidence and relatively long prodromal phase of methotrexate pneumonitis demands that patients should always be informed of the possibility of developing methotrexate lung, and the need to seek prompt evaluation of unexplained cough and dyspnea. Methotrexate lung was recognized more than 30 years ago (Sostman et al., 1976), and there are almost 200 published cases (Massin et al., 1990; Salaffi et al., 1997; Imokawa et al., 2000; Zisman et al., 2001). The disease is characterized by insidious dry cough, fever and dyspnea lasting for 1–4 weeks (Kremer et al., 1997), followed by the rapid and unexpected development of diffuse pulmonary infiltrates, variably progressing to dense bilateral infiltrates and acute respiratory failure (Sostman et al., 1976; Hargreaves et al., 1992). It is essential to rule out an opportunistic infection, which can be similar to methotrexate lung, with no reliable clinical or radiological discriminators (Logan et al., 1995; Cleverley et al., 2002). *Pneumocystis carinii*, CMV, *Cryptococcus*, *Herpes-zoster* and *Nocardia* have been particularly associated with treatments with methotrexate in isolated reports (Carmichael and Ryatt, 1990; Antonelli et al., 1991; Clerc et al., 1991; Kuitert and Harrison, 1991; Wollner et al., 1991; Kerstens et al., 1992; Vallerand et al., 1992; Kane et al., 1993; LeMense and Sahn, 1994; Aglas et al., 1995; Thomas et al., 1997). CD4+ lymphocytes below 150 per μl and cumulated doses of methotrexate >700 mg may increase the risk of *Pneumocystis carinii* pneumonia (Kane et al., 1993). Patients having received high cumulated doses of methotrexate, and who have low CD4+ counts, are considered for *Pneumocystis carinii* pneumonia prophylaxis, especially if their background disease impacts on immune defenses (Huynh-Do et al., 1995; Guillevin et al., 1997; Chung et al., 2000; Ullmer et al., 2000; Russian and Levine, 2001). Clusters of *Pneumocystis carinii* pneumonia in immunosuppressed patients suggest nosocomial transmission of the disease (Huynh-Do et al., 1995). By contrast, it is seldom difficult to distinguish between acute methotrexate pneumonitis and fibrosis due to rheumatoid lung, which is radiologically overt in up to 25% of RA patients receiving the drug (Dawson et al., 2002). Although the combination of drug withdrawal and high-dose intravenous corticosteroid therapy is usually associated with a favorable outcome without sequellae, a mortality of 15% in a recent series underlines the need for careful management (Kremer et al., 1997). Although methotrexate has been successfully reintroduced following an episode of methotrexate pneumonitis (Fehr et al., 2003), relapse will occur in at least 50% of those rechallenged with the drug, with a fatality rate of around 50% (Kremer et al., 1997).

Life-threatening methotrexate pneumonitis was first described in children with hematologic malignancies in clinical remission, and in these cases, open lung biopsy showed cellular interstitial pneumonitis and granulomas (Clarysse et al., 1969). Cessation of the drug and corticosteroid therapy were effective, although methotrexate was continued in some patients without harm (Clarysse et al., 1969). The 123 and 189 cases in the literature were reviewed recently by Imokawa et al. (2000) and by Zisman et al. (2001), respectively. While methotrexate pneumonitis can develop in various disease states (leukemia, solid tumors, primary biliary cirrhosis, asthma, and molar or ectopic pregnancy), most recent cases have occurred with chronic therapy for RA or, less often, psoriasis or unspecified arthritis. Methotrexate pneumonitis does not differ according to the background disease, and the majority of patients are women (62%). Methotrexate pneumonitis developed after administration of doses ranging from 2.5 to 1400 mg/week via the oral, parenteral or intrathecal route. The duration of treatment is diverse, ranging from a single exposure to 5 years of treatment, although half developed methotrexate pneumonitis within the first 32 weeks of treatment (Kremer and Joong, 1986). The development of methotrexate pneumonitis is largely unpredictable, with no correlation between the dose and time to onset or clinical severity. Fatal methotrexate lung can occur with low-dose methotrexate, as exemplified in RA (Newman and Harrington, 1988). Some investigators report that male gender and prior pulmonary disease may predispose to methotrexate lung (Searles and McKendry, 1987), but these findings are not consistent (Cottin et al., 1996). The risk may increase with the concomitant use of drugs that decrease MTX protein binding (e.g. aspirin, NSAID, sulfonamides). Recently, methotrexate lung has coincided with the introduction of infliximab (Kramer et al., 2002). Prospective evaluation of patients on the drug has shown that there is no consistent decrease in lung volumes (Wall et al., 1979; Camiciottoli et al., 1998) or the diffusing capacity (Cottin et al., 1996). Serial pulmonary function testing does not allow for the early detection of methotrexate pneumonitis (Cottin et al., 1996). Follow-up of imaging has also not shown consistent changes during long-term methotrexate use (Belzunegui et al., 2001; Dawson et al., 2002). Almost all patients are still on the drug at the time of onset, with only a handful of reported cases with delayed onset (Elsasser et al., 1989; Pourel et al., 1991).

The diagnostic criteria of Clearkin et al. (1997) include an acute onset of dyspnea, fever above 38 °C, respiratory rate greater than 28 per min, the presence of radiographic abnormalities, a white blood cell count above 15,000 per μl, negative blood and sputum cultures, a restrictive lung function defect with reduced diffusing capacity, a PaO_2 below 50 mmHg on room air, and evidence for ILD on a lung biopsy specimen. The disease is deemed definite, probable or possible if six, five or four criteria are fulfilled, respectively (Clearkin et al., 1997).

Unusual patterns of methotrexate lung include a subacute presentation (Kremer et al., 1997), pulmonary fibrosis (Kaplan and Waite, 1978), and an isolated cough, which is not a precursor of methotrexate pneumonitis (Schnabel et al., 1996). Mild peripheral eosinophilia is present in about a third (Zisman et al., 2001) to 40% of patients (Imokawa et al., 2000), however, methotrexate pneumonitis is not an eosinophilic pneumonia. Radiographic studies show a diffuse and symmetrical interstitial opacification of both lung fields, which predominates in the bases or, less often, in the apices (Imokawa et al., 2000; Zisman et al., 2001). In severe cases, a pattern of dense bilateral alveolar opacities with air bronchograms may develop (Everts et al., 1973). On HRCT, ground-glass, interstitial infiltrates, septal lines and intralobular septal thickening or widespread consolidation are present (Zisman et al., 2001; Erasmus et al., 2002b). A diffuse miliary pattern has been reported in a few patients (Ellis et al., 2000). BAL is highly useful in the diagnosis of methotrexate lung, and can be performed in nearly all patients, if provision is made to correct the hypoxemia, which invariably occurs during the procedure (Verra et al., 1992). Total BAL cellularity is increased in 60% of the patients, in part due to a lymphocytosis of the CD4 + or CD8 + phenotype (Akoun et al., 1987; White et al., 1989; Fuhrman et al., 2001; Zisman et al., 2001), depending on when BAL is performed with respect to the onset of disease, and whether corticosteroids have been given before BAL (Akoun et al., 1987; White et al., 1989; Fuhrman et al., 2001).

Histological findings were available in 49 of the 123 reports reviewed by Imokawa et al. (2000), and included interstitial inflammation or fibrosis, granuloma formation, and increased tissue eosinophils in 71, 59, 35 and 18%, of cases, respectively. Although eosinophils are present, they are not a predominant feature (Imokawa et al., 1996). Granulomas are typically small and ill defined, and central sterile necrosis is unusual (Imokawa et al., 2000). In predominantly granulomatous disease, the involvement is patchy, with intervening areas of normal lung tissue, or tissue showing moderate cellular interstitial pneumonia (Imokawa et al., 1996). Type 2 cell hyperplasia is a notable feature of methotrexate lung, as it is in other forms of chemotherapy-induced lung disease (Imokawa et al., 2000). However, dysplastic changes are less prominent with methotrexate than with other alkylating agents. Alveolar edema, DAD, hyaline membranes, and DAH are unusual features, and are preferentially seen in patients with severe disease (Imokawa et al., 2000). Rare appearances include desquamative interstitial pneumonia- or sarcoidosis-like patterns, or an acute interstitial pneumonia pattern (Hamman–Rich-like) (Bedrossian et al., 1979).

The differential diagnosis of methotrexate lung is complex. Firstly, the symptoms and imaging of methotrexate pneumonitis cannot be distinguished from those of opportunistic infections, which methotrexate can predispose to (White, 2004). Thus, in considering the diagnosis of methotrexate pneumonitis, a meticulous workup for opportunistic infection is required. Secondly, other pneumotoxic drugs in addition to methotrexate may have been used (e.g. NSAIDs). However, the clinical-pathologic pattern of a rapidly evolving granulomatous pneumonitis with mild blood eosinophilia is distinctive, as opposed to that of other drugs or NSAIDs, which typically produce an eosinophilic pneumonia pattern (Imokawa et al., 2000). Finally, some background diseases such as inflammatory bowel disease may also acutely involve the lung (Camus et al., 1993). In contrast, most cases of rheumatoid lung have an indolent course (Freemer and King, 2003).

The management of methotrexate pneumonitis includes drug discontinuation and, generally, corticosteroid therapy (Imokawa et al., 2000; Zisman et al., 2001), although the disease may clear without corticosteroids (Berkani et al., 2003). Neither the optimal dose nor the correct duration of corticosteroid treatment have been determined; both are likely to depend upon the early clinical, physiologic and radiographic response in individual cases. A lack of response to conventional dosages of corticosteroid requires increase in dosage (in the order of 240–480 mg methylprednisolone per day) until a response is observed. Radiographic regression of disease is paralleled by functional improvement, which may require up to several months to be complete. Eighty-five percent of patients recover fully, but up to 15% die from progressive respiratory failure (Newman and Harrington, 1988). In some patients, methotrexate pneumonitis has responded to corticosteroids despite continuation of treatment (Massin et al., 1990; Imokawa et al., 2000). Daunorubicin (Pasquinucci et al., 1971) and cyclophosphamide (Suwa et al., 1999) have been used in methotrexate lung resistant to drug withdrawal and corticosteroid therapy. Methotrexate does not produce chronic ILD or pulmonary fibrosis (Dawson et al., 2002).

5.9. Minocycline

Minocycline has been used to treat RA. The drug can produce many systemic conditions (*lupus*, hypersensitivity syndrome, vasculitis), and the syndrome of pulmonary infiltrates with eosinophilia (Sitbon et al., 1994; Clayton et al., 1999; Elkayam et al., 1999; Schrodt and Callen, 1999; Rosen, 2000; Schlienger et al., 2000; Gordon and Porter, 2001; Marzo-Ortega et al., 2001; Marai and Shoenfeld, 2002; Settgast et al., 2003; Wolthuis et al., 2003). See appropriate sections above.

5.10. Nonsteroidal anti-inflammatory agents

Most adverse effects of NSAIDs involve the gastrointestinal tract (about 40%), whereas adverse effects in the respiratory system represent less than 3% of the total (Figueras et al., 1994). Oral, parenteral, and topical (dermal, rectal, or ophthalmologic) application of NSAIDs can produce acute life-threatening bronchospasm (Ibanez et al., 1991), which is clinically similar to the bronchospasm following exposure to aspirin or β-blockers (see above).

NSAIDs can produce anaphylaxis, with or without associated bronchospasm. It is estimated that NSAIDs account for approximately 10% of anaphylaxis episodes (Kemp et al., 1995). Patients who develop anaphylaxis during treatments with COX-1 inhibitors can be given COX-2 inhibitors (Berkes, 2003). However, post-marketing surveillance of COX-2 inhibitors is still limited, and a few patients have developed anaphylaxis during treatments with COX-2 inhibitors as well (Layton et al., 2003).

NSAIDs can also produce eosinophilic pneumonia (see above) (Pfitzenmeyer et al., 1994; http://www.pneumotox.com, 1997), enlargement of mediastinal lymph nodes (Oishi et al., 2001), pulmonary edema (Chetty et al., 1993), the DHS (Le et al., 1994), and severe allergic vasculitis (Schneider et al., 2002).

5.11. Penicillamine

Few drugs can induce so many distinctive adverse pulmonary and systemic reactions as penicillamine. These include asthma, BO, several types of ILD including nonspecific interstitial pneumonia, PIE, acute interstitial pneumonia, OP, polymyositis, *myasthenia gravis* and the drug-induced *lupus* (Geddes et al., 1977; Epler et al., 1979; Matloff and Kaplan, 1980; Camus et al., 1982; Louie et al., 1986; Cannon, 1990; Boehler et al., 1996; Karkos et al., 1996; Lohr et al., 1997; Perez et al., 1997; Lin et al., 2000; Derk and Jimenez, 2003).

A Goodpasture-like syndrome is a distinctive pattern of adverse reaction to penicillamine (see also under drug-induced vasculitis). Derk and Jimenez described one patient with penicillamine-induced DAH, and reviewed 13 earlier cases (Derk and Jimenez, 2003). The patients presented with rapidly progressive glomerulonephritis and DAH. Anti-GBM antibodies were present in only one patient, ANA were present in six, and in one patient anti-MPO p-ANCA were present. However, most patients with this entity were seen before 1990, at a time when ANCA testing was not generally available. Currently, testing for ANA, anti-ds-DNA, ANCAs, and anti-GBM should be done routinely in patients presenting glomerulonephritis and DAH due to d-penicillamine or other drugs, as the condition may be ANCA-mediated (Choi et al., 2000a). Despite corticosteroids, plasmapheresis, azathioprine, and cyclophosphamide, six of 14 patients studied by Derk and Jimenez (2003), and two of two in the series by Choi et al., died. Penicillamine is used much less now, and this type of adverse reaction is likely to continue to decline in frequency.

5.12. Sulfamides

Adverse effects of sulfonamide were described in the 1940s (Ellis and McKinlay, 1941). Sulfasalazine was introduced in 1941 in the treatment of RA and inflammatory bowel disease by Svartz, and this was followed by reports of adverse effects (Collins, 1968), including 'allergic pneumonia' with, often, an eosinophilic pattern (Jones and Malone, 1972). It was soon recognized that adverse reactions to sulfasalazine were temporally associated with exposure to the drug, improved upon drug withdrawal and relapsed after rechallenge. Patients with the slow acetylator phenotype have a higher risk of developing sulfasalazine-associated adverse effects, presumably reflecting increased levels of sulfasalazine metabolites, including 5-aminosalicylate (now synthesized and used as the drug mesalazine) (Schröder and Price Evans, 1972; Das et al., 1973). Desensitization with sulfasalazine usually can be achieved by incremental dosages.

Forty cases of adverse pulmonary effects of sulfasalazine were reviewed in 1993 (Camus et al., 1993), and a few further cases have been described subsequently (Salerno et al., 1996; Peters et al., 1997; Manchanda and Rees, 1999; Nanayakkara and Postmus, 1999; Bielecki et al., 2000; Woltsche et al., 2001; Parry et al., 2002), with most patients receiving sulfasalazine for inflammatory bowel disease (mostly ulcerative colitis) or RA. Daily dosage ranged between 1.5 and 8.0 g, duration of treatment with sulfasalazine between 2 weeks and 8 years, and total dose between 24 and 11,520 g. Symptoms at presentation include fever and a skin rash. Pulmonary involvement takes the form of the PIE syndrome in approximately half the patients, and unspecified ILD in about a third. Other less common patterns included BOOP, pulmonary granulomas, pulmonary fibrosis (Camus et al., 1993), or a Wegener's-like picture with histopathologic demonstration of angiitis and alveolar hemorrhage (Salerno et al., 1996). The opacities have a predilection for the apices, often with a sub-pleural distribution consistent with PIE. Other less frequent imaging patterns include involvement of middle or basal lung regions and diffuse shadowing. BAL findings are variable, with increases in lymphocytes, neutrophils or eosinophils. The prognosis is good in most of patients: irreversible lung fibrosis, rapidly progressive ILD and death remain unusual (Camus et al., 1993). Rechallenge has confirmed the diagnosis in ten reported cases, including eight presenting with the pattern of PIE. In some patients, desensitization was successfully achieved, whereas others were switched to mesalazine, 5-ASA, or azodisalicylate without relapse of pulmonary symptoms. The distinction between rheumatoid lung and sulfasalazine pneumonitis is often straightforward, because rheumatoid lung rarely demonstrates an accelerated course responding to corticosteroids. The distinction can be more difficult in patients with inflammatory bowel disease, as the background disease can also manifest with acute ILD (Camus et al., 1993). A meticulous history, timely withdrawal of sulfasalazine, and judicious use of corticosteroids will elucitate the question in most cases (Camus et al., 1993).

The sulfamethoxazole moiety in trimethoprime-sulfamethoxazole can produce eosinophilic pneumonia (Guérin et al., 1980; Hashizume et al., 2001), pulmonary edema (Silvestri et al., 1987), or anaphylaxis (Schuster and Wüthrich, 2003).

6. Conclusion

Drugs used in CTDs can produce a constellation of pulmonary and systemic reactions. These can mimic pulmonary involvement from CTD, a systemic disease, or an infection, and are difficult to prevent, predict, and diagnose. Maintaining a high index of suspicion will enable earlier recognition of drug-induced diseases, and early drug withdrawal. This should translate into improved prognosis. The field of drug-induced respiratory disease is moving fast, and a permanently updated website (http://www.pneumotox.com) is available.

Acknowledgements

The author thanks Clio Camus, for her constant help and support throughout the stages of this manuscript, Adeline Metchedjin, for her input in the drug-induced *lupus*, Pascal Foucher, with whom we built Pneumotox® (http://www.pneumotox.com, 1997), and who maintains and updates the website.

Key points

- Classic and novel drugs used to treat connective tissue disease produce varied patterns of respiratory involvement, including parenchymal, circulatory, pleural and airway changes. Also, drugs can produce systemic illnesses which can involve the lung in a manner similar to naturally-occurring diseases.
- Drug-induced disease often remits after drug discontinuation.
- It is important to rule out an infection, which can mimic and are difficult to differentiate from the drug-induced condition.

References

Abbondazo, S.L., Irey, N.S., Frizzera, G. 1995. Am. J. Surg. Pathol. 19, 675–686.

Abbondazo, S.L., Rush, W., Bijwaard, K.E., Koss, M.N. 2000. Am. J. Surg. Pathol. 24, 587–597.

Abdel Karim, F.W., Ayash, R.E., Allam, C., Salem, P.A. 1983. Oncology 40, 174–176.

Abdi, E.A., Nguyen, G.K., Ludwig, R.N., Dickout, W.J. 1987. Cancer 59, 896–900.

Abi-Nassif, S., Mark, E.J., Fogel, R.B., Hallisey, R.K. 2003. Chest 124, 406–410.

Adachi, M., Saito, H., Kobayashi, H., Horie, Y., Kato, S., Yoshioka, M., Ishii, H. 2003. Ann. Intern. Med. 139, 488–492.

Adkinson, N.F.J., Essayan, D., Gruchalla, R., Haggerty, H., Kawabata, T., Sandler, J.D., Updyke, L., Shear, N.H., Wierda, D. 2002. J. Allergy Clin. Immunol. 109, S461–S478.

Agarwal, A., Azim, A., Ambesh, S., Bose, N., Dhiraj, S., Sahu, D., Singh, U. 2003. Can. J. Anaesthesia 50, 297–300.

Aglas, F., Rainer, F., Hermann, J., Gretler, J., Hüttl, E., Domej, W., Krejs, G.J. 1995. Arthritis Rheum. 38, 291–292.

Agusti, C., Rano, A., Filella, X., Gonzalez, J., Moreno, A., Xaubet, A., Torres, A. 2003. Chest 123, 488–498.

Aithal, G.P., Mansfield, J.C. 2001. Aliment. Pharmacol. Ther. 15, 1101–1108.

Akira, M., Ishikawa, H., Yamamoto, S. 2002. Radiology 224, 852–860.

Akoun, G.M., Mayaud, C.M., Touboul, J.L., Denis, M. 1986. Arch. Intern. Med. 146, 804–805.

Akoun, G.M., Mayaud, C.M., Touboul, J.L., Denis, M.F., Milleron, B.J., Perrot, B.J. 1987. Thorax 42, 652–655.

Albertson, T.E., Walby, W.F., Derlet, R.W. 1995. Chest 108, 1140–1149.

Alkins, S.A., Byrd, J.C., Morgan, S.K., Ward, F.T., Weiss, R.B. 1996. Cancer 77, 2123–2126.

Almoosa, K.F. 1999. South. Med. J. 92, 1100–1102.

Alvarado, C.S., Boat, T.F., Newman, A.J. 1978. J. Pediatr. 92, 443–446.

Anderson, R.J., Potts, D.E., Gabow, P.A., Rumack, B.H., Schrier, R.W. 1976. Ann. Intern. Med. 85, 745–748.

Anderson, P., Höglund, M., Rödjer, S. 2003. Am. J. Hematol. 73, 54–58.

Anonymous, 1972. N. Engl. J. Med. 286, 1405–1411.

Anonymous, 1978. N. Engl. J. Med. 298, 729–736.

Anonymous, 1984. N. Engl. J. Med. 311, 585–593.

Anonymous, 1996. N. Engl. J. Med. 335, 577–584.

Anonymous, 2002. Ann. Intern. Med. 2002, 1–31.http://www.annals.org.

Ansell, G. 1969. Clin. Radiol. 20, 133–148.

Anthony, J.J. 1970. Arch. Neurol. 22, 450–454.

Antonelli, M.S., Moreland, L.W., Brick, J.E. 1991. Am. J. Med. 90, 295–298.

Antoniou, K.M., Ferdoutsis, E., Bouros, D. 2003. Chest 123, 209–216.

Ashar, B.H., Miller, R.G., Getz, K.J., Pichard, C.P. 2003. Mayo Clin. Proc. 78, 944–946.

Asherson, R.A., Zulman, J., Hugues, G.R.V. 1989. Ann. Rheum. Dis. 48, 232–235.

Assadi, F.K., Wang, H.E., Lawless, S., McKay, C.P., Hopp, L., Fattori, D. 1999. Pediatr. Nephrol. 13, 917–919.

Assem, E.S. 1976. Agents Actions 6, 212–218.

Attila, T., Prajapati, D.N., Otterson, M.F., Binion, D.G. 2002. Am. J. Gastroenterol. 97, S226.

Autran, P., Garbe, L., Pommier de Santi, P., Baralis, G., Charpin, J. 1978. Revue Francaise des Maladies Respiratoires 6, 183–190.

Avitzur, Y., Jimenez-Rivera, C., Fecteau, A., Jones, N., Ngan, B.Y., Ng, V.L. 2003. J. Pediatr. Gastroenterol. Nutr. 37, 91–94.

Baethge, B.A., Wolf, R.E. 1988. J. Louisiana State Med. Soc. 140, 37–39.

Bagshaw, S.M., Cload, B., Gilmour, J., Leung, S.T., Bowen, T.J. 2003. Ann. Allergy Asthma Immunol. 90, 572–575.

Bando, T., Fujimura, M., Noda, Y., Hirose, J., Ohta, G., Matsuda, T. 1994. Intern. Med. 33, 177–179.

Banka, R., Ward, M.J. 2002. Postgrad. Med. J. 78, 621–622.

Baratz, K.H., Hattenhauer, M.G. 1999. Mayo Clin. Proc. 74, 362–366.

Bargon, G. 1984. Röntgenblatter 37, 261–265.

Basoglu, T., Erkan, L., Canbaz, F., Bernay, I., Onen, T., Sahin, M., Furtun, F., Yalin, T. 1997. Ann. Nucl. Med. 11, 271–274.

Bayliff, C.D., Sobiera, C.J., Paterson, N.A.M. 1997. Can. J. Hosp. Pharm. 50, 247.

Beasley, M.B., Franks, T.J., Galvin, J.R., Gochuico, B., Travis, W.D. 2002. Arch. Pathol. Lab. Med. 126, 1064–1070.

Bedrossian, C.W.M., Miller, W.C., Luna, M.A. 1979. South. Med. J. 72, 313–318.

Bedrossian, C.W.M., Sussman, J., Conklin, R.H., Kahan, B. 1984. Am. J. Clin. Pathol. 82, 148–154.

Beji, M., Louzir, B., Mahouachi, R., El Mekki, F., Laribi, H., Daghfous, J. 1995. Revue des Maladies Respiratoires 12 (Suppl. 2), R97–R98.

Belzunegui, J., Intxausti, J.J., De Dios, J.R., Lopez-Dominguez, L., Queiro, R., Gonzalez, C., Figueroa, M. 2001. Clin. Exp. Rheumatol. 19, 727–730.

Bentur, L., Bar-Kana, Y., Livni, E., Finkelstein, R., Ben-Izhak, O., Keidar, S., Bentur, Y. 1997. Ann. Pharmacother. 31, 733–735.

Benz, J., Oshrain, C., Henry, D., Avery, C., Chiang, Y.T., Gatlin, M. 1997. J. Clin. Pharmacol. 37, 101–107.

Benzaquen-Forner, H., Dournovo, P., Tandjaoui-Lambiotte, H., Sullerot, A., Mahé, C., Bonnin, A., Camus, P., Valeyre, D. 1998. Revue des Maladies Respiratoires 15, 804–810.

Beretta, L., Vanoli, M., Caronni, M., Scorza, R. 2001. Clin. Exp. Rheumatol. 19, 757.

Berges-Gimeno, M.P., Simon, R.A., Stevenson, D.D. 2003. J. Allergy Clin. Immunol. 111, 180–186.

Berkani, K., Bayle, J.Y., Perol, M., Bejui-Thivolet, F., Perrot, D., Guérin, J.C. 2003. Revue de Pneumologie Clinique 59, 301–305.

Berkes, E.A. 2003. Clin. Rev. Allergy Immunol. 24, 137–147.

Bernal, C., Patarca, R. 1999. Ann. Pharmacother. 33, 172–174.

Beskow, C.O., Drachenberg, C.B., Bourquin, P.M., Britt, E.J., Simsir, A., Gunev, I., Papadimitriou, J.C. 2000. Acta Cytol. 44, 640–646.

Bielecki, J.W., Avar, S., Joss, R. 2000. Schweiz Med Wochenschr 130, 1078–1083.

Bijl, A.M., Van der Klauw, M.M., Van Vliet, A.C., Stricker, B.H. 1998. Clin. Exp. Allergy 28, 510–512.

Bini, E.J., Weinshel, E.H. 1999. Mayo Clin. Proc. 74, 367–370.

Biron, P., Dessureault, J., Napke, E. 1991. Can. Med. Assoc. J. 145, 28–34.

Birring, S.S., Brightling, C.E., Symon, F.A., Barlow, S.G., Wardlaw, A.J., Pavord, I.D. 2003. Thorax 58, 1066–1070.

Bleumink, G.S., van der Molen-Eijgenraam, M., Strijbos, J.H., Sanwikarja, S., van Puijenbroek, E.P., Stricker, B.H.C. 2002. Clin. Neuropharmacol. 25, 290–293.

Bochner, B.S., Lichtenstein, L.M. 1991. N. Engl. J. Med. 324, 1785–1790.

Bocquet, H., Bagot, M., Roujeau, J.C. 1996. Semin. Cutaneous Med. Surg. 15, 250–257.

Boehler, A., Vogt, P., Speich, R., Weder, W., Russi, E.W. 1996. Eur. Respir. J. 9, 1317–1319.

Boissier, M.C., Sansonetti, P., Dupont, B., Lapresle, C. 1983. Semaine des Hopitaux de Paris 59, 2989–2990.

Bone, R.C., Wolfe, J., Sobonya, R.E., Kerby, G.R., Stechschulte, D., Ruth, W.E., Welch, M. 1976. Chest 69, 296–297.

Bourezane, Y., Salard, D., Hoen, B., Vandel, S., Drobacheff, C., Laurent, R. 1998. Clin. Infect. Dis. 27, 1321–1322.

Brain, C., Mac Ardle, B., Levin, S. 1984. Br. Med. J. 289, 354.

Brander, L., Selroos, O. 1969. Acta Med. Scand. 185, 215–220.

Braun, D., Tréchot, P., Netter, P., Danloy, V., Anthoine, D., Vaillant, G. 1993. Chest 103, 1927.

Bravo, J.F., Jacobson, M.P., Mertens, B.F. 1977. Ann. Intern. Med. 87, 200–201.

Bristedt, P., Tylén, U. 1998. Acta Radiol. 39, 81–83.

Broadfoot, A., Gillis, D., Heddle, R., Smith, W., Kette, F. 2002. Intern. Med. J. 32, 271–272.

Brogan, B.L., Olsen, N.J. 2003. Curr. Opin. Rheumatol. 15, 76–80.

Bruera, E., Miller, M.J. 1989. Pain 39, 297–300.

Bruyn, G.A., Veenstra, R.P., Halma, C., Grond, J. 2003. Arthritis Rheum. 48, 1164–1165.

Bucknall, C.E., Adamson, M.R., Banham, S.W. 1987. Thorax 42, 475–476.

Burke, D.A., Stoddart, J.C., Ward, M.K., Simpson, C.G.B. 1982. Br. Med. J. ii, 696.

Buse, J.B. 2003. Circulation 108, e57.

Buss, W.C., Stepanek, J., Bankhurst, A.D., Mayeno, A.N., Pastuszyn, A., Peabody, D. 1996. Autoimmunity 25, 33–45.

Cacatian, A.A., Rando, J. 1981. NY State J. Med. 81, 1085–1087.

Cacoub, P., Sbaï, A., Azizi, P., Gatfosse, M., Godeau, P., Piette, J.-C. 1999. Presse Medicale 28, 911–912.

Cafri, C., Gilutz, H., Ilia, R., Abu-ful, A., Battler, A. 1997. Angiology 48, 925–928.

Calabrese, L.H., Duna, G.F. 1996. Curr. Opin. Rheumatol. 8, 34–40.

Cameron, R.J., Kolbe, J., Wilsher, M.L., Lambie, N. 2000. Thorax 55, 249–251.

Camiciottoli, G., Trapani, S., Castellani, W., Ginanni, R., Ermini, M., Falcini, F. 1998. Rheumatol. Int. 18, 11–16.

Camus, P. 1982. Revue Française des Maladies Respiratoires 10, 7–20.

Camus, P. 2003. In: M.I. Schwarz, T.E. King, Jr. (Eds.), Infiltrative Lung Diseases. B C Dekker, Hamilton, ON, pp. 485–534.

Camus, P. 2004. In: D. Bouros, C. Lenfant (Eds.), Pleural Disorders. Marcel Dekker, New York, pp. 317–352.

Camus, P., Gibson, G.J. 2003. In: G.J. Gibson, D.M. Geddes, U. Costabel, P.J. Sterk, B. Corrin (Eds.), Respir. Med., vol. 1. Harcourt Health Sciences, London, pp. 764–806, chapter 22.

Camus, P., Reybet-Degat, O., Justrabo, E., Jeannin, L. 1982. Chest 81, 376–378.

Camus, P., Lombard, J.N., Perrichon, M., Guerin, J.C., Bejui-Thivolet, F., Piard, F., Jeannin, L. 1989. Thorax 44, 711–715.

Camus, P., Piard, F., Ashcroft, T., Gal, A.A., Colby, T.V. 1993. Medicine (Baltimore) 72, 151–183.

Camus, P., Martin, W.J.I., Rosenow, E.C.I. 2004. Clin. Chest Med. 25, 65–76.

Cannon, G.W. 1990. Semin. Arthritis Rheum. 19, 353–354.

Cannon, G.W. 1997. Rheum. Dis. Clin. N. Am. 23, 917–937.

Carlson, E., Rothfield, N. 2003. Arthritis Rheum. 48, 1165–1166.

Carlson, R.W., Schaeffer, R.C., Puri, V.K., Brennan, A.P., Weil, M.H. 1981. Crit. Care Med. 9, 883–885.

Carmichael, A.J., Ryatt, K.S. 1990. Br. J. Dermatol. 122, 291.

Carter, J.D., Valeriano-Marcet, J., Kanik, K.S., Vasey, F.B. 2001. South. Med. J. 94, 1122–1123.

Cassorla, F.G., Finegold, D.N., Parks, J.S., Tenore, A., Thawenari, H., Baker, L. 1983. Am. J. Dis. Children 137, 118–122.

Cauchie, M., Lafitte, J.J., Fortin, F., Tsicopoulos, A., Piette, F., Degreef, M. 1989. Revue Francaise des Maladies Respiratoires 6, R131.

Chafin, C.C., Soberman, J.E., Demerkan, K., Self, T. 1999. Cardiology 92, 99–105.

Chamberlain, D.W., Hyland, R.H., Ross, D.J. 1986. Chest 90, 458–460.

Chandrasekhar, A.J., Robinson, J., Barr, L. 1978. J. Allergy Clin. Immunol. 61, 399–402.

Chang, Y.L., Yao, Y.T., Wang, N.S., Lee, Y.C. 1998. Am. J. Respir. Crit. Care Med. 157, 594–598.

Chaouat, A., Kessler, R., Weitzenblum, E. 1996. Heart 75, 383.

Chastain, M.A., Russo, G.G., Boh, E.E., Chastain, J.B., Falabella, A., Millikan, L.E. 1999. J. Am. Acad. Dermatol. 41, 757–764.

Chatzigiannis, I., Schmidt, K.L., Stambolis, C. 1984. Zeitschrift für Rheumatologie 43, 49–58.

Chen, J., Radford, M.J., Wang, Y., Marciniak, T.A., Krumholz, H.M. 2001. J. Am. Coll. Cardiol. 37, 1950–1956.

Chetty, K.G., Ramirez, M.M., Mahutte, C.K. 1993. Chest 104, 967–969.

Chevrolet, J.C., Guelpa, G., Schifferli, J.A. 1991. Eur. Respir. J. 4, 899–901.

Chin, H.L., Buchan, D.A. 1990. Ann. Intern. Med. 112, 312–313.

Chin, K., Tabata, C., Satake, N., Nagai, S., Moriyasu, F., Kuno, K. 1994. Chest 105, 939–941.

Chiu, A.G., Krowiak, E.J., Deeb, Z.E. 2001a. Laryngoscope 111, 1729–1731.

Chiu, A.G., Newkirk, K.A., Davidson, B.J., Burningham, A.R., Krowiak, E.J., Deeb, Z.E. 2001b. Ann. Otol. Rhinol. Laryngol. 110, 834–840.

Chiyo, M., Sekine, Y., Iwata, T., Tatsumi, K., Yasufuku, K., Iyoda, A., Otsuji, M., Yoshida, S., Shibuya, K., Iizasa, T., Saitoh, Y., Fujisawa, T. 2003. J. Thorac. Cardiovasc. Surg. 126, 1141–1146.

Choi, H.K., Merkel, P.A., Niles, J.L. 1998. Clin. Exp. Rheumatol. 16, 743–744.

Choi, H.K., Merkel, P.A., Cohen-Tervaert, J.W., Black, R.M., McCluskey, R.T., Niles, J.L. 1999. Arthritis Rheum. 42, 384–388.

Choi, H.K., Merkel, P.A., Walker, A.M., Niles, J.L. 2000a. Arthritis Rheum. 43, 405–413.

Choi, H.K., Slot, M.C., Pan, G.L., Weissbach, C.A., Niles, J.L., Merkel, P.A. 2000b. Arthritis Rheum. 43, 2488–2492.

Christ, E., Linka, A., Jacky, E., Speich, R., Marincek, B., Schaffner, A. 1996. Leukemia 10, 731–734.

Chung, J.B., Armstrong, K., Schwartz, J.S., Albert, D. 2000. Arthritis Rheum. 43, 1841–1848.

Churg, A., Brallas, M., Cronin, S.R., Churg, J. 1995. Chest 108, 320–323.

Clarysse, A.M., Cathey, W.J., Cartwright, G.E., Wintrobe, M.M. 1969. JAMA 209, 1861–1864.

Clayton, B.D., Hitchcock, M.G., Williford, P.M. 1999. Arch. Dermatol. 135, 139–140.

Clearkin, R., Corris, P.A., Thomas, S.H.L. 1997. Postgrad. Med. J. 73, 603–604.

Clerc, D., Brousse, C., Mariette, X., Bennet, P., Bisson, M. 1991. Ann. Rheum. Dis. 50, 67.

Cleverley, J.R., Screaton, N.J., Hiorns, M.P., Flint, J.D., Müller, N.L. 2002. Clin. Radiol. 57, 292–299.

Coblyn, J.S., Weinblatt, M. 1981. Med. Times 109, 53–62.

Cockcroft, D.W., Fisher, K.L. 1999. Respir. Med. 93, 597–600.

Cohen, M.G., Prowse, M.V. 1989. Med. Toxicol. 4, 199–218.

Cohen, A.J., King, T.E. Jr., Downey, G.P. 1994. Am. J. Respir. Crit. Care Med. 149, 1670–1675.

Colby, T.V. 2000. Mod. Pathol. 13, 343–358.

Colby, T.V., Lombard, C., Yousem, S.A., Kitaichi, M. 1991. Atlas of Pulmonary Surgical Pathology. WB Saunders/Harcourt Brace, Jovanovich/Philadelphia.

Collins, J.R. 1968. South. Med. J. 61, 354–358.

Collins, J. 2001. Radiol. Clin. N. Am. 39, 1115–1135.

Conigliaro, R.L., Gleason, P.P. 1999. Am. J. Health—Syst. Pharm. 56, 914–915.

Conigliaro, R.L., Gleason, P.P. 2000. Am. J. Health—Syst. Pharm. 57, 996–997.

Cooke, N., Bamji, A. 1981. Rheumatol. Rehabil. 20, 129–135.

Cooper, S.M., Libman, B.S., Lazarovich, M. 2002. J. Rheumatol. 29, 2651–2652.

Cordier, J.F. 2000. Thorax 55, 318–328.

Corp, C.C., Ghishan, F.K. 1998. J. Pediatr. Gastroenterol. Nutr. 26, 103–105.

Costabel, U., Teschler, H., Schoenfeld, B., Hartung, W., Nusch, A., Guzman, J., Greschuchna, D., Konietzko, N. 1992. Chest 102 (Suppl.), 14S–20S.

Costabel, U., Uzaslan, E., Guzman, J. 2004. Clin. Chest Med. 25, 25–36.

Cottin, V., Tébib, J., Massonnet, B., Souquet, P.J., Bernard, J.-P. 1996. Chest 109, 933–938.

Cuguillière, A., Bérard, H., N'Guyen, G., Miltgen, J. Martert, G., Eskandari, J., Bonnet, D. 1999. Revue de Pneumologie Clinique 55, 100–104.

Cush, J.J., Goldings, E.A. 1985. Am. J. Med. Sci. 290, 36.

Dahlén, B., Nizankowska, E., Szczeklik, A. 1998. Am. J. Respir. Crit. Care Med. 157, 1187–1194.

Dajani, B.M., Sliman, N.A., Shubair, K.S., Hamzeh, Y.S. 1981. J. Allergy Clin. Immunol. 68, 201–204.

Dalakas, M.C., Hohlfeld, R. 2003. Lancet 362, 971–982.

Das, K.M., Eastwood, M.A., McManus, J.P.A., Sircus, W. 1973. N. Engl. J. Med. 289, 491–495.

Daumal, M., Gillon, J.C., Guilbert, J.M., Line, B., Manoury, B., Pila, Y. 1984. Cahiers d'Anesthésiologie 32, 313–315.

Dawson, J.K., Graham, D.R., Desmond, J., Fewins, H.E., Lynch, M.P. 2002. Rheumatology (Oxford) 41, 262–267.

Day, R. 2002. Lancet 359, 540–541.

D'Cruz, D., Chesser, A.M.S., Lightowler, C., Comer, M., Hurst, M.J., Baker, L.R.I., Raine, A.E.G. 1995. Br. J. Rheumatol. 34, 1090–1091.

de Swert, L.F., Ceuppens, J.L., Wijndaele, L., Casaer, P., Casteels-van Daele, M. 1984. Acta Paediatr. Scand. 73, 285–288.

De Vriese, A.S.P., Philippe, J., Van Renterghem, D.M., De Cuyper, C.A., Hindryckx, P.H.F., Matthys, E.G.J., Louagie, A. 1995. Medicine (Baltimore) 74, 144–150.

Deamer, R.L., Prichard, J.G., Loman, G.J. 1992. Ann. Pharmacother. 26, 1081–1084.

Decramer, M., De Bock, V., Dom, R. 1996. Am. J. Respir. Crit. Care Med. 154, 1958–1964.

Delage, C., Irey, N.S. 1972. J. Forensic Sci. 17, 525–540.

Demaziere, A., Maugars, Y., Chollet, S., Prost, A. 1993. Br. J. Rheumatol. 32, 172–174.

Denman, E.J., Denman, A.M. 1968. Ann. Rheum. Dis. 27, 582–589.

Derk, C.T., Jimenez, S.A. 2003. J. Rheumatol. 30, 1616–1620.

Descamps, V., Collot, S., Mahe, E., Houhou, N., Crickx, B., Ranger-Rogez, S. 2003. J. Invest. Dermatol. 121, 215–216.

Dhillon, S.S., Singh, D., Doe, N., Qadri, A.M., Ricciardi, S., Schwarz, M.I. 1999. Chest 116, 1485–1488.

Diaz-Gonzalez, F., Castaneda-Sanz, S., Lopez-Robledillo, J.C., Garcia-Vicuna, R. 1992. J. Rheumatol. 19, 325–327.

Diffee, J.J. III, Hayes, J.M., Montesi, S.A., Green, W.L., Milnor, P. Jr. 1986. J. Tenn. Med. Assoc. 79, 82–84.

Diggory, P., Franks, W. 1994. J. R. Soc. Med. 87, 575–576.

Dinmezel, S., Ogus, C., Ozdemir, T. 2003. Clin. Drug Invest. 23, 817–821.

Doherty, N.E., Siegel, R.J. 1985. Am. Heart J. 110, 1257–1265.

Dolman, K.M., Gans, R.O., Vervaat, T.J., Zevenbergen, G., Maingay, D., Nikkels, R.E., Donker, A.J., Von dem Borne, A.E., Goldschmeding, R. 1993. Lancet 342, 651–652.

Dominguez-Ortega, J., Martinez-Alonso, J.C., Dominguez-Ortega, C., Fuentes, M.J., Frades, A., Fernandez-Colino, T. 2003. Allergol. Immunopathol. (Madr.) 31, 345–347.

Dongay, G., Levade, T., Caratero, A., Salvayre, R., Lauque, D., Carles, P. 1986. Presse Médicale 15, 1863–1868.

Doniach, I., Morrison, B., Steiner, R.E. 1954. Br. Heart J. 16, 101–108.

Dosch, H.M., Jason, J., Gelfand, E.W. 1982. N. Engl. J. Med. 306, 406–409.

Dourmishev, A.L., Dourmishev, L.A. 1999. Adv. Exp. Biol. Med. 455, 187–191.

Doyle, M.K., Cuellar, M.L. 2003. Expert Opin. Drug Safety 2, 401–409.

Drazen, J.M. 2003. N. Engl. J. Med. 348, 777–778.

Drory, V.E., Korczyn, A.D. 1993. Clin. Neuropharmacol. 16, 19–29.

Dupon, M., Malou, M., Rogues, A.M., Lacut, J.Y. 1993. Br. Med. J. 306, 109.

Dustan, H.P., Taylor, R.D., Corcoran, A.C., Page, I.H. 1954. JAMA 154, 23–29.

Eberlein-König, B., Hein, R., Abeck, D., Engst, R., Ring, J. 1999. Br. J. Dermatol. 140, 370–372.

Egermayer, P. 2000. J. Intern. Med. 247, 11–17.

Eland, I.A., Dofferhoff, A.S.M., Vink, R., Zondervan, P.E., Stricker, B.H.C. 1999. Epilepsia 40, 1780–1783.

Elkayam, O., Yaron, M., Caspi, D. 1996. Ann. Rheum. Dis. 55, 769–771.

Elkayam, O., Yaron, M., Caspi, D. 1999. Semin. Arthritis Rheum. 28, 392–397.

Ellis, R.V., McKinlay, C.A. 1941. J. Lab. Clin. Med. 26, 1427–1432.

Ellis, S.J., Cleverley, J.R., Müller, N.L. 2000. Am. J. Roentgenol. 175, 1019–1024.

Elsasser, S., Dalquen, P., Soler, M., Perruchoud, A. 1989. Am. Rev. Respir. Dis. 140, 1089–1092.

Enrique, E., Garcia-Ortega, P., Gaig, P., San Miguel, M.M. 1999. Allergy 54, 529–530.

Epler, G.R. 2001. Arch. Intern. Med. 161, 158–164.

Epler, G.R. 2004. Clin. Chest Med. 25, 89–94.

Epler, G.R., Snider, G.L., Gaensler, E.A., Cathcart, E.S., FitzGerald, M.X., Carrington, C.B. 1979. JAMA 242, 528–532.

Erasmus, J.J., McAdams, H.P., Rossi, S.E. 2002a. Semin. Roentgenol. 37, 72–81.

Erasmus, J.J., McAdams, H.P., Rossi, S.E. 2002b. Radiol. Clin. N. Am. 40, 61–72.

Ernst, E. 1998. Am. J. Med. 104, 170–178.

Ersoz, N., Finestone, S.C. 1971. Br. J. Anaesthesia 43, 709–712.

Erten, Y., Bodur, H., Sahiner, S., Tolunay, O., Akkaya, V., Canbakan, B., Bali, M. 2002. Clin. Endocrinol. (Oxford) 57, 699–700.

Evans, W.E., McLeod, H.L. 2003. N. Engl. J. Med. 348, 538–549.

Everts, C.S., Wescott, J.L., Bragg, D.G. 1973. Radiology 107, 539–543.

Fairfax, A.J., David, V., Douce, G. 1999. Thorax 54, 860–861.

Faller, M., Quoix, E., Popin, E., Gangi, A., Gasser, B., Mathelin, C., Pauli, G. 1997. Eur. Respir. J. 10, 2159–2162.

Fallowfield, J.M., Marlow, H.F. 1996. Br. Med. J. 313, 1486.

Farber, H.W., Graven, K.K., Kokolski, G., Korn, J.H. 1999. J. Rheumatol. 26, 1195–1196.

Favalli, E.G., Sinigaglia, L., Varenna, M., Arnoldi, C. 2002. Lupus 11, 753–755.

Fawcett, I.W., Ibrahim, N.B.N. 2001. Thorax 56, 161.

Fehr, T., Jacky, E., Bachli, E.B. 2003. Ann. Hematol. 82, 193–196.

Fenoglio, J.J. Jr., McAllister, H.A., Mullick, F.G. 1981. Hum. Pathol. 12, 900–907.

Ferriby, D., Stojkovic, T. 2001. Lancet 357, 751.

Fiegenberg, D.S., Weiss, H., Kirshman, H. 1967. Arch. Intern. Med. 120, 85–89.

Figueras, A., Capella, D., Castel, J.M., Laorte, J.R. 1994. Eur. J. Clin. Pharmacol. 47, 297–303.
Fischer, T.J., Guilfoile, T.D., Kesarwala, H.H., Winant, J.G., Kearns, G.L., Gartside, P.S., Moomaw, C.J. 1983. Pediatrics 71, 313–318.
FitzGerald, G.A., Patrono, C. 2001. N. Engl. J. Med. 345, 433–442.
Flacke, J.W., Flacke, W.E., Williams, G.D. 1977. Anesthesiology 47, 376–378.
Fleisch, M.C., Blauer, F., Gubler, J.G.H., Kuhn, M., Scherer, T.A. 2000. Eur. Respir. J. 15, 205–208.
Flieder, D.B., Travis, W.D. 2004. Clin. Chest Med. 25, 37–46.
Fontenot, A.P., Schwarz, M.I. 2003. In: M.I. Schwarz, T.E. King, Jr. (Eds.), Infiltrative Lung Diseases. B C Dekker, Hamilton, ON, pp. 632–656.
Formgren, H., Lindgren, S., Ahlstedt, S., Zettergren, L., Hanson, L.A. 1980. Histopathological Findings and Immune Response Against Nitrofurantoin in Drug Intolerance Pneumonitis. Karger, Basel.
Frankenfeld, R.H. 1967. Ann. Intern. Med. 66, 1055.
Franquet, T. 2001. Radiol. Clin. N. Am. 39, 1171–1187.
Freemer, M.M., King, T.E. Jr. 2003. In: M.I. Schwarz, T.E. King, Jr. (Eds.), Infiltrative Lung Diseases. B C Dekker, Inc., Hamilton, Ont., pp. 535–598.
Fruehauf, S., Steiger, S., Topaly, J., Ho, A.D. 2001. Ann. Hematol. 80, 308–310.
Fuhrman, C., Parrot, A., Wislez, M., Prigent, H., Boussaud, V., Bernaudin, J.F., Mayaud, C., Cadranel, J. 2001. Am. J. Respir. Crit. Care Med. 164, 1186–1191.
Fujimori, K., Shimatsu, Y., Suzuki, E., Gejyo, F., Arakawa, M. 1999. Nihon Kokyuki Gakkai Zasshi 37, 401–405.
Fujimura, M., Yasui, M., Shinagawa, S., Nomura, M., Matsuda, T. 1998. Respir. Med. 92, 743–749.
Gaensler, E.A., Carrington, C.B. 1977. Am. J. Roentgenol. 128, 1–13.
Gaffey, C.M., Chun, B., Harvey, J.C., Manz, H.J. 1986 Arch. Pathol. Lab. Med. 110, 131–135.
Gagnon, R., Julien, M., Gold, P. 2003. J. Allergy Clin. Immunol. 111, 1404–1405.
Gaine, S.P., Rubin, L.J., Kmetzo, J.J., Palevsky, H.I., Traill, T.A. 2000. Chest 118, 1496–1500.
Gams, R.A., Neal, J.A., Conrad, F.G. 1968. Ann. Intern. Med. 69, 557–568.
Gardam, M., Iverson, K. 2003. J. Rheumatol. 30, 1397–1399.
Gardam, M.A., Keystone, E.C., Menzies, R., Manners, S., Skamene, E., Long, R., Vinh, D.C. 2003. Lancet Infect. Dis. 3, 148–155.
Garrell, M. 1960. Arch. Intern. Med. 106, 874–877.
Gearhart, M.O., Bhutani, M.S. 1992. Chest 102, 1891–1892.
Geddes, D.M., Corrin, B., Brewerton, D.A., Davies, R.J., Turner-Warwick, M. 1977. Q. J. Med. 46, 427–444.
Geller, M., Dickie, H.A., Kass, D.A., Hafez, G.R., Gillepsie, J.J. 1976. Ann. Allergy 37, 275–279.
Gerson, W.T., Fine, D.G., Spielberg, S.P., Sensenbrenner, L.L. 1983. Blood 61, 889–893.
Giannocarro, P.J., Wallace, G.J., Higginson, L.A., Williams, W.L. 1989. Can. J. Cardiol. 5, 335–336.
Gibbs, M.W., Kuczkowski, K.M., Benumof, J.L. 2003. Acta Anaesthesiol. Scand. 47, 230–232.
Glauser, F.L., Egan, P., Millen, J.E., Fisher, P., Propst, K., Lewis, J.W., Chetty, K. 1978. Crit. Care Med. 6, 181–184.
Goldberg, M.J., Husain, M., Wajszczuk, W.J., Rubenfire, M. 1980. Am. J. Med. 69, 159–162.
Goldstein, G. 1963. Ann. Intern. Med. 59, 97–100.
Gomez, J.L., Dupont, A., Cusan, L., Tremblay, M., Tremblay, M., Labrie, F. 1992. Am. J. Med. 92, 563–566.
Gomez-Reino, J.J., Carmona, L., Valverde, V.R., Mola, E.M., Montero, M.D. 2003. Arthritis Rheum. 48, 2122–2127.
Gondouin, A., Manzoni, P., Ranfaing, E., Brun, J., Cadranel, J., Sadoun, D., Cordier, J.F., Depierre, A., Dalphin, J.C. 1996. Eur. Respir. J. 9, 1463–1469.
Gonzalo Hernandez, C., Hernandez Caballero, A., Bello Dronda, S., Lucia Cuesta, J.F. 1987. Sangre 32, 762–763.
Gonzolez, E.R., Cole, T., Grimes, M.M., Fink, R.A., Fowler, A.A.I. 1998. Chest 114, 919–922.
Good, J.T. Jr., King, T.E. Jr., Antony, V.B., Sahn, S.A. 1983. Chest 84, 714–718.
Goodwin, S.D., Glenny, R.W. 1992. Arch. Intern. Med. 152, 1521–1524.
Gopalakrishnan, D., Tioran, T., Emanuel, C., Clark, V.L. 1997. Clin. Cardiol. 20, 298–300.
Gordon, M.M., Porter, D. 2001. J. Rheumatol. 28, 1004–1006.
Grabe, D.W., Manley, H.J., Kim, J.S., McGoldrick, M.D., Bailie, G.R. 1999. Clin. Drug Invest. 17, 79–81.
Grcevska, L., Polenakovic, M., Breskowska, G. 1993. Nephron 64, 325–326.
Green, R.L., Vayonis, A.G. 1999. Lancet 353, 729–730.
Greenberger, P. 2000. Ann. Allergy Asthma Immunol. 85, 250–251.
Gregory, K.W.P., Davis, R.C. 1996. N. Engl. J. Med. 334, 1641
Gromnica-Ihle, K.E. 2000. Zeitschrift für Rheumatologie 59, III/46.
Gross, T.J., Hunninghake, G.W. 2001. N. Engl. J. Med. 345, 517–525.
Guérin, J.C., Kofman, J., Chevalier, J.P., Perrin-Fayolle, M., Kalb, J.C. 1980. Revue Francaise des Maladies Respiratoires 8, 406–407.
Gugnani, M.K., Pierson, C., Vanderheide, R., Girgis, R.E. 2000. Arthritis Rheum. 43, 699–703.
Guillevin, L., Cordier, J.F., Lhote, F., Cohen, P., Jarrousse, B., Royer, I., Lesavre, P., Jacquot, C., Bind, P., Bielefeld, P., Desson, J.F., Detree, F., Dubois, A., Hachulla, E., Hoen, B., Jacomy, D., Seigneuric, C., Lauque, D., Stern, M., Longy-Boursier, M. 1997. Arthritis Rheum. 40, 2187–2198.
Gunton, J.E., Stiel, J., Caterson, R.J., McElduff, A. 1999. J. Clin. Endocrinol. Metab. 84, 13–16.
Gupta, M.K., McClymont, L.G., El-Hakim, H. 2003. Med. Sci. Monitor 9, CS95–CS97.
Hailemeskel, B., Namanny, M.D., Metzger, S.D. 1997. Am. J. Health—Syst. Pharm. 54, 199–200.
Hamada, K., Nagai, S., Kitaichi, M., Jin, G., Shigematsu, M., Nagao, T., Sato, A., Mishima, M. 2003. Intern. Med. 42, 82–87.
Hamel, H., Bonniaud, P., Sgro, C., Foucher, P., Camus, P. 2000. Presse Medicale 29, 1045.
Hamilton, C.D. 2003. Arthritis Rheum. 48, 2085–2091.
Handschin, A.E., Lardinois, D., Schneiter, D., Bloch, K.E., Weder, W. 2003. Respiration 70, 310–312.

Hannhahs Hahn, B. 1998. N. Engl. J. Med. 338, 1359–1368.
Hara, H., Fujitsuka, A., Morishima, C., Kurihara, N., Yamaguchi, Z.I., Morishima, T. 1998. Acta Dermato—Venereologica 78, 393–394.
Hargreaves, M.R., Mowat, A.G., Benson, M.K. 1992. Thorax 47, 628–633.
Hashizume, T., Numata, H., Matsushita, K. 2001. Nihon Kokyuki Gakkai Zasshi 39, 664–667.
Hayashi, S., Furuya, S., Imamura, H. 2001. Heart 86, E7.
Hedberg, K., Urbach, D., Slutsker, L., Matson, P., Fleming, D. 1992. Arch. Intern. Med. 152, 1889–1892.
Heffner, J.E., Sahn, S.A. 1981. Ann. Intern. Med. 95, 405–409.
Heitzman, E.R. 1967. Radiology 89, 311–312.
Hellebrand, J., Buytendijk, H.J., Maesen, F. 1979. Acta Tuberculosica Pneumologica Belgica 70, 203–214.
Hertl, M., Jugert, F., Merk, H.F. 1995. Br. J. Dermatol. 132, 215–220.
Hertzman, P.A., Clauw, D.J., Kaufman, L.D., Varga, J., Silver, R.M., Thacker, H.L., Mease, P., Espinoza, L.R., Pincus, T. 1995. Arch. Intern. Med. 122, 851–855.
Hess E.V. (Ed.), 1981. Arthritis Rheum., vol. 24, pp. 979–1111, Santa Ynez Valley, CA.
Hicks, K., Peng, D., Gajewski, J.L. 2002. Bone Marrow Transplant. 30, 975–978.
Higenbottam, T.W. 1997. Thorax 52, S68–S72.
Hill, R.N., Spragg, R.G., Wedel, M.K., Moser, K.M. 1975. Ann. Intern. Med. 83, 523–524.
Hill, C., Zeitz, C., Kirkham, B. 1995. Aust. NZ J. Med. 25, 745–746.
Hill, R.B., Rowlands, D.T., Rifkind, D. 1999. Rev. Med. Virol. 9, 5–10.
Hiraoka, K., Nagata, N., Kawajiri, T., Suzuki, K., Kurokawa, S., Kido, M., Sakamoto, N. 1998. Respiration 65, 152–155.
Hirsch, I.B., Kelly, J., Cooper, S. 1999. Arch. Intern. Med. 159, 1811.
Hoegholm, A., Rasmussen, S.W., Kristensen, K.S. 1990. Br. Heart J. 63, 186.
Hoffman, B.J. 1945. Arch. Dermatol. Syphilogr. 51, 190–192.
Hoffmann, R.M., Jung, M.-C., Motz, R., Gössl, C., Emslander, H.-P., Zachoval, R., Pape, G.R. 1998. J. Hepatol. 28, 1058–1063.
Hoffman, S.D., Hammadeh, R., Shah, N. 2003. Am. J. Gastroenterol. 98, S152.
Hofstra, A.H. 1994. Drug Metabol. Rev. 26, 485–505.
Hoigné, R.V., Braunschweig, S., Zehnder, D., Kuenzi, U.P., Hess, T., Leuenberger, P. 1997. Eur. J. Clin. Pharmacol. 53, 81–82.
Hollingsworth, H.M. 1994. In: G.R. Epler (Ed.), Diseases of the Bronchioles. Raven Press, New York, pp. 367–376.
Holmberg, L., Boman, G. 1981. Eur. J. Respir. Dis. 62, 180–189.
Hölz, W., Ludwig, A., Forst, H. 2002. Anaesthesist 51, 187–190.
Honoré, I., Nunes, H., Groussard, O., Kambouchner, M., Chambellan, A., Aubier, M., Valeyre, D., Crestani, B. 2003. Am. J. Respir. Crit. Care Med. 167, 953–957.
Horiki, T., Fuyuno, G., Ishii, M., Sasao, T., Shibuya, M., Yanagimachi, N., Ichikawa, Y. 1998. Intern. Med. 37, 554–560.
Horneff, G., Lenard, H.G., Wahn, V. 1992. Neuropediatrics 23, 272–275.
Houwerzijl, J., De Gast, G.C., Nater, J.P., Esselink, M.T., Nieweg, H.O. 1977. Clin. Exp. Immunol. 29, 272–277.
Hsu, H., Chang, H., Goan, Y. 2000. Transplant. Proc. 32, 2422–2423.
http://www.pneumotox.com (1997), Vol. 1997 Producers: P Foucher-Ph. Camus.
Hübner, C., Dietz, A., Stremmel, W., Stiehl, A., Andrassy, K. 1997. Lancet ii, 1552.
Hübscher, O., Re, R., Iotti, R. 2003. Arthritis Rheum. 48, 2077–2078.
Huggins, J.T., Sahn, S.A. 2004. Clin. Chest Med. 25, 141–154.
Humbert, V.H., Munn, N.J., Hawkins, R.F. 1991. Chest 99, 258–260.
Humbert, M., Sanchez, O., Fartoukh, M., Jagot, J.L., Le Gall, C., Sitbon, O., Parent, F., Simonneau, G. 1999. Eur. Respir. J. 13, 1351–1356.
Hutter, C. 2003. Anaesthesia 58, 285–286.
Huynh-Do, U., Gantenbein, H., Binswanger, U. 1995. Arch. Intern. Med. 155, 872–874.
Hyman, G.A., Sommers, S.C. 1966. Blood 28, 416–427.
Ibanez, L., Laporte, J.R., Carne, X. 1991. Drug Safety 6, 450–459.
Idris, I., Gray, S., Donnelly, R. 2003. Diabetologia 46, 288–290.
Im Hof, V.I. 1995. Schweizerische Rundschau für Medizin Praxis 84, 319–320.
Imokawa, S., Sato, A., Hayakawa, H., Toyoshima, M., Taniguchi, M., Chida, K. 1996. Ann. Allergy Asthma Immunol. 76, 419–422.
Imokawa, S., Colby, T.V., Leslie, K.O., Helmers, R.A. 2000. Eur. Respir. J. 15, 373–381.
Inoue, K., Sano, H. 2000. Arch. Intern. Med. 160, 871.
Irey, N.S. 1976a. JAMA 236, 575–578.
Irey, N.S. 1976b. Am. J. Pathol. 82, 613–647.
Ishizaki, T., Sasaki, F., Ameshima, S., Shiozaki, K., Takahashi, H., Abe, Y., Ito, S., Kuriyama, M., Nakai, T., Kitagawa, M. 1996. Eur. Respir. J. 9, 2691–2696.
Ishizuka, S., Yanai, M., Yamaya, M., Ohrui, T., Sekizawa, K., Sasaki, H. 2000. Chest 118, 279.
Israili, Z.H., Hall, W.D. 1992. Ann. Intern. Med. 117, 234–242.
Jacobs, S. 1975. J. Louisiana State Med. Soc. 127, 311–315.
James, L.P., Austen, K.F. 1964. N. Engl. J. Med. 270, 597–603.
Jara Chinarro, B., de Miguel Diez, J., Garcia Satue, J.L., Juretschke Moragues, M.A., Serrano Iglesias, J.A. 2003. Archivos De Bronconeumologia 39, 91–93.
Jarrett, S.J., Cunnane, G., Conaghan, P.G., Bingham, S.J., Buch, M.H., Quinn, M.A., Emery, P. 2003. J. Rheumatol. 30, 2287–2291.
Jarzobski, J., Ferry, J., Wombolt, D., Fitch, D.M., Egan, J.D. 1970. Am. Heart J. 79, 116–121.
Jedynak, U., Ciezarek, M., Kopinski, P. 1997. Pol. J. Pathol. 48, 63–67.
Johnson, M.P., Goodwin, S.D., Shands, J.W. Jr. 1990. Pharmacotherapy 10, 413–416.
Jones, G.R., Malone, D.N.S. 1972. Thorax 27, 713–717.
Jones, G., Mierins, E., Karsh, J. 1991. Am. Rev. Respir. Dis. 143, 179–181.
Jungling, A.S., Shangraw, R.E. 2000. Anesthesiology 92, 888–890.
Kahn, J. 1998. Am. J. Roentgenol. 171, 261.

Kalra, S., Bell, M.R., Rihal, C.S. 2001. Chest 120, 126–131.
Kamisako, T., Adachi, Y., Chihara, J., Yamamoto, T. 1993. Br. Med. J. 306, 896.
Kanda, T., Yokosuka, O., Tada, M., Kurihara, T., Yoshida, S., Suzuki, Y., Nagao, K., Saisho, H. 2003. J. Gastroenterol. Hepatol. 18, 999–1001.
Kane, G.C., Troshinsky, M.B., Peters, S.P., Israel, H.L. 1993. Respir. Med. 87, 153–155.
Kaplan, R.L., Waite, D.H. 1978. Arch. Dermatol. 114, 1800–1812.
Kaplan, A.I., Zakher, F., Sabin, S. 1978. Chest 73, 875–876.
Karkos, C., Moore, A., Manche, A., Thorpe, J.A.C. 1996. J. Clin. Pharmacol. Therapeut. 21, 15–17.
Kashiwabara, K., Nakamura, H. 2001. Intern. Med. 40, 124–126.
Kasper, L., Sladek, K., Duplaga, M., Bochenek, G., Liebhart, J., Gladysz, U., Malolepszy, J., Szczeklik, A. 2003. Allergy 58, 1064–1116.
Katayama, K., Hata, C., Kagawa, K., Noda, M., Nakamura, K., Shimizu, H., Fujimoto, M. 2002. Respiration 69, 473.
Kattwinkel, N., Cook, L., Agnello, V. 1991. J. Rheumatol. 18, 79–81.
Katzenstein, A.L.A. 2000. Am. J. Clin. Pathol. 114, 767–772.
Katzman, M., Meade, W., Iglar, K., Rachlis, A., Berger, P., Chan, C.K. 1992. Chest 101, 79–81.
Keane, J., Gershon, S., Wise, R.P., Mirabile-Levens, E., Kasznica, J., Schwieterman, W.D., Siegel, J.N., Braun, M.M. 2001. N. Engl. J. Med. 345, 1098–1104.
Kelly, J., Hirsch, I.B., Cooper, S. 2000. Arch. Intern. Med. 160, 871–872.
Kelly, C.A., Upex, A., Spencer, E.P., Flanagan, R.J., Bateman, D.N. 2003. Hum. Exp. Toxicol. 22, 103–105.
Kemp, S.F., Lockey, R.F., Wolf, B.L., Lieberman, P. 1995. Arch. Intern. Med. 155, 1749–1754.
Keogh, K.A., Specks, U. 2003. Am. J. Med. 115, 284–290.
Kermani, A., Garg, A. 2003. Mayo Clin. Proc. 78, 1088–1091.
Kerstens, P.J.S.M., Van Loenhout, J.W.A., Boerbooms, A.M.T., Van de Putte, L.B.A. 1992. Ann. Rheum. Dis. 51, 1179.
Kessler, D.A. 2000. N. Engl. J. Med. 342, 1742–1743.
Kharabsheh, S., Abendroth, C.S., Kozak, M. 2002. Am. J. Cardiol. 89, 896–898.
Khosla, R., Butman, A.N., Hammer, D.F. 1998. South. Med. J. 91, 873–874.
Kilbourne, E.M. 1992. Epidemiol. Rev. 14, 16–36.
Kilbourne, E.M., Philen, R.M., Kamb, M.L., Falk, H. 1996. J. Rheumatol. 23, 81–88.
Kilpiö, K., Hannuksela, M. 2003. Allergy 58, 1131–1135.
Kilraru, P.K., Schweiger, M.J., Hozman, H.A., Weil, T.R. 2001. J. Invasive Cardiol. 13, 535–537.
Kitson, G.E., Wauchob, T.D. 1988. Anaesthesia 43, 967–969.
Kleckner, H.B., Yakulis, V., Heller, P. 1975. Ann. Intern. Med. 83, 522–523.
Kluth, D.C., Rees, A.J. 1999. J. Am. Soc. Nephrol. 10, 2446–2453.
Knoell, D.L., Lucas, J., Allen, J.N. 1998. Chest 114, 332–334.
Knowles, S.R., Shapiro, L., Shear, N.H. 1996. Arch. Dermatol. 132, 934–939.
Kohlhäufl, M., Weber, N., Morressi-Hauf, A., geiger, D., Raith, H., Häusinger, K. 2003. Pneumologie 57, S30.
Kokelj, F., Plozzer, C., Muzzi, A., Ciani, F. 1999. J. Dermatol. Treat. 10, 67–69.
Kormano, M. 1974. Duodecim 90, 1129–1133.
Koselj-Kajtna, M., Koselj, M., Rott, T., Kandus, A., Bren, A. 2002. Transplant. Proc. 34, 3001–3002.
Kowalski, M.L., Ptasinska, A., Bienkiewicz, B., Pawliczak R., DuBuske, L. 2003. J. Allergy Clin. Immunol. 112 505–512.
Kramer, N., Chuzhin, Y., Kaufman, L.D., Ritter, J.M., Rosenstein, E.D. 2002. Arthritis Rheum. 47, 670–671.
Kramer, N., Chuzhin, Y., Kaufman, L.D., Ritter, J.M., Rosenstein, E.D. 2003. Arthritis Rheum. 49, 617–618.
Krantz, M.J., Dart, R.C., Mehler, P.S. 2002. Pharmacotherapy 22, 775–778.
Krasnowska, M., Malolepszy, J., Liebhart, E. 1992. Pneumonol. Allergol. Pol. 60, 22–25.
Kremer, J.M., Joong, K.L. 1986. Arthritis Rheum. 29, 822–831.
Kremer, J.M., Alarcon, G.S., Weinblatt, M.E., Kaymakcian, M.V., Macaluso, M., Cannon, G.W., Palmer, W.R., Sundy, J.S., St Clair, E.W., Alexander, R.W., Walker-Smith, G.J., Axiotis, C.A. 1997. Arthritis Rheum. 40, 1829–1837.
Kuhlman, J.E. 1991. J. Thorac. Imag. 6, 52–61.
Kuhlman, J.E., Scatarige, J.C., Fishman, E.K., Siegelman, S.S. 1987. J. Comput. Assist. Tomogr. 11, 160–162.
Kuitert, L.M., Harrison, A.C. 1991. Thorax 46, 936–937.
Kulke, M.H., Vance, E.A. 1997. Clin. Infect. Dis. 25, 215–218.
Kumar, K.S., Russo, M.W., Esposito, S., Borczuk, A., Jacobson, I., et al. 2001. Am. J. Gastroenterol. 96, 127.
Kumar, K.S., Russo, M.W., Borczuk, A.C., Brown, M., Esposito, S.P., Lobritto, S.J., Jacobson, I.M., Brown, R.S. Jr 2002a. Am. J. Gastroenterol. 97, 2432–2440.
Kumar, N.P., Wild, G., Ramasamy, K.A., Snape, J. 2002b. Postgrad. Med. J. 78, 439–440.
Kwon, H.J., Cote, T.R., Cuffe, M.S., Kramer, J.M., Braun, M.M. 2003. Ann. Intern. Med. 138, 807–811.
Lamson, R.W. 1929. JAMA 93, 1775–1778.
Lang, D.M., Alpern, M.B., Visintainer, P.F., Smith, S.T. 1991. Ann. Intern. Med. 115, 270–276.
Lao, P.N. 1997. Clin. Rev. Allergy Immunol. 15, 291–305.
Larsen, K. 1996. Allergy Asthma Proc. 17, 243–249.
Lascari, A.D., Strano, A.J., Johnson, W.W., Collins, J.G.P. 1977. Cancer 40, 1393–1397.
Layton, D., Riley, J., Wilton, L.V., Shakir, S.A. 2003. Br. J. Clin. Pharmacol. 55, 166–174.
Le, H.T., Bosse, G.M., Tsai, Y.Y. 1994. Clin. Toxicol. 32, 315–320.
Le Loet, X., Ozenne, G., Pinel, B., Deshayes, P. 1983. Rhumatologie 35, 19–21.
Le Quintrec, J.S., Le Quintrec, J.L. 1991. Baillieres Clin. Rheumatol. 5, 21–38.
Leatherman, J.W., Schmitz, P.G. 1991. Chest 100, 1391–1396.
Leav, B.A., Fanburg, B., Hadley, S. 2000. N. Engl. J. Med. 343, 586.
LeBlanc, K.E. 1980. Arch. Intern. Med. 140, 1250–1251.
Leduc, D., De Vuyst, P., Lheureux, P., Gevenois, P.-A., Jacobovitz, D., Yernault, J.-C. 1993. Chest 104, 1620–1623.
Lee, Y.J., Chiang, Y.F., Tsai, J.C.R. 2000. Diabetes Care 23, 427–428.

LeMense, G.P., Sahn, S.A. 1994. Am. J. Respir. Crit. Care Med. 150, 258–260.

Lentle, B.C., Starreveld, E., Catz, Z., Penney, H., Turner, A.R. 1983. J. Can. Assoc. Radiol. 34, 114–115.

Lepore, L., Leone, V., Marchetti, F., Ventura, A., Facchini, S. 2003. Clin. Exp. Rheumatol. 21, 276–277.

Leuppi, J.D., Schnyder, P., Hartmann, K., Reinhart, W.H., Kuhn, M. 2001. Respiration 68, 341–351.

Leveque, L., de Boulard, A., Bielefeld, P., Sgro, C., Hillon, P., Gabreau, T., Champigneulle, B., Makki, H., Besancenot, J.F. 2001. Revue Medecine Interne 22, 1248–1252.

Levinson, M.L., Lynch, J.P.R., Bower, J.S. 1981. Am. J. Med. 71, 908–912.

Lévy, A., Mal, H., Roué, C., Crestani, B., Fournier, M., Pariente, R. 1997. Presse Medicale 26, 1671–1672.

Lewis, I.J., Rosenbloom, L. 1982. Postgrad. Med. J. 58, 100–101.

Lewis, M.J., Cameron, A.H., Stah, K.J., Purdham, D.R., Mann, J.R. 1978. Br. Med. J. i, 330–331.

Li, C., Gefter, W.B. 1992. Chest 101, 102–104.

Libby, D., White, D.A. 1998. Clin. Chest Med. 19, 809–821.

Lichtenstein, L., Fox, L.J. 1946. Am. J. Pathol. 22, 665–671.

Lieberman, P.L., Seigle, R.L. 1999. Clin. Rev. Allergy Immunol. 17, 469–496.

Liebhaber, M.I., Wright, R.S., Gelberg, H.J., Dyer, Z., Kupperman, J.L. 1999. Chest 115, 886–889.

Lillie, M.A., Yang, L.C., Honig, P.J., August, C.S. 1983. Arch. Dermatol. 119, 415–418.

Lilly, C.M., Churg, A., Lazarovich, M., Pauwels, R., Hendeles, L., Rosenwasser, L.J., Ledford, D., Wechsler, M.E. 2002. J. Allergy Clin. Immunol. 109, S1–S19.

Limper, A.H. 2004. Clin. Chest Med. 25, 53–64.

Lin, H.C., Hwang, K.C., Lee, H.J., Tsai, M.J., Ni, Y.H., Chiang, B.L. 2000. J. Microbiol. Immunol. Infect. 33, 202–204.

Lindell, R.M., Hartman, T.E. 2004. Clin. Chest Med. 25, 15–24.

Lionakis, M.S., Kontoyiannis, D.P. 2003. Lancet 362, 1828–1838.

Lisbona, A., Schwartz, J., Lachance, C., Frank, H., Palayew, M.J. 1973. J. Can. Assoc. Radiol. 24, 215–220.

Liverani, E., Armuzzi, A., Mormile, F., Anti, M., Gasbarrini, G., Gentiloni, N. 2001. J. Intern. Med. 249, 565–566.

Lock, B.J., Eggert, M., Cooper, J.A.D. Jr. 2004. Clin. Chest Med. 25, 47–52.

Lockie, L.M., Smith, D.M. 1985. Semin. Arthritis Rheum. 14, 238–246.

Logan, P.M., Primack, S.L., Staples, C., Miller, R.R., Müller, N.L. 1995. Chest 108, 1283–1287.

Lohr, R.H., Boland, B.J., Douglas, W.W., Dockrell, D.H., Colby, T.V., Swensen, S.J., Wollan, P.C., Silverstein, M.D. 1997. Arch. Intern. Med. 157, 1323–1329.

Lontos, S., Jones, R.M., Angus, P.W., Gow, P.J. 2003. Med. J. Aust. 179, 390–391.

Loorand-Stiver, L., Murty, M. 2002. Can. Adverse React. Newslett. 12, 2–3.

Louie, S., Gamble, C.N., Cross, C.E. 1986. J. Rheumatol. 13, 963–966.

Lunde, H., Hedner, T., Samuelsson, O., Lötvall, J., Andrén, L., Lindholm, L., Wiholm, B.-E. 1994. Br. Med. J. 308, 18–21.

Mackay, F.J., Pearce, G.L., Mann, R.D. 1999. Br. J. Clin. Pharmacol. 47, 111–114.

MacLaren, R., Shields, C.A. 1998. Ann. Pharmacother. 32, 1017–1020.

Mahatma, M., Haponik, E.F., Nelson, S., Lopez, A., Summer, W.R. 1989. Am. J. Med. 87, 93–94.

Maillard, N., Foucher, P., Caillot, D., Durand, C., Sgro, C., Camus, P. 1999. Respiration 66, 279–282.

Majori, M., Poletti, V., Curti, A., Corradi, M., Falcone, F., Pesci, A. 2000. J. Allergy Clin. Immunol. 105, 239–244.

Malhorta, A., Muse, V.V., Mark, E.J. 2003. N. Engl. J. Med. 348, 1574–1585.

Malik, S.W., Myers, J.L., DeRemee, R.A., Specks, U. 1996. Am. J. Respir. Crit. Care Med. 154, 1851–1856.

Manchanda, S., Rees, P.J. 1999. Int. J. Clin. Pract. 53, 233–235.

Marai, I., Shoenfeld, Y. 2002. Harefuah 141, 151–152.

Marchlinski, F.E., Gansler, T.S., Waxman, H.L., Josephson, M.E. 1982. Ann. Intern. Med. 97, 839–845.

Marik, P. 1999. Pharmacotherapy 19, 346–348.

Mark, E.J., Ramirez, J.F. 1985. Arch. Pathol. Lab. Med. 109, 413–418.

Mark, G.J., Lehimgar-Zadeh, A., Ragsdale, B.D. 1978. Thorax 33, 89–93.

Marks, F., Harrell, K., Fischer, R. 2001. South. Med. J. 94, 256–257.

Marquette, C.H., Saulnier, F., Leroy, O., Wallaert, B., Chopin, C., Demarcq, J.M., Durocher, A., Tonnel, A.B. 1992. Am. Rev. Respir. Dis. 146, 76–81.

Marshall, A., Moore, K. 1973. Br. Med. J. i, 716–717.

Martin, W.J.I., Rosenow, E.C.I. 1988a. Chest 93, 1067–1075.

Martin, W.J.I., Rosenow, E.C.I. 1988b. Chest 93, 1242–1248.

Martin, R.M., Wilson, L.V., Mann, R.D. 1999. Pharmacoepidemiol. Drug Safety 8, 179–189.

Martinez-Vea, A., Ferrer, I., Carcia, C., Mayayo, E., Oliver, J.A., Richart, C. 1987. Am. J. Nephrol. 7, 71–73.

Marzo-Ortega, H., Misbah, S., Emery, P. 2001. J. Rheumatol. 28, 377–378.

Massin, F., Coudert, B., Marot, J.P., Foucher, P., Camus, P., Jeannin, L. 1990. Revue des Maladies Respiratoires 7, 5–15.

Matloff, D., Kaplan, M. 1980. Gastroenterology 78, 1046–1049.

Matsushima, H., Takayanagi, N., Ubukata, M., Tokunaga, D., Mori, S., Sato, N., Kurashima, K., Yanagisawa, T., Sugita, Y., Kawabata, Y., Kanazawa, M. 2002. Nihon Kokyuki Gakkai Zasshi 40, 955–959.

Matuschak, G.M. 1991. Chest 100, 1188–1189.

Mauri-Hellweg, D., Bettens, F., Mauri, D., Brander, C., Hunziker, T., Pichler, W.J. 1995. J. Immunol. 155, 462–472.

Mayberry, J.P., Primack, S.L., Müller, N.L. 2000. RadioGraphics 20, 1623–1635.

McCormick, J., Cole, S., Lahirir, B., Knauft, F., Cohens, S., Yoshida, T. 1980. Am. Rev. Respir. Dis. 122, 145–152.

McFadden, R.G., Fraher, L.J., Thompson, J.M. 1989. Chest 96, 216–218.

Mchaourab, A., Sarantopoulos, C., Stowe, D.F. 1999. Can. J. Anaesthesia 46, 975–978.

Medrano San Ildefonso, M., Mauri Llerda, J.A., Calabozo Raluy, M., Barrio, J., Orte Martinez, J., Beltran Gutierrez, J. 1986. Revista Espanola de Reumatologia 13, 130–132.

Mehandru, S., Smith, R.L., Sidhu, G.S., Cassai, N., Aranda, C.P. 2002. Thorax 57, 465–467.
Melloni, B., Vergnenègre, A., Bonnaud, F., Antonini, M.T., Gaillard, S., Touraine, F., Germouty, J. 1994. Revue des Maladies Respiratoires 11, 308–311.
Menéndez, R., Venzor, J., Ortiz, G. 1998. Ann. Allergy Asthma Immunol. 80, 225–226.
Merigian, K., Blaho, K. 1995. J. Anal. Toxicol. 19, 522–528.
Merkel, P.A. 1998. Curr. Opin. Rheumatol. 10, 45–50.
Merkel, P.A., Polisson, R.P., Chang, Y., Skates, S.J., Niles, J.L. 1997. Ann. Intern. Med. 126, 866–873.
Metzler, C., Fink, C., Lamprecht, P., Gross, W.L., Reinhold-Keller, E. 2004. Rheumatology (Oxford) 43, 315–320.
Meyer, M.M., Meyer, R.J. 1994. J. Urol. 152, 938–940.
Michael, J.R., Rudin, M.L. 1981. Ann. Intern. Med. 95, 452–454.
Milesi-Lecat, A.-M., Schmidt, J., Aumaître, O., Kemeny, J.-L., Moinard, J., Piette, J.-C. 1997. Mayo Clin. Proc. 72, 1145–1147.
Milewski, M., Mastalerz, L., Nizankowska, E., Szczeklik, A. 1998. J. Allergy Clin. Immunol. 101, 581–586.
Miller, F.F., Green, R.A. 1962. Dis. Chest 42, 100–103.
Min, D.I., Monaco, A.P. 1991. Pharmacotherapy 11, 119S–125S.
Minai, O.A., Dweik, R.A., Arroliga, A.C. 1998. Clin. Chest Med. 19, 713–731.
Moder, K.G., Miller, T.D., Tazelaar, H.D. 1999. Mayo Clin. Proc. 74, 275–284.
Mohty, R., Chaby, G., Pannier, M., Defossez, C., Denoeux, J.P., Lok, C. 2003. Ann. Dermatol. Venereol. 130, 551–552
Mommens, V., Just, N., Ngo, M.T., Cotte, L., GFournier, C., Wallaert, B. 2003. Revue Française d'Allergologie et d Immunologie Clinique 43, 393–396.
Mooren, F.C., Lerch, M.M., Ullerich, H., Bürger, H., Domschke, W. 2000. Br. Med. J. 320, 219.
Morcos, S.K. 2003. Br. J. Radiol. 76, 290–295.
Moreau, L., Quoix, E., Vandevenne, A., Dietemann, A., Kessler, R., Weitzenblum, E., Pauli, G. 1998. Revue de Pneumologie Clinique 54, 136–143.
Morelock, S.Y., Sahn, S.A. 1999. Chest 116, 212–221.
Morita, S., Ueda, Y., Eguchi, K. 2000. Endocrine J. 47, 467–470.
Moriya, K., Yasuda, K., Koike, K., Ichinose, Y., Yotsuyanagi, H., Kurokawa, K., Iino, S. 1994. J. Gastroenterol. 29, 514–517.
Morley, T.F., Komansky, H.J., Adelizzi, R.A., Giudice, J.C. 1984. Eur. J. Respir. Dis. 65, 627–632.
Morrison, D.A., Goldman, A.L. 1979. Radiology 131, 299–304.
Morrow, P.L., Hardin, N.J., Bonadies, J. 1989. J. Forensic Sci. 34, 1016–1020.
M'Raihi, M.L., Zegaya, M. 1990. Rev. Mal. Respir. 7, 75–78.
Mukhopadhyay, S.A., Stanley, N.N. 2001. Postgrad. Med. J. 77, 390–391.
Mullick, F.G., McAllister, H.A. Jr., Wagner, B.M., Fenoglio, J.J. Jr. 1979. Hum. Pathol. 10, 313–325.
Murin, S., Wiedemann, H.P., Matthay, R.A. 1998. Clin. Chest Med. 19, 641–665.
Murray, M.J., Kronenberg, R. 1965. N. Engl. J. Med. 273, 1185–1187.
Myers, J.L. 1993. Monogr. Pathol. 36, 32–53.
Myers, J.L., Colby, T.V. 1993. Clin. Chest Med. 14, 611–622.
Myers, J.L., Kennedy, J.I., Plumb, V.J. 1987. Hum. Pathol 18, 349–354.
Nakanishi, M., Okamura, S., Demura, Y., Ishizaki, T., Miyamori, I., Itoh, H. 2001. Nihon Kokyuki Gakkai Zasshi 39, 357–362.
Nakelchik, M., Mangino, J.E. 2002. Am. J. Med. 112, 78–79.
Namazy, J.A., Simon, R.A. 2002. Ann. Allergy Asthma Immunol. 89, 542–550.quiz 550, 605.
Nanayakkara, P.W.B., Postmus, P.E. 1999. Netherland J. Med. 54, A16.
Nässberger, L., Johansson, A.C., Bjorck, S., Sjoholm, A.G. 1991. J. Intern. Med. 229, 261–265.
Nathan, S.D., Barnett, S.D., Moran, B., Helman, D.L., Nicholson, K., Ahmad, S., Shorr, A.F. 2004. Respiration 71, 77–82.
Newman, E.D., Harrington, T.M. 1988. Arthritis Rheum. 31, 1585–1586.
Nizami, I.Y., Kissner, D.G., Vissher, D.W., Dubaybo, B.A. 1995. Chest 108, 271–277.
Nizankowska, E., Bestynska-krypel, A., Cmiel, A., Szczeklik, A. 2000. Eur. Respir. J. 15, 863–869.
Noh, J.Y., Asari, T., Hamada, N., Makino, F., Ishikawa, N., Abe, Y., Ito, K. 2001. Clin. Endocrinol. 54, 651–654.
Nomura, M., Fujimura, M., Matsuda, T., Kitagawa, M. 1997. Nihon Kyobu Shikkan Gakkai Zasshi 35, 72–76.
Noseworthy, T.W., Davey, R.S., Percy, J.S., King, E.G. 1983. Crit. Care Med. 11, 761–762.
Novack, G.D., O'Donnell, M.J., Molloy, D.W. 2002. J. Am. Geriatr. Soc. 50, 956–962.
Nyvad, O., Jensen, P.H. 1987. Ugeskrift for Laeger 149, 851–852.
Oermann, C.M., Panesar, K.S., Langston, C., Larsen, G.L., Menendez, A.A., Schofield, D.E., Cosio, C. 2000. J. Pediatr. 136, 351–358.
Ogata, K., Koga, T., Yagawa, K. 1994. Chest 106, 612–613.
Ohar, J.A., Jackson, F., Redd, R.M., Evans, G.R., Bedrossian, C.W. 1989. Am. J. Cardiol. 64, 1322–1326.
Ohtsuka, M., Yamashita, Y., Doi, M., Hasegawa, S. 1997. Eur. Respir. J. 10, 1405–1407.
Oishi, Y., Sando, Y., Tajima, S., Maeno, T., Maeno, Y., Sato M., Hosono, T., Suga, T., Kurabayashi, M., Nagai, R. 2001. Respirology 6, 57–60.
Olmer, J., Paillas, J., Roger, J., Muratore, R., Badier, M. 1952. Presse Medicale 11, 1748–1750.
Olshansky, B. 1997. N. Engl. J. Med. 337, 1814.
O'Reilly, S.C., Taylor, P.M., O'Driscoll, B.R. 1994. Respir. Med. 88, 393–395.
Oshitani, N., Matsumoto, T., Moriyama, Y., Kudoh, S., Hirata, K., Kuroki, T. 1998. J. Gastroenterol. 33, 578–581.
Otte, H.G., Hartig, C., Stalder, R. 1997. Hautarzt 48, 482–487.
Özkan, M., Dweik, R.A., Ahmad, M. 2001. Cleveland Clin. J. Med. 68, 782–795.
Padley, S.P.G., Adler, B., Hansell, D.M., Müller, N.L. 1992. Clin. Radiol. 46, 232–236.
Paganin, F., Poubeau, P., Yvin, J.L., Arvin-Berod, C. 2003. Presse Medicale 32, 978–984.
Paladini, G., Tonazzi, C., Marinig, L. 1982. Int. J. Clin. Pharmaceut. Res. 2, 43–45.
Palmer, S.M., Robinson, L.J., Wang, A.D., Gossage, J.R., Bashore, T., Tapson, S.F. 1998. Chest 113, 237–240.

Pape, L., Strehlau, J., Latta, K., Ehrich, J.H., Offner, G. 2002. Pediatr. Transplant. 6, 337–339.
Parry, S.D., Barbatzas, C., Peel, E.T., Barton, J.R. 2002. Eur. Respir. J. 19, 756–764.
Partanen, J., van Assendelft, A.H.W., Koskimies, S., Forsberg, S., Hakala, M., Ilonen, J. 1987. Chest 92, 277–281.
Partridge, M.R., Gibson, G.J. 1978. Br. Med. J. i, 1521–1522.
Partridge, B.L., Ward, C.F. 1986. Anesthesiology 65, 709–710.
Pasquinucci, G., Ferrara, P., Castellari, R. 1971. JAMA 216, 2017.
Patel, M., Ezzat, W., Pauw, K.L., Lowsky, R. 2001. Eur. J. Haematol. 67, 318–321.
Pearsall, H.R., Ewalt, J., Tsoi, M.S., Backus, S.D., Winterbauer, R.H., Webb, D.R., Jones, H. 1974. J. Lab. Clin. Med. 83, 728–737.
Pedvis, S., Anastakis, D., Inman, R. 1999. J. Rheumatol. 26, 1630.
Pei, Y.P.C., Thompson, D.A. 1987. Am. J. Med. 82, 381–382.
Peno-Green, L., Lluberas, G., Kingsley, T., Brantley, S. 2002. Chest 122, 1858–1860.
Perez, G.M.G.R., Bragado, F.G., Gil, A.M.P. 1997. Pathol. Int. 47, 692–697.
Perreaux, F., Zenaty, D., Capron, F., Trioche, P., Odièvre, M., Labrune, P. 2000. J. Pediatr. Gastroenterol. Nutr. 31, 190–192.
Perrone, M.R., Artesani, M.C., Viola, M., Gaeta, F., Caringi, M., Quaratino, D., Romano, A. 2003. Int. Arch. Allergy Immunol. 132, 82–86.
Persoz, C.F., Cornella, F., Kaeser, P., Rochat, T. 2001. Chest 119, 1963–1965.
Peter, E., Bakri, F., Ball, D.M., Cheney, R.T., Segal, B.H. 2002. Clin. Infect. Dis. 35, e54–e56.
Peters, F.P., Engels, L.G., Moers, A.M. 1997. Postgrad. Med. J. 73, 99–100.
Pfitzenmeyer, P., Foucher, P., Piard, F., Coudert, B., Braud, M.L., Gabez, P., Lacroix, S., Mabille, J.P., Camus, P. 1992. Thorax 47, 622–627.
Pfitzenmeyer, P., Meier, M., Zuck, P., Peiffer, G., Masson, P., Turcu, A., Piard, F., Camus, P. 1994. J. Rheumatol. 21, 1573–1577.
Pfitzenmeyer, P., Foucher, P., Dennewald, G., Chevalon, B., Debieuvre, D., Bensa, P., Piard, F., Camus, P. 1996. Eur. Respir. J. 9, 1013–1019.
Phillips, D., Phillips, B., Mannino, D. 1998. J. Womens Health 7, 1099–1104.
Piastra, M., Barbaro, R., Chiaretti, A., Tempera, A., Pulitano, S., Polidori, G. 2002. Arch. Dis. Childhood 86, 302–303.
Pichler, W.J. 2003. Ann. Intern. Med. 139, 683–693.
Pietra, G.G. 1991. J. Thorac. Imag. 6, 1–7.
Pileire, G., Leclerc, P., Hermant, P., Meeus, E., Camus, P. 1999. Presse Medicale 28, 913.
Pincus, T. 1996. J. Rheumatol. 23 Suppl 46, 19–24.
Pirmohamed, M., Graham, A., Roberts, P., Smith, D., Chadwick, D., Breckenridge, A.M., Park, B.K. 1991. Br. J. Clin. Pharmacol. 32, 741–749.
Pirmohamed, M., Naisbitt, D.J., Gordon, F., Park, B.K. 2002. Toxicology 181–182, 55–63.
Plaza, V., Serrano, J., Picado, C., Sanchis, J. 2002. Eur. Respir. J. 19, 846–852.
Pleskow, W.W., Stevenson, D.D., Mathison, D.A., Simon, R.A., Schatz, M., Zeiger, R.S. 1982. J. Allergy Clin. Immunol. 69, 11–19.
Podell, T.E., Klinenberg, J.R., Kramer, L.S., Brown, H.V. 1980. Arthritis Rheum. 23, 347–350.
Polman, A.J., van der Werf, T.S., Tiebosch, A.T.M.C., Zijlstra, J.G. 1998. Eur. Respir. J. 11, 501–503.
Poole, M.D., Postma, D.S. 1991. Otolaryngol. Head Neck Surg. 105, 714–716.
Portanova, J.P., Arndt, R.E., Tan, E.M., Kotzin, B.L. 1987. J. Immunol. 138, 446–451.
Portel, L., Hilbert, G., Gruson, D., Gbikpi-Benissan, G., Cardinaud, J.-P. 1998. Eur. Respir. J. 12, 259–260.
Pourel, J., Guillemin, F., Fener, P., Webanck, L., Bene, M.-C., Delorme, N. 1991. J. Rheumatol. 18, 303–304.
Prakash, U.B. 1984. Postgrad. Med. 76, 119–125. See also pp. 129–142; 143–152.
Prasse, A., Muller, K.M., Kurz, C., Hamm, H., Virchow, J.C. 2003. Eur. Respir. J. 22, 906–911.
Pratt, D.S., Schwartz, M.I., May, J.J., Dreisin, R.B. 1979. Thorax 34, 587–593.
Price, E.J., Venables, P.J. 1995. Drug Safety 12, 283–290.
Primack, S.L., Muller, N.L. 1998. Clin. Chest Med. 19, 573–586.
Propst, A., Propst, T., Dietze, O., Kathrein, H., Judmeier, G., Vogel, W. 1995. Digest. Dis. Sci. 40, 2117–2118.
Pumphrey, R.S.H. 2000. Clin. Exp. Allergy 30, 1144–1150.
Quinn, M.W., Dillard, T.A. 1999. Chest 116, 257–260.
Rachappa, B., Murthy, H.S., Rogers, W.F. 1984. The Practitioner 228, 519–522.
Rademaker, M., Maling, T. 2003. www.medsafe.govt.nz: 2003. Producers Information for Health Professionals. Last update: October 2003.
Raghu, G., Brown, K.K., Bradford, W.Z., Starko, K., Noble, P.W., Schwartz, D.A., King, T.E. Jr. 2004. N. Engl. J. Med. 350, 125–133.
Ravenel, J.G., McAdams, H.P., Plankeel, J.F., Butnor, K.J., Sporn, T.A. 2001. Am. J. Roentgenol. 177, 199–201.
Ray-Chaudhuri, K., Pye, I.F., Boggild, M. 1989. Neurology 39, 436–438.
Reed, C.R., Glauser, F.L. 1991. Chest 100, 1120–1124.
Reid, M.J., Lockey, R.F., Turkeltaub, P.C., Platts-Mills, T.A. 1993. J. Allergy Clin. Immunol. 92, 6–15.
Ren, H., Kuhlman, J.E., Hruban, R.H., Fishman, E.K., Wheeler, P.S., Hutchins, G.M. 1990. J. Comput. Assist. Tomogr. 14, 760–765.
Resta, O., Foschino Barbaro, M.P., Guido, P., Tozzi, C., Damiano, M., Pietrafesa, G., Talamo, S. 1999. Clin. Drug Invest. 18, 239–241.
Rich, A.R. 1942. Bull. Johns Hospkins Hosp. 71, 123–140.
Rich, M.W., Thomas, R.A. 1997. Chest 111, 1767–1769.
Riegert-Johnson, D.L., Godfrey, J.A., Myers, J.L., Hubmayr, R.D., Sandborn, W.J., Loftus, E.V. Jr. 2002. Inflamm. Bowel Dis. 8, 186–191.
Ripps, C.S., Fellner, M.J. 1966. Lancet ii, 803.
Robinson, N.M.K., Thomas, M.R., Jewitt, D.E. 1995. Respir. Med. 89, 629–630.

Rocca, P., Dumortier, J., Taniere, P., Duperret, S., Vial, T., Cottin, V., Delafosse, B., Scoazec, J.Y., Boillot, O. 2002. Gastroenterologie Clinique et Biologique 26, 405–408.

Rolston, K.V.I. 2001. Curr. Opin. Oncol. 13, 218–223.

Romano, A., Mondino, C., Viola, M., Montuschi, P. 2003. Int. J. Immunopathol. Pharmacol. 16, 19–23.

Rosado, A., Vives, R., Gonzalez, R., Rodriguez, J. 2003. Allergy 58, 689–690.

Rosen, E. 2000. Harefuah 139, 438–440. See also p. 494.

Rosenbaum, L., Thurman, P., Krantz, S. 1979. Arch. Intern. Med. 139, 1151–1153.

Rosketh, R., Storstein, O. 1960. Acta Med. Scand. 167, 23–27.

Rossi, S.E., Erasmus, J.J., McAdams, P., Sporn, T.A., Goodman, P.C. 2000. Radiographics 5, 1245–1259.

Rostand, R.A., Feldman, R.L., Block, E.R. 1977. South. Med. J. 70, 1128–1130.

Roujeau, J.C., Stern, R.S. 1994. N. Engl. J. Med. 331, 1272–1285.

Roux, F., Zitnik, R.J. 1997. J. Respir. Dis. 18, 431–446.

Rubin, G., Baume, P., Vandenberg, R. 1972. Aust. NZ J. Med. 3, 272–274.

Rubin, R.L., Nusinow, S.R., Johnson, A.D., Rubenson, D.S., Curd, J.G., Tan, E.M. 1986. Am. J. Med. 80, 999–1002.

Rubinstein, I., Langevitz, P., Shibi, G. 1985. Oncology 42, 104–106.

Rubinstein, I., Baum, G.L., Hiss, Y., Goldhammer, Y. 1986. Eur. Neurol. 25, 281–284.

Russian, D.A., Levine, S.J. 2001. Am. J. Med. Sci. 321, 56–65.

Ryu, J.H., Myers, J., Swenson, S.J. 2003. Am. J. Respir. Crit. Care Med. 168, 1277–1292.

Sabio, J.M., Jimenez-Alonso, J., Gonzalez-Crespo, F. 2001. Chest 120, 2114.

Sahn, S.A. 1988. Am. Rev. Respir. Dis. 138, 184–234.

Salaffi, F., Manganelli, P., Carotti, M., Subiaco, S., Lamanna, G., Cervini, C. 1997. Clin. Rheumatol. 16, 296–304.

Salama, A.D., Levy, J.B., Lightstone, L., Pusey, C.D. 2001. Lancet 358, 917–920.

Salerno, S.M., Ormseth, E.J., Roth, B.J., Meyer, C.A., Christensen, E.D., Dillard, T.A. 1996. Chest 110, 556–559.

Salles, G., Vial, T., Archimbaud, E. 1991. Ann. Haematol. 62, 74–75.

Salpeter, S., Ormiston, T., Salpeter, E. 2002. Ann. Intern. Med. 137, 715–725.

Salpeter, S.R., Ormiston, T.M., Salpeter, E.E., Poole, P.J., Cates, C.J. 2003. Respir. Med. 97, 1094–1101.

Saltzstein, S.L., Ackerman, L.V. 1959. Cancer 12, 164–182.

Salzman, M.B., Valderrama, E., Sood, S.K. 1997. N. Engl. J. Med. 336, 878–879.

Samenuk, D., Link, M.S., Homoud, M.K., Contreras, R., Theohardes, T.C., Wang, P.J., Estes, N.A.M. III 2002. Mayo Clin. Proc. 77, 12–16.

Samter, M., Beers, R.F. Jr. 1968. Ann. Intern. Med. 68, 975–983.

Santo-Ocampo, A.S., Mandell, B.F., Fessler, B.J. 2000. Chest 118, 1083–1090.

Santrach, P.J., Askin, F.B., Wells, R.J., Azizkhan, R.G., Merten, D.F. 1989. Cancer 64, 806–811.

Sarkany, I. 1967. Lancet i, 743–745.

Savici, D., Katzenstein, A.L.A. 2001. Hum. Pathol. 32, 1398–1402.

Schattner, A., Gilad, A., Cohen, J. 2002. J. Intern. Med. 251, 272–277.

Scheinman, J.I., Stamler, F.W. 1969. J. Pediatr. 74, 117–119.

Schlienger, R.G., Bircher, A.J., Meier, C.R. 2000. Dermatology 200, 223–231.

Schmitz Schumann, M., Palca, A., Simon, U., Blaser, K. 1998. Eur. J. Clin. Invest. 28 (Suppl. 1), A49.

Schnabel, A., Dalhoff, K., Bauerfeind, S., Barth, J., Gross, W.L. 1996. Clin. Rheumatol. 15, 277–282.

Schneider, F., Meziani, F., Chartier, C., Jaeger, A. 2002. Lancet 359, 852–853.

Schooley, R.T., Wagley, P.F., Lietman, P.S. 1977. JAMA 237, 1716–1717.

Schreiber, M.M., McGregor, J.G. 1968. Arch. Dermatol. 97, 297–300.

Schreiber, J., Zissel, G., Greinert, U., Schlaak, M., Muller-Quernheim, J. 1999. Eur. J. Med. Res. 4, 67–71.

Schröder, H., Price Evans, D. 1972. Gut 13, 278–284.

Schrodt, B.J., Callen, J.P. 1999. Pediatrics 103, 503–505.

Schuster, C., Wüthrich, B. 2003. Allergy 58, 1072.

Schuster, C., Reinhart, W.H., Hartmann, K., Kuhn, M. 1999. Schweizerische Medizinische Wochenschrift 129, 362–369.

Schwartzman, K.J., Bowie, D.M., Yeadon, C., Fraser, R., Sutton, E.D., Levy, R.D. 1995. Eur. Respir. J. 8, 2191–2193.

Schwarz, M.I. 1998. Clin. Chest Med. 19, 701–712.

Schwarz, M.I., Fontenot, A.P. 2004. Clin. Chest Med. 25, 133–140.

Searles, G., McKendry, R.J.R. 1987. J. Rheumatol. 14, 1164–1171.

Seidman, M.D., Lewandowski, C.A., Sarpa, J.R., Potesta, E., Schweitzer, V.G. 1990. Otolaryngol. Head Neck Surg. 102, 727–731.

Settgast, A.M., Groth, T., Gertner, E. 2003. Int. J. Dermatol. 42, 316–317.

Settipane, R.A., Shrank, P.J., Simon, R.A., Mathison, D.A., Christensen, S.C., Stevenson, D.D. 1995. J. Allergy Clin. Immunol. 96, 480–485.

Shakoor, N., Michalska, M., Harris, C.A., Block, J.A. 2002. Lancet 359, 579–580.

Shaw, E.G., Deming, R.L., Creagan, E.T., Nair, S., Levitt, R., Steen, P.D., Wiesenfeld, M., Mailliard, J.A. 1995. Int. J. Radiat. Oncol. Biol. Phys. 31, 827–831.

Shear, N.H., Spielberg, S.P. 1988. J. Clin. Invest. 82, 1826–1832.

Sheikhzadeh, A., Schafer, U., Schnabel, A. 2002. Arch. Intern. Med. 162, 834–836.

Shelhamer, J.H., Gill, V.J., Quinn, T.C., Crawford, S.W., Kovacs, J.A., Masur, H., Ognibene, F.P. 1996. Ann. Intern. Med. 124, 585–599.

Shepherd, G.M. 2003. Mt Sinai J. Med. 70, 113–125.

Shkutin, A.E., Naresheva, K.A., Donchenko, V.S. 1989. Arkh. Patol. 51, 48–54.

Shore, E.T. 1990. Chest 98, 1540.

Shulan, D., Katlan, M., Lavsky-Shulan, M. 2003. Ann. Intern. Med. 139, 304.

Sicherer, S.H. 2003. J. Allergy Clin. Immunol. 111, S829–S834.

Siddiqui, M.A., Khan, I.A. 2002. Am. J. Therapeut. 9, 163–165.

Sidransky, H. 1994. Mod. Pathol. 7, 806–810.

Siegel, M., Lee, S.L., Peress, N.S. 1967. Arthritis Rheum. 10, 407–415.
Silvestri, R.C., Jensen, W.A., Zibrak, J.D., Alexander, R.C., Rose, R.M. 1987. Am. Rev. Respir. Dis. 136, 1003–1004.
Similowski, T., Strauss, C. 2004. Clin. Chest Med. 25, 155–166.
Simon, H.B., Dagett, W.M., DeSanctis, R.W. 1969. JAMA 208, 1830–1834.
Siniakowicz, R.M., Narula, D., Suster, B., Steinberg, J.S. 2001. J. Cardiovasc. Electrophysiol. 12, 431–436.
Sinnige, H.A.M., Boender, C.A., Kuypers, E.W., Ruitenberg, H.M. 1990. J. Intern. Med. 227, 355–358.
Sitbon, O., Bidel, N., Dussopt, C., Azarian, R., Braud, M.L., Lebargy, F., Fourme, T., Piard, F., Camus, P. 1994. Arch. Intern. Med. 154, 1633–1640.
Skaer, T.L. 1992. Clin. Therapeut. 14, 496–506.
Slingerland, R., Hoogsteden, H.C., Adriaansen, H.J., van der Kwast, T.H., Hilvering, C. 1987. Respiration 52, 232–236.
Smith, D., Letendre, S. 2002. Ann. Intern. Med. 136, 174.
Smith, P.R., Nacht, R.I. 1992. Chest 101, 268–269.
Smith, R.L., Alexander, R.F., Aranda, C.P. 1993. Cancer 71, 1846–1847.
Solans, R., Bosch, J.A., Selva, A., Orriols, R., Vilardell, M. 2002. Thorax 57, 183–185.
Sorell, T.C., Forbes, I.J. 1975. Aust. NZ J. Med. 5, 144–147.
Sorhage, F., Stover, D.E., Mortazavi, A. 1996. Chest 110, 852–854.
Sostman, H.D., Matthay, R.A., Putman, C.E., Walker Smith, G.J. 1976. Medicine (Baltimore) 55, 371–388.
Sovijärvi, A.R.A., Lemola, M., Stenius, B., Idänpään-Heikkilä, J. 1977. Scand. J. Respir. Dis. 58, 41–50.
Spielberg, S.P., Gordon, G.B., Blake, D.A., Goldstein, D.A., Herlong, H.F. 1981. N. Engl. J. Med. 305, 722–727.
Sporer, K.A., Dorn, E. 2001. Chest 120, 1628–1632.
Sridhar, M.K., Abdulla, A. 1998. Lancet 352, 114.
Stadnyk, A., Grossman, R.F. 1986. Chest 90, 773–774.
Stankus, S.J., Johnson, N.T. 1992. Chest 102, 1595–1596.
Starzl, T.E. 1999a. Rev. Med. Virol. 9, 10–14.
Starzl, T.E. 1999b. Rev. Med. Virol. 9, 3–5.
Stentoft, J. 1987. Acta Med. Scand. 221, 403–407.
Stephan, W.C., Parks, R.D., Tempest, B. 1978. Chest 74, 463–464.
Stetter, M., Schmidli, M., Krapf, R. 1994. Am. J. Kidney Dis. 23, 874–877.
Stevens, M.B. 1992. Hosp. Pract. 27, 27–36.
Stevenson, D.D. 1998. Immunol. Allergy Clin. North Am. 18, 773–798.
Stevenson, D.D. 2003. Clin. Rev. Allergy Immunol. 24, 159–167.
Stevenson, D.D., Zuraw, B.L. 2003. Clin. Rev. Allergy Immunol. 24, 169–187.
Stirling, R.G., Chung, K.F. 1999. Thorax 54, 865–866.
Stoloff, S., Stempel, D.A. 2000. Chest 118, 1515.
Strom, B.L., Schinnar, R., Apter, A.J., Margolis, D.J., Lautenbach, E., Hennessy, S., Bilker, W.B., Pettitt, D. 2003. N. Engl. J. Med. 349, 1628–1635.
Sturtevant, J. 1999. NZ Dent. J. 95, 84.
Suarez, M., Krieger, B.P. 1986. Chest 90, 452–453.
Sullivan, S.N. 1987. J. Clin. Gastroenterol. 9, 461–463.
Sullivan, E.J., Hoffman, G.S. 1998. Clin. Chest Med. 19, 759–776.
Suratt, B.T., Lynch, D.A., Cool, C.D., Jones, R.B., Brown, K.K. 2003. Bone Marrow Transplant. 31, 939–941.
Suwa, A., Hirakata, M., Satoh, S., Mimori, T., Utsumi, K., Inada, S. 1999. Clin. Exp. Rheumatol. 17, 355–358.
Sweet, J.M., Stevenson, D.D., Simon, R.A., Mathison, D.A. 1990. J. Allergy Clin. Immunol. 85, 59–65.
Szczeklik, A., Sanak, M. 2000. Am. J. Respir. Crit. Care Med. 161, S142–S146.
Szczeklik, A., Stevenson, D.D. 2003. J. Allergy Clin. Immunol. 111, 913–921.
Szczeklik, A., Sladek, K., Dworski, R., Nizankowska, E., Soja, J., Sheller, J., Oates, J. 1996. Am. J. Respir. Crit. Care Med. 154, 1608–1614.
Szczeklik, A., Nizankowska, E., Duplaga, M. 2000. Eur. Respir. J. 16, 432–438.
Szczeklik, A., Nizankowska, E., Bochenek, G., Nagraba, K., Mejza, F., Swierczynska, M. 2001. Clin. Exp. Allergy 31, 219–225.
Tahan, V., Ozseker, F., Guneylioglu, D., Baran, A., Ozaras, R., Mert, A., Ucisik, A.C., Cagatay, T., Yilmazbayhan, D., Senturk, H. 2003. Digest. Dis. Sci. 48, 169–173.
Taillé, C., Fartoukh, M., Houël, R., Kobeiter, H., Rémy, P., Lemaire, F. 2001. Chest 120, 311–313.
Takahashi, T., Yamaguchi, E., Furuya, K., Kawakami, Y. 2001. Respir. Med. 95, 130–135.
Takeda, A., Ikegame, K., Kimura, Y., Ogawa, H., Kanazawa, S., Nakamura, H. 2000. Hepato-Gastroenterology 47, 1431–1435.
Tang, M.B.Y., Yosipovitch, G. 2003. Arch. Dermatol. 139, 715–718.
Tanoue, L.T. 1998. Clin. Chest Med. 19, 667–685.
Tatsis, E., Schnabel, A., Gross, W.L. 1998. Ann. Intern. Med. 129, 370–374.
Taylor, C.R. 1990. Clin. Chest Med. 11, 87–94.
Tazelaar, H.D., Myers, J.L., Drage, C.W., King, T.E. Jr., Aguayo, S., Colby, T.V. 1990. Chest 97, 1032–1036.
Tazelaar, H.D., Myers, J.L., Strickler, J.G., Colby, T.V., Duffy, J. 1993. Mod. Pathol. 6, 56–60.
Terho, E.O., Torkko, M., Valta, R. 1979. Scand. J. Respir. Dis. 60, 345–349.
Thickett, D.R., Millar, A.B. 1997. Postgrad. Med. J. 73, 165–166.
Thomas, E., Mazyad, H., Olive, P., Blotman, F. 1997. Clin. Exp. Rheumatol. 15, 583–584.
Thomeer, M., Demedts, M., Vandeurzen, K. 2001a. Acta Clinica Belgica 56, 163–172.
Thomeer, M.J., Costabel, U., Rizzato, G., Poletti, V., Demedts, M. 2001b. Eur. Respir. J. 18, 114s–118s.
Thompson, J., Chengappa, K.N.R., Good, C.B., Baker, R.W., Kiewe, R.P., Bezner, J., Schooler, N.R. 1998. Int. Clin. Psychopharmacol. 13, 95–98.
Tohyama, M., Tamaki, Y., Toyama, M., Ishimine, T., Miyazato, A., Nakamoto, A., Miyara, T., Higa, F., Tateyama, M., Kawakami, K., Nakamura, H., Saito, A. 2002. Nihon Kokyuki Gakkai Zasshi 40, 123–128.
Tomioka, H., King, T.E. Jr. 1997. Am. J. Respir. Crit. Care Med. 155, 1011–1020.
Tompson, R.T., Zeek, P.M. 1945. Ohio State Med. J. 41, 824–825.
Topilow, A.A., Rothenberg, S.P., Cottrell, T.S. 1973. Am. Rev. Respir. Dis. 108, 114–117.

Toyoshima, M., Sato, A., Hayakawa, H., Taniguchi, M., Imokawa, S., Chida, K. 1996. Intern. Med. 35, 176–179.

Tucker, A.S., Newman, A.J., Alvorado, C. 1977. Radiology 125, 805–809.

Tuggey, J.M., Hosker, H.S.R. 2000. Thorax 55, 805–806.

Tweed, W.A., Dakin, D. 2001. Anesthesia Analgesia 92, 1442–1443.

Ueda, K., Sakano, H., Tanaka, T., Hayashi, M., Fujita, N., Zempo, N. 2002. Ann. Thorac. Surg. 74, 2176–2177.

Ulmer, J.L., Garvey, M.J. 1992. Ann. Pharmacother. 26, 1245–1246.

Ullmer, E., Mayr, M., Binet, I., Ebnother-Staub, C., Dalquen, P., Soler, M., Tamm, M. 2000. Eur. Respir. J. 15, 213–216.

Usuba, Y., Aiba, S., Hashimoto, K., Tanita, Y., Sakai, K. 1989. Nippon Hifuka Gakkai Zasshi 99, 725–730.

Vaccarezza, R.F., Pavlovsky, A. 1945. Anales de la Catedra de Patologia y Clinica Tuberculosa Buenos Aires 7, 164–174.

Vallerand, H., Cossart, C., Milosevic, D., Lavaud, F., Leone, J. 1992. Lancet 339, 1551.

Vally, H., Taylor, M.L., Thompson, P.J. 2002. Thorax 57, 569–574.

van Arsdel, P.P.J. 1984. J. Allergy Clin. Immunol. 73, 431–434.

van de Laar, M.A.F.J., Westermann, C.J.J., Wagenaar, S.S., Dinant, H.J. 1985. Arthritis Rheum. 28, 93–97.

van der Geld, Y.M., Simpelaar, A., van der Zee, R., Cohen-Tervaert, J.W., Stegeman, C.A., Limburg, P.C., Kallenberg, C.G.M. 2001. Kidney Int. 59, 147–159.

van der Klauw, M.M., Stricker, B.H.C., Herings, R.M.C., Cost, W.S., Valkenburg, H.A., Wilson, J.H.P. 1993. Br. J. Clin. Pharmacol. 35, 400–408.

van der Klauw, M.M., Wilson, J.H., Stricker, B.H. 1996. Clin. Exp. Allergy 26, 1355–1363.

van der Veen, M.J., Dekker, J.J., Dinant, H.J., Van Soesbergen, R.M., Bijlsma, J.W.J. 1995. J. Rheumatol. 22, 1766–1768.

van Mieghem, W., Coolen, L., Malysse, I., Lacquet, L.M., Deneffe, G.J.D., Demedts, M.G.P. 1994. Chest 105, 1642–1645.

van Sonnenberg, E., Wittich, G. 1998. Am. J. Roentgenol. 171, 261.

Vandenplas, O., Hanston, P., Dive, A., Mahieu, P. 1990. Acta Clinica Belgica 45, 334–339.

Varnell, R.M., Godwin, J.D., Richardson, M.L., Vincent, J.M. 1989. Radiology 170, 667–670.

Vavricka, S.R., Wettstein, T., Speich, R., Gaspert, A., Bachli, E.B. 2003. Thorax 58, 278–279.

Veerabagu, M.P., Finkelstein, S.D., Rabinovitz, M. 1997. Digest. Dis. Sci. 42, 1445–1448.

Verdich, J., Christensen, A.L. 1979. Acta Dermato-Venereologica (Stockholm) 59, 471–473.

Verma, S.P., Yunis, N., Lekos, A., Crausman, R.S. 2000. Chest 117, 597–598.

Vernhet, H., Bousquet, C., Cover, S., Giron, J., Gruson, C., Senac, J.P. 1995. Revue des Maladies Respiratoires 12, 317–319.

Vernhet, H., Bousquet, C., Durand, G., Giron, J., Senac, J.P. 2001. Eur. Radiol. 11, 1697–1703.

Verra, F., Hmouda, H., Rauss, A., Lebargy, F., Cordonnier, C., Bignon, J., Lemaire, F., Brochard, L. 1992. Chest 101, 1215–1220.

Virolainen, M. 1971. Clin. Exp. Immunol. 9, 429–435.

Vischer, T.L. 1966. Lancet ii, 467–469.

Volk, B.W., Nathanson, L., Losner, S., Slade, W.R., Jacobi, M. 1951. Am. J. Med. 10, 316–324.

Volkman, J.A., Pontikes, P.J. 2002. Ann. Pharmacother. 36, 1457–1461.

Vucicevic, Z., Suskoovic, T. 1997. Ann. Pharmacother. 37, 429–432.

Wagner, R., von Hundelshausen, B., Tempel, G., Schneck, H.J., Pichlmeier, R., Hipp, R. 1994. Anaesthesiologie et Reanimation 19, 159–161.

Walker-Smith, G.J. 1990. Clin. Chest Med. 31, 95–118.

Wall, M.A., Wall, M.E.B., Jaffe, N., Strieder, D.J. 1979. Pediatrics 63, 741–746.

Wallis, J.P. 2003. Br. J. Anaesthesia 90, 573–576.

Walzer, R.A., Feinstein, R., Shapiro, C., Einbinder, J. 1972. Arch. Dermatol. 106, 231–234.

Wandl, U.B., Kloke, O., Nagel-Hiemke, M., Moritz, T., Becher, R., Opalka, B., Holtkamp, W., Bartels, H., Seeber, S., Niederle, N. 1992. Br. J. Haematol. 81, 516–519.

Wang, J.S., Tseng, H.H., Lai, R.S., Hsu, H.K., Ger, L.P. 2000. Histopathology 37, 402–410.

Wang, F., Aleksunes, L.M., Reagan, L.A., Vergara, C.M. 2002. Diabetes Technol. Ther. 4, 505–514.

Ward, M.M., Donald, F. 1999. Arthritis Rheum. 42, 780–789.

Warris, A., Bjorneklett, A., Gaustad, P. 2001. N. Engl. J. Med. 344, 1099–1100.

Weaver, L.T., Law, J.S. 1978. Br. J. Dis. Chest 72, 247–250.

Wechsler, M.E., Drazen, J.M. 2000. Chest 118, 1515–1516.

Wechsler, M.E., Garpestad, E., Flier, S.R., Kocher, O., Weiland, D.A., Polito, A.J., Klinek, M.M., Bigby, T.D., Wong, G.A., Helmers, R.A., Drazen, J.M. 1998. JAMA 279, 455–457.

Wechsler, M.E., Pauwels, R., Drazen, J.M. 1999. Drug Safety 21, 241–251.

Weller, P.F., Plaut, M., Taggart, V., Trontell, A. 2001. J. Allergy Clin. Immunol. 108, 175–183.

White, D.A. 2004. Clin. Chest Med. 25, 179–188.

White, J.P., Ward, M.J. 1985. Adv. Drug React. Acute Poison. Rev. 4, 183–211.

White, D.A., Rankin, J.A., Stover, D.E., Gellene, R.A., Gupta, S. 1989. Am. Rev. Respir. Dis. 139, 18–21.

Williams, I.P., Millard, F.J.C. 1980. Thorax 35, 160.

Wilschut, F.A., Cobben, N.A.M., Thunnissen, F.B.J.M., Lammers, L.J.S., Wouters, E.F.M., Drent, M. 1997. Eur. Respir. J. 10, 2163–2165.

Wing, S.S., Fantus, I.G. 1987. Can. Med. Assoc. J. 136, 121–127.

Winterbauer, R.H., Wilske, K.R., Wheelis, R.F. 1976. N. Engl. J. Med. 294, 919–921.

Woessner, K.M., Simon, R.A., Stevenson, D.D. 2002. Arthritis Rheum. 46, 2201–2206.

Wolf, Y., Haddad, R., Jossipov, J., Werbin, N. 1997. J. Toxicol. Clin. Toxicol. 35, 113–114.

Wolff, A.J., O'Donnell, A.E. 2004. Clin. Chest Med. 25, 203–216.

Wollner, A., Mohle-Boetani, J., Lambert, R.E., Perruquet, J.L., Raffin, T.A., McGuire, J.L. 1991. Thorax 46, 205–207.

Wolthuis, A., Nackaerts, K., Guffens, P., Jousten, P., Demedts, M. 2003. Acta Clinica Belgica 58, 50–53.

Woltsche, M., Woltsche Karhr, I., Roeger, G.M. 2001. Allergologie 24, 171.
Wong, D.T., Gadsden, J.C. 2003. Can. J. Anaesthesia 50, 900–903.
Woolley, J., Collett, J., Goldstein, D. 1997. Aust. NZ J. Med. 27, 605–606.
Yalçin, S., Sahin, A., Yalçin, B., Altinok, G. 1997. Liver 17, 166–167.
Yale, S.H., Limper, A.H. 1996. Mayo Clin. Proc. 71, 5–13.
Yamaguchi, S., Kubo, K., Fujimoto, K., Honda, T., Sekiguchi, M., Sodeyama, T. 1997. Thorax 52, 33–37.
Yamaoka, K.A., Miyasaka, N., Inuo, G., Saito, I., Komb, J.P., Fujita, K., Kashiwazaki, S. 1994. J. Clin. Immunol. 14, 50–60.
Yamawaki, I., Katsura, H., Taira, M., Kadoriku, C., Hashimoto, I., Chiyotani, A., Kondo, M., Tamaoki, J., Nagai, A., Konno, K. 1996. Nihon Kyobu Shikkan Gakkai Zasshi 34, 1331–1336.
Yavorkovsky, L.L., Carrum, G., Bruce, S., McCarthy, P.L. 1998. Am. J. Hematol. 58, 80–81.
Yee, A.M.F., Pochapin, M.B. 2001. Ann. Intern. Med. 135, 27–31.
Yel, L., Chen, W., Gupta, S. 2004. Ann. Allergy Asthma Immunol. 92, 88–91.
Yermakov, V.M., Hitti, I.F., Sutton, A.L. 1983. Hum. Pathol. 14, 182–184.
Yokoi, T., Hirabayashi, N., Ito, M., Uno, Y., Tsuzuki, T., Yatabe, Y., Kodera, Y. 1997. Virchows Arch. Int. J. Pathol. 431, 275–282.
Yoshida, Y. 2003. Nihon Kokyuki Gakkai Zasshi 41, 300–303.
Youlten, L.J.F. 1989. Clin. Exp. Allergy 19, 233–235.
Zaacks, S.M., Klein, L., Tan, C.D., Rodriguez, E.R., Leikin, J.B. 1999. J. Toxicol. Clin. Toxicol. 37, 485–489.
Zamarron, C., Maceiras, F., Gonzalez, J., Gomez-Reino, J.J. 2004. Respir. Med. 98, 123–125.
Zanoletti, E., Bertino, G., Malvezzi, L., Benazzo, M., Mira, E. 2003. Acta Oto—Laryngologica 123, 960–964.
Zhou, C.H., Asuncion, A., Love, G.L. 2003. Arch. Pathol. Lab. Med. 127, 893–894.
Zisman, D.A., McCune, W.J., Tino, G., Lynch, J.P.I. 2001. Sarcoidosis Vasc. Diffuse Lung Dis. 18, 243–252.
Zitnik, R.J. 1996. J. Respir. Dis. 17, 254–270.
Zitnik, R.J., Cooper, J.A.D. 1990. Clin. Chest Med. 11, 139–150.
Zucker, A.R., Meadow, W.L. 1995. Crit. Care Med. 23, 767–772.
Zuckner, J. 1994. Rheum. Dis. Clin. North Am. 20, 1017–1032.

Index

F

G

H

I

L

M

N

O

P

CPSIA information can be obtained at www.ICGtesting.com
Printed in the USA
LVOW03*0839150114

369447LV00009B/102/P

9 780444 516527